Biological Monitoring
An Introduction

Edited by
Shane Que Hee

Department of Environmental Health Sciences
UCLA School of Public Health

Library of Congress Catalog Card Number 92-27823
ISBN 0-442-23677-8

I(T)P Van Nostrand Reinhhold is a division of International Thomson Publishing. ITP logo is a trademark under license.

Printed in the United States of America

Van Nostrand Reinhold
115 Fifth Avenue
New York, NY 10003

International Thomson Publishing
Berkshire House
168-173 High Holborn
London WC1V 7AA, England

Thomas Nelson Australia
102 Dodds Street
South Melbourne 3205
Victoria, Australia

Nelson Canada
1120 Birchmount Road
Scarborough, Ontario
M1K 5G4, Canada

16 15 14 13 12 11 10 9 8 7 6 5 4 3 2 1

Library of Congress Cataloging-in-Publication Data
Que Hee, Shane S.
Biological monitoring: an introduction/by Shane S. Que Hee.
p. cm.
Includes bibliographical references and index.
ISBN 0-442-23677-8
1. Biological monitoring. I. Title.
RA1223.B54Q4 1993
614.4—dc20 92-27823
CIP

Preface

There has been a need for a basic introduction to biological monitoring that covers the fundamentals of the field and that can be used as the basis for a graduate one-semester or one-quarter course. This need has become increasingly important in the United States because of the publication of the Biological Exposure Indices (BEIs) of the American Conference of Governmental Industrial Hygienists (ACGIH) for workplace exposures, the public furor concerning exposures to hazardous wastes, the significant home pollution detected in the Total Exposure Assessment Methodology (TEAM) studies sponsored by the U.S. EPA, urine monitoring tests for drugs mandated by the U.S. government and in sports, and the use of blood/urine/breath tests to assess health. No basic textbook has appeared abroad either, in spite of the fact that the importance of biological monitoring in Japan, Germany, Sweden, and other European countries has been long acknowledged. There, traditional biological monitoring is a part of occupational medicine, which also includes medical monitoring/medical–health surveillance.

Since biological monitoring is interfaced with such diverse fields as health and safety, analytical chemistry, biology, molecular biology, biochemistry, clinical chemistry, human toxicology, environmental health, public health, pharmacokinetics, physiology, toxicokinetics, epidemiology, risk assessment, pharmaceutics, laboratory sciences, nursing, and medicine, the publication of such a basic introduction is long overdue.

Some will disagree with my broad application of the term "biological monitoring" to mean monitoring of any chemical marker for humans associated with dose of a chemical or a physical agent (biological monitoring for exposure), and/or associated in the past, present, or future with any adverse effect (medical monitoring and medical–health surveillance). All the factors that influence medical monitoring markers related to adverse health effects also may influence biological monitoring markers of exposure. Beyond critical concentrations of biological monitoring markers of exposure, adverse health effects may also be observed. These are ample reasons to validate the connection.

In most countries outside the United States, both traditional biological and medical monitoring decisions are usually determined by physicians. In the United States there are only about 1000 certified occupational physicians, and much of the traditional biological monitoring sampling (but not interpretation) is actually done by industrial/environmental hygienists or nurses. The latter need to be able to talk knowledgeably with physicians and vice versa. One reason for this book is to bridge that gap.

This book has been written to introduce people with a first-year university science background (biology, chemistry, physics, and mathematics) to the basic concepts of biological monitoring in humans. This means that the essentials of chemistry and biochemistry are the starting points, as these fields are the major foundations of biological monitoring. Chemical equations, however, have been kept to a minimum. Only a thorough understanding of the basic concepts allows valid interpretation of biological monitoring data, probably the biggest problem in the field. Thus students in medicine, nursing, pharmacy, dentistry, industrial/environmental hygiene, public health, medical and laboratory technology, toxicology, health and safety, laboratory sciences, biotechnology, and epidemiology should find this book useful, in addition to environmentalists, people concerned with detecting exposures to hazardous chemicals and wastes, and those just wanting to know what biological monitoring is. Thus the book attempts to be truly interdisciplinary and to be a reference compendium and text.

The book grew out of a course I taught at the University of Cincinnati from 1987 to 1989 and am still teaching, with considerable modifications, at the UCLA School of Public Health. The broad format is based on the first short course ever offered on biological monitoring in the United States, which I organized in 1986 through 1989 at the University of Cincinnati.

The book is organized into five major sections: (1) introductory material (Chapters 1 and 2) on chemistry and biochemistry, where basic concepts associated with biochemical processes in humans are explained, leading to an overview at the end of Chapter 2 on how xenobiotics are processed after they are absorbed; (2) four chapters (Chapters 3–6) describing in detail the roles of exposure route, distribution, metabolism, and excretion in the processing of xenobiotics by the body, with special attention paid to the excretion routes because these are the usual media for noninvasive biological monitoring; (3) three chapters (Chapters 7–9) on medical monitoring/health/medical surveillance, where selected nonspecific markers of adverse effect are explained with consideration of factors associated with life-style and long-term/medical parameters along with applications to programs for the workplace, hazardous waste sites, nursing situations, pharmacies, dental surgeries, and laboratories; (4) a section on adducts, immunology, and AIDS, including three chapters on adducts (Chapters 10–12) and seven chapters on the immune system and AIDS (Chapters 13–19); and (5) special topics, including an introduction to quantitative posturography and its correlation to biological monitoring (Chapter 20), the Biological Monitoring Exposure Indices (BEIs) and their non-U.S. analogs (Chapter 21), biological monitoring for pesticides (Chapter 22), and biological monitoring data around and at hazardous waste sites, in homes, and in the ambient environment (Chapter 23). Of necessity I have not emphasized the purely clinical use of markers relative to therapeutic ranges and toxic ranges although a summary table in Appendix B has been provided. There are already many books available for that purpose.

The books cited as "Further Reading" at the ends of many of the chapters are the major sources and the backup reading for those chapters. This book refers to humans and not animals unless so stated. Because of the huge breadth of the material it was impossible to provide "cutting-edge" references for many chapters. I have opted for a clear exposition of basic concepts and representative examples rather than completeness in references. The understanding of concepts is more important than the tabulation of recent data. Another book is needed for advanced interpretation of biological monitoring data, but it would be impossible to use without an understanding of the basic concepts presented in this book.

The fact that traditional biological monitoring markers may indicate exposure intensity is also correlated with adverse effects of those exposures and with traditional medical monitoring markers. Sometimes, as for urinary cadmium, the marker is both a traditional biological monitoring marker of exposure and a medical monitoring marker. There is no need to compartmentalize knowledge in terms of physician areas and nonphysician areas, or environmental and nonenvironmental areas; "knowledge is power." Most businesses and people in the United States cannot afford the regular services of the few physicians with the appropriate training to interpret biological monitoring data; so prevention of adverse health effects by educating potential users and practitioners about biological monitoring is important, and is another reason for the writing of this book.

Indeed, the more direct the connection between adverse health effects and their markers, the more biological meaning a marker has. Surrogate marker critical concentrations of adverse effect, like most of the BEI marker concentrations recommended by the ACGIH, depend on the assumptions implicit in the establishment of recommended "safe" environmental levels of xenobiotics. In this case the BEIs are based on the ACGIH's Threshold Limit Value–Time-Weighted Average values (TLV-TWAs) for workplace air. The situation becomes even more confusing when analogous levels, the Permissible Exposure Limits (PELs), set by the Occupational Safety and Health Administration (OSHA) disagree for the same situation. When viewed from afar, disagreements in environmental and biological monitoring "safe" concentrations can be extremely confusing (see Section 21.1).

The uses of cholinesterase and methemoglobin as BEI markers illustrate that traditional medical monitoring markers have to be considered on a par with traditional biological monitoring markers of exposure because there may be no viable alternative, especially for multiple routes of exposure and for multicomponent chemical exposures. Thus I believe the division between traditional biological monitoring and medical monitoring is largely artificial and arbitrary and a hindrance to further progress. This is especially so if people still suffer adverse effects when exposed to supposedly "safe" levels as shown by biological or other monitoring, or if people are actually safe when the levels they are exposed to are deemed "unsafe" by biological or other monitoring. The broadened definition for biological monitoring does not restrict exposure situations to "occupational" and "nonoccupational" or "medical" and "nonmedical," but allows all exposures and all factors influencing biological monitoring marker concentrations to be better considered on their merits and according to the data for each individual or group.

The broadened definition of biological monitoring has allowed me to include an apparent anomaly such as quantitative posturography, which is a noninvasive technique analogous in information to the traditional nonspecific medical monitoring marker. The same can also be said for the treatment of AIDS in this book. No one would dispute that the HIV-1 antibody test is a medical monitoring test. Yet it also is a traditional specific biological monitoring marker of exposure because a dose-effect relative to serum antibody concentration can be demonstrated even though the test as utilized is deemed "positive" above a critical concentration of antibodies. The only difference is that the antibodies detected are not metabolites of the exposing viral antigens, though they are raised by the host human in response to these antigens, a common property of immunoassays based on host antibody production. The interpretation of such a test must be understood in terms of the purity of the original isolates used to produce the reagents in the available test kits, which are supposed to be specific (Chapter 15). The hygienic considerations of personal protection against HIV via condoms (Chapter 17) and the universal medical safety precautions for laboratory/hospital personnel handling biological media (Chapter 18) have their counterparts in respirator and garment/glove protections against toxic chemical exposure in the occupational environment. In the latter situation, the use of biological monitoring to assess the degree of protection is well known, just as the occurrence of a positive HIV-1 test may be related also to the protectiveness of condoms. Safety, as it relates to exposure to biological and chemical agents, is equally important to the researcher, the laboratory technician, the student, the dentist, the physician, the nurse, and the pharmacist.

The postulated interaction between nitrites (for which few biological monitoring techniques have been developed) and susceptibility to HIV-1–mediated breakdown of the immune system has its analogy in the many known interactions between chemicals relative to biological monitoring marker concentrations, as, for example, trichloroethylene metabolite excretion and retention on alcohol ingestion. Unfortunately, as Chapter 19 tells us, there are few biological monitoring methods to indicate exposure to volatile nitrites.

There is another reason to emphasize immunologic methods. They represent the future of biological monitoring because of their sensitivity and specificity. They are already being utilized for the detection of many xenobiotics and to detect disease states before the latter become uncontrolled.

I want to thank my long-suffering editorial friends at Van Nostrand Reinhold, Steve Zollo, Pamela Touboul and Cindy Savaglio, for their kindness and understanding during the writing of the book.

This book is dedicated to my long-time companion, Bob McNee, who died January 8, 1992.

Shane Que Hee

Department of Environmental Health Sciences
UCLA School of Public Health
Los Angeles, California 90024-1772

Brief Table of Contents

Contents

PART 1

Basic Mechanisms

1

Concepts in Chemistry

1.0 INTRODUCTION

Biological monitoring as used in this book is the relationship between chemical parameters measured in the biological media of humans to past exposures to chemicals or physical factors. The parameters used in this analysis are called biological monitoring markers when the markers are correlated to the occurrences of these past exposures. They are called biological monitoring markers of exposure when the concentrations of the markers are correlated ("dose effect") to the amount(s) of exposing chemical(s) or physical factor(s). Biochemical markers are those reflecting perturbation of biochemical processes; they may or may not show a dose effect with exposure. The term "biomarkers" is a much broader one that can include the responses of animals, plants, invertebrates, or microorganisms to physical or chemical stresses.

Biological monitoring markers may be organ-specific, tissue-specific, media-specific, or nonspecific. If the marker is related to an adverse effect, the biological marker is one of adverse effect. Such markers are commonly part of a medical surveillance program (the collection, analysis, or evaluation of data to suggest adverse human health effects or further research on adverse human health effects). Medical monitoring is defined as the collection, analysis, or evaluation of data using markers reflecting dysfunction in humans. These markers are definitely known to be related to adverse effects in humans. Medical monitoring markers are commonly interpreted by physicians after blood, urine, breath, or other biological fluid analysis.

When the data associated with all these areas are subjected to analysis on a human population basis through epidemiological and biostatistical methods, the resultant field of endeavor is biochemical epidemiology. Whereas biological monitoring, medical surveillance, and medical monitoring are generally applied to individuals, biochemical epidemiology relates to populations. The relationship of the population-based information to the state of health of the individual is often hard to interrelate.

The most difficult basic sciences required to understand biological monitoring are probably the ones involving chemistry rather than biology, physics, or mathematics. Physics and higher mathematics than calculus generally are not required to any great extent for this interpretation. Biology is intrinsically more approachable than chemistry, hence the focus on chemistry concepts in this chapter.

1.1 CHEMISTRY AND BIOLOGICAL MONITORING

Chemistry is the fundamental discipline that explores the structure and composition of matter, and the latter's reactions and transformations. The smallest quantity of matter of defined atomic composition that exhibits unique properties is a molecule. Specific chemicals or chemical substances are aggregates of molecules of the same kind. Biochemistry is the subbranch of chemistry pertaining to biological systems, which additionally includes mechanisms of maintenance of those systems.

The basic concepts in chemistry will now be discussed because chemical transformation of xenobiotics (compounds not made naturally by the body) occurs in humans. It is assumed that a first-year chemistry course at a university has been completed so that the following is a refresher of the salient concepts.

1.2 ATOMS

Atoms are comprised of elementary particles in motion. The atom consists of the nucleus, which contains over 99% of the mass of any atom, and the electrons, which orbit the nucleus. The nuclear particles are the massive protons (with a unit of positive charge for each proton, which is 1836.15 times heavier in mass than an electron) and the neutrons (each having about 0.14% more mass than a proton but bearing no charge). The nucleus does not participate in chemical reactions. Though all atoms of a particular element have the same number of protons, atoms of an element do not necessarily have the same number of neutrons. The entities with different numbers of neutrons are called isotopes. The atoms of a specific isotope all have the same numbers of protons and neutrons. Because the isotopes of an element have the same number of electrons, their chemical reactions are the same except for those of hydrogen.

The remaining elementary particles, the electrons, orbit the nucleus. Each electron bears a unit negative charge and has an electron spin defined as being "up" (spin quantum number of $+\frac{1}{2}$) or "down" (spin quantum number of $-\frac{1}{2}$). The electrons move around the nucleus such that the attractive force of the nucleus is balanced by the centripetal force due to each moving electron. There are different types of electrons, as characterized by the shape of their orbitals (where they are most likely to be found) around their nuclei and by the most likely distance from their nuclei. Because the electrons would not be stable in the same location as the protons (positive and negative charges react), the electrons stay out of the nucleus most of the time, their speed allowing them to survive any rare collisions with the nuclear particles.

The number of protons equals the number of electrons in an atom, and defines the atomic number of the atom. The combined mass of the neutrons and the protons determines the atomic weight of each isotope. The atomic weight of each element is the sum total of the atomic weights for all the isotopes of the element, each weighted by their natural abundance. The reference isotope atomic weight is that for the most abundant isotope of carbon ($^{12}C_6$), which is defined as having an atomic weight of 12 atomic mass units (amu or daltons). The atomic weight of the element carbon then is 12.001 amu. All atomic weights of the elements are scaled relative to that for $^{12}C_6$.

Physicists do not believe that protons and neutrons are elementary particles. The latter are postulated to be comprised of quarks. Quarks have not been detected in their free state yet, and there are six categories of them: up, down, charm, strange, top, and bottom. The proton is thought to be composed of two up and one down quarks; the neutron consists of two down quarks and one up quark. Physicists also think the electron is but one of a family of elementary particles called leptons. These consist of the electron, the muon, and the tauon, each with a corresponding neutrino (no charge, no rest energy). All of these particles are part of a general class of particles called fermions.

Because the application of electrons-neutrinos, muons, and tauons to chemistry has no supporting literature, we will consider the traditional picture henceforth, in terms only of electrons.

1.3 ELECTRONIC STRUCTURE

The electrons of atoms are defined in a manner consistent with the periodic table (Figure 1.1). The table contains seven horizontal periods of atoms, each period starting with a highly reactive atom (hydrogen, lithium, sodium, potassium, rubidium, cesium, and francium), and ending with an inert (not reactive) gas atom (helium, neon, argon, krypton, xenon, and radon, respectively), with the last period incomplete. Each period is characterized by a principal quantum number that increases by one for the next element after each inert gas. The chemical inertness of an inert gas is explained by the spherical electron density geometry together with maximum paired-electron occupancy.

Each orbital or preferred energy state in an atom can contain two electrons. For a given quantum number there can be one spherically shaped *s* orbital, three dumbbell-shaped *p* orbitals (starting with principal quantum number of 2), five double-dumbbell-shaped *d* orbitals (starting with principal quantum number of 3), and seven triple-dumbbell-shaped *f* orbitals (starting with a principal quantum number of 4). Some of the *d* (for example, $d_z{}^2$) and *f* orbitals have unique shapes.

The electrons of an atom occupy the orbitals nearest to the nucleus first (Aufbau principle). Singly occupied orbitals are preferred (Hund's rule) if double occupancy with electrons of opposite spins is not possible (Pauli exclusion principle). Double occupancy occurs when the electron cloud becomes spherical, as for *s* orbitals, or when the electron density in orbitals other than *s* for a given quantum number attains a spherical shape. Double

Group Number

1	2	3	4	5	6	7	8	9	10	11	12	13	14	15	16	17	18
s-Block		Transition Elements (*d*-Block)										*p*-Block					VIIIA
IA	IIA	IIIB	IVB	VB	VIB	VIIB	VIIIB			IB	IIB	IIIA	IVA	VA	VIA	VIIA	
1 H																	2 He
3 Li	4 Be											5 B	6 C	7 N	8 O	9 F	10 Ne
11 Na	12 Mg											13 Al	14 Si	15 P	16 S	17 Cl	18 Ar
19 K	20 Ca	21 Sc	22 Ti	23 V	24 Cr	25 Mn	26 Fe	27 Co	28 Ni	29 Cu	30 Zn	31 Ga	32 Ge	33 As	34 Se	35 Br	36 Kr
37 Rb	38 Sr	39 Y	40 Zr	41 Nb	42 Mo	43 Tc	44 Ru	45 Rh	46 Pd	47 Ag	48 Cd	49 In	50 Sn	51 Sb	52 Te	53 I	54 Xe
55 Cs	56 Ba	57 La	72 Hf	73 Ta	74 W	75 Re	76 Os	77 Ir	78 Pt	79 Au	80 Hg	81 Tl	82 Pb	83 Bi	84 Po	85 At	86 Rn
87 Fr	88 Ra	89 Ac	104 Rf	105 Ha	106												

Lanthanides	58 Ce	59 Pr	60 Nd	61 Pm	62 Sm	63 Eu	64 Gd	65 Tb	66 Dy	67 Ho	68 Er	69 Tm	70 Yb	71 Lu
Actinides	90 Th	91 Pa	92 U	93 Np	94 Pu	95 Am	96 Cm	97 Bk	98 Cf	99 Es	100 Fm	101 Md	102 No	103 Lr

NOTE: The group numbers in Arabic numerals are those presently recommended by IUPAC. The Roman numerals are those generally used in North America until 1984. *Some pseudonyms for certain groups of elements:* Group 1: Alkali metals. Group 2: Alkaline earth metals. Group 15: Pnictogens. Group 16: Chalcogens. Group 17: Halogens. Group 18: Noble gases, inert gases, rare gases. Group 11: Coinage metals. Elements 44–46 and 76–78: Platinum metals. Groups 4, 5, and 6 are sometimes referred to as the refractory metals. The term *noble metal* is applied to those elements that are less electropositive than hydrogen—that is, the platinum metals, the coinage metals, and mercury.

FIGURE 1.1. The modern periodic table.

occupancy of orbitals therefore begins once all the orbitals characterized by the same principal quantum number and shape are singly occupied (one for *s*, three for *p*, five for *d*, and seven for *f*). Complete single occupancy of such orbitals with electrons confers relative inertness and spherical shape on the electron density cloud.

The electrons occupying the orbitals of highest principal quantum number (valence electrons) are the least strongly held by the nuclear forces and are the most exposed so that interaction with other valence electrons can occur. Each column of the periodic table contains elements of the same number of valence electrons; those of *p* orbitals are specified with an "A" after the column number, and those of *d* orbitals are specified with a "B" after the column number. Thus atomic size increases down each column of the periodic table, and the nuclear forces experienced by the valence electrons become progressively weaker also.

All chemical and biochemical reactions are considered to involve only interactions between valence electrons, generally on different atoms and molecules but sometimes on the same molecule. Disruption of the nucleus does not occur in nearly all chemical or biochemical reactions because the energy required for this usually is not available.

1.4 BONDING AND MOLECULES

When atoms share electrons, covalent bonds (as in organic compounds) are formed, there being more electron density in the area between the participating nuclei than before the sharing. The stable entity of more than one atom produced after the interaction is called a molecule. Each constituent atom retains its characteristic number of protons and inert gas electron core shell. To break covalent or coordinate bonds, more energy is required for small atoms bonded to a given atom than large ones because of the greater strength of the nucleus–electron interactions in the original molecule. More energy also is required to break the covalent bonds of atoms of equal electronegativity (charge to mass ratio) than of unlike electronegativity where ionic covalent bonds of asymmetric electron density are present. Every covalent bond contains two shared electrons. A dative covalent bond exists when one atom donates two electrons and the other participating atom donates none. In inorganics, this bond is called a coordinate link.

If one covalent bond exists between two atoms, the covalent bond is called sigma. If another covalent bond is formed between the same two atoms, it is called pi and surrounds the first sigma bond. The two bonds together are called a double bond, even though the two are independent bonds sharing the same nuclei. If three covalent bonds exist between the same two atoms, the bond system is a triple bond. The outer pi bonds are more exposed to attack and are farther away from the nuclei than the inner sigma bond, so leading to lower bond dissociation energies (and hence greater reactivity) for pi relative to sigma bonds. The outermost pi bond is always more reactive and exposed to attack than an inner pi bond.

Bonds between one atom and an atom greater in atomic number, for example C–Cl, are weaker than same-atom (homonuclear) sigma bonds, for example, C–C. The major exception is for covalent bonds with F, for example, C–F. This is also true for the pi bonds. Conversely, bonds between an atom and one smaller in atomic number, for example, C–H, are stronger than homonuclear bonds. The types and numbers of functional groups (characteristic grouping of adjacent atoms within the same molecule characterized by distinctive reactions) affect bond strengths; so do atoms substituted on the participating atoms in a covalent bond, and, to a lesser extent, those one atom removed. Table 1.1 gives the bond strengths of isolated bonds. Bond strengths can vary within 15 kcal/mole of the value quoted.

The weakest bonds are broken first in any molecule. Similarly, the most exposed electrons and those less bound to the nuclear and inert-gas electron core also will react first. Often the latter are the nonbonded electrons in the valence shell of heteronuclear functional groups (atoms other than carbon and hydrogen, also called "heteroatoms"). Because carbon is generally tetravalent (four valence electrons bond fully) in all its compounds (except in carbon monoxide and as the element), it has no nonbonded electrons in its valence shell. This is also true for hydrogen, whose one electron is always shared in a covalent bond. Nitrogen is generally trivalent, thus allowing two valence shell *s* electrons to remain as nonbonded electrons for potential initial reaction or for further coordinate linking (nitrogen (V) compounds). Oxygen is usually divalent and so has two each of nonbonded *s* and *p* electrons; sulfur in its divalent states shows the same behavior. However, sulfur can also show stable tetravalent and hexavalent states through coordinate links where the nonbonded electrons are two and zero, respectively. Phosphorus exhibits trivalent and pentavalent states, the nonbonded electrons being two and zero, respectively. Halogens, being monovalent, have six nonbonded electrons after covalent bonding.

TABLE 1.1. Bond energy *E* values for some important bond types. *E* values are arranged within each group in order of decreasing strength. The mean values are averaged over a large senes of compounds. The calculated values are computed for just one compound using values for other bonds from earlier values in the table.*

Bond	Mean value of *E* at 25°C, kcal/mol	Value	Calculated from	Bond	Mean value of *E* at 25°C, kcal/mol	Value	Calculated from
O—H	110–111	110.6	H_2O	C—S	66	64	C_2H_5SH
C—H	96–99	99.5	CH_4	C—I	52	50.1	CH_3I
N—H	93	93.4	NH_3				
S—H	82	83	H_2S	C≡C	199–200	194.4	C_2H_2
				C═C	146–151	141.3	C_2H_4
C—F	. . .	116	CF_4	C—C	83–85	79.1	C_2H_6
C—H	96–99	99.5	CH_4				
C—O	85–91	76.8	CH_3OH	C≡N	204	206.1	HCN
		84.2	C_2H_5OH	C═O	173–81	164	HCHO
C—C	83–85	79.1	C_2H_6			192	CO_2
C—Cl	79	78.3	CCl_4	C═N	143		
C—N	69–75	66.5	CH_3NH_2				
C—Br	66	69	CBr_4				
		65	$CHBr_3$				

* O. Norch, *Advanced Organic Chemistry: Reactions, Mechanisms, dur Structure*, 3rd ed., p. 23.

When there are only small differences in energy between the valence orbitals (for example, the 2*s* and 2*p* orbitals, and the 4*s* and 3*d* orbitals), the energy levels tend to be evened-out to be able to produce a relatively stable spherical electron density cloud. This is "hybridization" of the orbitals. Thus, although the carbon atom has two 2*s* and two 2*p* valence electrons, this evening-out produces four equivalent sp^3 hybrids for end-on overlap to produce the sigma framework of saturated organic compounds. For organic hydrocarbons containing a double bond, each of the two carbons in the bond donates three valence electrons to create the sigma framework (sp^2 hybrids) through end-on overlap of the hybrids with the appropriate valence electron orbitals. The pi bond between the two carbons of the double bond then is visualized to form through sideways overlap of the remaining unhybridized *p* orbital.

For triple bonds in an organic hydrocarbon, the two carbon atoms have *sp* hybrids, the sigma framework being formed first by end-on overlap of the hybrids with the appropriate valence electron orbitals. The two pi bonds are then produced by two sideways overlaps of the remaining unhybridized *p* orbitals.

Under practical conditions we generally use quantities of chemicals for synthesis or reactions. The molecular weight in amu is defined as one mole of the chemical and contains an Avogadro number of molecules, 6.0234×10^{23}.

1.5 IONIZATION

When an atom or a molecule loses an electron through energy input by physical or chemical means, a positive ion is formed. For atoms, the positive ion is a cation. For molecules, the name depends on which atom carries the positive charge. For a carbon atom attached only to sigma bonds, the moiety is called a carbonium ion. For nitrogen, the analog is an ammonium ion. Conversely, when an atom or a molecule gains an electron, a negative ion is formed. For atoms the negative ion is an anion. For molecules where only the carbon attached to sigma bonds carries the negative charge, the species is called a carbanion. Sometimes, atoms can share the negative charge (signaled when resonance structures—theoretical structures with the same sigma bond framework but with different electronic configurations—can be written). Such a case is a carboxylate anion where a negative charge is shared by a carbon and two oxygen atoms.

Ions in the gas phase differ from those in the liquid or solid phases. A hydrogen ion in the gas phase consists of one proton and no electrons. A hydrogen ion in the aqueous phase consists of one proton surrounded by four water molecules attached via the nonbonded electrons of the oxygen atoms to create a solvated proton, commonly called the hydronium ion. The concentration of this hydronium ion is related to acidity through the definition of pH as the negative logarithm to the base ten of the hydronium ion concentration in dilute solution or of the hydronium ion activity in concentrated solution. Ions in nonaqueous liquids also exist as solvated species.

Ions in solids are surrounded by other oppositely charged ions and/or molecules. These ions do not tumble as occurs in liquids but only vibrate or rotate, and cannot convect as in the liquid phase or translate as in the gaseous phase. Electrons also can be solvated in the liquid phase, as, for example, in liquid ammonia.

Ions of different charge-to-mass ratio at a liquid–solid phase interface can set up a potential difference called a redox potential, in which one ionic species is more likely to donate or accept a solvated electron than the other. Electron transfer also can occur in the solid phase.

Oppositely charged ions in solution, in the gas phase, or in solids can react to form solid ionic compounds where oppositely charged ions are often clustered around one another in an ordered fashion to preserve electrical neutrality. Liquid solutions of ionic compounds also show clustering but much less order than solids because the Brownian motion of the solvent molecules precludes the attainment of regular structures. Solid ionic compounds show much greater water solubility and polarity than the molecules possessing the same elements but linked covalently.

One function of the active site of enzymes implicated in biological electron transfers is to provide a relatively rigid site to limit the motions of the substrate, to orient it relative to the reactants and cofactors so as to provide efficient reaction and/or electron transfer even against an unfavorable energy gradient. Biochemical systems often require the simultaneous use of high energy compounds such as adenosine triphosphate (ATP) to overcome thermodynamically unfavorable energy gradients.

1.6 ACIDS AND BASES

Species such as cations that attract electrons are called Lewis acids; more generally they are termed "electrophiles" because they "love" negatively charged or electron-rich species. Electrophiles do not have to bear a formal positive charge. The sites of electrophilic attack may be at the sites of smallest electron density. Conversely, species such as anions that may donate electrons are called Lewis bases; they are more generally termed "nucleophiles" because they "love" positively charged species in terms of reaction. Free radicals (species with unbonded electrons that are usually covalently bonded) are also nucleophiles. Under the Lewis scale of acidity and those of electrophilicity or nucleophilicity, the hardness or the softness of the philicity and the degree of acidity or basicity are relative and depend on the components of the system being studied. An example is that nitric acid is an acid in the presence of sodium hydroxide but acts as a base when in the presence of sulfuric acid.

A more familiar definition of an acid (the Lowry–Bronsted definition) defines it as the species that produces a hydronium ion, whereas a base produces a hydroxyl ion, both being in aqueous solution. The product of a chemical reaction is the focus here rather than the original compound itself. Such reactions always occur along stoichiometric lines.

When the salts and their corresponding weak acids or weak bases (those that do not dissociate into their full complement of hydronium or hydroxide ions) are present together, buffer solutions (which resist pH change) are produced. The major buffer systems in the human body are the monohydrogen phosphate–dihydrogen phosphate and the carbonate-bicarbonate systems. No simple buffer systems in the body are based on chloride, nitrate, and sulfate because their corresponding acids are all strong.

The Henderson-Hasselbach equation, which is written as follows for dilute solutions:

$$\text{pH} = \text{p}K_a + \log\text{ (equilibrium salt concentration/equilibrium acid concentration)} \tag{1.1}$$

expresses the relationship between the buffer salt and acid in terms of pH, the concentrations of acid and base, and the negative logarithm to the base ten of the dissociation constant of the acid at specified conditions (pK_a). When the concentrations of acid and base are equal, the pH defines the pK_a.

The body processes that regulate properties such as pH, temperature, osmolarity, density, redox potential, and concentrations of essential elements and vitamins (essential organic compounds), and those indices having characteristic constant values in each organ or tissue are termed "homeostatic" for each individual. Group homeostatic values are termed "reference ranges" ("normal values" in the older literature). When regular variations occur within this homeostasis, a circadian rhythm may be observable. Different people may have different circadian rhythms.

1.7 OXIDATION AND REDUCTION

When there is a loss of electrons from one species, that species is said to be oxidized. The species that gains electrons is said to be reduced. The redox potential (E) is the measure of how much electromotive force is required to effect the oxidation/reduction and is related to the equilibrium constant (K) for the reaction through the Nernst equation:

$$E = E^0 - (RT/nF)(\ln K) \tag{1.2}$$

where R is the gas constant (8.3143 joules (J) $mol^{-1}K^{-1}$), T is the absolute temperature, n is the number of electrons transferred in the oxidation or reduction process, F is a constant called the Faraday constant (96,487 coulombs per equivalent), and E^0 is the redox potential at 25°C, and one atmosphere pressure relative to a hydrogen reference electrode at unit activity (idealized concentration) of hydrogen ions, whose potential at all temperatures is defined as zero.

Alternative definitions of oxidation include addition of oxygen, loss of hydrogen, or increase in oxidation number. Conversely, reduction is also defined as loss of oxygen, gain of hydrogen, or decrease in oxidation number.

In a situation where a nonpolar low molecular weight xenobiotic is absorbed through inhalation, oral ingestion, or skin absorption, it may have to be oxidized enough that the products are sufficiently water-soluble to be excreted in the urine in conjugated or free form. If the molecular weight is high (>320–340), elimination occurs in the bile from the gall bladder and thence in the feces. If the molecular weight is low enough and the compound also has a high vapor pressure and is nonpolar, the compound and its volatile nonpolar metabolites may also be expired in the breath unchanged. All of these stable end products constitute potential biological monitoring markers.

Under oxygen-deficient (anaerobic) conditions, reduction to more volatile compounds may occur as in anaerobic symbiotic microorganisms, many of which live in the human gastrointestinal tract and in the lungs. All of these processes may occur simultaneously and competitively so that only a small fraction of usable markers may be excreted in the urine or in the other excretion pathways. Any biological monitoring marker, however generated, ought to be a sensitive index; so the pathway of greatest excretion potential must first be known before the marker itself can be chosen for a given excretion medium. This involves defining how fast the marker is excreted (kinetics).

1.8 KINETICS

The kinetics of reactions and processes determine when to sample the biological medium and for how long.

The most general kinetic expression relates the mass absorbed (m) to its whole body disappearance rate, at a given time t, $-dm/dt$. The rate $-dm/dt$ is proportional to m raised to a power n:

$$-dm/dt = k_n m^n \tag{1.3}$$

where k_n is the rate constant, and n is a real number called the order of the process. This equation can be integrated with respect to time and solved generally. However the physical interpretation may only be clear for n values of 0, 1, and 2 where the processes are zero-, first-, and second-order, respectively.

For zero-order processes characteristic of kinetic steady states:

$$X[\text{excreted}] = 1 - X[\text{in body}] = k_0 t/m_0 \tag{1.4}$$

where X[excreted] is the mass fraction excreted of the initial mass[m_0] at time t after absorption, and X[in body] is the mass fraction of the initial mass still in the body at time t after absorption.

For first-order processes characteristic of radioactivity, photochemistry, and a rate-limiting reactant ("pseudo first order"):

$$-\log X[\text{in body}] = k_1 t/2.303 \tag{1.5}$$

For second-order processes where there are two slow processes involving the same reactant:

$$X[\text{excreted}]/X[\text{in body}] = k m_0 t \tag{1.6}$$

Only the first-order process has a half-life that is independent of m_0. It is equal to $0.693/k_1$.

The order of the process if signified by linear relations between:

- X[excreted] and time for a zero-order process with slope k_0/m_0.
- $-\log(1 - X$[excreted]) and time for a first-order process with slope $k_1/2.303$.
- X[excreted]/X[in body] and time for a second-order process with a slope of km_0.

The distinction between equilibrium and steady state is important. Equilibrium occurs when the rates of the forward and the back processes of a reversible process are the same at defined conditions of temperature, pressure, and other characteristic variables. This means that a plot of the concentrations of both reactants and products relative to time will be constant and independent of time; that is, the slope is zero. Steady state occurs when the rate of disappearance and/or appearance of a marker at defined conditions is constant whether the process is reversible or not. Steady states describe kinetic situations solely and not equilibrium conditions. Steady states are not unique at the prevailing conditions, unlike equilibrium.

1.9 CATALYSTS AND ENZYMES

It is important to realize that kinetics is a descriptive, empirical approach, influenced by such things as the conditions and biological integrity of the system under study as well as mechanism and geometry. This can be compared with the thermodynamic approach, which considers only the initial and final states of systems and does not consider time as a variable. The presence of catalysts in chemical systems and enzymes in biological systems illustrates that time is a crucial variable. Both terms describe a situation where an agent that is regenerated completely decreases the reaction time for the process relative to when the agent is not present. The original definition of catalysis included both increasing and decreasing reaction rates, but the property of decreasing reaction rates is now defined to be exerted by the agents called inhibitors rather than catalysts.

Biological processes occur in systems that include the serum, the red blood cells, cell membranes, the cell cytosol, and cell organelles as well as different organs subject to hormonal control. Kinetics measured under such conditions reflect heterogeneous conditions because more than one phase (chemical systems) or compartment (biological systems) is involved. For one-phase or one-compartment processes, the kinetics are termed homogeneous. The above discussion of the order of different processes is interpretable mostly for homogeneous processes.

However, if one step is slower than the rest, homogeneous first-order kinetics ("pseudo first-order") may be applicable. If there are two slow steps for the same component, "pseudo second-order" kinetics based on homogeneous second-order kinetics may be descriptive. The simplicity is still illusory, however, for biological markers because all that such measurements can hope to characterize are net, overall trends, which by definition are empirical and which may not hold from person to person. Fortunately, homeostatic mechanisms are common to many people so that some generalizations can be made for a given human population of relatively homogeneous ancestry, diet, and social habits.

Because temperature is important to reaction rates, the constancy of body temperature in mammals signifies that temperature will not be an important variable in biological processes for humans who are healthy. Thus, there is no temperature dependence of activation energy (the energy input required to make a reaction or process proceed at a measurable rate) as expressed by the Arrhenius equation for chemical reactions in the liquid and solid phases:

$$d \ln k/dT = E/RT^2 \tag{1.7}$$

or:

$$\log k = -E/2.303RT + C \tag{1.8}$$

where k is a unitless rate constant, E is the activation energy, T is the absolute temperature, and C is an arbitrary constant.

The function of enzymes in biological systems is to supply the activation energy of the process to be facilitated without increasing or decreasing body temperature. The extra energy needed to overcome any activation energy comes from the solvation energy linked with "high-energy" phosphate compounds, with any required "cofactors," and the existence of complex templates of low entropy.

1.10 MICHAELIS–MENTEN KINETICS

Homogeneous kinetics can also be obeyed when reactants are rate-limiting, that is, when one or two reactants are in low enough concentration to control the reaction rate. For example, in the process $aA + bB$ to give cC, using k_1 to denote the rate constant of the forward reaction and k_2 for the rate constant of the back reaction, the rate expression can be written:

$$-dA/dt = k_1 aA^aB^b - k_2 aC^c \tag{1.9}$$

where t is the time, and A, B, C represent molar concentrations. When B is large and k_2aC^c is small, equation (1.9) changes to:

$$-dA/dt = k_1'A^a \tag{1.10}$$

where k_1' is a new rate constant equal to k_1aB^b, which appears to be constant because B is large. The process becomes "pseudo first-order" to A when a equals one, and "pseudo second-order" when a equals two, even though the reaction does not really involve A alone. This approach is often used in chemically defined processes but generally is harder to apply and interpret in biological systems where the major entity to be measured is a product rather than a reactant.

Another way to see how the mechanism of a process can affect this same sequence is to write the same process as $aA + bB$ to give an activated complex (AB) by a slow reaction with forward and back reaction rate constants k_1 and k_2, respectively, with subsequent fast reaction of rate constant k_3 to provide the product C and to regenerate B in the mechanism:

$$aA + bB \rightarrow (AB) \rightarrow cC + bB \tag{1.11}$$

If a, b, and c are equal to one, equation (1.11) becomes:

$$A + B \rightarrow (AB) \rightarrow C + B \tag{1.12}$$

$$-dA/dt = -dB/dt = dC/dt = dB/dt = k_3(AB) - k_2(AB) + k_1AB \tag{1.13}$$

where A, B, and (AB) are in molar concentration units.

If the rate of formation of (AB) equals the rate of depletion [(AB) is in steady state], then:

$$k_1AB = k_2(AB) + k_3(AB) \tag{1.14}$$

Rearranging equation (1.14) gives:

$$(AB) = \frac{AB}{[k_2 + k_3]/k_1} \tag{1.15}$$

where $[k_2 + k_3]/k_1 = K_m$, the Michaelis constant, so that equation (1.15) becomes:

$$(AB) = AB/K_m \tag{1.16}$$

If A is nearly equal to A_0, the initial concentration of A, and B is very much less than A with B also being nearly equal to B_0, then:

$$B = B_0 - (AB) \tag{1.17}$$

On substituting for B in equation (1.16):

$$(AB) = [B_0 - (AB)]A/K_m \tag{1.18}$$

Solving equation (1.18) for (AB) gives:

$$(AB) = B_0A/K_m \times 1/[1 + A/K_m] \quad (1.19)$$

$$= B_0A/[A + K_m] \quad (1.20)$$

Since:

$$dC/dt = V = k_3(AB) \quad (1.21)$$

We obtain:

$$dC/dt = V = k_3B_0A/[A + K_m] \quad (1.22)$$

If A is much greater than K_m so that $A/[A + K_m]$ approaches one, then:

$$[dC/dt]_{max} = V_{max} = k_3B_0 \quad (1.23)$$

where "max" denotes a maximum because one of the reactants is large.

Substituting equation (1.23) into equation (1.22) yields the famous Michaelis–Menton equation, which describes enzyme kinetics (replace A with substrate concentration S and B with enzyme concentration E):

$$V = V_{max}\,A/[A + K_m] \quad (1.24)$$

At low A when A is much less than K_m:

$$V = AV_{max}/K_m \quad (1.25)$$

This means that the velocity of the reaction with respect to product C or reactant A is directly related to A, so obeying a first-order process.

At high A when A is much greater than K_m, $V = V_{max}$ or the rate is independent of A, so obeying a zero-order process.

When $A = K_m$, $V = V_{max}/2$ so that K_m is equal to the A at which the reaction rate is half its maximum value.

When equation (1.25) is transformed into the following expression:

$$1/V = 1/V_{max} + (K_m/V_{max})\,(1/A) \quad (1.26)$$

a linear plot of $1/V$ versus $1/A$ (a Lineweaver–Burk plot) indicates that the process obeys Michaelis–Menton kinetics characterized by a $1/V$ intercept of $1/V_{max}$, a $1/A$ intercept of $-1/K_m$, and a slope of K_m/V_{max}.

For most enzymes, K_m values range between 0.1 M and 100 nM. Most biochemistry texts interpret K_m to be related to the concentration of A at which half of the active sites of an enzyme are filled. A kinetic interpretation is that K_m is equal to k_2/k_1, the dissociation constant of the complex (AB), when k_3 is small relative to k_2 in $K_m = [k_2 + k_3]/k_1$, so that K_m becomes a measure of the strength of the (AB) complex. However, if k_1 and k_2 are both similar, and k_1 is also small, K_m becomes a measure of how difficult it is to form (AB).

Clearly the interpretation of K_m depends on the system, a characteristic of a kinetic model.

Even though k_3 may be large, the largest value it can have is defined by diffusion control. This limit can be partly overcome by confining substrates and products in the limited volume of a multienzyme complex where the product of one enzyme is very rapidly found by the next enzyme of the complex, so that an assembly line of reactions can be performed with the rate-determining step being effectively the formation of the first enzyme–substrate complex, a common feature in many mammalian systems. The cytochrome P-450 entity, which catalyzes complicated reductions and oxidations in the mammalian endoplasmic reticulum, is such a multienzyme complex.

Inhibition of enzymatic activity can be reversible or irreversible. Irreversible inhibition generally results when the inhibitor–enzyme complex is much more stable than the substrate–enzyme complex so that a favorable substrate–inhibitor ratio does not restore the activity quickly. An example is the relatively irreversible action of organophosphorus pesticides and nerve gases on cholinesterase activity, as compared with the action of the organocarbamate pesticides, which are reversible inhibitors of cholinesterase activity.

Reversible inhibition can be competitive or noncompetitive. A competitive inhibitor may resemble the substrate and so bind at the same enzyme sites but with less affinity than the substrate. The substrate cannot bind at these occupied sites, and so the rate of catalysis is reduced and the K_m is changed. The $V_{\max}$ is not affected. Increasing the substrate concentration to beyond a critical value will overcome competitive inhibition. In noncompetitive inhibition, both the inhibitor and the substrate can bind simultaneously to the enzyme, causing a changed substrate–enzyme complex that reduces the efficiency of product molecule release. However, the K_m is not changed while the $V_{\max}$ is. Such an inhibition cannot be reversed by increasing substrate concentration. When substrate binding and product release are both affected, the inhibition is termed "mixed."

The Michaelis–Menton model is not obeyed by all enzymes, particularly those with sigmoidal velocity versus substrate concentration plots rather than the expected hyperbolic ones. When there are interactions between different binding sites on the same enzyme complex, the binding sites are no longer equivalent, and a Gaussian distribution of affinities for the sites may produce the sigmoidal plot. Such enzymes are called allosteric.

1.11 REACTION TYPES

Chemical reactions involve the breaking and re-forming of bonds. The reaction producing the largest quantity of product is the main reaction, with the others called competing reactions. Test tube reactions often form several products, whereas enzymic reactions are generally more specific than that. Each reaction will have its own stoichiometry, that is, the number of reactant molecules required to create product molecules. Each reaction will have its own equilibrium constant, defined by the product of the concentrations of the products relative to those of the reactants and allowing for stoichiometry. The main reaction will have the largest equilibrium constant, whereas the competing reactions will have much smaller equilibrium constants under the conditions of the reaction. When there are many competitive reactions, yields of the various products are more important than the stoichiometry of the individual reactions. Markers excreted into biological media may not be practical if the overall yields are too small.

There are four basic types of nonpolymeric reactions for organic compounds: substitution, elimination, addition, and condensation. Substitution (S) involves the exchange of one functional group with another. Elimination (E) involves the net removal of one functional group each from two atoms of a molecule, with the appearance of a new bond between the two participating atoms. Elimination of the two groups from the same atom is alpha elimination to produce a carbene. Elimination between two adjacent atoms is beta elimination. In gamma elimination a three-membered ring is formed. 1,4-Eliminations have also been observed. Addition to a pi bond is the reverse of a beta-elimination reaction. Condensation reactions involve the insertion (but not an exchange) of a new group with the production of two stable uncharged molecules. All can be first- or second-order in kinetics. Usually the molecularity of the reaction (the number of the molecules important in the rate-determining step) is indicated.

Substitution by nucleophiles (N) is termed an SN process, commonly unimolecular (SN_1) or bimolecular (SN_2). The latter involves backside nucleophilic attack relative to the leaving group so that the bonds are broken and formed simultaneously in a concerted process involving both nucleophile and substrate. The SN_1 reaction consists of a slow reversible first step where the leaving group is detached by solvolysis to produce a solvated intermediate carbonium ion, and then a fast step involving the nucleophile. Elimination is a competing reaction for the carbonium ion. Similarly, elimination can be E_1 or E_2.

Substitution is found in many inorganic systems, an example being the reaction of an acid and a base to produce a salt and water. Electrophilic substitution occurs in substituted benzene rings, to carbanions, and to the lone pairs of heteronuclear atoms. Addition at unsymmetrical double bonds is Markownikoff or anti-Markownikoff. Markownikoff addition occurs when an unsymmetrical alkene adds a hydrogen to the atom in the double bond with the greatest number of hydrogens. Anti-Markownikoff addition is the reverse. Symmetrical double bonds produce mixtures of products on addition. Double bonds, being electron-rich, act like Lewis bases. More generally, the type of substitution on double bonds or benzene rings determines the products of electrophilic or nucleophilic addition and substitution, respectively, in addition to the type of attacking species. Thus electron-donating functional groups such as alkyl and amino groups promote electrophilic substitution at the *ortho-* and *para-* positions of a benzene ring, whereas they promote Markownikoff addition to asymmetric double bonds. Electron-withdrawing groups such as nitro-, carboxylic, or carbonyl groups promote electrophilic substitution at the *meta-* position of the benzene ring and promote anti-Markownikoff addition to asymmetric double bonds.

Intermolecular condensation reactions generally produce small stable molecules such as water and ammonia as well as a much higher molecular weight product that has the molecular weight of the sum of the two reactants minus the molecular weight of the small molecule produced, as, for example, the amide of an amine and a carboxylic acid. Intramolecular condensations also produce small stable molecules, but the product has a molecular weight less than the molecular weight of the original molecule, as, for example, in the dehydration of phthalic acid to phthalic anhydride.

Free radicals may also be produced as activated intermediates in addition to anions and cations. All of these species are reactive, and in biological systems, when their concentrations are not controlled, may cause organelle, cellular, or tissue damage.

Further Reading

Chemistry

Butler, I. S., and Harrod, J. F. 1989. *Inorganic Chemistry: Principles and Applications*, Benjamin/Cummings Publishing, Redwood City, CA.

Holum, J. R. 1990. *Fundamentals of General, Organic, and Biological Chemistry*, 4th ed., John Wiley and Sons, New York.

March, J. 1985. *Advanced Organic Chemistry*, 3rd ed., Wiley-Interscience, New York.

Maron, S. H., and Prutton, C. F. 1967. *Principles of Physical Chemistry*, 4th ed., Macmillan, New York.

Physics

Halliday, D.; Resnick, R.; and Merrill, J. 1988. *Fundamentals of Physics*, 3rd ed. extended, John Wiley and Sons, New York.

2

Concepts in Biochemistry

It is not the intent here to provide an exhaustive introduction to biochemistry in humans. What will be emphasized are the general concepts important to general metabolism (breakdown and biosynthetic processes).

2.0 MACROMOLECULES

The large molecules (macromolecules) important to biochemistry are proteins, lipids, polysaccharides, and nucleic acids. Not only is primary structure important (the sequence of the fundamental building blocks: amino acids through amide links for proteins, fatty acids in lipids through phosphate ester links, sugars through alpha or beta links in polysaccharides, and purine/pyrimidine bases in nucleic acids through phosphate ester/N-ether links), but also higher-order structures contribute. Secondary structure is the spatial geometry of the primary structure (helical or otherwise for proteins and polysaccharides; double helix for nuclear DNA). Tertiary structure is the spatial arrangement of nonadjacent fundamental building blocks to one another (for example, the amino acids in the primary sequence of a protein, which form the active site of an enzyme and which, though distant in terms of primary sequence, are in close proximity spatially, often through the agency of disulfide links; another example is the pairing of purines and pyrimidines in separate DNA strands through hydrogen bonds). Quaternary structure occurs in super macromolecules where there are repeating macromolecular subunits, as, for example, in certain enzymes that have well-defined protein or polypeptide subunits, and in chromosomes which are bundles of DNA and protein.

The higher-order structures are a result of the hydrophobic and hydrophilic forces characteristic of the building blocks and hydrogen bonding of the aqueous solvent. Higher-order structures can be interpreted as a kind of self-aggregation to produce a thermodynamically stable entity. Many higher structures remain to be discovered.

The fundamental building blocks and cofactors for macromolecule synthesis that must be supplied through the diet (because they cannot be synthesized by the organism) are termed "essential." These often change from one species to another; for example, ascorbic acid (vitamin C) is essential for humans and guinea pigs but not for rats or mice. Essential organic compounds are termed "vitamins," and essential inorganics are called "essential elements." The processes of anabolism (synthesis of compounds of higher molecular weights than those of the original constituents), catabolism (endogenous degradative processes), and metabolism (redox processes in organisms concerned with energy acquisition and synthesis of the basic building blocks of molecules) are dependent on endogenous processes also. All of these processes require a steady state supply of energy and conditions (homeostasis) that is characteristic of a kinetic system rather than one at equilibrium. This is so because most metabolic pathways are irreversible. Usually an early step is the rate-determining one (committed step), which is often the one under genetic control. In addition, not all the reactions in a given metabolic cycle will occur in one cellular compartment; so heterogeneous kinetics operate. The kinds of reactions that occur are common to *in vitro* chemistry (Section 1.11): group transfers or nucleophilic substitution (most often acyl, phosphoryl, and glycosyl groups); redox (via NAD, FAD, molecular oxygen, and cytochrome chain participation); eliminations, isomerizations, and rearrangements (the maintenance of stereochemistry is often important here); and making or breaking of carbon–carbon bonds involving substitution, condensation, addition, and elimination.

2.1 GLYCOLYSIS AND THE CITRIC ACID CYCLE

Glycolysis is the process of ten cytosolic reactions that convert the aldohexose sugar glucose (C_6) into two molecules of pyruvate (C_3) with the production (Figure 2.1) of two molecules of adenosine triphosphate (ATP). There are two rate-determining reactions, one being the conversion of fructose-6-phosphate to fructose-1,6-diphosphate via phosphofructokinase and the other being the transformation of phosphoenolpyruvate to pyruvate via pyruvate kinase. When glycogen is the source of glucose, the hexokinase step is not rate-limiting. Glycolysis occurs even in the absence of oxygen, and the pyruvate is converted to lactate in muscle, which stores this acid and also allows the anaerobic process to continue. In aerobic processes, the ATP and pyruvate generated through glycolysis feed into the citric acid or Krebs cycle inside the matrix of mitochondria [the pyruvate is esterified into acetyl coenzyme A (acetyl CoA) to produce citrate from oxaloacetate, which is then sent through eight other reactions that finally regenerate oxaloacetate (Figure 2.2)]. The enzymes catalyzing the rate-determining steps are citrate synthase, isocitrate dehydrogenase, and α-ketoglutarate dehydrogenase. The citric acid cycle generates reduced nicotinamide adenine dinucleotide (NADH) and reduced flavin adenine dinucleotide ($FADH_2$), which are further used in the electron-transport chain to produce three ATPs per NADH, and two ATPs per $FADH_2$. Only one high energy phosphate bond as guanosine triphosphate (GTP) is formed directly. The cycle provides building blocks for macro-

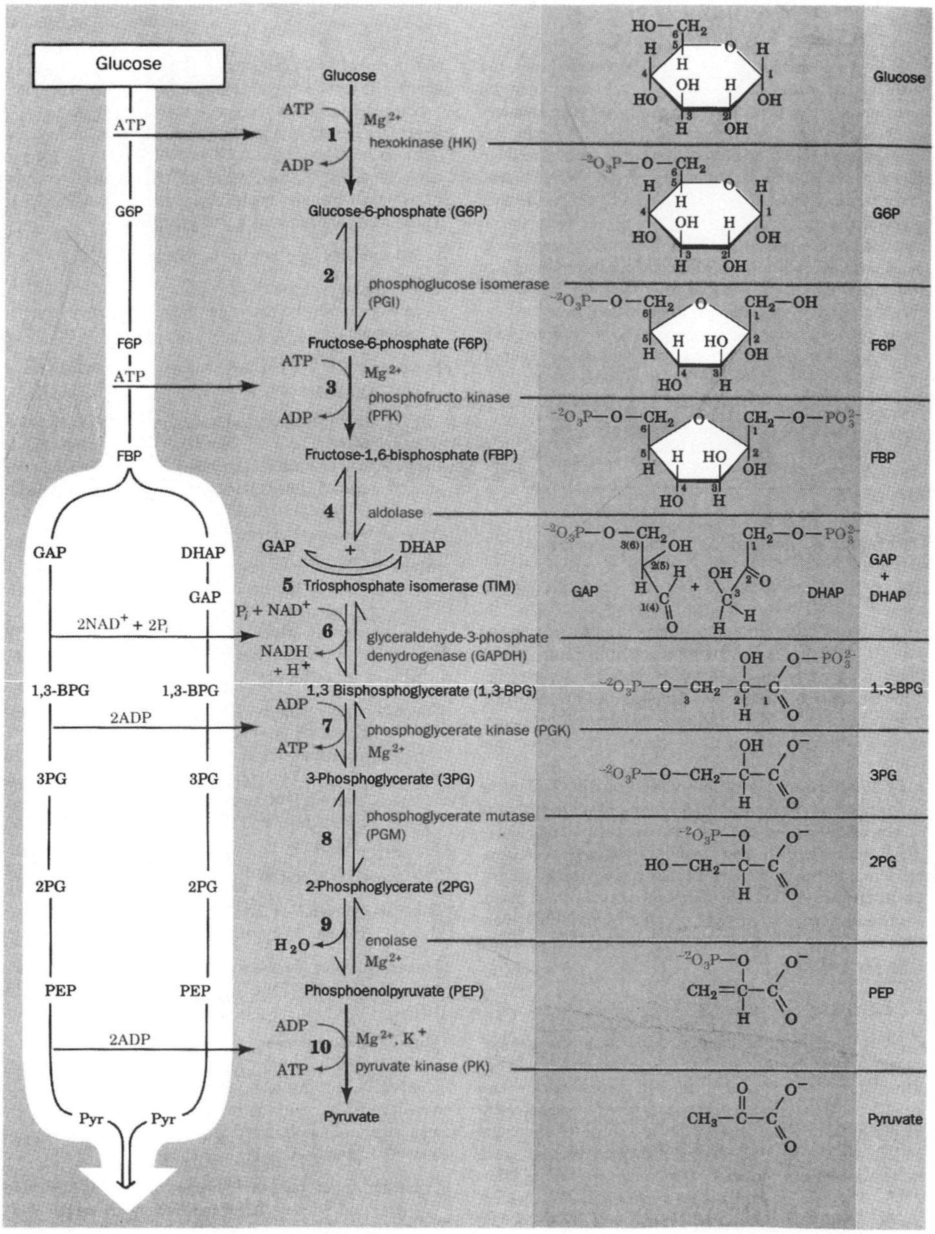

FIGURE 2.1. The degradation of glucose via the glycolytic pathway. Glycolysis may be considered to occur in two stages. Stage I (Reactions 1–5): Glucose is phosphorylated and cleaved to form two molecules of the triose glyceraldehyde-3-phosphate. This requires the expenditure of two ATPs in an "energy investment" (Reactions 1 and 3). Stage II (Reactions 6–10): The two molecules of glyceraldehyde-3-phosphate are converted to pyruvate with the concomitant generation of four ATPs (Reactions 7 and 10). (Courtesy of *Biochemistry*, Voet/Voet, J. Wiley & Sons.)

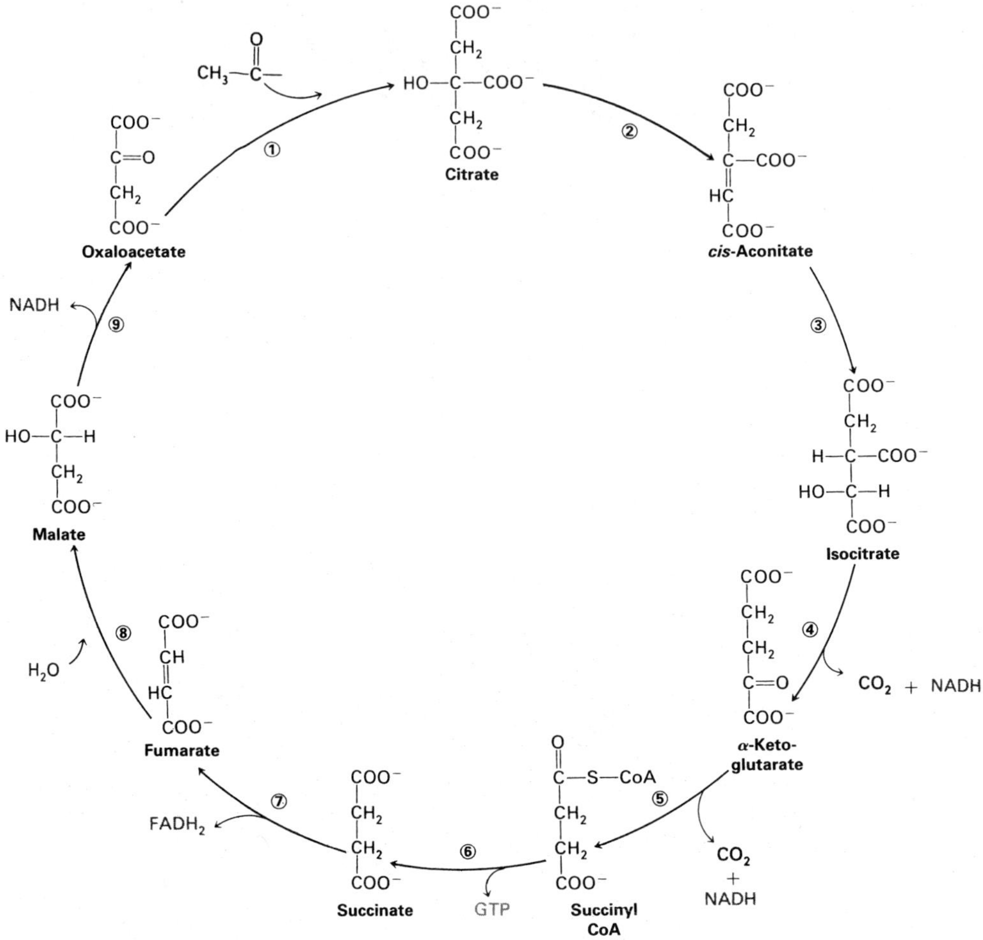

Citric acid cycle

Step	Reaction	Enzyme	Prosthetic group	Type*	$\Delta G^{\circ\prime}$
1	Acetyl CoA + oxaloacetate + H_2O $\longrightarrow$ citrate + CoA + H^+	Citrate synthetase		a	−7.5
2	Citrate $\rightleftharpoons$ *cis*-aconitate + H_2O	Aconitase	Fe-S	b	+2.0
3	*cis*-Aconitate + H_2O $\rightleftharpoons$ isocitrate	Aconitase	Fe-S	c	−0.5
4	Isocitrate + NAD^+ $\rightleftharpoons$ α-ketoglutarate + CO_2 + NADH	Isocitrate dehydrogenase	Lipoic acid FAD	d + e	−2.0
5	α-Ketoglutarate + NAD^+ + CoA $\rightleftharpoons$ succinyl CoA + CO_2 + NADH	α-Ketoglutarate dehydrogenase complex	TPP	d + e	−7.2
6	Succinyl CoA + P_i + GDP $\rightleftharpoons$ succinate + GTP + CoA	Succinyl CoA synthetase		f	−0.8
7	Succinate + FAD (enzyme-bound) $\rightleftharpoons$ fumarate + $FADH_2$ (enzyme-bound)	Succinate dehydrogenase	FAD Fe-S	e	~0
8	Fumarate + H_2O $\rightleftharpoons$ L-malate	Fumarase		c	−0.9
9	L-Malate + NAD^+ $\rightleftharpoons$ oxaloacetate + NADH + H^+	Malate dehydrogenase		e	+7.1

*Reaction type: (a) Condensation (b) Dehydration (c) Hydration (d) Decarboxylation (e) Oxidation (f) Substrate-level phosphorylation

FIGURE 2.2. The citric acid cycle. (Courtesy of *Biochemistry*, third edition, Stryer, Freeman.)

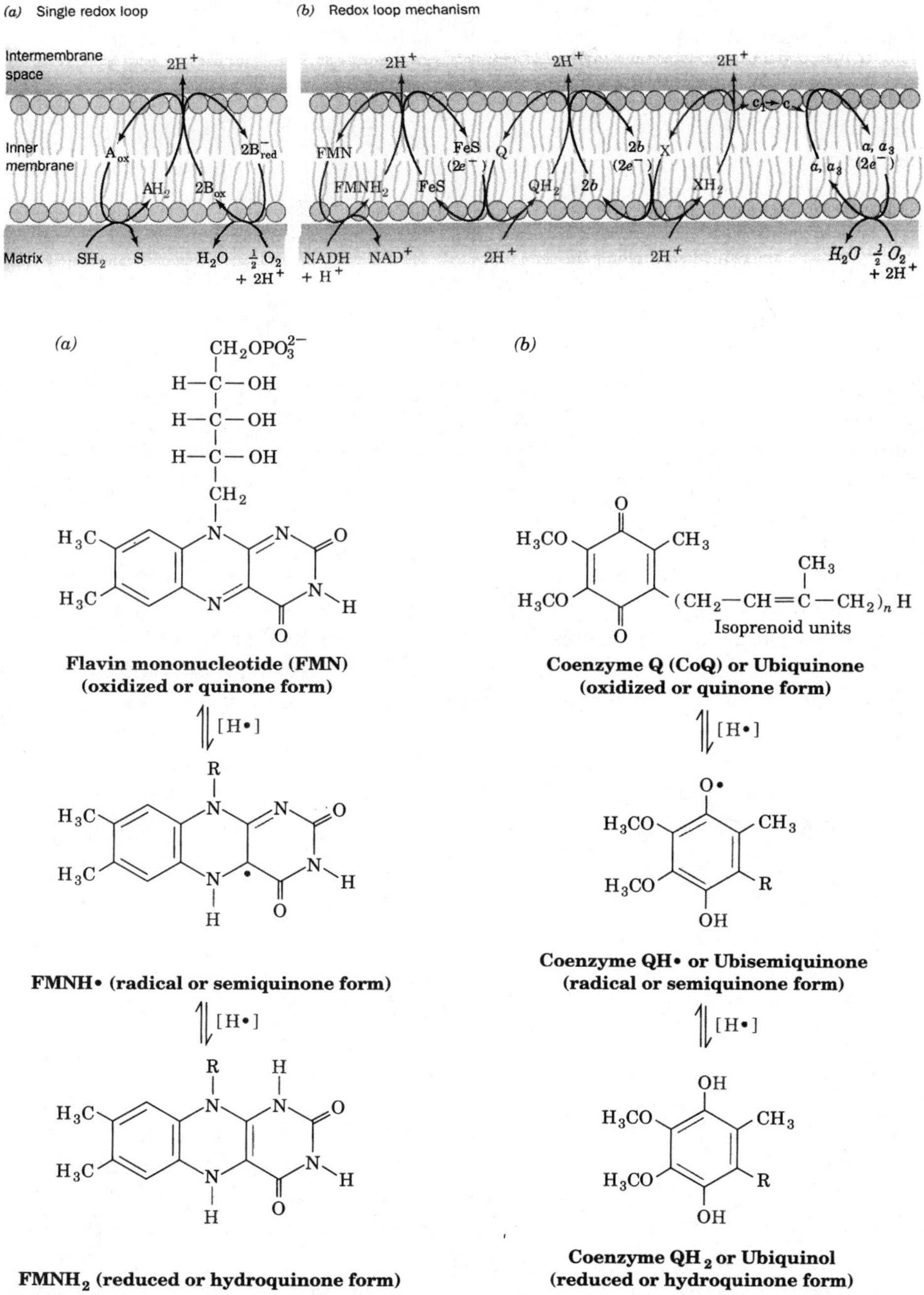

FIGURE 2.3. The redox loop mechanism. (a) A single redox loop for electron-transport-linked H^+ translocation. (b) The proposed redox loop mechanism of electron-transport-linked proton translocation in mitochondria. FMN and CoQ function as ($H^+ + e^-$) carriers while the iron–sulfur clusters and the cytochromes function as pure e^- carriers. These components are so arranged as to require that electron transport be accompanied by H^+ translocation. Note that a mystery ($H^+ + e^-$) carrier, X, is included to account for a third H^+ translocation site. Inset: The oxidation states of (a) FMN and (b) CoQ. Both coenzymes form stable semiquinone free radical states. (Courtesy of *Biochemistry*, Voet/Voet, J. Wiley & Sons.)

molecules, for example, succinyl CoA for porphyrins, and α-ketoglutarate and oxaloacetate for nonessential amino acids. The cycle is the final common pathway for the oxidation of fuel molecules, commonly entering as two carbon fragments of acetyl CoA. In eucaryotes, the citric acid cycle operates in tandem with the electron-transport chain (oxidative phosphorylation) in aerobic biosynthetic processes.

2.2 OXIDATIVE PHOSPHORYLATION AND ELECTRON TRANSPORT

Oxidative phosphorylation in eucaryotes is the process by which ATP is formed as electrons are transferred from NADH or $FADH_2$ to oxygen by a series of electron carriers (such as the cytochromes) located in the invaginated inner membrane (cristae) of mitochondria (Figure 2.3). It generates 32 of the 36 molecules of ATP that are produced when glucose is completely oxidized to carbon dioxide and water. Under normal physiological conditions, electron transport is tightly coupled to phosphorylation, and precise electrical potential as maintained by a homeostatic proton potential across the inner mitochondrial membrane is linked to the regulation of body temperature. The inner gel-like mitochondrial compartment, the "matrix" with $<50\%$ water, has high concentrations of the soluble enzymes of oxidative metabolism such as the citric acid cycle enzymes and the unique mitochondrial DNA, RNA, and ribosomes. The outer mitochondrial membrane permits diffusion in of molecules of up to 10,000 molecular weight, whereas the inner membrane has a much more tightly controlled access by transport systems only, except for oxygen and carbon dioxide. This allows compartmentalization of mitochondrial functions in a highly regulated manner.

2.3 PENTOSE PHOSPHATE PATHWAY

Reducing power is as important as the generation of ATP in glycolysis, the citric acid cycle, and oxidative phosphorylation. The concentration of reduced nicotinamide adenine dinucleotide phosphate (NADPH) determines cellular reducing power by serving as an electron donor source in reductive biosyntheses. The pentose phosphate pathway (also the hexose monophosphate shunt or phosphogluconate pathway) generates up to 12 molecules of NADPH and ribose-5-phosphate in the cell cytosol. The NADPH is an essential cofactor in nullifying the buildup of oxidative byproducts, through abetting the action of glutathione peroxidase by reducing oxidized glutathione, together with glutathione reductase. The ribose-5-phosphate is utilized in the synthesis of RNA, DNA, and nucleotide coenzymes.

The pentose phosphate pathway starts with the dehydrogenation of glucose-6-phosphate and ends with the production of ribose-5-phosphate via four different types of processes (Figure 2.4). All of these processes constitute a controlled interplay between glycolysis and the pentose phosphate pathway. NAPH and NADH, though they differ only by a phosphate group at the 2′-OH group of the adenosine moiety, are not interchangeable sources of reducing power. NADH participates in utilizing the free energy of metabolite oxidation to synthesize ATP, whereas NADPH is involved in using this free energy for

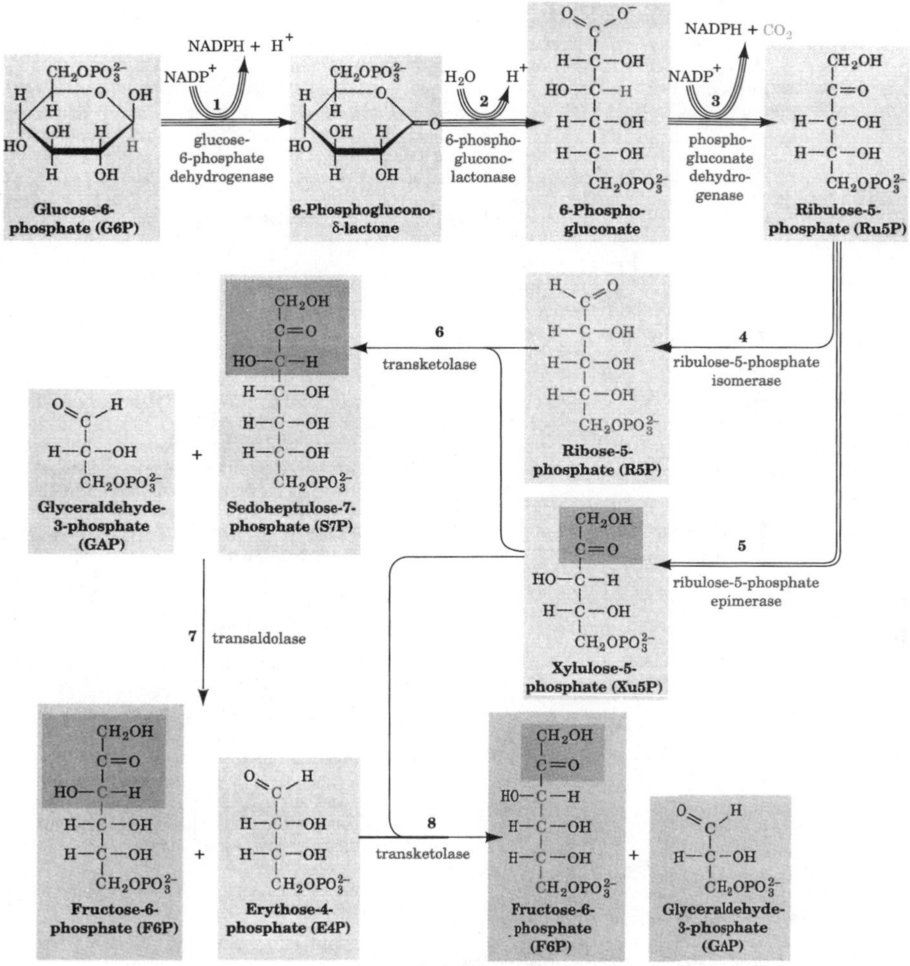

FIGURE 2.4. The pentose phosphate pathway. The number of lines in an arrow represents the number of molecules reacting in one turn of the pathway so as to convert three G6Ps to three CO_2s, two F6Ps, and one GAP. For the sake of clarity, sugars from reaction 3 onward are shown in their linear forms. The C_2 units are transferred by transketolase. C_3 units are transferred by transaldolase. (Courtesy of *Biochemistry*, Voet/Voet, J. Wiley & Sons.)

otherwise energy-requiring reductive biosyntheses. The rate-determining step is the glucose-6-phosphate dehydrogenase reaction.

2.4 GLUCONEOGENESIS

Glucose can be produced through catabolism of tissue glycogen (only about a half-day's supply) or via synthesis from noncarbohydrate sources (gluconeogenesis) such as lactate, amino acids, and glycerol, especially in muscles, the liver, and red blood cells. The brain and the red blood cells are almost totally dependent on glucose as an energy source. Gluconeogenesis occurs predominantly in the liver and, to a lesser extent, in the kidney.

Pyruvate (formed from lactate and some amino acids) is converted into

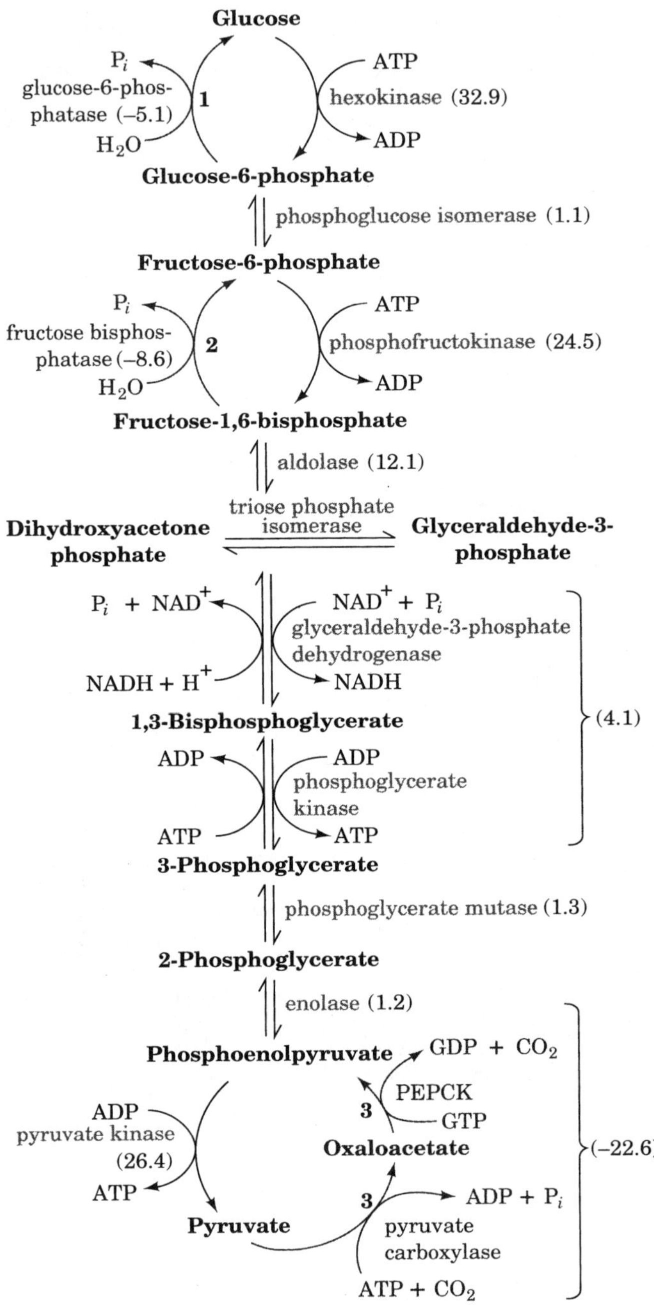

FIGURE 2.5. The pathways of gluconeogenesis and glycolysis. All enzymes are cytosolic except for pyruvate carboxylase which is mitochondrial, and except for glucose-6-phosphatase which is membrane-bound inside the endoplasmic reticulum. The three numbered steps are catalyzed by different enzymes in gluconeogenesis. The changes in Gibbs free energies for the reactions in the direction of gluconeogenesis are given in parentheses in kJ/mol. (These energies were obtained from E. A. Newsholme and A. R. Leech, *Biochemistry for the Medical Sciences*, Wiley, 1983, p. 448.) (Courtesy of *Biochemistry*, Voet/Voet, J. Wiley & Sons.)

glucose, bypassing the three essentially irreversible reactions of glycolysis (catalyzed by hexokinase, phosphofructokinase and pyruvate kinase) and utilizing the early reversible reactions of glycolysis (Figure 2.5). Six high-energy phosphate bonds are consumed. Glycerol can enter the gluconeogenesis cycle via formation of dihydroxyacetone phosphate. Any xenobiotics that ultimately produce pyruvate, lactate, alanine, or glycerol as metabolites can act as carbon sources. However, whatever the ultimate carbon source, oxaloacetate needs to be produced for gluconeogenesis to be a committed process. All amino acids except leucine and lysine can act as carbon sources for the process in animals. These latter two amino acids are converted to acetyl coenzyme A, which cannot be further converted in animals to oxalacetate. In the same vein, fatty acids cannot act as carbon sources for oxaloacetate either.

2.5 FATTY ACID DEGRADATION

Fatty acids (carboxylic acids with more than six carbon atoms) are building blocks of phospholipids and glycolipids, both important components of biological membranes as well as precursors of hormones and intracellular messengers. They can be saturated or unsaturated (generally *cis*-hydrogen substituted double bonds beyond C9). They usually have even-numbered carbon atoms, generally between 12 and 24 with the 16- and 18-carbon fatty acids the most common. The chain is generally unbranched in animals. Any double bonds are separated by at least one methylene group. Unsaturated fatty acids have lower melting points than their saturated analogs and therefore confer "fluidity". The shorter the chain and the greater the unsaturation, the more fluidity is conferred, an important consideration for membranes which consist of lipid bilayer–protein aggregates and also for the fatty acid composition on external (compared with internal) cell and organelle membranes.

Triacylglycerols are energy-rich forms of calories relative to proteins and carbohydrates, which is the reason why they predominate in the fat stores. They also constitute about 90% of dietary lipids and supply about 90% of metabolic storage energy in humans. The triacylglycerols are hydrolyzed by lipases (under hormonal control) to their three constituent fatty acids and glycerol, at lipid–water interfaces. The glycerol is phosphorylated and oxidized to dihydroxyacetone phosphate, a key intermediate in glycolysis and in gluconeogenesis. The released fatty acids can be incorporated elsewhere or undergo beta-oxidation.

2.6 BETA-OXIDATION

Beta-oxidation is the progressive removal of two-carbon fragments from the terminal carboxylate group in a fatty acid. All saturated fatty acids with an odd number n of carbon atoms ultimately produce $n/2 - 1$ units of acetyl CoA and one molecule of propionyl CoA. The acetyl CoA enters the citric acid cycle; the propionyl CoA also enters the citric acid cycle after conversion of succinyl CoA. All saturated fatty acids with an even number n of carbon atoms yield $n/2$ units of acetyl CoA. Activations of saturated fatty acids to the acetyl CoA derivatives occur on the outer membrane of mitochondria via an acyl adenylate

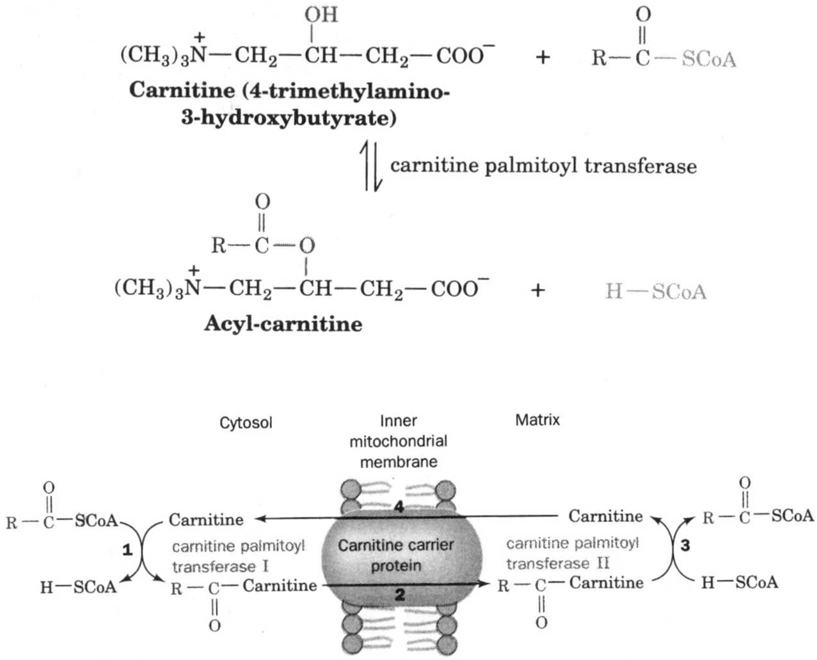

FIGURE 2.6. The transport of fatty acids into the mitochondrion. The flow of acyl carnitine from the cytosolic side of the mitochondrial membrane into the mitochondrial matrix is mediated by a translocase enzyme (step 2). The fatty acid must first be activated to its coenzyme A derivative R–CO–SCoA (step 1). Inset: The acylation of carnitine in step 1 is catalyzed by carnitine palmitoyl transferase. CoA is released to the cytosol. Step 3 involves transfer of the acyl group to CoA in the mitochondrial matrix. Step 4 shows the return of the product carnitine to the cytosol. (Courtesy of *Biochemistry*, Voet/Voet, J. Wiley & Sons.)

intermediate (a common feature of activation of carboxylate groups for biochemical purposes). The activated saturated fatty acids are carried into the mitochondrial matrix from the external membrane on the hydroxy group of carnitine (derived from lysine) in a chemical carrier process, and the acyl group is transferred back to CoA in the mitochondrial matrix (Figure 2.6). This shows that the complexity of many physiological processes is due to the heterogeneous nature of the blood–cell–cytosol–organelle processes, which involve transport through multiple membranes and compartments.

The newly activated saturated CoA derivative is then progressively oxidized to a *trans*-enoyl CoA, an L-hydroxyacyl CoA, a ketoacyl CoA, and the next acyl CoA shortened by two carbon atoms (steps 1 to 4 in Figure 2.7), in a process resembling the last steps in the citric acid cycle. Step 1 in Figure 2.7 is coupled to the mitochondrial electron transport chain (steps 5 to 8 in Figure 2.7). The shortened saturated acyl CoA then undergoes further cycling. For palmitoyl CoA, seven cycles are required for degradation, consuming two high energy phosphate bonds. Generations of 7 $FADH_2$ (equivalent to 14 ATP), 7 NADH (equivalent to 21 ATP), and 8 acetyl CoA (equivalent to 96 ATP) occur with a net production of 129 ATP. The biological efficiency of the process is actually about 40%, a value similar to that for glycolysis, the citric acid cycle, and oxidative phosphorylation.

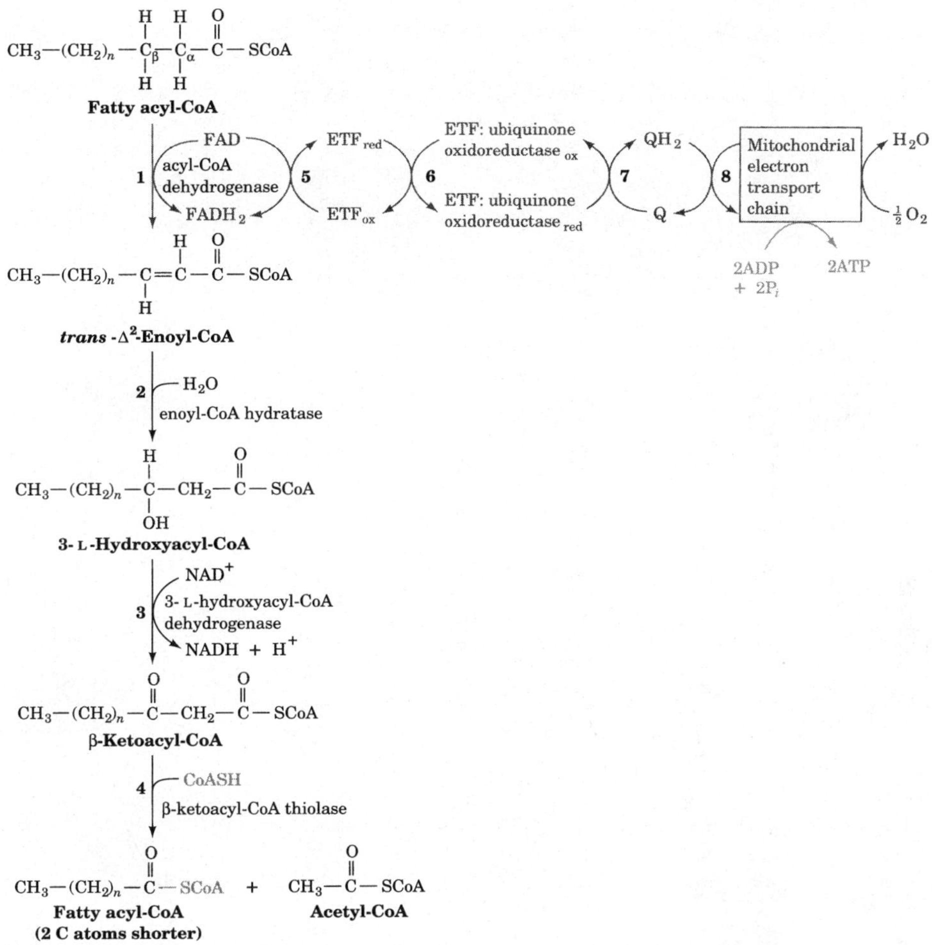

FIGURE 2.7. The β-oxidation pathway of fatty acyl-CoA. (Courtesy of *Biochemistry*, Voet/Voet, J. Wiley & Sons.)

The beta-oxidation of unsaturated fatty acids shares many of the same reactions as discussed for saturated fatty acids. Activation and transport into mitochondria are identical. Removal of two-carbon fragments occurs until a carbon–carbon double bond occurs between carbon atoms 2 and 3 or 3 and 4 of the unsaturated enoyl CoA. Generally the first double bond encountered in the original fatty acid, which usually has an even number of carbon atoms, is *cis* and between carbon atoms 9 and 10. Thus the usual first unsaturated shortened enoyl CoA resistant to direct beta-oxidation contains a *cis* double bond between carbon atoms 3 and 4. An isomerase enzyme allows the double bond to be shifted to between carbon atoms 2 and 3 with the hydrogens across the bond in a *trans* configuration. This *trans*-enoyl CoA is the normal substrate for further oxidation, and further cycling of shortened derivatives. For polyunsaturated fatty acids where the *cis* double bonds are separated by a methylene group, the double bond closest to the activated end is hydrated to a D-3-hydroxy-*cis*-enoyl CoA, which is not a substrate for the dehydrogenase enzyme

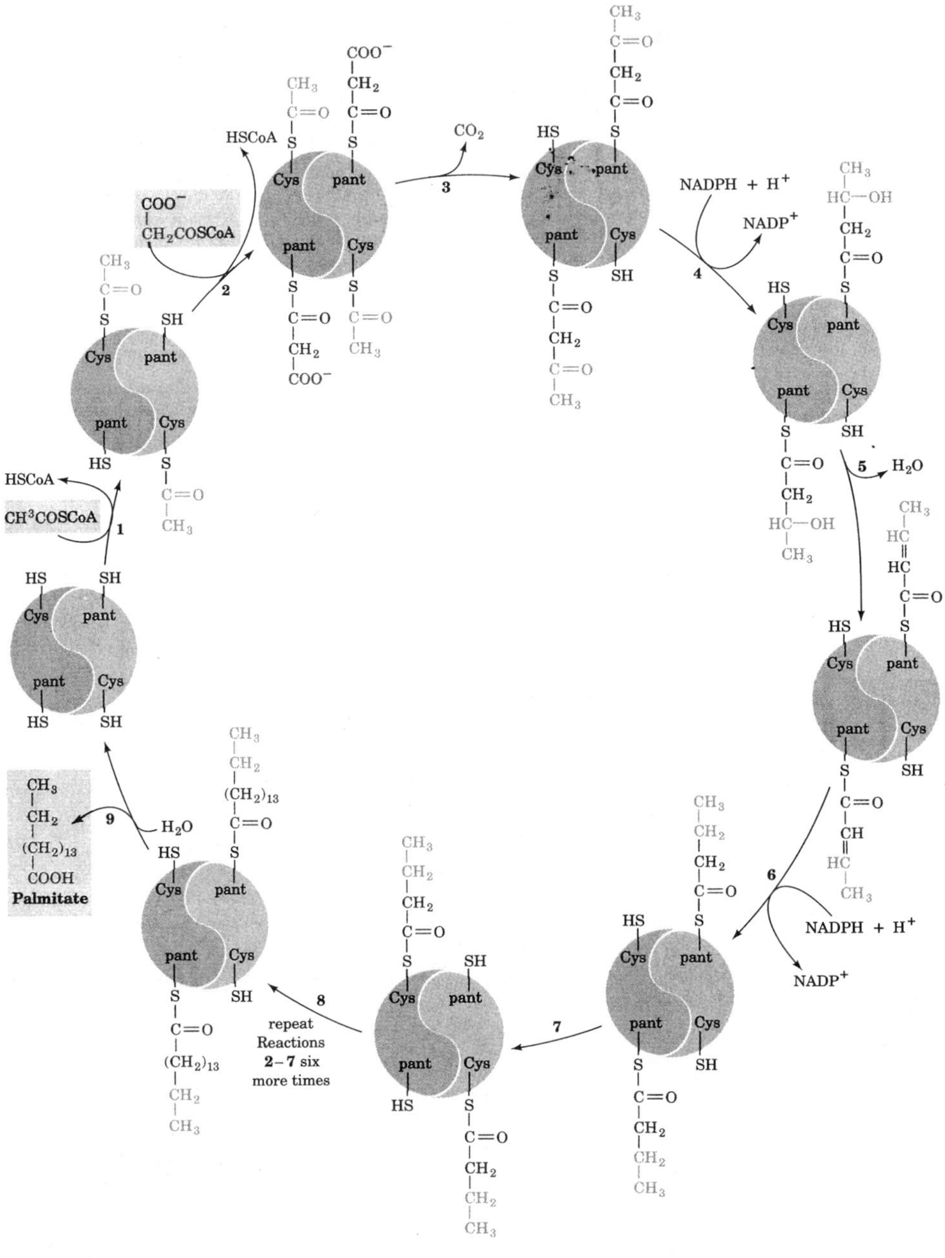

FIGURE 2.8. Fatty acid synthase and the chain-lengthening process in fatty acid biosynthesis. The identical chains of fatty acid synthase each contain three domains. Domain 1 contains acetyl transferase, malonyl transferase, and condensing enzyme (CE). Domain 2 contains acyl carrier protein (ACP), β-ketoacyl reductase, dehydratase, and enoyl reductase. Domain 3 contains thioesterase. The flexible phosphopantetheinyl group (pant-SH) that carries the fatty acid acyl chain from one catalytic site to the other is attached to ACP. The elongating fatty acyl chain translocates between the active cysteine sulfhydryl group of the beta-ketoacyl-ACP synthase CE (Cys-SH) and the pant-SH. The circles represent the multifunctional dimer of fatty acid synthase. The other catalytic domains are not shown but are present in both subunits of the dimer. Palmitate is the final product. (After S. J. Stoops, J. K. Stoops, and V. C. Joshi, *Ann. Rev. Biochem.* **52**: 568, 1983.) (Courtesy of *Biochemistry*, Voet/Voet, J. Wiley & Sons.)

which attacks only L-configurations. The L-configuration is attained, however, through an epimerase that inverts the configuration of the hydroxyl group at C3. Further oxidation can then occur, with other double bonds being accommodated in the same manner.

The utilization of acetyl CoA from the beta-oxidation of fats occurs in the citric acid cycle only if fat and carbohydrate degradation are balanced. Because oxaloacetate level depends on carbohydrate availability and proper utilization, lack of oxaloacetate prevents acetyl CoA entry into the citric acid cycle. The acetyl CoA in this situation (as in fasting or diabetes) dimerizes into acetoacetyl CoA (with loss of CoA), and then successively into 3-hydroxy-3-methylglutaryl CoA and acetoacetate, finally ending up as either acetone or D-3-hydroxybutyrate, the last three compounds being called ketone bodies. The major site of production of acetoacetate and 3-hydroxybutyrate is liver mitochondria. These end products diffuse into the blood to be transported to other tissues, where they act as sources of energy and fuels of respiration. Acetoacetate is so used predominantly in the heart and renal cortex under normal conditions, and in the brain when glucose is scarce. The excretion of acetone in the breath drives the whole process. Many xenobiotic organics ultimately are oxidized to carboxylic acids, which, if aliphatic, can be used directly as carbon sources through beta-oxidation via production of acetyl CoA (even chain length) and propionyl CoA (odd chain length).

The rate of fatty acid oxidation is determined by the availability of the substrates. During fasting or starvation, the levels of free fatty acids increase because adipose-cell lipase is stimulated by hormones such as epinephrine and glucagon. Fatty acid CoA molecules do not have ready access to the mitochondrial matrix under normal conditions.

2.7 FATTY ACID BIOSYNTHESIS

Fatty acid biosynthesis in animals (Figure 2.8) occurs in the cell cytosol rather than in the mitochondria where fatty acids are degraded. The activated intermediate for fatty acid biosynthesis is linked to the sulfhydryl groups of an acyl carrier protein (ACP) rather than through the sulfhydryl group of coenzyme A. Biosynthesis occurs on a multienzyme assembly called fatty acid synthase. Degradative enzymes are not associated because the products of degradation are common building blocks of macromolecules. The growing fatty acid chain is elongated to the final product palmitate (C_{16}) by the sequential addition of two-carbon units derived from acetyl CoA, the actual activated donor being malonyl-ACP with the process driven by release of carbon dioxide gas and the availability of bicarbonate.

The reductant used in biosynthesis is NADPH, whereas NAD^+ or FAD are the oxidizing agents in beta-oxidation. The initial step forming malonyl CoA from acetyl CoA and bicarbonate requires powering by ATP and the activation of the acetyl CoA carboxylase enzyme into its active filamentous form by the allosteric activator citrate, which also carries the acetyl groups from acetyl CoA from inside the mitochondria to the cell cytosol (in contrast, the end product palmitoyl CoA deactivates the filamentous form of the enzyme back to its inactive protomeric form). The biosynthesis of palmitate requires 8 acetyl CoA, 14 NADPH, and 7 ATP.

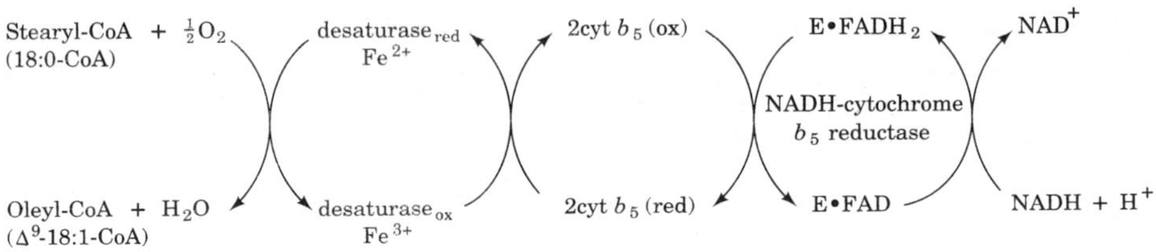

FIGURE 2.9. The electron transport chain involvement in the desaturation of stearoyl CoA to oleoyl CoA. The process is mediated by a fatty acyl–CoA desaturase complex. Its three proteins—desaturase, cytochrome b_5, and NADH-cytochrome b_5 reductase—are situated in the endoplasmic reticulum membrane. (After R. Jeffcoat, *Essays Biochem.* **15**: 19, 1979.) (Courtesy of *Biochemistry*, Voet/Voet, J. Wiley & Sons.)

Fatty acids longer than palmitate are manufactured from palmitate on the cytosolic face of the endoplasmic reticulum membranes, through sequential two-carbon elongation at the carboxyl end using malonyl CoA as donor, the evolution of carbon dioxide again driving the process. Double bonds can be introduced here, also using molecular oxygen and NADH or NADPH, and involving an enzyme complex consisting of two cytochromes and a non-heme iron-containing desaturase (Figure 2.9). Unsaturated fatty acids in mammals are derived from either palmitoleate, oleate, linoleate, or linolenate. Mammals lack the ability to introduce carbon-carbon double bonds beyond C_9 in fatty acid chains. Thus linoleate and linolenate are essential fatty acids. Arachidonic acid (C_{20}) with four double bonds, the source of many important signal molecules such as prostaglandin hormones, is derived from linolenate.

There are many interlocking controls between fatty acid degradation and biosynthesis. Malonyl CoA inhibits carnitine transferase I when biosynthesis is required. Excess NADH inhibits 3-hydroxyacyl CoA dehydrogenase, and excess acetyl CoA inhibits thiolase. Increasing citrate concentration in the cytosol enhances biosynthesis, and increasing palmitoyl CoA concentration inhibits it. The latter also inhibits the translocase that transfers citrate from the mitochondria to the cytosol, as well as glucose-6-phosphate dehydrogenase which produces NADPH. Acetyl CoA carboxylase activity is also regulated by reversible phosphorylation. When blood glucose is lowered past a critical point, glucagon is released and binds to receptors on the plasma membrane of liver cells. This triggers the ultimate formation of cyclic adenosine monophosphate (cAMP) and hence the phosphorylating enzyme protein kinase, which controls glycogen metabolism. Acetyl CoA carboxylase is also inhibited by phosphorylation, but this inhibition is reversed by the release of insulin.

2.8 MEMBRANE LIPIDS AND STEROIDAL HORMONES

2.8.1 Phosphoglycerides and Triacylglycerols

The starting compound is glycerol-3-phosphate, which is formed mainly by reduction of dihydroxyacetone phosphate. Some is formed by phosphorylation of glycerol. Acyl CoA (usually saturated) reacts to form a lysophosphatide (a monoacylglycerol-3-phosphate), and then another acyl CoA (generally unsaturated if the lysophosphatide is saturated) reacts via the same glycerol-phosphate acyl transferase enzyme to form a phosphatide (a diacylglycerol-3-phosphate). This is the common precursor to phospholipids and triacylglycerols. To form the latter, the phosphatide is dephosphorylated to produce a diacylglycerol, which is then acylated by acyl CoA to form the triacyl glycerol, all operations being performed on a triacylglycerol synthetase complex bound to the endoplasmic reticulum.

A couple of routes are possible for phosphoglyceride synthesis (Figure 2.10): (a) Cytidine triphosphate (CTP) reacts with phosphatide to form cytidine diphosphodiacylglycerol (CDP-diacylglycerol) driven by pyrophosphate formation. The activated unit can react with the hydroxy group of a polar alcohol: if serine, then phosphatidyl serine and cytidine monophosphate (CMP) are formed; if inositol, the phosphoglyceride formed is phosphatidyl inositol, which, when phosphorylated to phosphatidyl inositol-4,5-biphosphate, is a key molecule in signal transduction. (b) A diacylglycerol can react with CDP-choline or CDP-ethanolamine (choline is a vitamin for mammals) to form phosphatidyl choline and phosphatidyl ethanolamine, respectively. The latter can also be made from phosphatidyl serine by transesterification. Other related phospholipids are glyceryl ether phospholipids, starting from dihydroxy acetone phosphate, and plasmalogens (alpha, beta-unsaturated C_1 ether phospholipids).

Several specific phospholipases have been isolated, and they are grouped according to the bonds they attack (Figure 2.11). The phospholipases can be digestive enzymes, and they can participate in enzymatic cascades to release active lipids or transduce signals. They are also used in studies on DNA adducts.

2.8.2 Other Lipids

The backbone of a sphingolipid is sphingosine (made from palmitoyl CoA and serine) rather than glycerol. The amino group of sphingosine is acylated by acetyl CoA to form a ceramide. When the terminal hydroxy group is also substituted with phosphorylcholine (by CDP-choline), the sphingolipid is a sphingomyelin; when the hydroxy group is also substituted with glucose or galactose [by uridine diphosphate (UDP)-sugar], a cerebroside results. When a ceramide is linked to an oligosaccharide by a glucose moiety, the sphingolipid is a ganglioside. When at least one acidic sugar, *N*-acetylneuraminate or *N*-glycolylneuraminate, is part of the oligosaccharide, the ganglioside is a sialic acid. More than 15 different gangliosides have been characterized. They are found mostly in the nervous system but particularly in gray matter, where they undergo continual turnover. Lysosomes contain enzymes that can break down gangliosides.

Cholesterol is a steroid that modulates the fluidity of eucaryotic membranes. It is also the precursor of steroid hormones such as progesterone, testosterone, estradiol, and cortisol. All 27 carbon atoms of cholesterol are derived from acetyl CoA, with isopentenyl pyrophosphate (C_5) being the activated synthon and the production of mevalonate the key step (Figure 2.12).

Bile salts are excretion products of cholesterol that are made in the liver, stored and concentrated in the gallbladder, and then released into the small

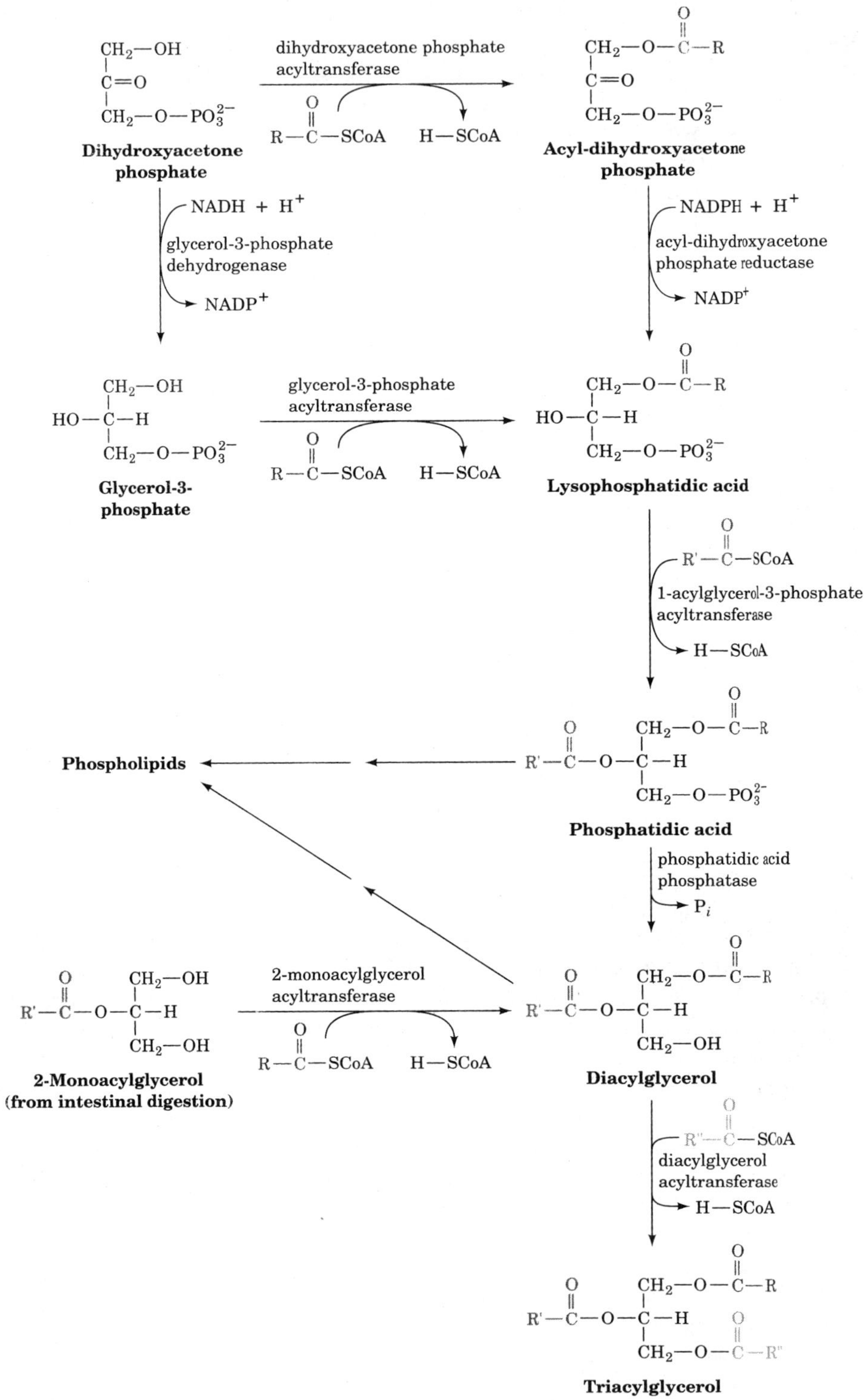

Dihydroxyacetone phosphate
dihydroxyacetone phosphate acyltransferase
R—C(=O)—SCoA
H—SCoA
Acyl-dihydroxyacetone phosphate
NADH + H+
glycerol-3-phosphate dehydrogenase
NADP+
NADPH + H+
acyl-dihydroxyacetone phosphate reductase
NADP+
Glycerol-3-phosphate
glycerol-3-phosphate acyltransferase
Lysophosphatidic acid
R'—C(=O)—SCoA
1-acylglycerol-3-phosphate acyltransferase
H—SCoA
Phospholipids
Phosphatidic acid
phosphatidic acid phosphatase
Pi
2-Monoacylglycerol (from intestinal digestion)
2-monoacylglycerol acyltransferase
Diacylglycerol
R''—C(=O)—SCoA
diacylglycerol acyltransferase
H—SCoA
Triacylglycerol

FIGURE 2.10.

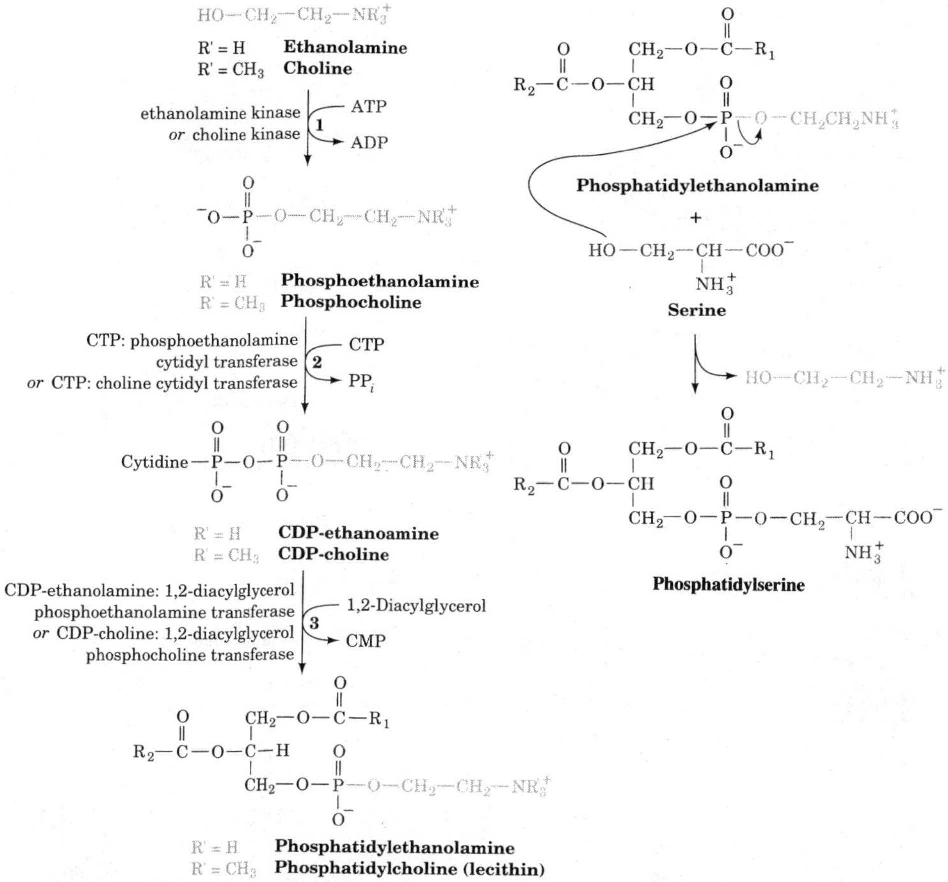

FIGURE 2.10. Some reactions of triacylglycerol and phosphatidyl glyceride biosynthesis. The biosyntheses of phosphatidylethanolamine and phosphatidylcholine involve CDP-ethanolamine and CDP-choline, respectively. Phosphatidylserine synthesis from phosphatidylethanolamine occurs by a head group exchange reaction. (Courtesy of *Biochemistry*, Voet/Voet, J. Wiley & Sons.)

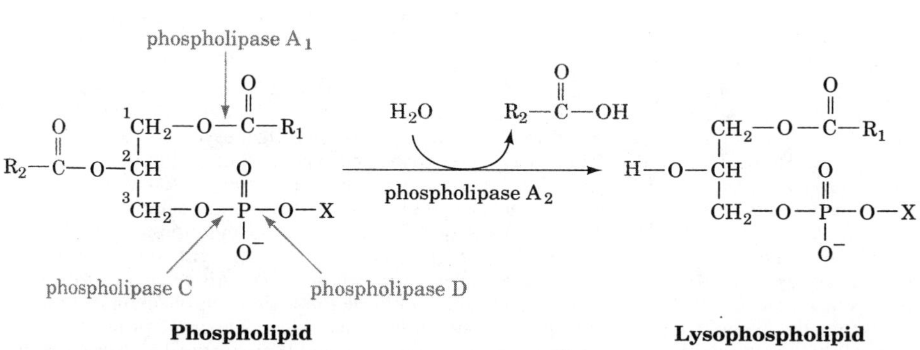

FIGURE 2.11. Cleavage sites for phospholipases. Phospholipase A_2 hydrolytically excises the C_2 fatty acid residue from a triacylglycerol to yield the corresponding lysophospholipid. The bonds hydrolyzed by other specific lipases are also indicated. (Courtesy of *Biochemistry*, Voet/Voet, J. Wiley & Sons.)

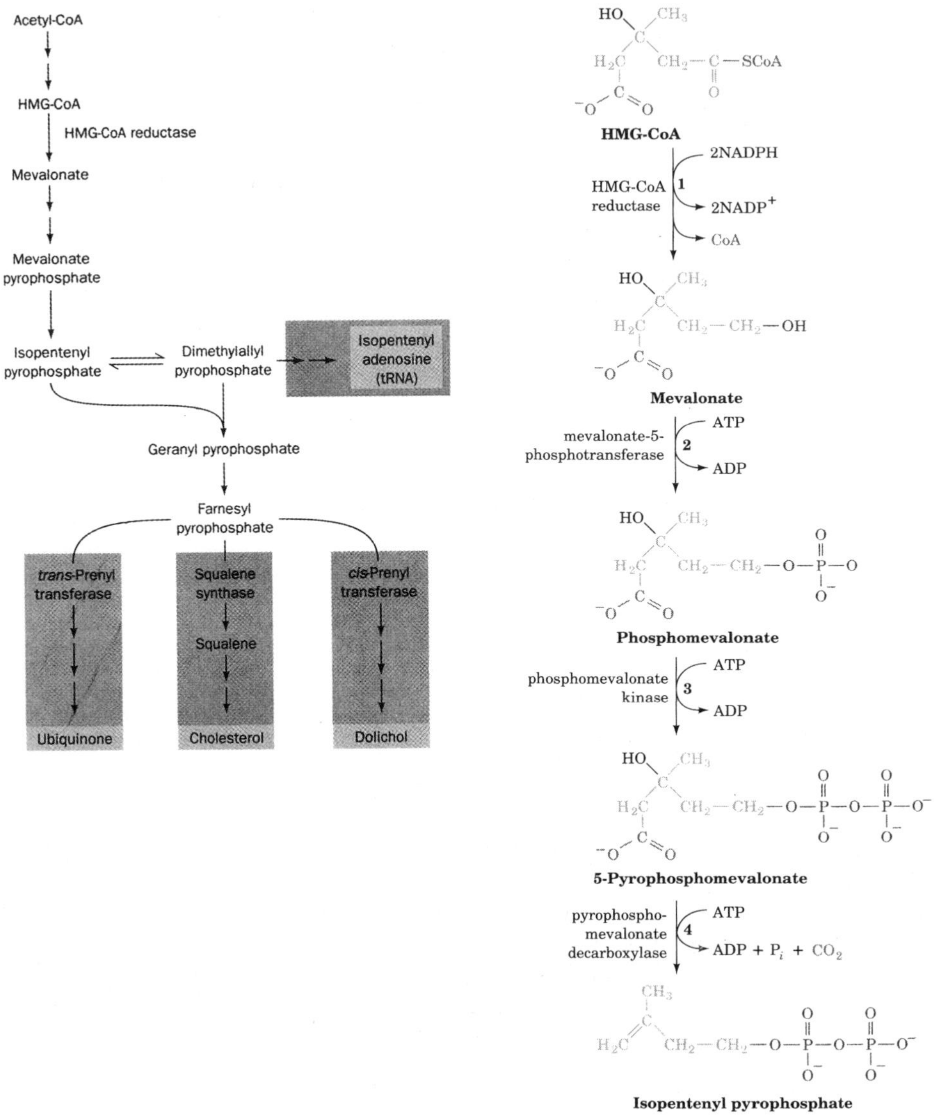

FIGURE 2.12. The branched pathway of isoprenoid metabolism in mammalian cells. The pathway produces ubiquinone, dolichol, and isopentenyl adenosine, a modified tRNA base, in addition to cholesterol. There are six main stages to the biosynthesis of cholesterol. Stage I involves formation of isopentenyl pyrophosphate from hydroxymethylglutaryl-CoA (HMG-CoA) in the cytosol. Stage II consists of isopentenyl pyrophosphate isomerase interconverting isopentenyl pyrophosphate and dimethylallyl pyrophosphate by a concerted protonation/deprotonation reaction. Stage III involves the formation of squalene from isopentenyl pyrophosphate and dimethylallyl pyrophosphate by two head-to-tail condensations catalyzed by prenyl transferase, and a head-to-head condensation mediated by squalene synthase. Stage IV has the squalene epoxidized at the 2,3-position by squalene epoxidase. Stage V is a complex squalene oxidocyclase reaction where: (a) 2,3-oxidosqualene is cyclized to the protosterol cation in a process that is initiated by the enzyme-assisted protonation of the squalene epoxide oxygen while this extended molecule is folded in the manner predicted by Bloch and Woodward (the opening of the epoxide leaves an electron-deficient center whose migration drives the series of cyclizations that form the protosterol cation); and (b) the elimination of a proton occurs from C_9 of the sterol to form a double bond with a series of methyl and hydride migrations to produce neutral lanosterol. Stage VI is the 19-reaction conversion of lanosterol to cholesterol. (After H. C. Rilling and L. T. Chayet in H. Danielsson and J. Sjovall, eds., *Sterols and Bile Acids*, Elsevier, 1985, p. 33.) (Courtesy of *Biochemistry*, Voet/Voet, J. Wiley & Sons.)

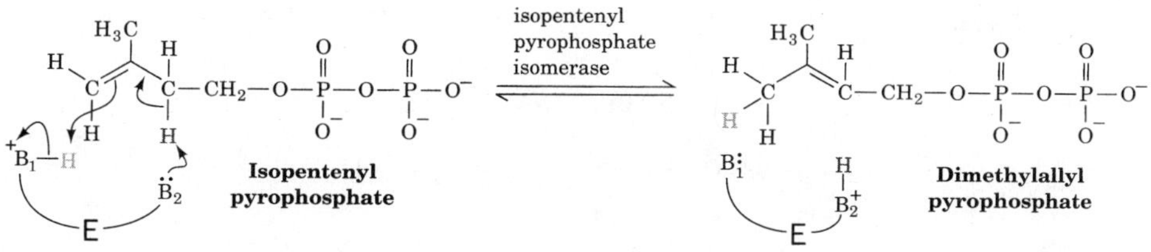

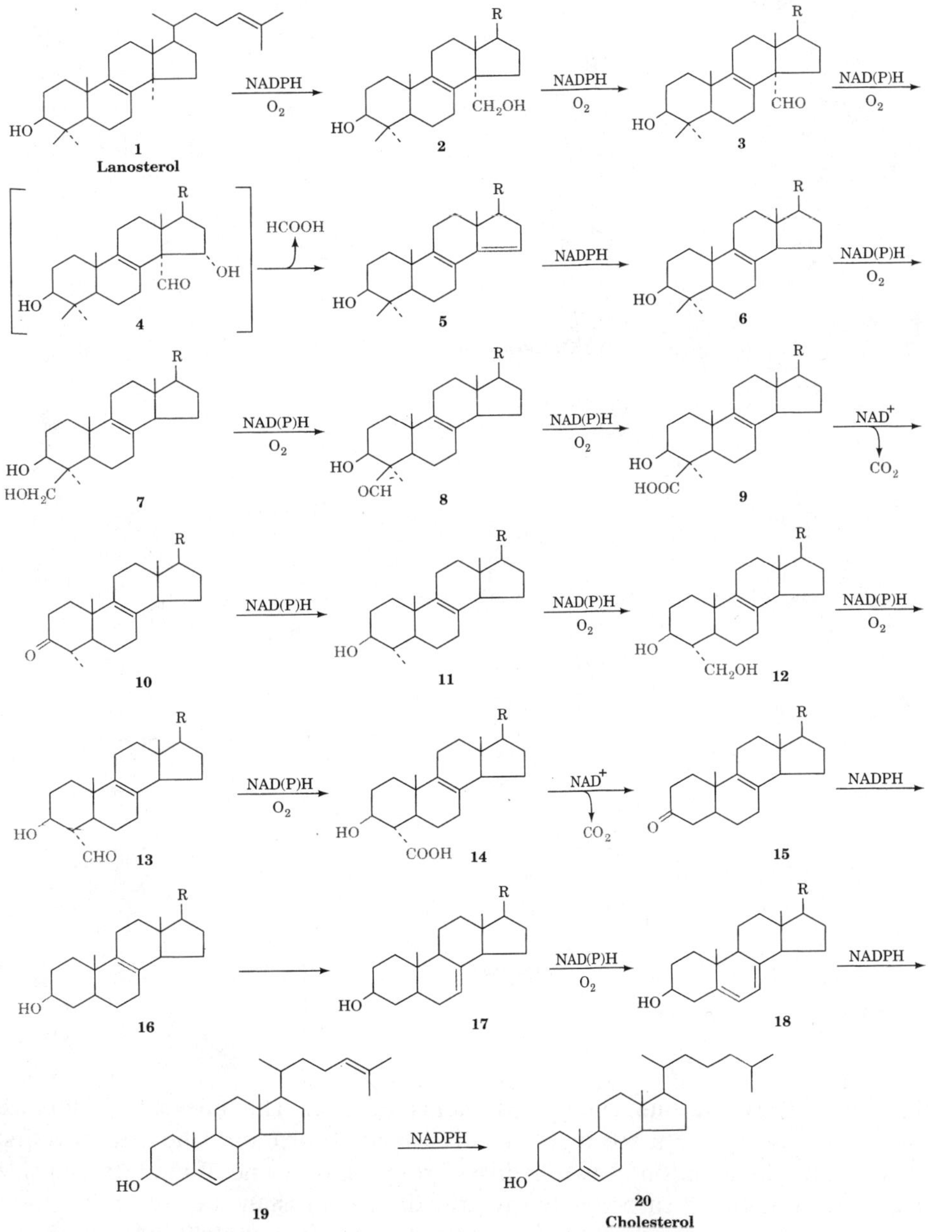

FIGURE 2.12. *Continued*

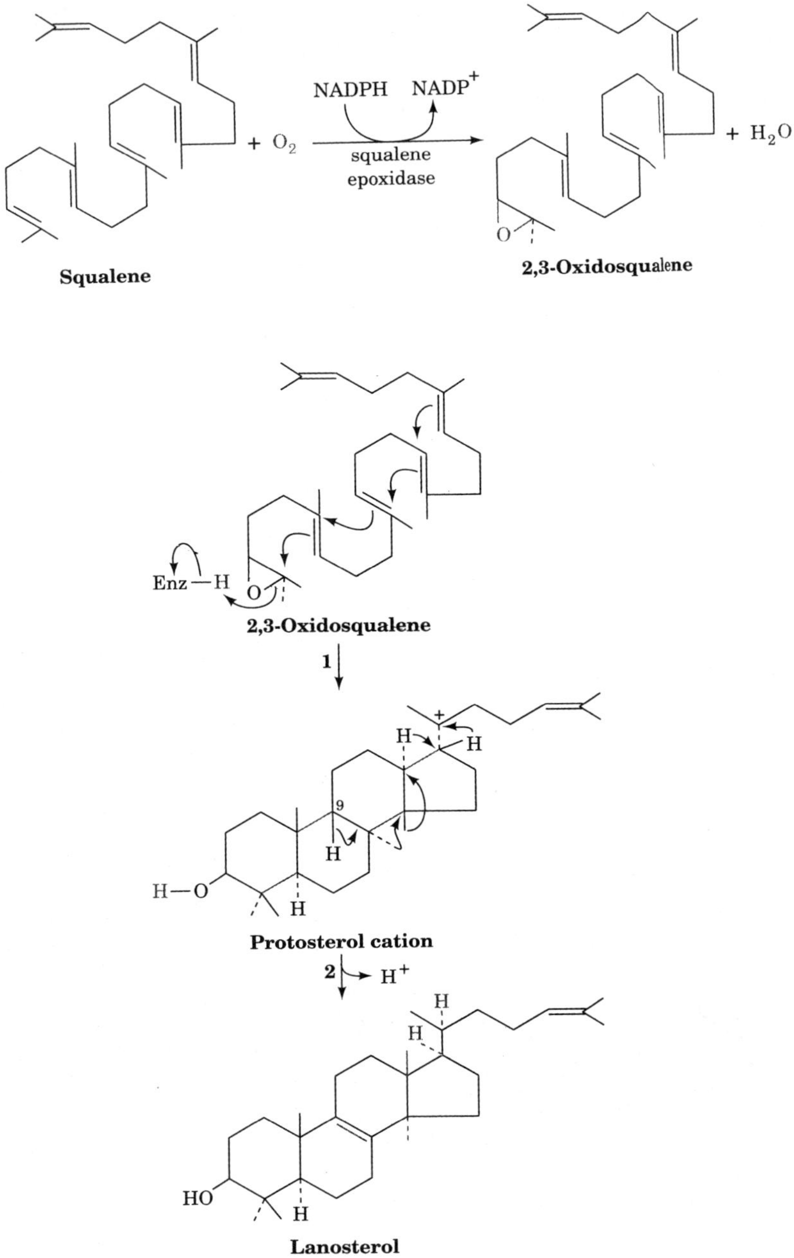

FIGURE 2.12. *Continued*

intestine. They are the chief constituents of bile. The bile salts solubilize dietary lipids, and enhance their hydrolysis and absorption. Cholesterol is first oxidized by the addition of two hydroxy groups and by one of the terminal side chain carbons being carboxylated to trihydroxycoprostanoate; the latter loses three carbon atoms in its activation with CoA to yield cholyl CoA, which, on reaction with glycine and taurine, forms glycocholate (major) and taurocholate,

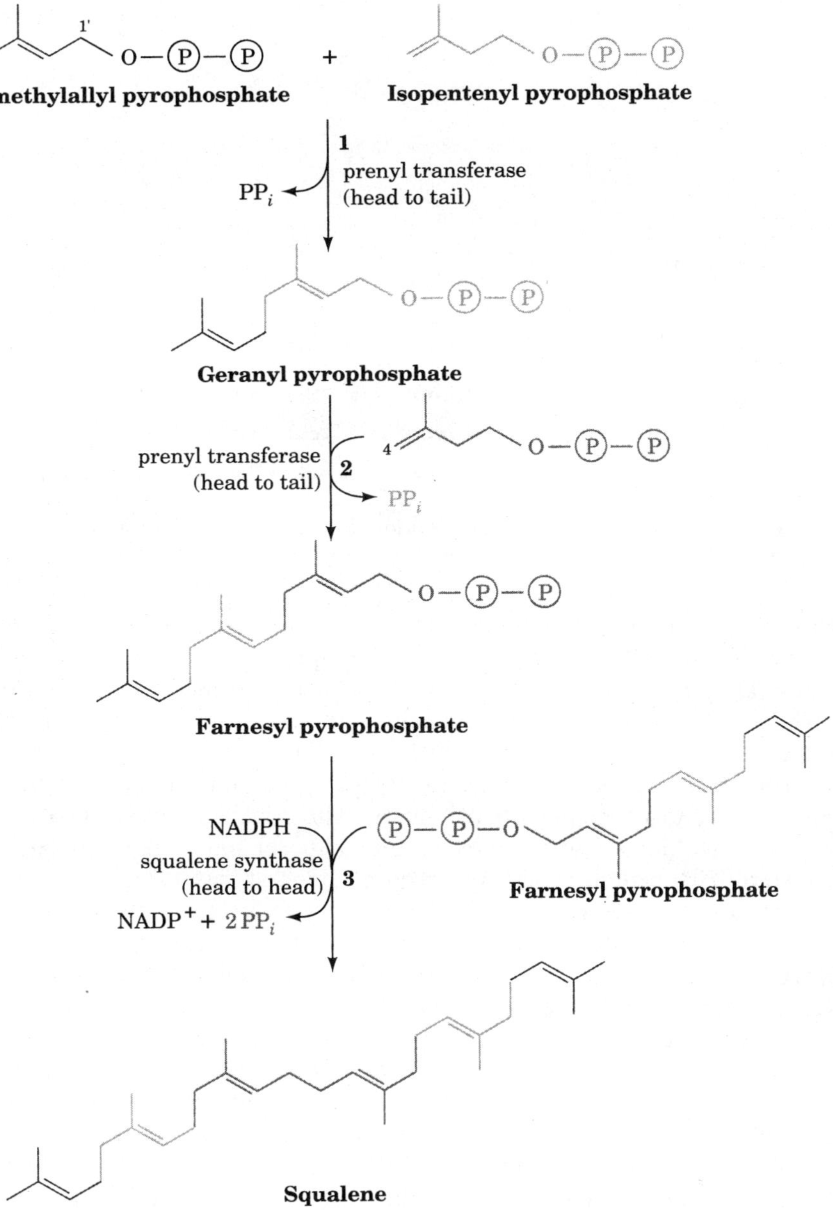

FIGURE 2.12. *Continued*

respectively (Figure 2.13). The levels of blood and urine bile salts have been utilized as medical surveillance markers.

The transport of lipids in body fluids is done by lipoproteins classified according to increasing density: chylomicra, chylomicron remnants, very low-density lipoproteins (VLDL), intermediate-density lipoproteins (IDL), low-density lipoproteins (LDL), and high-density lipoproteins (HDL). These lipoproteins have cores of hydrophobic lipids surrounded by hydrophilic polar

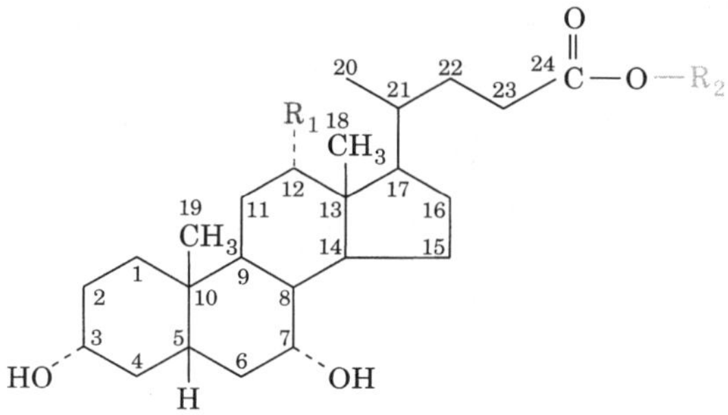

	R_1 = OH	R_1 = H
R_2 = H	**Cholic acid**	**Chenodeoxycholic acid**
R_2 = NH—CH_2—COOH	**Glycocholic acid**	**Glycochenodeoxycholic acid**
R_2 = NH—CH_2—CH_2—SO_3H	**Taurocholic acid**	**Taurochenodeoxycholic acid**

FIGURE 2.13. Structures of the major bile acids and their glycine and taurine conjugates. (Courtesy of *Biochemistry*, Voet/Voet, J. Wiley & Sons.)

lipids and apoproteins. Their function is to solubilize lipids, and to facilitate the chemical messengers necessary to move lipids in and out of target cells and tissues. Dietary lipids are first solubilized in the stomach in the chylomicra, which, on absorption from the intestine, are carried in the blood to adipose tissue and the liver in lipoidal material with diameters of 80 to 500 nm, density $<0.94\,g/cm^3$, and protein content less than 2%, and containing triacylglycerols, cholesterol, and other absorbable lipids. The triacylglycerols are hydrolyzed by lipases within a few minutes in the adipose and organ capillaries. The cholesterol-rich residues, the chylomicron remnants, are taken up by receptor-mediated endocytosis in the liver. Nondietary triacylglycerols are transported by the VLDL, produced primarily by the liver. After lipase action on the VLDL, the residue rich in cholesterol esters is the IDL. Half is taken up by the liver, and the other half is converted into the LDL, the major carrier of blood cholesterol. The LDL has a diameter of 22 nm, and a mass of 3×10^6 amu. A core of hydrophobic esterified cholesterol is dominated by linoleate surrounded by a shell of hydrophilic phospholipids, a specific B-100 apoprotein, and unesterified cholesterol. The LDL transports cholesterol, and regulates cholesterol synthesis at target sites. Both the IDL and the LDL deliver lipids by receptor-mediated endocytosis in the liver and other organs. Inside the cell, lysosomal action hydrolyzes the protein to free amino acids, and lipases release free cholesterols. The LDL receptor returns intact to the plasma membrane in about 10 minutes, ready for more transfer. The receptor's lifetime is about one day.

HDL, density $>1.06\,g/cm^3$, picks up cholesterol released in the plasma from dying cells and from membranes undergoing turnover. The HDL contains an acyl transferase that esterifies these cholesterols, which are quickly transported to the VLDL or LDL by a transfer protein.

Cholesterol is the precursor for vitamin D, which regulates calcium and phosphorus metabolism. 7-Dehydrocholesterol or provitamin D_3 reacts with ultraviolet light to form previtamin D_3 (cholecalciferol), which is then converted

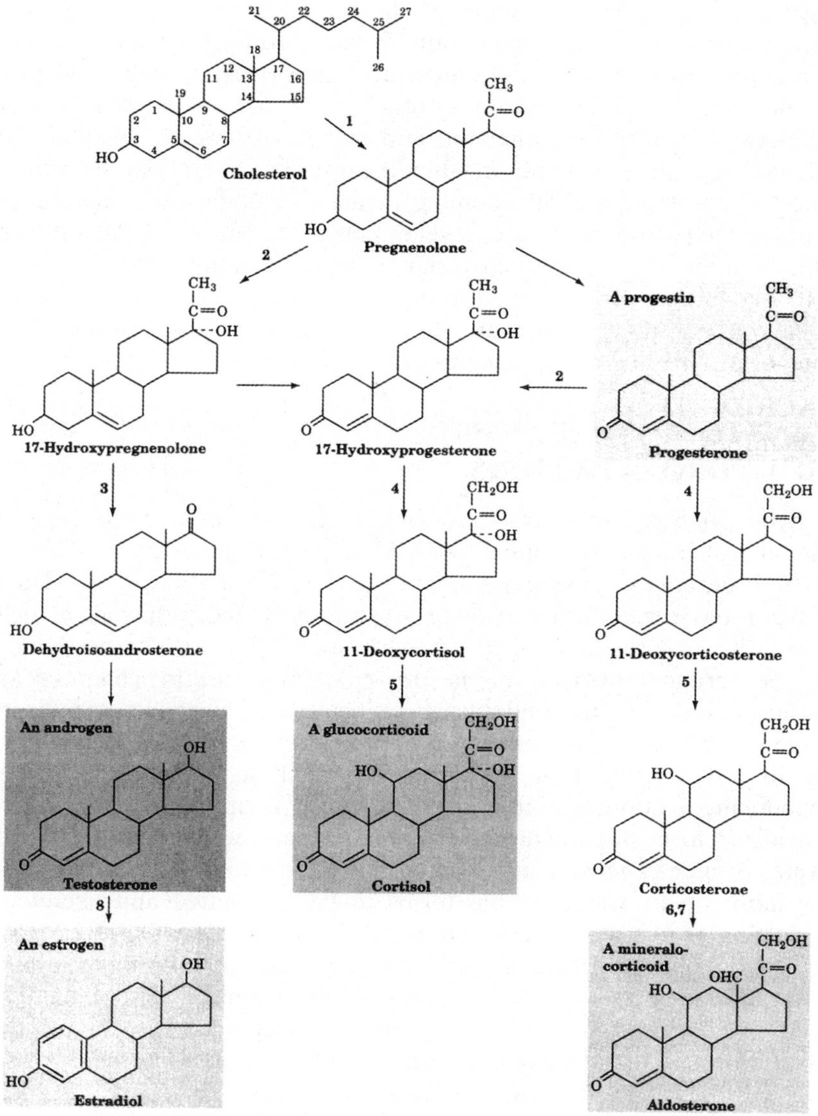

FIGURE 2.14. Biosynthetic relations of some steroid hormones and the synthesis of progesterone, corticoids, aldosterone, androgens, and estrogens. The enzymes involved are: (1) the cholesterol side chain cleavage enzyme; (2) steroid C17 hydroxylase; (3) steroid C17, C20 lyase; (4) steroid C21 hydroxylase; (5) steroid 11-beta-hydroxylase; (6) steroid C18 hydroxylase; (7) 18-hydroxysteroid oxidase; and (8) aromatase. (Courtesy of *Biochemistry*, Voet/Voet, J. Wiley & Sons.)

into calcitriol (1,25-dihydroxycholecalciferol) which is the active hormone through hydroxylation in the liver and the kidneys. Vitamin D_2 (ergocalciferol) can be formed in a similar manner, starting from ergosterol. Vitamin D_2 is the same as vitamin D_3 except for having a C22–C23 double bond and a C24 methyl group.

Cholesterol (which contains 27 carbon atoms) also gives rise to five major types of steroid hormones (which contain fewer than 22 carbons): progestagens (progesterone prepares the lining of the uterus for ovum implantation and maintains pregnancy); glucocorticoids (which promote gluconeogenesis and the formation of glycogen, and enhance the degradation of fat and protein); mineralocorticoids, primarily aldosterone (which act on the distal tubules of the kidney to reabsorb sodium ion and excrete potassium ion and protons, which increase blood volume and blood pressure); androgens such as testosterone (which affect the development of male secondary sex characteristics); and estrogens (which affect the development of female secondary sex characteristics and the integrity of the ovarian cycle). The major sites of synthesis are corpus luteum, adrenal cortex, adrenal cortex, testis, and ovary, respectively. The biosynthetic relationships are shown in Figure 2.14. All of these markers are important medical monitoring markers for hormonal status.

2.9 CYTOCHROME P-450 AND HYDROXYLATIONS

The hydroxylation oxidations necessary in the synthesis of the steroid hormones and of vitamin D require $NADPH_2$ and oxygen (the oxygen atom in the hydroxy group does not originate from water but from the oxygen of the air). Activation of oxygen occurs through cytochrome P-450, a specific cytochrome complex that absorbs light at 450 nm when complexed with carbon monoxide. It is the terminal cytochrome in the electron transport chain in adrenal mitochondria and in the endoplasmic reticulum of liver. Its specific role is hydroxylation rather than oxidative phosphorylation. NADPH donates electrons to a flavoprotein in the complex, which in turn transfers them to adrenodoxin, a non-heme iron protein, which then conveys an electron to the oxidized form of cytochrome P-450. The reduced cytochrome P-450 then activates oxygen. This system is responsible for the oxidation of xenobiotics to allow more polar, water-soluble forms to be eliminated and excreted. The introduction of hydroxy groups allows conjugation reactions to occur in otherwise hydrophobic compounds. Some reactive and carcinogenic intermediates result, however, for specific xenobiotics; for example, the epoxide intermediates of some aromatic systems. Another function of cytochrome P-450 is oxidation of a terminal carbon atom. This allows monocarboxylic acids to be converted to dicarboxylic acids. Hydroxylation occurs first as discussed above. Oxidation continues to a carboxylic acid moeity that is then converted to a CoA derivative at either end, and this molecule is then oxidized further through beta-oxidation.

In mammals, cytochrome P-450 enzymes originate from eight families of genes. Though the synthesis and degradation of fatty acids and steroids were probably cytochrome P-450's first functions in evolution, detoxification of organic compounds was added to its functions because of the similarity of the xenobiotics to some natural substrates, or because some of the metabolic products of xenobiotics often ended up as carbon sources in fatty acid biosynthesis. An important function of heme in liver is as the prosthetic group of cytochrome P-450.

Covalent Structures of the "Standard" Amino Acids of Proteins

Name	Structural Formula [a]	Residue Mass (D)	Average Occurrence in Proteins (%) [b]
Amino acids with nonpolar side chains			
Glycine	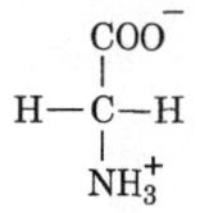	57.0	7.5
Alanine	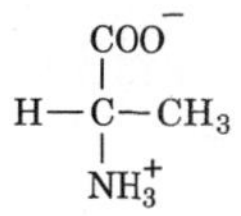	71.0	9.0
Valine	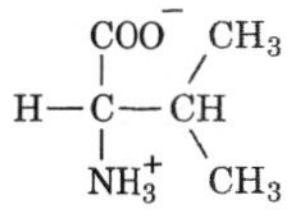	99.1	6.9
Leucine	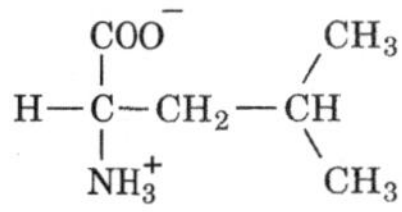	113.1	7.5
Isoleucine	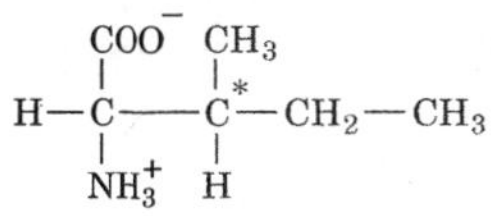	113.1	4.6
Methionine	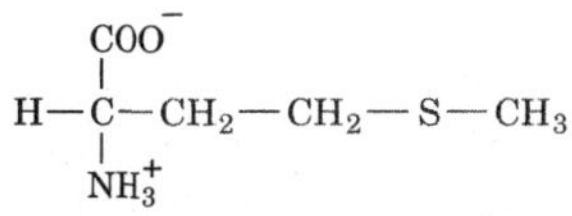	131.1	1.7
Proline	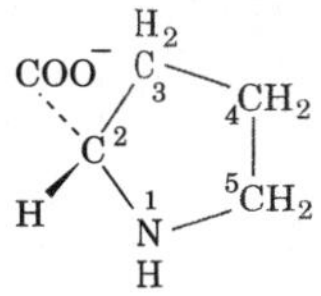	97.1	4.6
Phenylalanine	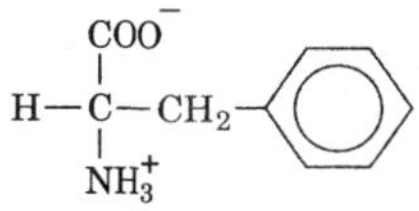	147.1	3.5
Tryptophan	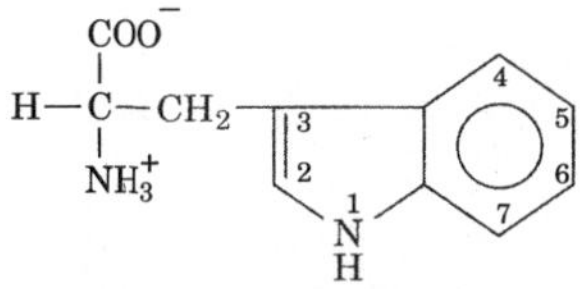	186.2	1.1

[a] The ionic forms shown are those predominating at pH 7.0. The C_α atoms, as well as those atoms marked with an asterisk, are chiral centers with configurations as indicated according to Fischer projection formulas. The standard organic numbering system is provided for heterocycles. For the molecular masses of the parent amino acids, add 18.0 D, the molecular mass of H_2O, to the residue masses. For side chain masses, subtract 56.0 D, the formula mass of a peptide group, from the residue masses.

[b] Estimated from the compositions of 207 unrelated proteins as compiled by Klapper, M. H., *Biochem. Biophys. Res. Commun.* **78,** 1020 (1977).

FIGURE 2.15.

Name	Structural Formula [a]	Residue Mass (D)	Average Occurrence in Proteins (%) [b]
Amino acids with uncharged polar side chains			
Serine	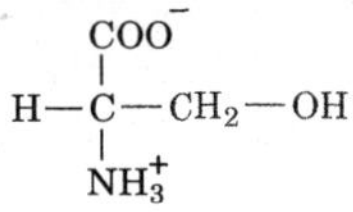	87.0	7.1
Threonine	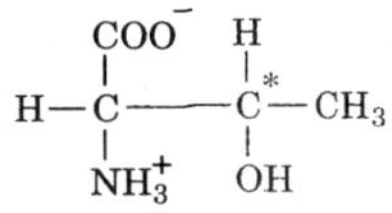	101.1	6.0
Asparagine	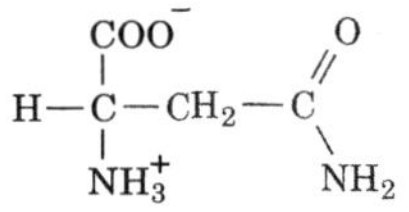	114.1	4.4
Glutamine	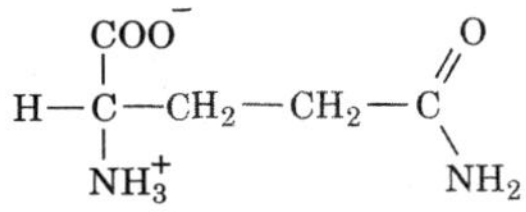	128.1	3.9
Tyrosine	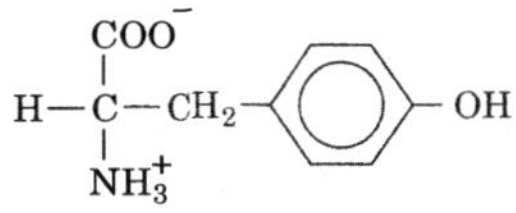	163.1	3.5
Cysteine	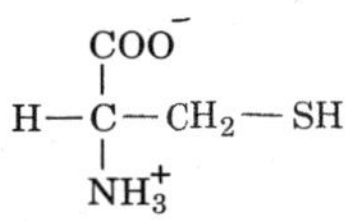	103.1	2.8
Amino acids with charged polar side chains			
Lysine	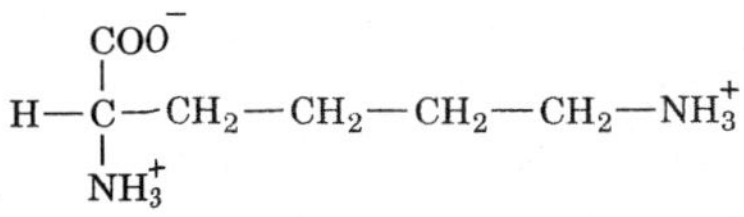	129.1	7.0
Arginine	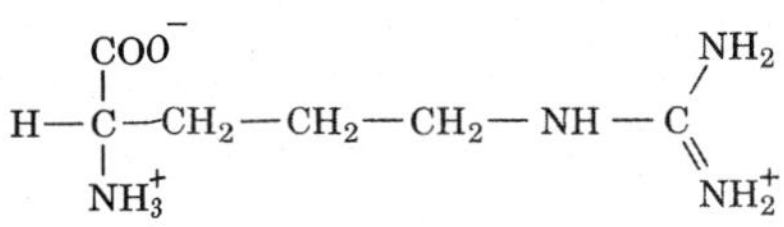	157.2	4.7
Histidine	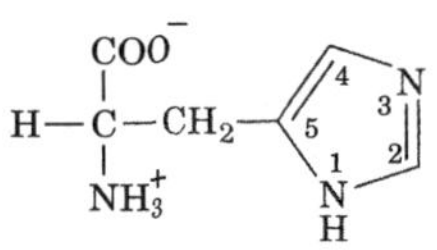	137.1	2.1
Aspartic acid	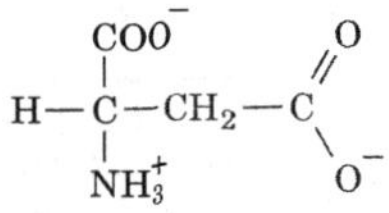	114.0	5.5
Glutamic acid	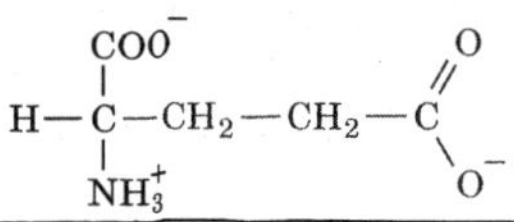	128.1	6.2

FIGURE 2.15.

Amino Acid	Three Letter Symbol	One Letter Symbol[a]
Alanine	Ala	A
Arginine	Arg	R
Asparagine	Asn	N
Aspartic acid	Asp	D
Asparagine *or* aspartic acid	Asx	B
Cysteine	Cys	C
Glutamic acid	Glu	E
Glutamine	Gln	Q
Glutamine *or* glutamic acid	Glx	Z
Glycine	Gly	G
Histidine	His	H
Isoleucine	Ile	I
Leucine	Leu	L
Lysine	Lys	K
Methionine	Met	M
Phenylalanine	Phe	F
Proline	Pro	P
Serine	Ser	S
Threonine	Thr	T
Tryptophan	Trp	W
Tyrosine	Tyr	Y
Valine	Val	V

[a] The one letter symbol for an undetermined or "nonstandard" amino acid is X.

FIGURE 2.15. Covalent structures of the "standard" amino acids of proteins and their abbreviations (inset). Gly, Ala, Val, Leu, and Ile have aliphatic side chains. Pro has a secondary amino group. Phe, Tyr, and Trp have aromatic side chains. Cys and Met have a side chain containing one sulfur. Ser and Thr contain aliphatic hydroxy side chains. Lys, Arg, and His have basic side chains. Asp and Glu are acidic amino acids with amide derivatives, Asn and Gln. Cystine has a disulfide link formed from two Cys residues. A more recent discovery has revealed that selenium instead of S in Cys is also a fundamental amino acid.

2.10 ISOPENTENYL PYROPHOSPHATE AS A SYNTHON

Many compounds are synthesized from the basic C_5 building block of isopentenyl pyrophosphate: squalene (Figure 2.12), the C_{30} hydrocarbon side chain of vitamin K_2 (a key molecule in the clotting process), the C_{50} side chain of coenzyme Q_{10} (in the mitochondrial respiratory chain), and the C_{40} carbon skeletons of carotenoids (essential for vision as retinal where beta-carotene is the precursor).

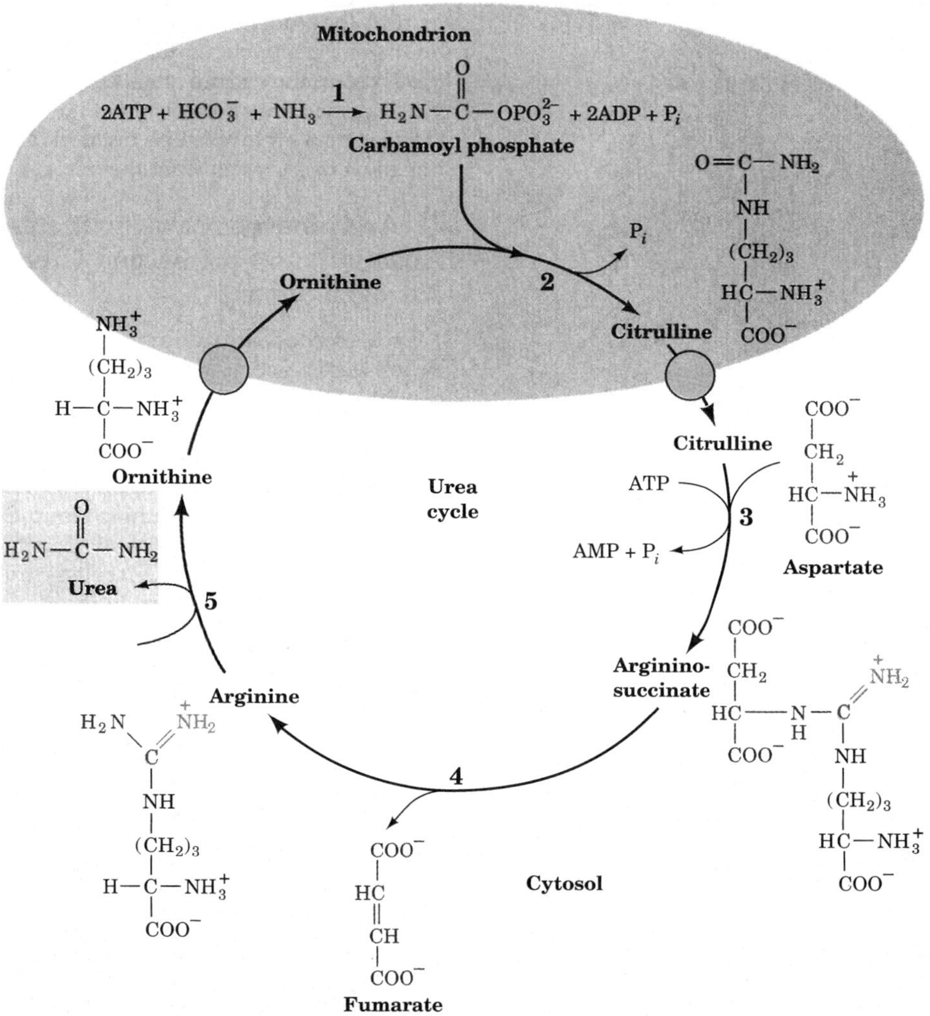

FIGURE 2.16. The urea cycle. The urea cycle occurs partially in the mitochondrion and partially in the cytosol, with ornithine and citrulline being transported across the mitochondrial membrane by specific transport systems. Five enzymes participate in the urea cycle: (1) carbamoyl phosphate synthetase, (2) ornithine transcarbamoylase, (3) argininosuccinate synthetase, (4) argininosuccinase, and (5) arginase. (Courtesy of *Biochemistry*, Voet/Voet, J. Wiley & Sons.)

2.11 NITROGEN COMPOUNDS

2.11.1 Degradation

Excess amino acids (Figure 2.15) above the needs for protein, polypeptide, or other biosyntheses cannot be stored or excreted but are used as metabolic carbon fuel in the cycles mentioned above, mostly in the liver of mammals. The α-amino group of many amino acids (for example, aspartate and alanine) is removed in the cell cytosol by transfer (transamination) to α-ketoglutarate to form glutamate, which is then oxidized by either NAD^+ or $NADP^+$ with deamination to ammonium ion and to α-ketoglutarate. The

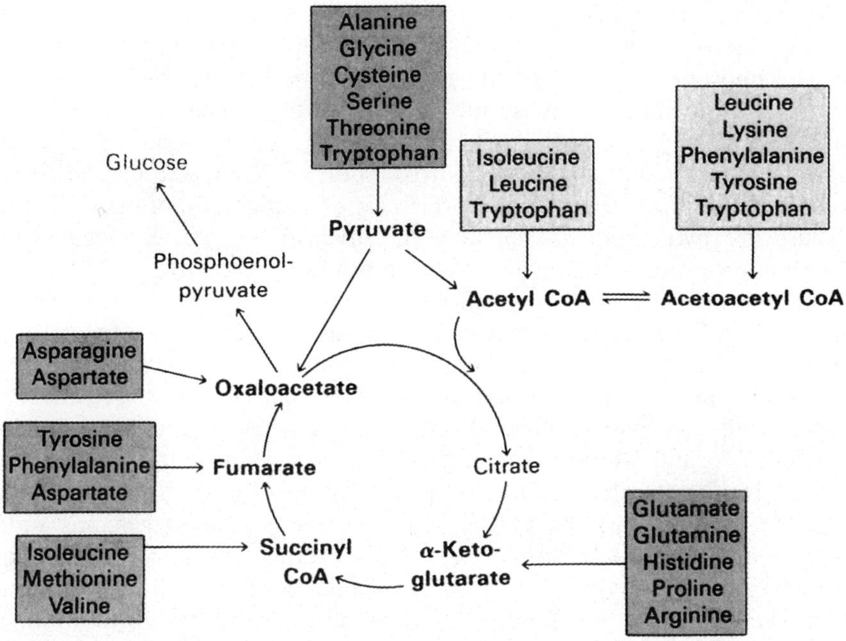

FIGURE 2.17. Fates of the carbon skeletons of amino acids. All are glucogenic apart from the three leading to acetyl CoA and the five yielding acetoacetyl CoA, which are ketogenic. (Courtesy of *Biochemistry*, third edition, Stryer, Freeman.)

latter reaction occurs in the matrix of mitochondria. The ammonium ion in terrestrial vertebrates is converted (Figure 2.16) into urea ($NH_2-CO-NH_2$), which is excreted in the urine (urotelic). The immediate precursor to urea is arginine. The urea cycle is linked to the citric acid cycle through the production of fumarate. The α-amino groups of serine and threonine can be directly converted into ammonium ion because of the presence of a hydroxy group on the beta-carbon atom. In birds and terrestrial reptiles, the ammonium ion is mostly transformed to uric acid (uricotelic). In many aquatic animals, ammonium ion itself is eliminated (ammonotelic).

The fates of the carbon skeletons of amino acids after removal of the alpha-amino group are depicted in Figure 2.17. The skeletons from 20 amino acids end up in only seven molecules, namely, pyruvate, acetyl CoA, acetoacetyl CoA, alpha-ketoglutarate, succinyl CoA, fumarate, and oxaloacetate.

2.11.2 Biosynthesis of Amino Acids

Nitrogen can come from dietary sources, or from N_2 fixed by symbiotic bacteria. Ammonium ion is then used to produce glutamate and glutamine via α-ketoglutarate. Glutamate production is a central control point in nitrogen metabolism. Eleven of the amino acids (alanine, arginine, asparagine, aspartate, cysteine, glutamate, glutamine, glycine, proline, serine, and tyrosine) are synthesized from the intermediates of the citric acid cycle and other metabolic pathways. The aromatic amino acids apart from tyrosine are essential. The demand for arginine usually is easily met by the urea cycle in adults but not in children, where it is essential. Glutamate donates its α-amino group to pyruvate to form alanine, to oxaloacetate to produce aspartate, and to 3-phosphohydroxypyruvate resulting from 3-phosphoglycerate to form 3-phosphoserine and finally serine. Serine is the precursor of glycine and cysteine. Asparagine receives its extra amino group from glutamine via aspartate. Tyrosine is made by hydroxylation of phenylalanine, an essential amino acid. Glutamate is also the precursor of proline and arginine.

There are two major C_1 carriers, tetrahydrofolate and *S*-adenosyl methionine, important in amino acid biosynthesis and degradation.

The pteridine ring of tetrahydrofolate comes from the diet or from symbiotic bacteria. The C_1 derivatives of tetrahydrofolate are responsible for methionine production from homocysteine, for glycine production from carbon dioxide and ammonium ion, for some carbon atoms of the purines of DNA, and for the methyl group of thymine. The C_1 fragments can be in the form of methyl, methylene, formyl, formimino, and methenyl, usually at the N^5 and/or N^{10} position. In turn tetrahydrofolate is an acceptor of C_1 fragments in biodegradations, the major source being the conversion of serine to glycine, and to a lesser extent the breakdown of histidine. Pterins are also redox cofactors resembling the N-containing rings of the flavins. Pterins tend to catalyze intramolecular shifts of hydrogen atoms on aromatics after epoxide formation during oxidative processes that require molecular oxygen. This intramolecular shift is called the NIH shift. Thus, the hydrogen atom on carbon atom 4 of the aromatic ring in phenylalanine is transferred to carbon atom 3 rather than being lost to the solvent by replacement with a hydroxy group. This reaction forms tyrosine in an enzyme complex consisting of phenylalanine hydroxylase, the cofactor 5,6,7,8-tetrahydrobiopterin, dihydropteridine reductase, and NADH. Another NIH shift-type reaction involving methyl group transfer is catalyzed in the phenylalanine degradative pathway for *p*-hydroxyphenylpyruvate to homogentisic acid by the copper-containing enzyme *p*-hydroxyphenylpyruvate dioxygenase, which involves oxidative decarboxylation of an α-keto acid as well as ring hydroxylation. Both hydride and methyl transfer-type NIH shift reactions have also been noted in aromatic xenobiotic metabolism, requiring molecular oxygen and featuring epoxide intermediate formation.

Methylations (for example, of adrenaline to form noradrenaline, and of a glutamate residue in the regulatory protein for chemotaxis) are usually performed with *S*-adenosylmethionine, with *S*-adenosylhomocysteine as the demethylation product from which homocysteine can be produced (Figure 2.18). The *S*-adenosyl group arises from ATP. This route is the almost exclusive one for methylations for xenobiotics.

Methionine can be regenerated from homocysteine by methylation by N^5-methyltetrahydrofolate and betaine (an oxidation product of choline). The homocysteine can react also with serine to form cystathione, which cleaves its sulfhydryl link to produce cysteine and α-ketobutyrate (Figure 2.18).

2.11.3 Amino Acids as Building Blocks

Amino acids are precursors for six of the nine atoms of purine rings and four out of the six atoms of the pyrimidines. Serine provides the reactive terminus of sphingosine; histidine is decarboxylated to form histamine; tyrosine is the

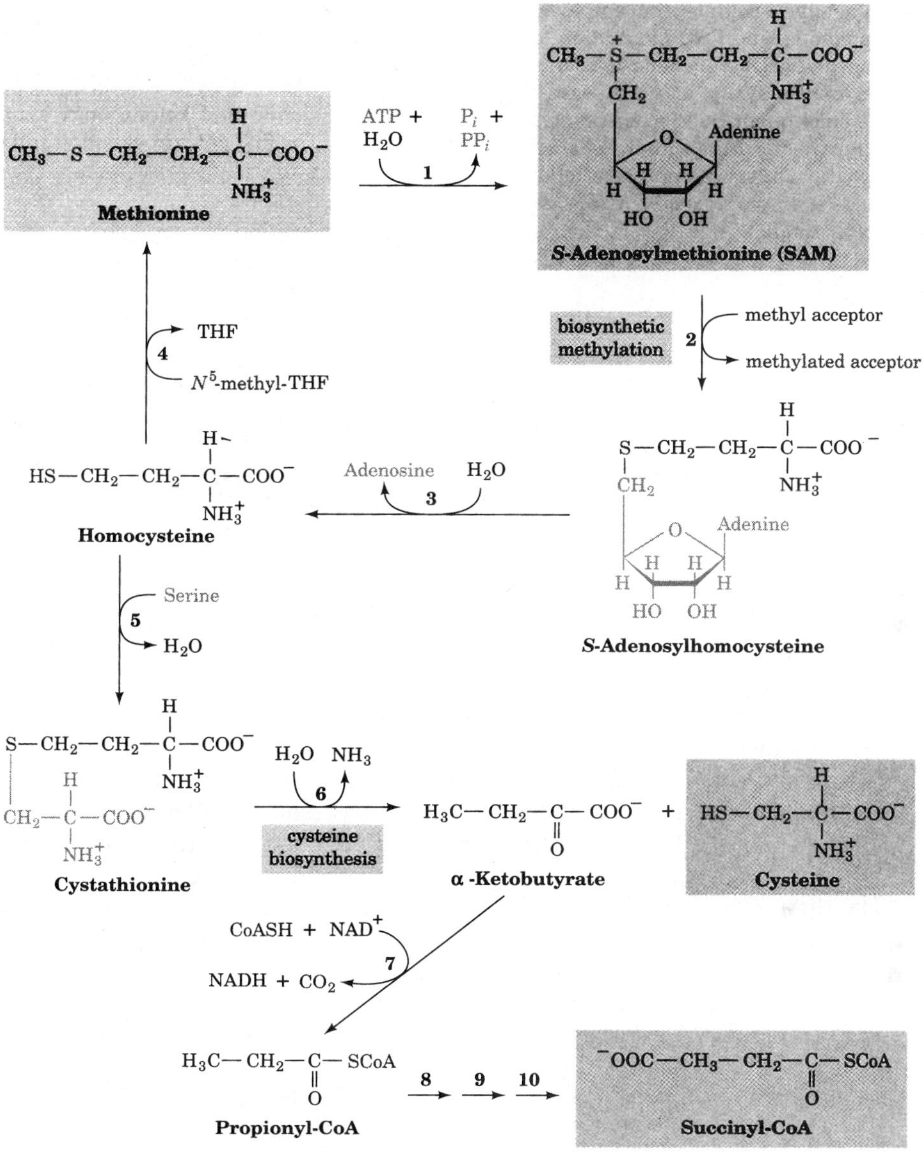

FIGURE 2.18. Donation of methyl groups from *S*-adenosylmethionine (SAM), which is derived from the essential amino acid methionine. The pathway of methionine degradation yields cysteine and succinyl-CoA as products. The enzymes involved are: (1) methionine adenosyl transferase; (2) methylase; (3) adenosylhomocysteinase; (4) homocysteine methyltransferase, a coenzyme B_{12}-dependent enzyme; (5) cystathionine β-synthase, a pyridoxal-5′-phosphate (PLP)-dependent enzyme; (6) cystathionine γ-lyase, a PLP-dependent enzyme; (7) α-keto acid dehydrogenase; (8) propionyl-CoA carboxylase; (9) methylmalonyl-CoA racemase; and (10) methylmalonyl-CoA mutase, a coenzyme B_{12}-dependent enzyme. (Courtesy of *Biochemistry*, Voet/Voet, J. Wiley & Sons.)

precursor of thyroxine, adrenaline, and melanin; tryptophan is the precursor for serotonin and the nicotinamide unit of NAD^+; glycine donates 8 out of the 34 carbon atoms of heme; and glutamine provides the amide group of the nicotinamide moiety.

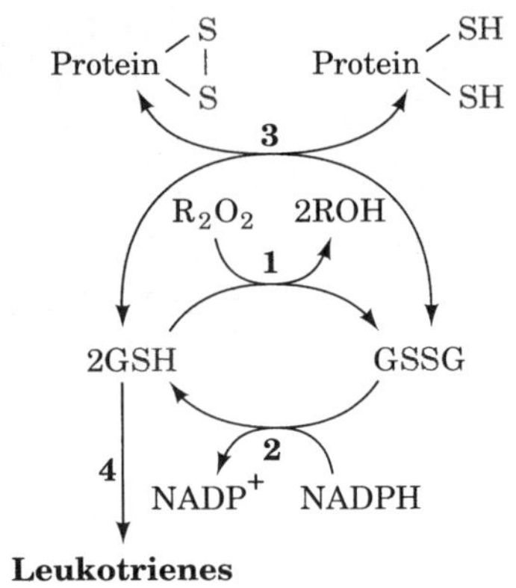

FIGURE 2.19. Some reactions involving glutathione: (1) peroxide detoxification by glutathione peroxidase, (2) regeneration of GSH from GSSG by glutathione reductase, (3) thiol transferase modulation of the protein thiol–disulfide balance, and (4) leukotriene biosynthesis by glutathione-*S*-transferase. GSH is reduced glutathione; GSSG is oxidized glutathione dimer; R_2O_2 is an organic peroxide; ROH is an organic alcohol. (Courtesy of *Biochemistry*, Voet/Voet, J. Wiley & Sons.)

2.11.4 Glutathione

Glutathione is a tripeptide, Glu–Cys–Gly. It protects red cells from oxidative damage; serves as a sulfhydryl buffer (it cycles between a reduced thiol form denoted by GSH and an oxidized disulfide form, GSSG, which is a dimer linked by a disulfide link, with the GSH/GSSG ratio usually being greater than 500); plays a key role in the detoxification of organic peroxides, hydrogen peroxide, and electrophiles; and transports amino acids through the membrane of kidney cells. It also has found much use as an agent to protect against the effects of ionizing radiation.

The first step in GSH synthesis is the condensation reaction between glutamate and cysteine with the aid of ATP and the γ-glutamyl cysteine synthetase to form Glu–Cys dipeptide, which then produces GSH after reaction with glycine, ATP, and glutathione synthetase. The oxidation step to GSSG requires NADPH and the enzyme glutathione reductase. GSSG is also formed when GSH reduces peroxides with the help of the selenium-containing enzyme glutathione peroxidase (Figure 2.19). The latter enzyme is the chief way that red blood cell membranes are kept from oxidizing.

The transport of γ-glutamyl groups from one side of a cell membrane to the other occurs through the agency of γ-glutamyl transpeptidase, which transfers the γ-glutamyl group of GSH on the extracellular side of the cell to the α-amino group of an acceptor amino acid such as glutamine or cysteine on the cytosol side of the cell membrane (Figure 2.20). Because glutamate is the source of many other amino acids, this allows these amino acids to be synthesized within cells in a regulated manner. Overstimulation of the activity of γ-glutamyl transpeptidase has been used as a medical surveillance marker for precarcinogenic events and as a similar tool in histopathology. GSH conjugation is a major metabolic fate for xenobiotics containing heteroatoms, but especially those with the halogens chlorine, bromine, and iodine (Section 9.3.7). Hydroxylated metabolic intermediates often are conjugated also by GSH, and thus this process competes with further oxidation.

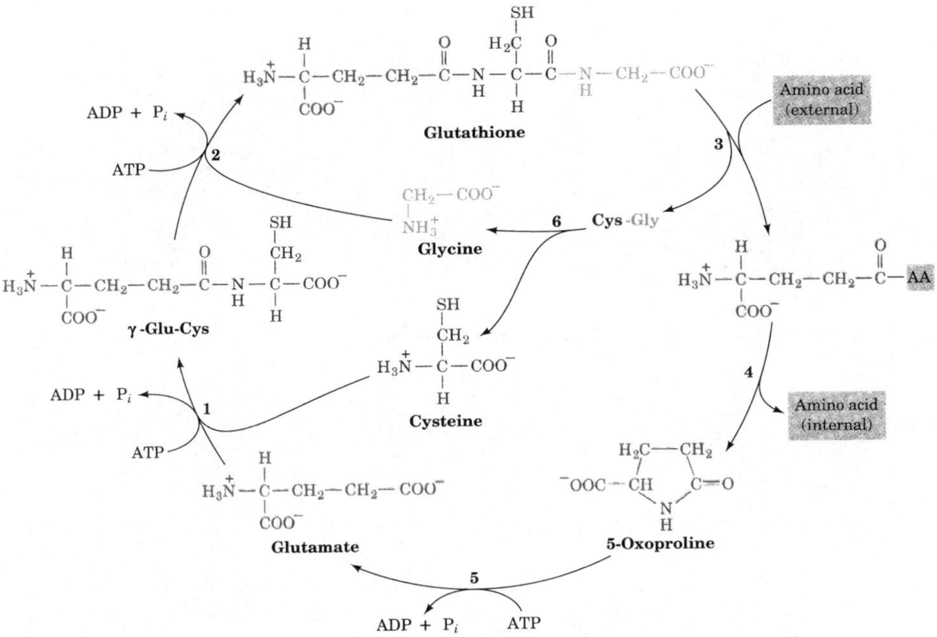

FIGURE 2.20. The γ-glutamyl cycle. An amino acid is carried from one cell to another as a γ-glutamyl derivative. All reactions are cytosolic except for the formation of the γ-glutamyl amino acid, which occurs on the extracellular face of the plasma membrane. The cycle's reactions are catalyzed by: (1) γ-glutamylcysteine synthetase, (2) glutathione synthetase, (3) γ-glutamyl transpeptidase, (4) γ-glutamyl cyclotransferase, (5) 5-oxoprolinase, and (6) an intracellular protease. (Courtesy of *Biochemistry*, Voet/Voet, J. Wiley & Sons.)

2.11.5 Porphyrins

^{14}C-label studies reveal that 8 carbon atoms of heme are derived from the α-carbon of glycine, with 24 from the methyl group of acetate and 2 from the carboxyl group of acetate. The first step of biosynthesis of porphyrins in mammals and the committed step of the pathway is the condensation of glycine and succinyl CoA to form δ-aminolevulinate with the aid of a zinc-dependent synthase in mitochondria. Two molecules of this product condense, catalyzed by a zinc-dependent dehydratase, to form porphobilinogen. In mammals both the synthase and dehydratase functions are carried out on the same enzyme complex. Four of these porphobilinogens condense head-to-tail to form a linear tetrapyrrole that is bound to the enzyme, which cyclizes by losing ammonium ions to create uroporphyrinogen III under the influence of a synthase and a cosynthase. If the latter is inhibited, uroporphyrinogen I accumulates. Further reactions alter the side chains and the degree of saturation in the porphyrin skeleton. When the acetate side chains are decarboxylated, coproporphyrinogen III is produced. Desaturation of the porphyrin ring and transformation of two propionate side chains to vinyl groups yield protoporphyrin IX. Insertion of iron in a four-coordinate link to the four pyrrole nitrogens gives heme, the prosthetic group for myoglobin, hemoglobin, catalase, peroxidase, and cytochrome c. The biosynthetic pathway is depicted in Figure 2.21. The insertion of Fe[II] is catalyzed by ferrochelatase, a zinc-dependent enzyme found in greatest quantity in bone marrow where red blood

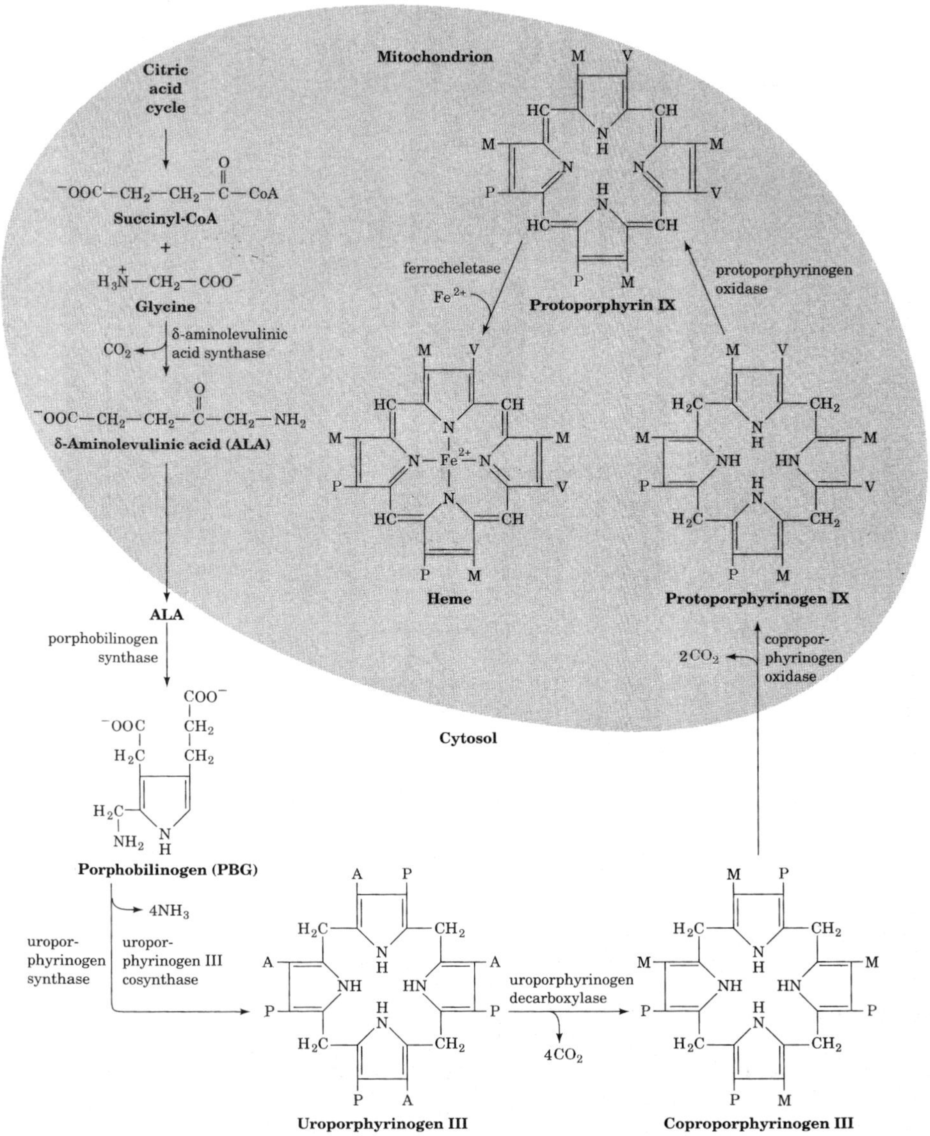

FIGURE 2.21. Synthesis of heme from succinyl-CoA and glycine. δ-aminolevulinic acid (ALA) is synthesized in the mitochondrion by ALA-synthase. ALA leaves the mitochondrion and is converted to porphobilinogen (PBG), four molecules of which condense to form a porphyrin ring. The next three reactions involve oxidation of the pyrrole ring substituents, yielding protoporphyrinogen IX, whose formation is accompanied by its transport back into the mitochondrion. After oxidation of the methylene groups linking the pyrroles to yield protoporphyrin IX, ferrochelatase catalyzes the insertion of Fe^{2+} to yield heme. A is acetate; M is methyl; P is propionate; V is vinyl. (Courtesy of *Biochemistry*, Voet/Voet, J. Wiley & Sons.)

cells are made. This is thought to be the rate-limiting step of heme synthesis in the presence of adequate iron in reticulocytes (immature red blood cells that synthesize hemoglobin in the bone) along with the action of uroporphyrin synthase.

Iron is transported in the plasma by transferrin, a protein that binds two ferric ions. Iron is stored in tissues inside ferritin, which can hold as many as

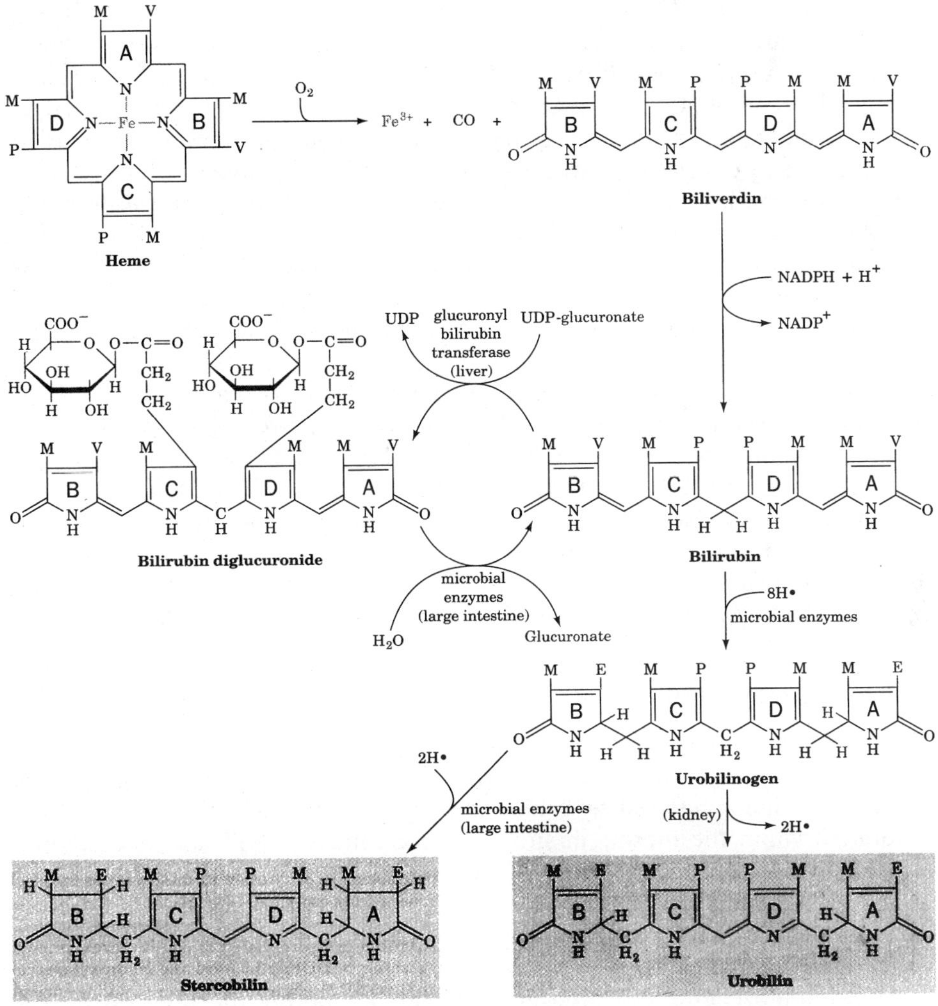

FIGURE 2.22. Degradation of heme to bilirubin. M, V, P, and E represent methyl, vinyl, propionyl, and ethyl groups, respectively. (Courtesy of *Biochemistry*, Voet/Voet, J. Wiley & Sons.)

4500 ferric ions. Cellular uptake of iron is also rate-limiting in reticulocytes and in the liver because the uptake is controlled by receptor-mediated endocytosis.

The detection of urinary porphyrins is a medical monitoring test of liver function and of inherited disorders, as well as for specific effects of certain xenobiotics, notably lead and hexachlorobenzene. Lead inhibits the enzymes requiring zinc, causing accumulation of the enzyme substrates in the blood and urine. The accumulation of zinc protoporphyrin in the blood has been used as a marker of chronic exposure to lead reflecting lead exposure over the previous 3 to 4 months. The accumulation of δ-aminolevulinic acid, which resembles the neurotransmitter γ-aminobutyric acid, is postulated to be responsible for the neurobehavioral effects of lead poisoning.

The lifetime for a red blood cell is about 120 days. Old cells are degraded in the spleen (Figure 2.22). First the apoprotein of hemoglobin is hydrolyzed to its amino acids. The heme group then cleaves at its α-methene bridge in the presence of heme oxygenase to form biliverdin, which is a linear tetrapyrrole. Oxygen and NADPH are required also. The α-methene bridge carbon is released as carbon monoxide, which is carried in the blood as carboxyhemoglobin. The latter is also the chief biological monitoring marker for exposure to exogenous carbon monoxide and to methylene chloride. The central methene bridge of biliverdin is reduced by a reductase in the presence of NADPH to form bilirubin, which is one of the three major plasma antioxidants along with urate and ascorbate and, in membranes, is as potent an antioxidant as vitamin E. The bilirubin is then transported by serum albumin to the liver and is glucuronidated at its two propionate side chains by UDP-glucuronate (derived from oxidized UDP-glucose) and secreted into the bile. The latter process is also a major pathway of processing hydroxylated xenobiotics. Bacterial symbionts in the large intestine hydrolyze the glucuronic acid groups and convert bilirubin to urobilinogen. Some of the latter is reabsorbed through the intestinal walls (enterohepatic circulation) and transported by the bloodstream to the kidney, where it is converted to the yellow urobilin, which provides the urine with its characteristic yellow color. Most of the urobilinogen in the large intestine suffers further microbial action to form the deep red-brown stercobilin, the major pigment of feces.

2.11.6 Creatine and Creatinine

ATP typically is a short-lived source of energy inside muscles. The major reservoir of energy for muscle contractile activity is creatine phosphate or phosphocreatine, catalyzed by a kinase in the presence of ADP. Thus ATP is generated within the muscle in situ. In resting muscle, typical concentrations of ATP, ADP, creatine phosphate, and creatine product are 4, 0.013, 25, and 13 mM, respectively. Creatine phosphate is produced by the phosphorylation of creatine, which is initially synthesized in the kidney, liver, and pancreas. Arginine and glycine react under the influence of an amidinotransferase to form guanidinoacetate and ornithine, the latter entering the urea cycle. The guanidinoacetate is methylated by *S*-adenosylmethionine and catalyzed by a transferase to produce creatine. Creatinine, the anhydride of creatine, forms spontaneously from both creatine and phosphocreatine (Figure 2.23). Creatinine is released into the bloodstream and is constant for a healthy individual of constant muscle weight; it is filtered by the kidney glomeruli into the urine and is used for normalization purposes to correct for urine dilution in the absence of glomerular damage.

2.11.7 Biosynthesis of Nucleotides

Nucleotides are the activated precursors of DNA and RNA, and are activated intermediates in many biosynthetic pathways. For example, UDP-glucose and CDP-diacylglycerol are precursors of glycogen and phosphoglycerides, respectively. *S*-Adenosylmethionine has an activated methyl group. ATP is the universal source of energy. GTP energizes macromolecule movements, for example, the activation of signal-coupling proteins. Adenine is essential to the coenzymes NAD^+, FAD, and CoA. Nucleotides are metabolic regulators:

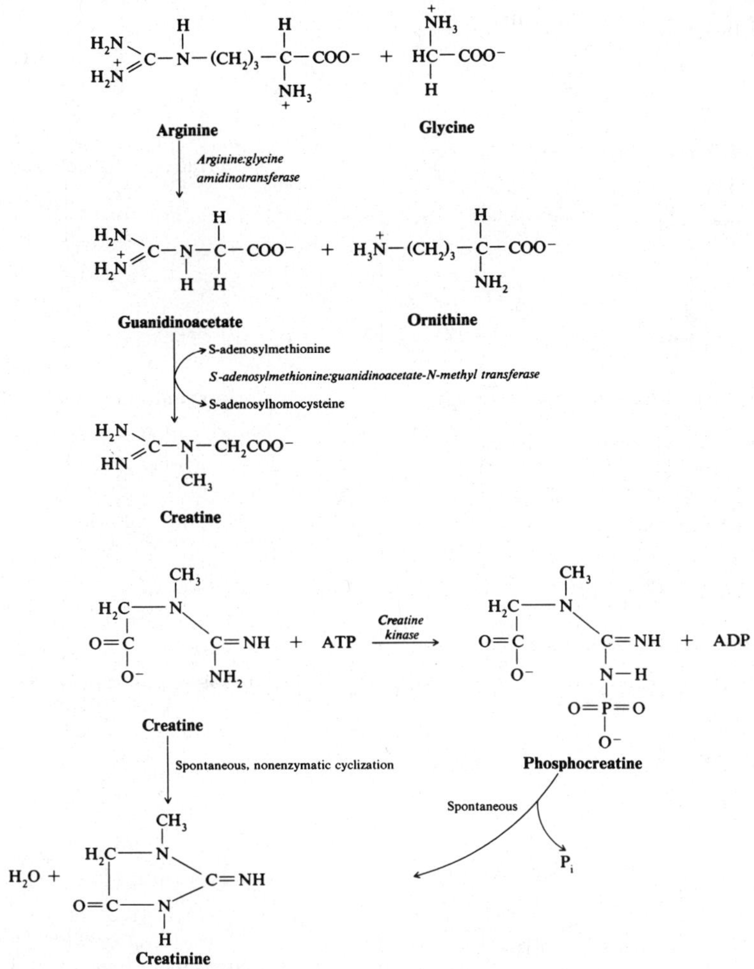

FIGURE 2.23. Formation of creatinine from arginine and glycine precursors.

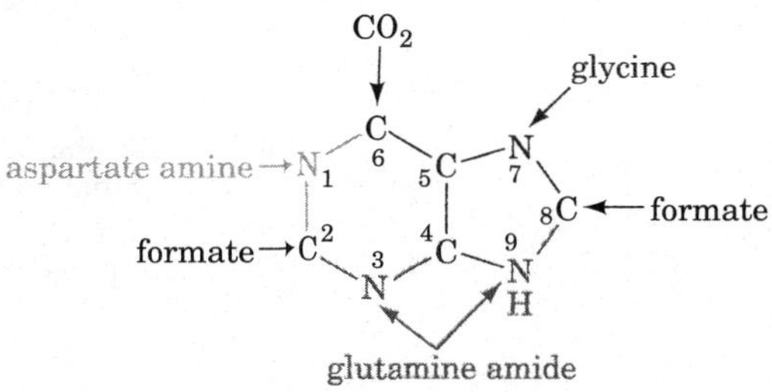

FIGURE 2.24.

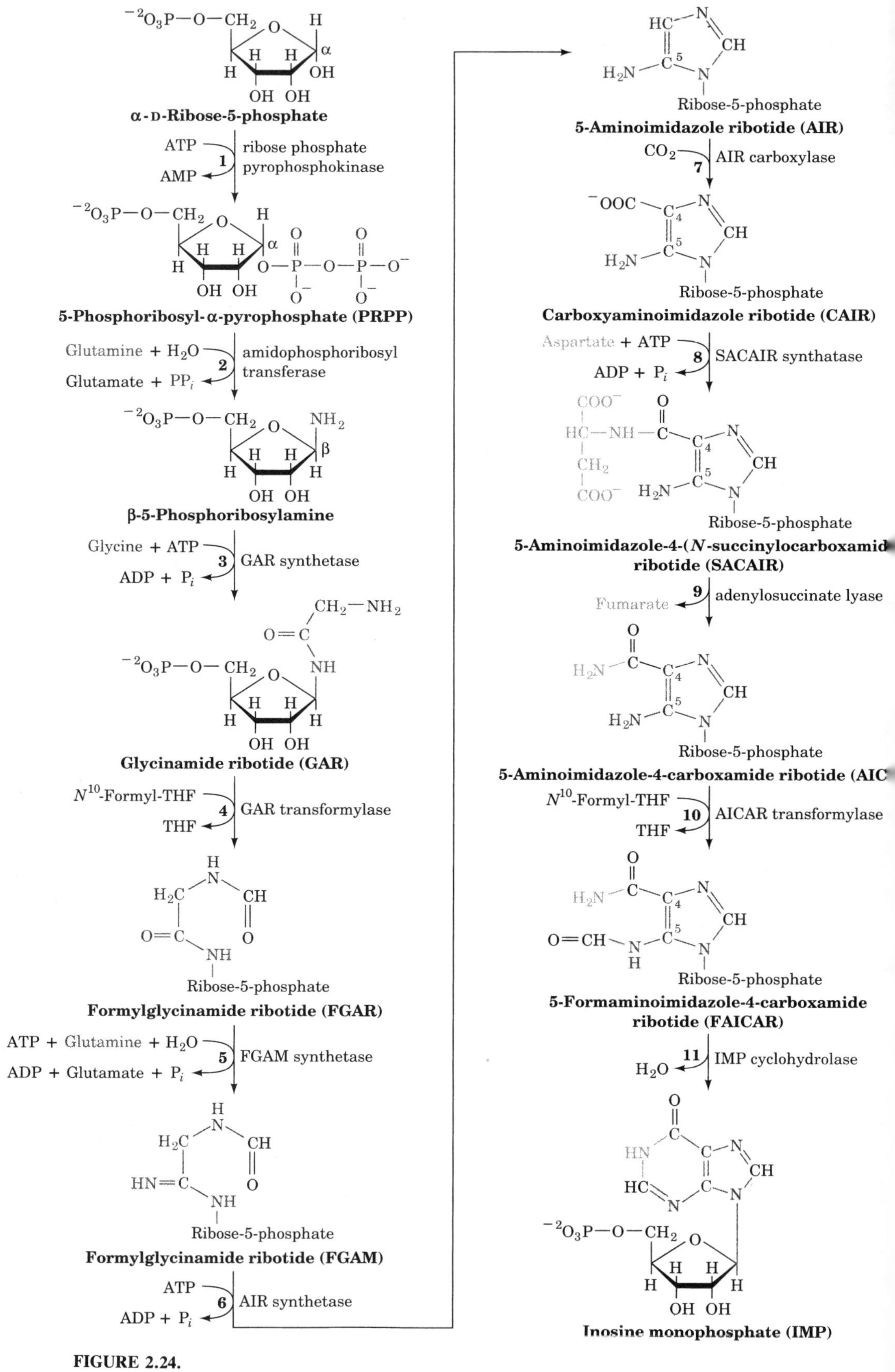

α-D-Ribose-5-phosphate
ATP
AMP
1
ribose phosphate pyrophosphokinase
5-Phosphoribosyl-α-pyrophosphate (PRPP)
Glutamine + H2O
Glutamate + PPi
2
amidophosphoribosyl transferase
β-5-Phosphoribosylamine
Glycine + ATP
ADP + Pi
3
GAR synthetase
Glycinamide ribotide (GAR)
N10-Formyl-THF
THF
4
GAR transformylase
Ribose-5-phosphate
Formylglycinamide ribotide (FGAR)
ATP + Glutamine + H2O
ADP + Glutamate + Pi
5
FGAM synthetase
Ribose-5-phosphate
Formylglycinamide ribotide (FGAM)
ATP
ADP + Pi
6
AIR synthetase
Ribose-5-phosphate
5-Aminoimidazole ribotide (AIR)
CO2
7
AIR carboxylase
Ribose-5-phosphate
Carboxyaminoimidazole ribotide (CAIR)
Aspartate + ATP
ADP + Pi
8
SACAIR synthatase
Ribose-5-phosphate
5-Aminoimidazole-4-(N-succinylocarboxamid
ribotide (SACAIR)
Fumarate
9
adenylosuccinate lyase
Ribose-5-phosphate
5-Aminoimidazole-4-carboxamide ribotide (AIC
N10-Formyl-THF
THF
10
AICAR transformylase
Ribose-5-phosphate
5-Formaminoimidazole-4-carboxamide ribotide (FAICAR)
H2O
11
IMP cyclohydrolase
Inosine monophosphate (IMP)

FIGURE 2.24.

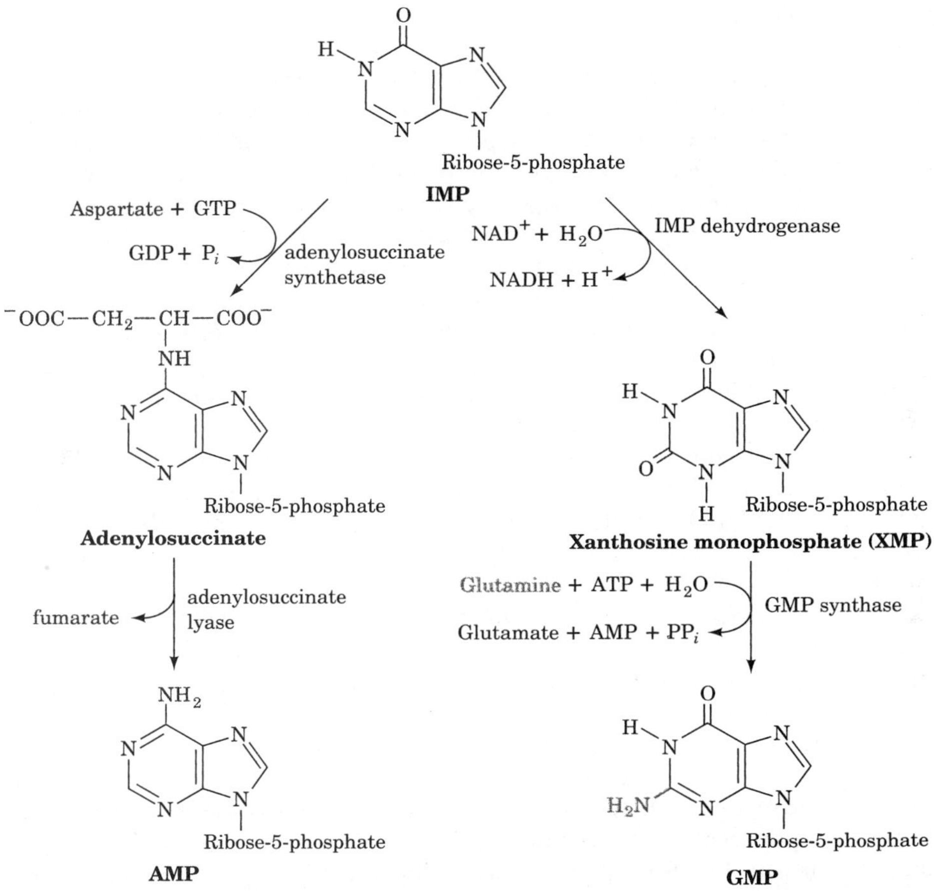

FIGURE 2.24. Biosynthesis of the purine ring, the origin of its atoms, and the nomenclature of bases, nucleosides, and nucleotides. Note that C4, C5, and N7 of the purine ring come from a single glycine molecule, but each of the other atoms are derived from independent precursors. The first stage of purine biosynthesis consists of production of inosine monophosphate (IMP) by (1) activation of ribose-5-phosphate with ATP, (2) acquisition of purine atom N9 with displacement of pyrophosphate (PP_i) by the side chain amino group of glutamine, the rate-determining step; (3) acquisition of purine atoms C4, C5, and N7 by addition of glycine; (4) acquisition of purine atom C8 by formylation by N^{10}-formyltetrahydrofolate; (5) acquisition of purine atom N3 by transfer of a nitrogen atom from glutamine; and (6) dehydration and formation of the purine imadazole ring. Vertebrates have reactions 3, 4, and 6 on a single polypeptide chain. The second stage of purine biosynthesis from 5-aminoimadazole ribotide is (7) acquisition of C6 by carboxylation; (8) acquisition of N1 by addition of aspartate; (9) elimination of fumarate, but leaving the amino group of aspartate; (10) acquisition of C2 by formylation by N^{10}-formyltetrahydrofolate; and (11) dehydration and ring closure to produce IMP, which is the precursor for AMP and GMP. The latter are produced in separate two-reaction pathways. (Courtesy of *Biochemistry*, Voet/Voet, J. Wiley & Sons.)

cAMP mediates the action of many hormones. ATP may mediate allosteric control (control other than through the active site) of enzyme activity, for example, the adenylation of glutamine synthase. A nucleoside consists of a purine or a pyrimidine base linked to a pentose; a nucleotide is a phosphate ester of a nucleoside. If the pentose is ribose, the base adenine has adenosine as its ribonucleoside and adenylate as its ribonucleotide (5′-monophosphate), used, for example, in RNA as building blocks. In DNA the pentose is deoxyribose.

Figure 2.24 gives the origins of the atoms in the purine ring (two carbons from N^{10}-formyltetrahydrofolate; two carbons and a nitrogen from glycine; two nitrogens from glutamine; one nitrogen from aspartate; and one carbon from carbon dioxide). The committed step is the formation of 5-phosphoribosylamine from 5-phosphoribosyl-1-pyrophosphate (PRPP) and glutamine in the presence of amidophosphoribosyl transferase. Similarly, Figure 2.25 provides the origins of the atoms in a pyrimidine ring (one carbon and one nitrogen from carbamoyl phosphate, and three carbons and one nitrogen from aspartate). The committed step for pyrimidine synthesis is the formation of *N*-carbamoylaspartate from aspartate and cytosolic carbamoyl phosphate catalyzed by aspartate transcarbamoylase. Five of the enzymes are associated in two complexes, one for the first three steps and another for the last two steps.

Deoxyribonucleotides are formed by reduction of ribonucleotides (Figure 2.26), where the 2′-hydroxy group on ribose is replaced by a hydrogen atom using NADPH as reductant and a sulfhydryl-containing reductase. This reductase is an allosteric enzyme that has an associated sulfhydryl electron carrier (thioredoxin for NADP reductant or glutaredoxin for GSH reductant).

Uracil is unique to RNA. Thymine, the methylated analog of uracil, is characteristic of DNA. Methylation of, and hydride transfer to, uracil occurs in the deoxyribonucleoside monophosphate form by N^5,N^{10}-methylenetetrahydrofolate aided by a synthase (Section 2.11.2).

Nucleotides in cells are degraded continously to nucleosides by nucleotidases. Phosphorylases degrade the nucleosides to free bases and ribose-1-phosphate or deoxyribose-1-phosphate. The former is isomerized by phosphoribomutase to ribose-5-phosphate, a precursor of PRPP. Free purine can also be salvaged by reaction with PRPP to form the nucleotide directly. AMP degradation also includes a deamination to IMP before formation of hypoxanthine, xanthine, and urate, the latter being excreted in the urine of primates (Figure 2.27). Urate is a very efficient antioxidant (on the order of vitamin C, ascorbic acid).

In pyrimidines, any carbon–carbon double bonds are first reduced, followed by breaking of the ring at the amide link closest to the now reduced double bond with subsequent liberation of ammonium ion (excreted as urea), carbon dioxide, and an amino acid, which is first transaminated, with the residue activated by CoA.

2.12 METABOLISM REGULATION

One of the recurring principles encountered in this brief survey of general metabolism is that biosynthetic and degradative biochemical pathways are nearly always distinct. This separation allows both processes to be operable simultaneously. Control points in these pathways often involve change in a cellular compartment. The enzymes catalyzing the committed step in specific processes are also major regulators of biosynthesis and degradation. They are generally allosterically controlled.

The key energy producing molecule ATP, the reductant NADPH, and the activator CoA are ubiquitous cofactors. The existence of key intermediates at the beginning of multiple pathways is also important: glucose-6-phosphate for

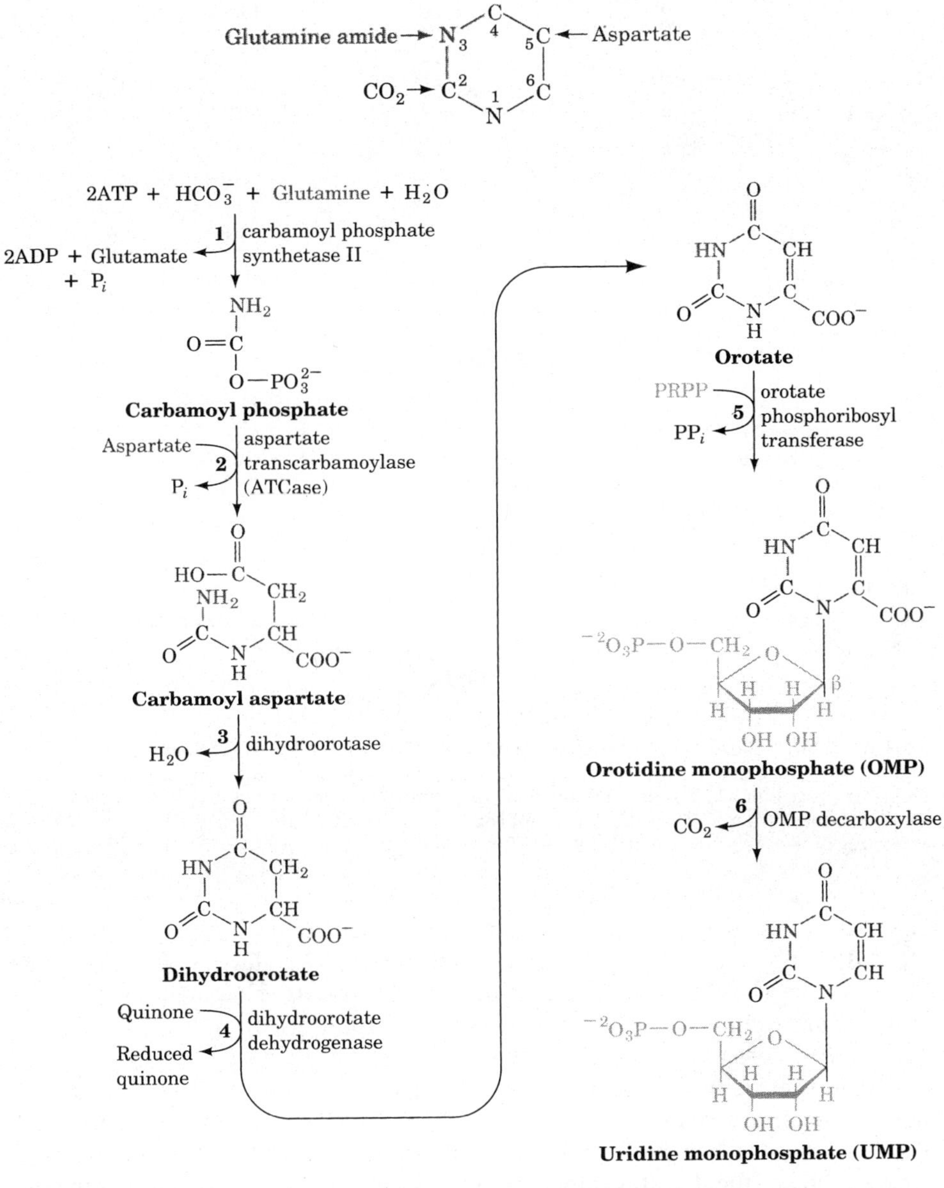

FIGURE 2.25. Biosynthesis of the pyrimidine ring in uridine monophosphate (UMP) and the origin of its atoms from *N*-carbamoylaspartate (N1, C4, C5, and C6) produced by carbamoyl phosphate and aspartate in the cytosol, in addition to N3 from glutamine amide and C2 from CO_2. The carbamoyl phosphate utilized in the urea cycle is activated in the mitochondria. There are six essential steps: (1) synthesis of carbamoyl phosphate in the cytosol via carbamoyl phosphate synthetase II; (2) synthesis of carbamoyl aspartate, the rate-determining step through the agency of a transcarbamoylase; (3) ring closure to form dihydroorotate mediated by dihydroorotase; (4) oxidation of dihydroorotate by a dehydrogenase; (5) acquisition of the ribose phosphate moiety via a transferase; and (6) decarboxylation to form UMP. Note that, in contrast to the case of purine biosynthesis (Figure 2.24), the pyrimidine ring is formed before its attachment to a ribose ring. (Courtesy of *Biochemistry*, Voet/Voet, J. Wiley & Sons.)

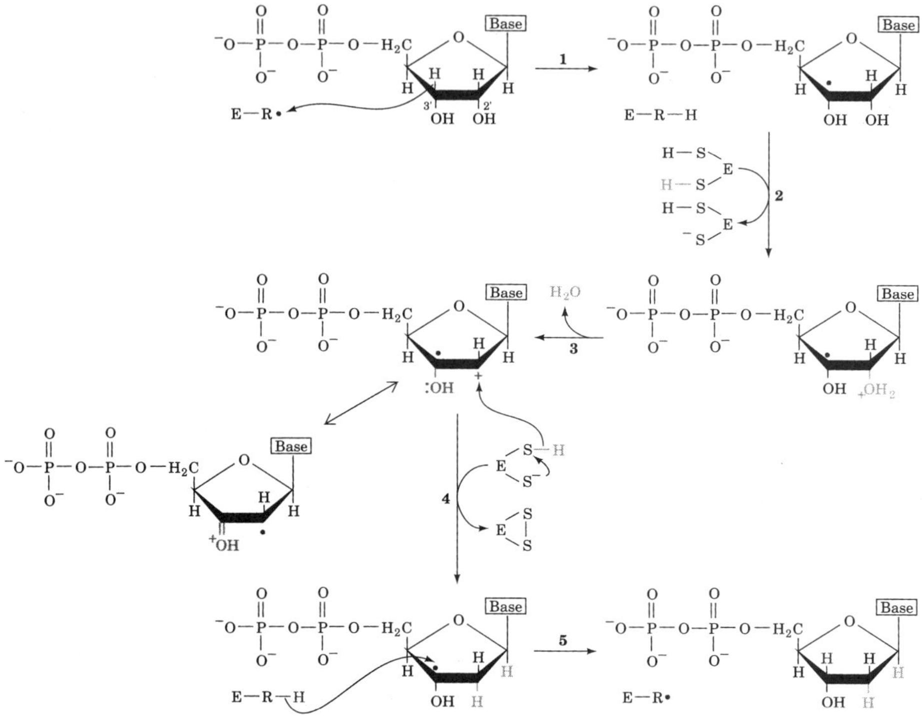

FIGURE 2.26. Biosynthesis of deoxyribonucleoside diphosphates from ribonucleoside diphosphates mediated by ribonucleotide reductase. The reaction occurs via a free radical–mediated process in which reducing equivalents are supplied by the formation of an enzyme disulfide bond. (After J. A. Stubbe, M. Ator, and T. Krenitsky, *J. Biol. Chem.* **258**: 1630, 1983.) (Courtesy of *Biochemistry*, Voet/Voet, J. Wiley & Sons.)

glycogen (glucose reservoir), pyruvate (ATP also), and ribose-5-phosphate (NADPH also); pyruvate for oxaloacetate (glycolysis/gluconeogenesis switch also), lactate (NAD^+ also), acetyl CoA (ATP, oxidation, lipid synthesis also), and alanine (amino acid synthesis and degradation also); and acetyl CoA for cholesterol, ketone bodies, carbon dioxide, and fatty acids.

Organ specificity in energy reservoirs is also apparent: the liver has approximately equal reserves of glucose and glycogen, triacylglycerols, and mobilizable proteins; muscle has predominantly mobilizable proteins but uses fatty acids when at rest; the heart prefers ketone bodies as fuel rather than glucose; adipose tissue has overwhelmingly triacylglycerol reserves; blood has little mobilizable protein; the brain has glucose as a source with ketone bodies as backup. The hormone regulators insulin (secreted from the pancreas to signal mostly the liver, muscle, and adipose tissues to store their major fuels), glucagon (secreted from the pancreas to direct mainly the liver to remedy low blood sugar), and adrenaline and noradrenaline (secreted from the adrenal medulla and sympathetic nerve endings to mobilize glycogen in the liver to break it down to glucose to export it mainly to muscle during physical activity) affect energy utilization and storage. During starvation the ketone bodies are the backup fuel in the brain, which is supplied mostly by the liver, with adipose tissue lipolysis more important than muscle-protein degradation.

DNA and RNA biosynthesis will be considered in Chapter 10.

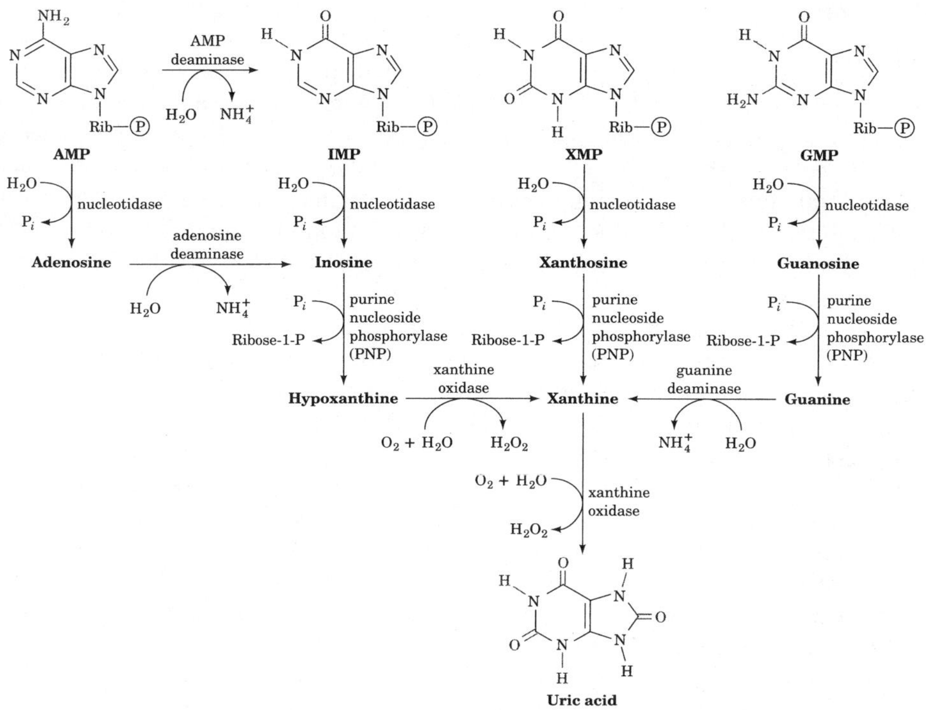

FIGURE 2.27. Degradation of purines to uric acid, which is excreted in the urine of humans. (Courtesy of *Biochemistry*, Voet/Voet, J. Wiley & Sons.)

2.13 GENERAL BODY HANDLING OF XENOBIOTICS

2.13.1 Biological Monitoring Markers and Oxidation/Reduction

Specific biological markers are often metabolites, conjugated or free, of the original exposing chemical. Some metabolites are redox products of the original compound that are not completely reduced or oxidized. The formation of metabolites allows the body to process the exposing chemical for excretion or elimination without harm. The completely oxidized products of organic chemicals are carbon dioxide, carbonate ion, and water, characteristic of aerobic (oxidation) processes. The completely reduced products of organics are methane and hydrogen, characteristic of anaerobic (oxygen-deficient) environs. For example, the stable incomplete oxidation products of methanol are formaldehyde, formic acid, formate ion, bicarbonate ion, and carbon monoxide, in order of formation.

When heteroatoms are present, their presence must also be considered. For example, for S, whose completely oxidized form is sulfur trioxide or sulfate ion, and whose completely reduced form is hydrogen sulfide or sulfide ion, stable incomplete oxidation forms include thiosulfate ion, sulfite ion, bisulfite ion, and bisulfate ion. Table 2.1 gives the various oxidation–reduction forms of different elemental combinations in organic compounds. In Table 2.1 the oxidized form has oxygen attached to the element, whereas the reduced form has hydrogen or multiple bonds. The compounds with multiple bonds are more oxidized than the analogs without them.

Most metallic elements will usually be found in their most oxidized anionic or cationic state in urine (for example, arsenates for arsenic; selenates for selenium; cations for alkali and alkaline earth metals) and the most reduced, volatile form in the breath (for example, methylated derivatives of selenium). In general, blood monitoring occurs for the original exposing chemical, as in fat analysis for hydrophobic compounds which bioaccumulate. Breath analysis is generally done for the original exposing compound if it is volatile, or for a volatile metabolite.

The stable intermediates named in Table 2.1 are called Phase I metabolic products. They are just the various stable redox states of the exposing compound subjected to oxidation and reduction and to the universe of chemical reactions noted in Section 1.11. However, these are the usual potential biological-monitoring candidate markers, as markers must be stable for measurement. In between each stable redox state are reactive intermediates that may cause local damage in the tissues and organelles where these intermediates form, or if they persist longer than they should (for example, when they are produced at such high concentrations that the detoxification systems cannot cope, or under multiexposure conditions where the cumulative effect is that the detoxification systems do not cope).

In biological systems redox reactions can occur in many organs—the chief occurring, however, in the liver, which is the major organ of detoxification. This does not mean that every organ can perform the same reactions or is equally efficient at the common processes; so knowledge of target organs and of their detoxification processes is important in biological monitoring for health effects (Chapter 5).

Most biochemical reactions are mediated by enzymes and their associated cofactors, but some processes are also nonenzymic. Increase (induction) and decrease (inhibition) of enzyme activities have been utilized as part of the medical monitoring armory, and this practice has given rise to recommended "reference ranges" for medical monitoring and medical surveillance markers (Appendix A; Chapters 7–9).

2.13.2 Phase II Reactions: Conjugations

A vital part of detoxification is an organ's ability to nullify the effect of reactive and stable intermediates by combining a specific cellular chemical to form new compounds, called conjugates, that can be more easily eliminated, processed, or excreted. These processes are called Phase II reactions, and are mediated generally by enzymes. The weakest bonds in molecules are generally those conjugated first. Thus halogen (not fluorine)–carbon sigma bonds break before carbon–carbon or carbon–hydrogen sigma bonds (Table 1.1). This is so also because the lone pairs of electrons on halogens facilitate attack, and the diffusion away of the stable leaving group (a halide ion) drives the reaction. Many types of conjugation are possible, with some backup pathways to accommodate high concentrations or multicomponent exposures. The conjugations may also compete.

Table 2.2 shows the major conjugating reactions and agents and the organic

TABLE 2.1. Oxidized and reduced stable forms of elements found for some organic elemental compositions.

Elements	Oxidized forms	Reduced forms
C	CO_2*, CO, CO_3^{2-}#	CH_4*, C, HCO_3^-#
H	H_2O_2, H_2O#, H^+	H_2*, H^-
O	O_2*, O_2^{2-}, O_2^-, O_3	H_2O#, H_2O_2, OH^-#
S	SO_3, SO_2*, SO_4^{2-}#, $S_2O_3^{2-}$, SO_3^{2-}	HSO_4^{2-}, HSO_3^-, HS^-#, S^{2-}, S, H_2S*
P	PO_4^{3-}#, P_2O_5, P_2O_3	HPO_4^{2-}, $H_2PO_4^-$#, PH_3
N	N_2O_4, N_2O_5, NO_2*, NO, N_2O, NO_3^-#, NO_2^-	N_2, NH_3*, NH_4^+#, NH_2NH_2, NH_2OH
Halogen (X)	XO_4^-, XO_3^-#, XO^-	HX*, X_2, X^-#, HOX, HXO_3, HXO_4
CS	COS*, sulfonic acids (R–OSO_2OH), sulfonates (R–OSO_2O^-)#, thiosulfonates (R–SO_2–S^-), thiolsulfonates (R_1–SO_2–S–R_2), sulfinates (R–SO_2^-), sulfone (R_1–SO_2–R_2), thiosulfate ester (R–S–SO_3^-), thiolsulfinate (R_1–SO–SR_2), sulfoxide (R_1–SO–R_2, sulfenic acid (R–SO–H)	CS_2*, thiols (RS–H)#, thioethers (R_1–S–R_2), *S*-glycoside (R–S–sugar), thiolesters (R_1–S–CO–R_2), persulfide (R–SS–H), disulfide (R_1–SS–R_2)
CN	Nitro (R–NO_2#), nitroso (R–NO), nitrones (R_1–C=(NO)–R_2), oximes (R–C=N–OH), *N*-oxides (R–C=NO), azoxy (R_1–N=(NO)–R_2), *N*-nitrosamines (R–NH–N=O)	HCN*, CN^-, ureas (NR_1R_2–CO–NR_3R_4)#, imino (R_1–HC=N–R_2), hydroxylamines (R_1–(NH)–OR_2), amines ($R_1R_2R_3N$), nitriles (R–CN), isonitriles (R–NC), urethanes (R_1–(CO)–$NHOR_2$), amides (R_1–(CO)–N–R_2R_3), azo (R_1–N=N–R_2), hydrazines (R_1R_2–N–NR_3R_4)
CH	Carboxylic acids (R–(C=O)–OH), carboxylates (R–(C=O)–O^-),# peracids (R–(C=O)–O–O–H), ketones (R_1–(C=O)–R_2), epoxides (R_1R_2–C(O)C–R_3R_4), furans (cyclic –C–O–C–), ethers (R_1–O–R_2), alcohols (R–O–H), aldehydes (R–(C=O)–H), peroxides (R_1–O–O–R_2)	Alkanes (contain sigma carbon/carbon bonds), alkenes (R_1R_2–C=C–R_3R_4), alkynes (R_1–C≡C–R_2), aromatics (cyclic, flat, alternating –C=C–), alicyclics (cyclic nonaromatic hydrocarbons)

* Major gas phase product; # major urinary product.

functional groups that are conjugated. The urinary products of glucuronidation are β-glucuronides (there are five types) and D-glucaric acid; the ultimate products of glutathione conjugation are thioethers or mercapturic acids; and the products of glucosidation are β-glucosides. Carboxylic acids are usually conjugated with an amino acid before urinary excretion. The major backup process for hydroxy- and amino- group conjugation is glucuronidation. The ultimate detoxification process for electrophiles (metals also) is glutathione conjugation. Many competing processes occur at each step in metabolism so that several products and hence biological markers are possible. The biological

TABLE 2.2. Major conjugating reactions, agents, and functional groups for conjugation of organics.

Conjugating reaction	Conjugating agent	Functional group
Acetylation	Acetyl coenzyme A	Hydroxy, amino
Amino acid conjugation	Alanine	Carboxyl
	Cysteine	Carboxyl
	Glutamic acid	Carboxyl
	Glutamine	Carboxyl
	Glycine	Carboxyl
	Ornithine	Carboxyl
	Serine	Carboxyl
	Taurine	Carboxyl
Glucosidation	Glucose	Hydroxy, thiol, carboxyl
Glucuronidation	D-Glucuronic acid	Hydroxy, carboxyl, amino, thiol
Glutathione conjugation	Glutathione (a tripeptide Glu–Cys–Gly)	Halides, epoxides, oxides, carbonium ions
Methylation (O and N)	Methyl group from 5-adenosylmethionine	Hydroxy, amino
Sulfation	Sulfate group from 3′-phosphoadenosine-5′-phosphosulfate	Hydroxy, amino

monitoring marker often chosen is the one produced in largest quantity because this allows maximum sensitivity. In some instances conjugates may be the predominant metabolites rather than the simple redox forms shown in Table 2.1. Thus conjugates may also be biological markers, for example, hippuric acid in urine for toluene.

Often it is advisable to quantitate a Phase I intermediate plus its conjugates to assess these candidates as potential markers. This allows greater sensitivity and a better correlation to the absorbed dose of the xenobiotic. This is at the cost of knowledge about the conjugate/free form ratio, which may be related to exposure concentration and the integrity of the conjugating system. Sometimes the analytical technique may automatically provide this information if alkaline or acid hydrolysis steps are a part of the analytical chemistry method. The danger is that the efficiency of these analytical chemistry steps may not be known, and interpretation of the results thus may be confounded. Partial hydrolysis of conjugates may also occur during sample transport and storage. Recovery studies with suspected conjugates must be performed to clarify these situations. This is especially important for metals and carboxylic acids.

2.13.3 Specificity of Biological Monitoring Markers

When organic xenobiotic molecules contain atoms in sigma bonds other than carbon, hydrogen, and oxygen, these atoms are often replaced by hydroxy groups through the agency of the cytochrome P-450 complex referred to in Section 2.9.

As discussed in Section 2.9, the oxygen atom in the hydroxyl group comes from molecular oxygen in the air, and not from water molecules in the surrounding tissues. The Phase I oxidation products of methyl halide (not fluorine) in the urine or blood could be:

$$CH_3{-}X \rightarrow CH_3{-}OH \rightarrow CH_2O \rightarrow H{-}(CO){-}OH \rightarrow H{-}(CO){-}OOH \\ \rightarrow HCO_3^- \rightarrow CO_3^{2-} \rightarrow HbCO_2 \rightarrow CO_2$$

where Hb signifies hemoglobin, and X is any halogen other than fluorine.

The Phase I oxidation products in the breath could be:

$$CH_3{-}X \rightarrow CH_3{-}OH \rightarrow CH_2O \rightarrow CO \rightarrow CO_2$$

or if reduction occurred:

$$CH_3{-}X \rightarrow CH_4 + HX$$

It will be observed that after the heteroatom is eliminated, the oxidation products are potentially the same as for other chemicals in the workplace. Thus urinary formate may arise from formaldehyde, formic acid, or methanol exposure, as well as from any halomethane (not fluoromethane) or C_1 compound that has a leaving group that can be easily oxidized. Urinary formate thus is a nonspecific marker. Formate, however, is more specific than carbon dioxide, carbon monoxide, carbonate ion, or bicarbonate ion. Another disadvantage of formate as a marker is that it is produced naturally by the body and so depends on the diet, on the basal metabolic rate, and on genetics. Table 2.3 lists some biological monitoring markers that have multiple sources. The advantage of such nonspecific markers is that they integrate the exposures of several exposing chemical sources by all routes of absorption—a disadvantage if a specific chemical is being investigated, but an advantage when multicomponent exposures are involved. However if there is receptor site preference for specific substrates, the integrated nature of the marker may not be observed, a characteristic of "wait-in-line" metabolism. The latter causes blood and urine concentrations of the chemicals waiting to be processed to be higher, compared with exposure situations where the more preferred substrate is not present.

For biological monitoring markers also produced endogenously, the contribution of the body can be found by taking a sample of biological medium before exposure under the same conditions as the sample after exposure and subtracting the amount of marker in this baseline sample from the amount of marker found after exposure. This assumes that no perturbation in baseline occurs in the sample taken after exposure except that caused by the exposure itself. Baseline sampling is an essential part of the validation of the practicability of any biological marker and also can be used to correct for unexpected exposures. Exposures due to life-style, medication usage, diet, and individual genetic variations from person to person can be detected and allowed for by baseline sampling.

Halogenated (not fluorine) compounds such as halomethanes will also undergo Phase II processes at the same time that Phase I processes are occurring. Thus reaction of glutathione with these compounds is likely (Table 2.2). Hydroxylated Phase I intermediates may also be acetylated, glucosidated,

TABLE 2.3. Some urinary biological markers with multiple sources.

Marker	Source
Acetate	Acetaldehyde, ethanol, substituted ethanes
p-Aminophenol	Acetanilide, aniline, Carbetamide, dimethylaniline, Fenuron, hydrazobenzene, *p*-nitroaniline, nitrobenzene, *p*-nitrophenol, phenazopyridine, phenacetin, *p*-phenetidine, Propham, Siduron, *p*-toluidine
Carboxyhemoglobin	Carbon monoxide, dihalomethane (not fluorine)
Haloacetic acid	1,2-Dihaloethane, haloacetaldehyde, haloethanol, haloethylenes
Formate	Formaldehyde, ethanol, substituted methanes
Hippuric acid	*n*-Alkylbenzenes, *n*-haloalkylbenzenes and *n*-carboxylic acid benzenes with an odd number of carbon atoms, benzoic acid, benzyl halides (not fluorine), ethylbenzene, quinic acid, sodium benzoate, styrene, toluene
Mandelic acid	Ethyl benzene, α-phenylaminoacetic acids, phenyl glycol, styrene, styrene glycol, styrene oxide
p-Nitrophenol	EPN, methylparathion, nitrobenzene, *p*-nitrophenol, parathion
Oxalic acid	Disubstituted ethanes, ethylene glycol, glyoxal
Phenol	Benzene, phenol, phenylsalicylate, sodium phenolate
Thiodiacetic acid	*S*-Carboxy-L-cysteine, *bis*-(2-chloroethyl) ether, 1,2-dihaloethane (not fluorine), 1,1,2-trihaloethane (not fluorine), vinyl chloride
2-Thiazolidine-4-carboxylic acid	Captan, carbon disulfide, Disulfiram, Thiram, formaldehyde
Trihaloacetic acid (not fluorine)	Methyl haloform, perhaloethylene, 1,1,1,2-tetrahaloethane, 1,1,2,2-tetrahaloethane, tetrahaloethylenes, trihaloacetaldehyde, 1,1,1-trihaloethane, trihaloethylene
Trihaloethanol (not fluorine)	Methyl haloform, perhaloethylene, 1,1,1,2-tetrahaloethane, 1,1,2,2-tetrahaloethane, tetrahaloethylenes, trihaloacetaldehyde, 1,1,1-trihaloethane, trihaloethylenes

glucuronidated, *O*- or *N*-methylated, or sulfated (Table 2.2). Phase I intermediates with carboxylic acid groups may also be conjugated with amino acids (eight possibilities), glucosidated, or glucuronidated (Table 2.2).

Nonaromatic aliphatic compounds with two or more carbon atoms or side chains of greater than two carbon atoms on aromatic compounds may act as carbon sources through β-oxidation of long chains (Section 2.6) or through fatty acid biosynthesis (Section 2.7) after any heteroatoms have been oxidized or reduced through Phase I processes and a carboxylic acid moiety has formed at a terminal carbon. This may mean that a definite threshold for adverse effects of the exposing compound may be related to the target organ's ability to use metabolites as carbon sources or in other biochemical pathways. Beta-oxidation for aromatic side chains stops at the benzylic carbon atom so that *n*-propylbenzene has the same biological monitoring markers as toluene, and *n*-butylbenzene has the same biological monitoring markers as ethylbenzene. Such markers are clearly nonspecific, and interpretation of their levels requires a knowledge of the exposing chemicals, their quantities, and the time/duration of exposures.

In analogy to the halomethanes, Phase I intermediates of monohaloethanes (not fluorine) are:

$$CH_3{-}CH_2{-}X \rightarrow CH_3{-}CH_2{-}OH \rightarrow CH_3{-}CHO \rightarrow CH_3{-}COOH$$

Acetaldehyde can be formed from pyruvate in yeast and other microorganisms, and acetaldehyde is also reduced to ethanol in the mammalian liver by alcohol dehydrogenase, which requires NADH and a proton pump. Ethanol can be breathed out or subjected to Phase II conjugation.

Ethanes substituted with one or more halogens on the second carbon atom will produce halosubstituted alcohols, aldehydes, and carboxylic acids as Phase I products, all of which are subject to reaction with glutathione and the Phase II processes experienced by the monohaloethanes. Ethylene glycol is another possible Phase I product formed from the monohaloethanol, as is oxalic acid; the intermediate mixed aldehydes are very reactive. The haloacetaldehyde may also produce $CHO{-}CH_2{-}OH$ as a Phase I product. Oxalic acid can be produced through four Phase I pathways.

$$X{-}CH_2{-}CH_2{-}X \rightarrow X{-}CH_2{-}CH_2{-}OH \rightarrow X{-}CH_2{-}CHO \rightarrow X{-}CH_2{-}COOH$$

$$X{-}CH_2{-}CH_2{-}OH \rightarrow HO{-}CH_2{-}CH_2{-}OH \rightarrow CHO{-}CH_2{-}OH \rightarrow CHO{-}CHO \rightarrow HOOC{-}CHO \rightarrow HOOC{-}COOH$$

$$X{-}CH_2{-}CHO \rightarrow HO{-}CH_2{-}CHO \text{ and so on}$$

$$X{-}CH_2{-}COOH \rightarrow HO{-}CH_2{-}COOH \rightarrow CHO{-}COOH \text{ and so on}$$

$$CHO{-}CH_2{-}OH \rightarrow COOH{-}CH_2{-}OH \text{ and so on}$$

Oxalic acid crystals which deposit in the kidney severely damage that organ, and many deaths have occurred through this mechanism when ethylene glycol (the major ingredient of permanent-type automobile antifreeze) has been ingested. Excess ethanol (intoxicating dose) inhibits this oxidation in a competitive manner in the same way that ethanol is used to counteract methanol (wood alcohol) or propanol (rubbing alcohol) poisoning.

Even for these comparatively simple molecules, there are many possible Phase I pathways and hence also Phase II processes. It can be seen that metabolism is a set of concurrent, sequential, and competitive processes. Which of the possibilities dominate often depends on where the original receptor site is located, the target organs, the exposing chemical, and which conjugation systems are present near the receptor site. It can be understood then that many potential biological markers may be produced from exposure to a single chemical or physical agent. Thus it is very unlikely that one mole of biological marker will be produced in the urine after absorption of one mole of compound.

Similarly, not all of a compound that is absorbed will be exhaled in the breath or will be found in the blood. The biological marker of choice must be of high molar yield relative to the exposing compound to ensure sensitivity, and must exhibit a dose effect over the exposure range of interest.

Sometimes at high concentrations of exposing chemical, another biological marker may have to be chosen if the low-concentration pathway saturates (a "capacity-limited process"). Thus the sulfate conjugate of phenol is the appropriate biological marker excreted in the urine after the glucuronide pathway becomes saturated at high exposures of air benzene. The glucuronide conjugation pathway is the usual overflow pathway for neutral hydroxylated species because tissue glycogen is a huge glucose source that can be utilized to produce β-glucuronic acid for Phase II conjugation purposes. However, phenol is acidic enough to be glucuronidated before it is sulfated.

In contrast to a biological monitoring marker, a biological marker of adverse health effect may be in a very minor pathway, but one that is responsible for the adverse health effect. Thus for investigators to be able to identify a biological marker of adverse health effect, the mechanism leading to the adverse effect must be known. Although a dose effect is expected, there may be a critical threshold dose above which the health effect is elicited. This may be so in the case of damage after saturation of low-concentration detoxification systems. On the other hand, the appearance of cadmium in the urine implies kidney damage and is automatically a biological marker of adverse health effect as well as a biological monitoring marker of exposure.

Xenobiotic molecules or derivative metabolites can react covalently with blood proteins and cellular DNA to produce modified macromolecules called adducts (Chapters 10 to 12). Not all adducts are related to an adverse health effect; only if the particular adduct is in the pathway to adverse effects is the marker one for adverse health effects. Thus a specific DNA adduct may be the crucial marker adduct for a particular cancer, but this adduct may not be the major one produced.

If it is known that an adverse effect occurs above a critical concentration of an exposing chemical, then an equivalent concentration of a biological marker that is not necessarily on the pathway to toxic effects can be selected to be a surrogate marker for adverse health effect. This is the situation (Chapter 21) for most biological limit values (BLVs) or biological exposure indices (BEIs).

Most of the BEIs recommended by the American Conference of Governmental Industrial Hygienists are of this category, as are similar recommendations in countries other than the United States. This procedure takes advantage of the sensitivity of the selected biological monitoring marker. It must be remembered, however, that this marker may not be related to the pathway responsible for the adverse health effect.

2.13.4 General Remarks on Metals and Their Markers

After absorption as ions, metals are transported as organic chelates in the bloodstream, carried across cell membranes as different organic chelates, and stored as other distinct organic chelates. Anions and cations may also have zwitterionic amino acids as carriers.

Phase II processes generally occur to cations that act as typical electrophiles by being detoxified by glutathione. Methylation and acetylation may also occur. For example, selenium and tellurium can be exhaled as methylated derivatives, and elemental mercury can be exhaled after absorption of mercury compounds. Redox states are important. For example, iron in ionic form is absorbed through the gastrointestinal tract only as Fe^{2+}. It is transported in the blood by transferrin (a β-globulin) in the Fe(III) form, and is stored in tissues as ferritin in the Fe(III) form and also as hemosiderin in the Fe(II) form. The redox cycling of iron in the cytochrome chain is absolutely essential.

The Fe(II) state is maintained in hemoglobin, deoxymyoglobin, and oxymyoglobin. The Fe(III) state is attained in ferrimyoglobin and methemoglobin.

Metal chelates are formed through coordinate links that do not affect the oxidation state. Because specific geometries are conferred by these links and bulky organic groups can add more uniqueness, a specific geometry can be created that is ideal for the exacting stereochemical requirements of the active sites of enzymes to recognize substrates. It is no wonder that many enzymes have a metal at active sites (for example, zinc for dehydrogenases) or metal cofactors to facilitate quick reactions (for example, magnesium ions for synthetase enzymic reactions which require ATP).

The excreted form in the urine is generally the most oxidized one (for example, selenate for selenium, arsenate for arsenic, and mercurates for mercury). Most toxic metals found in the blood are chelated by an organic ligand (for example, transferrin for iron). Lead, manganese, and cadmium are mostly bound in the red blood cells. Cadmium is transported by metallothionen. Manganese is transported in blood serum by a β-globulin, and some appears to be transported by transferrin as well.

Because analytical chemistry quantitation methods often employ digestions with nitric or nitric–perchloric acids, all metal speciation is forced to the most oxidized form. Thus total metal is generally reported unless specific forms are chromatographed. Analytical artifacts may mask a very complex metal speciation scheme even in the urine. Elements of long half-times such as lead and cadmium may accumulate in the bone or fat.

Further Reading

Stryer, L. 1988. *Biochemistry*, 3rd ed., W. H. Freeman, New York.

Tietz, N. W. (ed.) 1986. *Textbook of Clinical Chemistry*, W. B. Saunders, Philadelphia, PA.

Voet, D., and Voet, J. G. 1990. *Biochemistry*, John Wiley and Sons, New York.

PART 2

Routes of Exposure, Distribution, Metabolism, and Biological Monitoring Media

Chapters 3 through 6 are concerned with xenobiotic routes of exposure, absorption, distribution and redistribution, metabolism, and the media utilized for measurement of biological monitoring markers. The xenobiotic on absorption will be transported by the blood to organs and tissues to become a nutrient source and/or to be oxidized, reduced, conjugated, and excreted. The major advantage to biological monitoring as a technique is that marker concentration reflects absorption from all exposure routes, be they the lung after inhalation, the gastrointestinal tract after oral exposure, or the skin after dermal contact. The efficiency of absorption by each route also varies. The interpretation of the concentration of any marker depends on the xenobiotic, exposure routes, kinetics, and mechanisms involved. Complex interactions among the biochemical processes important in handling xenobiotics may result when multicomponent xenobiotic exposures, physical agents, and dietary and life-style factors simultaneously change. The relationships obtained on exposure to one chemical may not be valid when multicomponent exposures and other perturbing parameters are also present.

Ideally, the concentration of a biological monitoring marker should be related to the total exposure dose of the xenobiotic or physical agent by all routes, be noninvasive (i.e., no sampling of internal body fluids or tissues), be specific, and be of high sensitivity to make measurement easy. Moreover, the analysis should be inexpensive. Needless to say, no marker meets all these criteria.

The Biological Exposure Indices (BEI) Committee of the American Conference of Governmental Industrial Hygienists (ACGIH) has proposed that a biological monitoring marker is adequate for inhalation if the amount absorbed by other routes does not exceed 30% of the inhalation uptake, or if the arterial blood concentration is not similarly exceeded under TLV-TWA conditions for an 8-hour (h) day. By extension, the adequacy of markers for skin absorption and ingestion can be similarly defined for workers.

A 24-h critical value for each route can also be derived, assuming an equivalent risk assessment model, by dividing any recommended BEI or similar value by 4.2 $[(24 \times 7)/(8 \times 5)]$. However, the toxicology of continual 24-h exposures is different from that for intermittent exposures 8 h/day for 5 days/week. The toxic effects of exposures for 8 h/day for 5 days/week are mitigated by the weekend and overnight recovery periods, especially for agents with body residence half-times between 12 h and 3 days. Contributions from all exposure routes need also to be factored in as appropriate.

The references for Chapters 3 through 6 are located at the end of Chapter 6.

3

Exposure Routes

3.0 INHALATION

3.0.1 Gases and Vapors

Inhalation via the lung is important for a gas (the whole physical form of the chemical at 25°C and 760 mm Hg pressure) or vapor (the gaseous form of a chemical whose major physical form is not a gas at 25°C and 760 mm Hg). Thus while aliphatic chemicals from methane to *n*-butane are gases at 25°C and 760 mm Hg pressure, the term "vapor" is reserved for the gaseous state for chemicals whose predominant physical form for one mole of compound is a liquid or solid at 25°C and 760 mm Hg pressure, as, for example, benzene and naphthalene, respectively.

Most gases and vapors of less than 20 mm Hg pressure obey the ideal gas law (equation 3.1):

$$pV = \frac{mRT}{M} = nRT \tag{3.1}$$

where:

p = partial or vapor pressure of the chemical (Table 3.1)
V = volume of pure gas/vapor
m = mass of the vapor/gas in grams
T = absolute temperature in degrees Kelvin (°C plus 273.15)
M = molecular weight of the compound in the gas or vapor state in grams based on a scale where 1 mole of carbon-12 has a mass of 12 g exactly (Table 3.1)
n = number of moles of compound and is equal to m/M

The units of R, the gas constant, depend on the units used for p and V. The most common values used are 0.08205 liter-atmosphere per degree Kelvin per

TABLE 3.1. Some physical parameters of interest for selected organics relative to biological monitoring.

Chemical	M	log K_{ow}	s	K_{ba}	P	K_{fa}
Aniline	93.1	0.90	34		0.3	
Benzene	78.1	2.13	0.83	7.8	80.0	425
Carbon disulfide	76.1	2.00	2.94	2.2	300.0	
Chlorobenzene	112.6	2.46	0.50		8.8	
Dimethylacetamide	87.1	−0.77	943.00		1.3	
Dimethylformamide	73.1	−1.01	944.00		2.6	
Ethyl benzene	106.2	3.15	0.20	30.0	10.0	
Furfural	96.1	0.99	83.0		1.0	
n-Hexane	86.2	3.94	0.014	0.8–2.3	151.0	130–159
Methanol	32.0	−0.77	791.00	1625.0	92.0	231.0
Methyl chloroform	133.4	2.49	0.30	3.0	100	250.0
Methyl ethyl ketone	72.1	0.28	353.00	125.0	100	162.0
Nitrobenzene	123.1	1.85	1.9		1.0	
Parathion	291.3	3.81	0.024		3.8×10^{-5}	
Pentachlorophenol	266.4	5.01	0.0008		0.0001	
Perchloroethylene	165.8	2.60	0.40	9–15	19.0	10^3–2×10^3
Phenol	94.1	1.48	67.0		0.35	
Styrene	104.0	2.95	0.30	55.0	5.0	
Toluene	92.1	2.69	0.60	11–16	22.0	962
Trichloroethylene	131.5	2.29	1.10	9.5	60.0	600
Xylenes	106.2	3.14	0.18	26–38	8.3	3600
-ortho	106.2		0.175		5.0	
-meta	106.2	3.20			6.0	
para	106.2	3.15	0.198		6.5	

M is the molecular weight; log K_{ow} is the logarithm to base 10 of the octanol/water coefficient defined by equation (3.12); s is the solubility in water at 25°C in mg/mL; K_{ba} is the blood/air partition coefficient at 37°C; P is the vapor pressure at 20°C in torr; K_{fa} is the fat/air partition coefficient at 37°C.

The data for M, log K_{ow}, P, K_{ba}, K_{fa}, and s are from reference 8, apart for the data for the xylene isomers which are from reference 7.

Note that $K_{fb} = 70.9 \log K_{ow} - 127.0$ for brominated and chlorinated hydrocarbons and unsubstituted hydrocarbons where K_{fb} is the fat/blood partition coefficient [9].

gram-mole (L-atm K^{-1} g-mole^{-1}); 82.05 cubic centimeter-atmosphere per degree Kelvin per gram-mole (cm^3-atm K^{-1} g-mole^{-1}); 8.314 joule per degree Kelvin per gram-mole (J K^{-1} g-mole^{-1}); 8.314×10^7 erg per degree Kelvin per gram-mole (erg K^{-1} g-mole^{-1}); 1.987 calorie per degree Kelvin per gram-mole (cal K^{-1} g-mole^{-1}); 62,360 cubic centimeter-mm Hg per degree Kelvin per gram-mole (cm^3-mm Hg K^{-1} g-mole^{-1}).

Physically, the molecules of an ideal gas are defined as points having position and translational energy but no volume. No intermolecular forces are postulated to exist.

Suppose the concentration of carbon tetrachloride at 25°C and 760 mm Hg atmospheric pressure is required at its Threshold Limit Value–Time Weighted Average (TLV-TWA) value of 5 parts per million (ppm) as recommended by the ACGIH. The definition of 1 ppm (volume/volume) as 1 microliter (μL) of pure vapor of the chemical per liter of air mixture is the starting point. Thus 5 ppm means 5 μL of carbon tetrachloride vapor per liter of air mixture.

The next question is what volume does 1 mole of pure carbon tetrachloride vapor occupy at 25°C and 760 mm Hg? The pressure in mm Hg must be divided by 760 mm Hg to obtain p in atmospheres so as to use the R value in L atm^{-1} K^{-1} g-mole^{-1}.

Rearranging equation (3.1), we have:

$$\begin{aligned} V &= \frac{nRT}{p} \\ &= \frac{1 \times 0.08205 \times 298.15}{1} \\ &= 24.46\,\text{L} \end{aligned}$$

Thus if 1 mole (153.84 g) of carbon tetrachloride vapor occupies 24.46 L at 25°C and 760 mm Hg atmospheric pressure, what weight corresponds to 5 μL of carbon tetrachloride vapor?

$$\begin{aligned} \text{Weight of } 5\,\mu\text{L of } CCl_4 \text{ vapor} &= \frac{153.84 \times 5 \times 10^{-6}}{24.46} \\ &= 31.45\,\mu\text{g} \end{aligned}$$

This weight of carbon tetrachloride is contained in, and is spread evenly through, one liter of air. Therefore the concentration of carbon tetrachloride is 31.45 μg/L or 31.45 mg/m^3. This agrees with the 31 mg/m^3 given by ACGIH. Note that the conversion depends on the assumption of an ideal gas; that is, one mole of any ideal gas occupies 24.46 L at 25°C and 760 mm Hg.

It is instructive to determine what air concentration corresponds to 20 mm Hg at 25°C, the approximate upper pressure limit for most gases to act ideally. Rearranging equation (3.1) gives:

$$\begin{aligned} \frac{m}{V} &= \frac{pM}{RT} = \text{air concentration} \\ &= \frac{20 \times 153.84}{0.08205 \times 298.15 \times 760} \\ &= 0.166\,\text{g/L} = 166\,\text{g/m}^3 \end{aligned} \tag{3.2}$$

This concentration is 166,000/31 = 5354 times greater than the TLV-TWA. Nearly all gases and vapors at their TLV-TWA concentrations will act like ideal gases. This may not be so for explosive or inflammable concentrations, which are commonly above 1% (v/v) in concentration. Most inhalation LC_{50} values (the concentration that kills half the animals) are low enough that ideal gas behavior occurs during inhalation exposures in toxicology experiments.

If a man at rest breathes in 10 m^3 of air per 8-h workday (the approximate volume for a sedentary man), then at the TLV-TWA of carbon tetrachloride he would breathe in 31.45 × 10 = 314.5 mg per 8-h working day. Assuming this was all absorbed, then 314.5 mg is the mass that the blood has carried and which must be detoxified, or excreted. In practice a fraction will be breathed out. If metabolism occurs, the maximum moles of marker that can be excreted is:

$$\frac{314.5}{153.84} = 2.04 \text{ millimoles.}$$

If ideal gas behavior is not followed, the relationship that has been most used to describe a nonideal gas, the Van der Waals equation of state, can be used:

$$\left[p + \frac{n^2a}{V^2}\right][V - nb] = nRT \tag{3.3}$$

where p, V, n, R, and T are defined as in equation (3.1), a is a molecular characteristic for each gas/vapor related to the intermolecular forces, and b is a molecular characteristic that corrects for the finite volume of real gas/vapor molecules.

Therefore for 1 mole of carbon tetrachloride vapor at 1 atm and 25°C, what is V, the molar volume, using the Van der Waals equation of state?

Rearranging equation (3.3), we obtain:

$$pV - pnb + \frac{n^2a}{V} - \frac{n^3ab}{V^2} = nRT$$

Multiplying by V^2/p gives:

$$V^3 - nbV^2 + \frac{n^2aV}{p} - \frac{n^3ab}{p} = \frac{nRTV^2}{p}$$

$$V^3 - \left[nb + \frac{nRT}{p}\right]V^2 + \left[\frac{n^2a}{p}\right]V - \frac{n^3ab}{p} = 0 \tag{3.4}$$

Substituting for $n = 1$, we have $p = 1\,\text{atm}$; $R = 0.08205\,\text{L atm}^{-1}\,\text{K}^{-1}\,\text{mole}^{-1}$; $T = 298.15\,\text{K}$; $a = 20.39\,\text{atm-L}^{-2}\,\text{mole}^{-1}$; and $b = 0.1383\,\text{L mole}^{-1}$; thus:

$$V^3 - (0.1383 + [0.08205 \times 298.15])V^2 + 20.39V - [0.1383 \times 20.39] = 0$$

$$V^3 - 24.60V^2 + 20.39V - 2.82 = 0 \tag{3.5}$$

This equation can be solved iteratively to produce a V of approximately 23.75 L. The ideal gas treatment yielded 24.46 L. The absolute error for the latter is +0.71 L or a relative error of +3.0%. This is an acceptable error for the ideal gas treatment for carbon tetrachloride, but may not be so for other compounds or at higher p.

In practice, not all of a gas or vapor inhaled is ever absorbed. Some will be breathed out, especially if the blood/air partition coefficient is low. Some of the gases and vapors may be depleted if they are reactive, as for oxidant gases such as ozone and nitrogen dioxide or for reactive gases such as formaldehyde. Most organic solvent molecules are chemically inert.

Astrand et al. [1] showed that the 30-min uptake over a total exposure period of 2 h of such inert organic solvents as methylene chloride, trichloroethylene, aliphatic white spirit, aromatic white spirit, styrene, xylenes, and toluene obeyed equation (3.6):

TABLE 3.2. Influence of physical activity on some physiological parameters [8].

Physical workload (W)	Oxygen demand (L/min)	Alveolar ventilation (L air/min)	Heart pump rate (L/min)	Perfusion (L blood/min) Muscles	Liver	Brain
0	0.3	5.0	6.0	1.0	1.5	0.6
50	0.8	16.0	9.0	3.6	1.3	0.7
100	1.3	27.0	13.0	7.9	1.2	0.7
150	1.8	38.0	19.0	13.0	1.1	0.7

$$\%\ \text{uptake} = -86 \times \text{alveolar air concentration 20 to 30 min after exposure/inspired air concentration} + 79.3 \quad (3.6)$$

The correlation coefficient was −0.949 for 60 male subjects. Butyl alcohol did not obey this general relationship.

For xylene [mixture of *o*-, *m*-, and *p*-xylenes (8.8, 49.4, 1.4%, respectively) plus ethylbenzene (40.4%)], exposures of 200 ppm for 30 min over 2 h of total exposure at rest or for 90 min during light exercise on a bicycle ergometer [up to 50 watts (W) and corresponding [8] to a pulmonary ventilation of about 25 L/min (Table 3.2)], caused about 63% of inspired xylene to be absorbed [1]. The alveolar air concentration at 30–40 min after the beginning of exposure was 15% of the inspired concentration at rest. As the work load increased, % uptake decreased (but absolute uptake increased); for example, 50% at 55 *L*/min (150 W). The percent of alveolar air concentration measured 30–40 min after exposure relative to inspired air for at rest, for light exercise (50 W), and for heavy work (150 W) were 15, 20, and 30%, respectively. The absorption of benzene by inhalation was gender-dependent, males absorbing 20.3% and females, 41.6%; however, no correction was made for physical activity.

A commonly used marker of physiological capacity is the maximal oxygen uptake (VO_2 max) during physical work at sea level. Most of these values come from bicycle ergometer, step-test, or treadmill experiments. For lifting tasks for a 36.36 kg weight from 0 to 60 cm, the VO_2 max values found directly were about 54 to 80% of the values obtained from a bicycle ergometer experiment on the same persons [2]. For lifting a box 38.1 cm square and 25.4 cm deep equipped with side handles for loads varying from 6.82 to 40.91 kg from 0 to 76.2 cm (floor to knuckle), from 0 to 127 cm (floor to shoulder height), and from 76.2 to 127 cm, the VO_2 values plateaued consistently after 5 lifts/min and VO_2 values were again 57 to 91% of bicycle ergometer-derived values [3]. The lifting frequency was recommended to never exceed 10 lifts/min. Thus each type of job activity must be investigated individually to find human capacities. The maximal intake of xenobiotics would be presumably modeled by VO_2 max data because the maximum capacity for work is dependent on VO_2 max.

Because only a double membrane separates the bloodstream from the alveolar air spaces, transport into the blood is very efficient as long as the blood/air partition coefficient for the compound in blood is high (Table 3.1). For *m*-xylene this partition coefficient is 29 from *in vitro* experiments [4]. Nonchlorinated organic solvents generally have greater solubility in tissues than in blood, and so this also drives the tissue uptake process, as does fast metabolism. Blood saturation can occur at very high air concentrations but generally not for TLV-TWA conditions. Chlorinated solvents appear to have low solubility in tissues. The fat depots become important in removal of potentially dangerous chlorinated species from the blood, and in producing slow release of the stored xenobiotic to allow detoxification systems to cope. Gases such as sulfur dioxide and formaldehyde that are extremely soluble in the mucous linings of the upper airways are solubilized predominantly in the nose and upper airways, so creating a lower concentration in alveolar air than at the nose entrance. Gases of low solubility such as nitrogen dioxide and ozone affect the airways rather evenly along their entire length, but the concentration in alveoli air is still lower than at the nose entrance. Inert gases and vapors (hydrocarbon vapors, carbon monoxide, and nitrogen) will have similar alveolar air concentrations to those found at the entrance to the nose.

Solvents that are absorbed into the bloodstream can also be exhaled. For example, xylene is between 4 and 5% exhaled after 2 h once it is absorbed at TLV-TWA concentrations [1]. Exhalation is a more important elimination path for inert hydrocarbons with higher vapor pressures than xylene, such as toluene or benzene (Table 3.1).

The lung is a gas-exchanging organ consisting of two lobes opening to the trachea, which is connected to the pharnyx. The lung facilitates the uptake of air gases via the arterial route and the exhalation of excess carbon dioxide and other gaseous products of metabolism via the venous route. The gas-exchanging surface is comprised of blood capillaries overlain by a very thin single cell layer with an effective surface of about $70\,m^2$. Blood is brought to this membrane via the pulmonary arteries and conducted away via the pulmonary veins. A second major system of gas exchange, the bronchial system, conducts air to and from the gas phase contained in the alveoli, whose thin walls contain capillaries. The heart pumps blood through the system, and muscles connected to the flexible rib cage move the chest bellows in the breathing process.

In quiet breathing, a healthy human inspires and expires about 500 mL (tidal volume) about 15 times per minute, or about $11\,m^3$ daily or $3.6\,m^3$ per 8-h workday. Of the tidal volume only about 350 mL actually ventilates the alveoli for direct gas/vapor exchange, the rest being anatomical dead space. Sometimes the latter space is increased by the volume in contact with unperfused alveoli and the volume in excess required to saturate blood with oxygen; it is then called physiological dead space. The inspired air is then mixed with alveolar air ("mixed air"), which is about 2 L during normal breathing.

3.0.2 Aerosols and Alveolar Deposition

Aerosols (liquid or solid) of particle size less than 10 μm in aerodynamic diameter deposit in the alveoli of the deep lung. The formal definition of aerodynamic diameter (D_a) is: the diameter of a smooth sphere of unit density (that is, $1\,g/cm^3$) that has the same terminal velocity as the particle itself. The terminal velocity of a spherical particle falling freely in air is approximately 0.003 particle density times the square of the particle diameter in micrometers.

Originally, particle size was defined in terms of what was observed under a microscope with the aid of a micrometer scale. The term "diameter" implies a circle or a sphere. Thus in the definition for aerodynamic diameter, the shape of the aerosol particle is expressed as a sphere equivalent in volume to that of the actual particle itself after correction for density. The terminal velocity is the maximum velocity at which this sphere can travel after being released in stagnant air from rest. The velocity is the result of a steady state attained between gravitational forces and forces caused by the aerodynamic resistance of air. This velocity is therefore dependent on particle density (d), which is the total mass divided by the equivalent spherical volume. Hence, a lead fume (solid aerosol produced from a vapor) has a larger terminal velocity than a cotton dust (an aerosol produced from aerial dispersion of a solid). Other factors that influence terminal velocity of an aerosol particle are shape and size.

The general expression for D_a is:

$$D_a = \left(\frac{d \times C_p}{d_0 \times C_a}\right)^{0.5} \times D_p \tag{3.7}$$

where: d is particle density; d_0 is $1\,\text{g/cm}^3$; C_p and C_a are Cunningham slip factors for particle diameters D_p and D_a, respectively; and D_p is the diameter for spherical particles or the Stokes diameter for nonspherical particles (the diameter of a sphere, called a Stokes sphere, that has the same density and terminal velocity as the particle).

Slip factors account for the reduction of drag force on particles through the resistance caused by air molecules, and are important for particles smaller than $5\,\mu\text{m}$ in diameter. C_p is a function of the ratio between the particle diameter and the mean free path of the air:

$$C_p = 1 + \frac{f_p}{D_p}\left[2.514 + 0.8\exp\left(-0.55\frac{D_p}{f_p}\right)\right] \tag{3.8}$$

where f_p is the mean free path of the air, the average distance between collisions of air molecules:

$$f_p = \left[2^{0.5} \times \frac{22}{7} \times {d_m}^2 \times n\right]^{-1} = \frac{1.88 v_g}{v_d\left(\frac{RT}{M}\right)^{0.5}} \tag{3.9}$$

where d_m is the average gas molecular diameter, n is the number of molecules per cubic centimeter, v_g is the gas viscosity, and v_d is the vapor density of the gas.

At 20°C and 1 atm pressure in air, $f_p = 0.066\,\mu\text{m}$. For particles greater than D_p of 5 to $50\,\mu\text{m}$, $C_p = 1$; C_p is greater than 1 for D_p of less than $5\,\mu\text{m}$. For particle diameters much greater than f_p, equation (3.7) is approximated by:

$$D_a = \left(\frac{d}{d_0}\right)^{0.5} D_p \tag{3.10}$$

Equation (3.10) is also often used for particle diameters down to 0.5 μm when d is close to 1 g/cm^3.

When diameters are much smaller than f_p, the following equation holds:

$$D_a = \frac{d}{d_0} D_p \tag{3.11}$$

For an aerosol of particles of a pure liquid (a mist), the mass of one particle is equal to the particle equivalent volume times liquid density. For several nonreacting components in the liquid or solid particle (an "inert" aerosol particle), the total particle mass is the sum of the masses of the individual components. The particle density is largely determined by the predominant contributors to particle mass. In practice, the concept only works for particles not too far different from spheres.

A solid particle whose length is at least three times greater than its cross-sectional diameter is called a fiber (as for asbestos), and aerodynamic diameter is not a workable concept for such a particle. Lengths between the cross-sectional diameter and three times this diameter define a solid particle called a whisker.

Most aerosols do not consist of particles of identical size; they are polydisperse rather than monodisperse. In fact, a plot of number versus aerodynamic diameter is usually distributed in a lognormal manner (defined by a geometric mean and a geometric standard deviation), though multimodal distributions (defined through their modes and individual standard deviations) also occur. The total mass potentially deposited in the alveoli is calculated by finding the area under such curves for diameters below 10 μm after adjustment for material density.

3.0.3 Aerosols and Airways Deposition

Particles of aerodynamic diameter greater than 20 μm deposit in the turbulent airflow regions of the nose and upper respiratory tract (nasopharyngeal region, the trachea, and the lung bronchi). Smaller particles, from 20 to 0.5 μm, deposit in the smaller airways and alveoli. The ACGIH defines its "respirable" dust sampling upper aerodynamic diameter cut-off as 10 μm. Particles between 0.1 and 0.5 μm are mostly exhaled because their low terminal velocity does not allow enough time for deposition. The particles below 0.1 μm have many collisions and hence Brownian energy, which enables ready deposition in the alveoli. These deposition patterns also apply for clumps of small particles stuck together (agglomerations), which in extreme cases form clouds, as, for example, mainstream tobacco smoke.

The particle frequency versus diameter distributions measured outside the body may not be related to the particle size distribution. This is so because of effects of humidity, the higher body temperature, chemical reactions, agglomeration, and airways "wall effects." The effects of humidity are very important for deliquescent materials, and chemical reactions deplete oxidant gas concentrations of alveolar air relative to nasal concentrations of oxidants. Physical activity also plays a role because uptake is generally faster and more efficient at conditions of high physical activity than when one is sedentary.

Particles deposited in the nose and the upper respiratory tract are transported to the pharynx by the ciliary locomotor flow (the longest time for transport is about 30 min unless the flow is impaired), and then ingested through the gastrointestinal tract. The surface cells of the airways are protected from desiccation by a thin layer of aqueous fluid. A more viscous fluid is present in the upper respiratory tract down to the 15th or 16th generation of airway branching. A thinner film, replaced at a much slower rate than in the upper respiratory tract, is present in the distal airways down to the alveoli. These films also serve as carriers or vehicles to transport particles to the pharynx via the ciliary escalator, and they help cleanse the airways cilia. The major component of this "lung surfactant" is lysophosphatidylcholine in its palmitic acid manifestation. It will be remembered that palmitic acid is the major end product of fatty acid biosynthesis (Section 2.7).

The major removal mechanism for particles that are up to 15 μm in maximum length and that deposit in the alveoli and small airways involves the phagocytic pulmonary macrophages. The complex mechanisms involved in macrophage protection as part of the defense mechanism of innate immunity are discussed in Section 13.0.

A third mechanism of clearance in the lung is provided by the lymphatic system via the lymph, which fills the space between the capillaries and the surface of the alveoli. Gases/vapors and particles smaller than 0.1 μm must negotiate this barrier before absorption in the pulmonary bloodstream; that is, this barrier must essentially be saturated with the xenobiotic before transfer into the bloodstream is efficient. This is relatively easy because the lymph flow is slow in spite of the breathing motions, and the lymph barrier diameter in the alveoli is small.

The lymph also is the medium whereby macrophages are transported to their closest lymph nodes for filtering, reclamation, and processing of xenobiotics (Chapter 13). Lymph flow is directed toward the larger-diameter lymph tubes but parallel to the bronchi. The flow passes through lymphoid tissues and to the lymph nodes at the lung root, which act as large-particle and large-macrophage filters. The chemical processes further associated with the innate and the acquired immunity responses are discussed in Chapter 13. The lymph discharges finally into the venous system. This facilitates excretion by exhalation before the xenobiotic or its metabolites can exert any deleterious effects directly on any important organs other than the lung.

Lungs that are digested gently to remove organic tissue, to produce a particulate residual that represents particulate exposure over a lifetime, show that the average person's exposure to particulate matter is 50% represented by diameters less than 0.5 μm, a size range inaccessible to real-time direct-reading instruments as yet. Almost all the rest of the particulate burden is between 0.5 and 5 μm in diameter. Less than 0.2% of the residue is larger than 5 μm, and 0.002% is larger than 10 μm. Most fibers in the residue are generally less than 50 μm in length, though the largest ones may be 200 μm long. One of the functions of the tortuous nature of the lung's airways is to act as a giant impacter for particles, the largest depositing in the top half of the lung to be eventually transported to the pharnyx by the ciliary motor clearance process. This accounts for the small size of the particles and fibers actually found in the lung after a lifetime of exposure.

It has been postulated that particles larger than 10 μm in aerodynamic diameter are deposited completely in the nose and upper airways, and that particles between 5 and 10 μm are deposited in the airways cleansed by the mucociliary locomotor. Only particles of diameters less than 2 μm are thought to penetrate into the alveoli. These hypotheses have generally been confirmed for inert and microbiological aerosols, though some variation has been observed for reactive aerosols.

3.1 INGESTION

Industrial hygiene courses and texts often omit this route of exposure on the basis that most worker exposure is said to be through inhalation and, to a lesser extent, skin. We have already seen that particles of diameters of 5 to 10 μm deposited in the upper airways of the lung down to the 15th or 16th generation airway can be ingested by means of the ciliary locomotor clearance process of the lung. Deposition of particles in the nose and upper airways also may result in ingestion.

Hygienic considerations also determine the extent of workplace exposure through the ingestion route. Dusty air conditions may cause much dust to settle on the skin and lips of the mouth. Continual pursing, licking, and smacking of lips as well as talking or mouth breathing can lead to ingestion of all sizes of particles. This can be quite an important route of exposure in hot, dusty foundries, especially those with no showers as part of their industrial hygiene programs. The rate of licking of contaminated lips increases as the lips dry out under hot conditions. Another instance is the well-known ingestion of leaded paint chips or of polychlorinated dibenzo-*p*-dioxin (PCDD)–contaminated soils by children (pica). Tobacco smoking combines both inhalation and ingestion as exposure routes, both lung and oral cancers resulting from direct contact of the smoke or tobacco products.

Xenobiotics in food and drink are what people usually think of in relation to ingestion. Thus lead in drinking water that is acidic or of small buffering capacity is a well-known source of lead poisoning. Pesticides in foods, especially in fish, shellfish, and milk, are also well documented. The market-basket surveys provide such food data, and the STORET data base operated by the U.S. EPA contains ground and drinking water data for the United States.

Xenobiotics with high (greater than 10) octanol–water coefficients (K_{ow}; Table 3.1) have great affinity for lipid/bilayer membranes. K_{ow} is defined as follows:

$$K_{ow} = \frac{c_{\text{octanol}}}{c_{\text{water}}} \tag{3.12}$$

where c_{octanol} is the equilibrium isooctanol concentration in the isooctanol fraction and c_{water} is the equilibrium concentration in water in a water/isooctanol water system at 25°C.

Compounds with $K_{ow} > 10$ are absorbed efficiently through membranes and taken up by chylomicra (Section 2.8.2), whereas water-soluble species are not necessarily efficiently absorbed unless the compound is a vitamin, or contains an essential element, essential amino acid, or other needed carbon, nitrogen, sulfur, or phosphorus sources. Thus xenobiotics such as trichloroethylene, lead ion, polychlorinated biphenyls (PCBs), and PCDDs are almost completely absorbed on ingestion, but total ionic iron is not, the preference being for iron(II).

Ethanol is 90% absorbed within an hour after ingestion. It is distributed with body water and has high permeation ability through biological membranes. Ionized organics, for example, salts of carboxylic acids and bases, are poorly and variably absorbed. Many chelating agents for heavy metal poisoning [such as disodium ethylene diamminetetraacetic acid (EDTA) for lead] depend for their action on their relative inability to enter cells and yet be able to chelate the toxicant in the blood and noncellular fluids. The pK_a of a compound (Section 1.6) can also determine at what pH a compound might be absorbed. For example, at stomach pH values of about 1.4, organic acids are protonated and are quickly absorbed from the stomach, both through the intestinal wall and by chylomicra. Under these conditions weak bases are water-soluble, and are more readily absorbed in the small intestinal mucosa where the pH is about 5.3. The absorption efficiency for weak bases increases as the pH increases. Major absorptions of specific toxicants thus can occur soon after the point where gastrointestinal secretions enter, simply through the adjustment of pH, and independent of any additional enzymatic contribution.

Absorption of xenobiotics can vary from individual to individual. For example, the amount of ampicillin absorbed after oral administration to nine healthy men aged 20 to 40 years, varied between 32 and 64%. Access to the bloodstream in the gastrointestinal system is easy via the gumline of the mouth, but usually a short contact time ensures little absorption from this mechanism. However, the continued licking of contaminated lips (for example, of lead in dust for workers in nonferrous foundries or for workers in dusty trades who do not shower before they go home) may lead to high exposures from this mechanism.

The reader is referred to textbooks on physiology for a discussion of digestive enzymes important in releasing xenobiotics and their metabolites from their adducted forms (Chapter 10) in the diet. The function of the digestive system is to facilitate entry of the compounds necessary for human life into the circulatory system. The gastrointestinal system prepares foodstuffs, minerals, vitamins, and liquids for absorption and sends the absorbed entities into the circulatory system of capillaries, arteries, and lymphatics for transport to organs. It also aids in the excretion of many compounds.

After food is chewed in the mouth and some of the starches are hydrolyzed to disaccharides by amylases present in saliva, the gastric juices and enzymes of the acid milieu of the stomach break proteins down to polypeptides, and partition the available fat and fatty acids into the chylomicra (Section 2.8.2). Pancreatic and bile secretions promote further degradation of large molecules. Most digestion and absorption occur in the small intestine, with carbohydrates such as starches hydrolyzed to disaccharides and then to easily absorbed monosaccharides after further degradation by enzymes located in the small intestinal mucosa. Polypeptides are eventually broken down into their constituent amino acids, which are easily absorbed across the small intestine. Newborn children can absorb proteins directly in the absence of proteolytic enzymes. Pancreatic lipase and bile salt antioxidants and emulsifiers produce fatty acids that are resynthesized to triglycerides in intestinal cells, where they are secreted into the lymphatic system as small droplets of lipid. Metal ions are absorbed only in specific redox states, for example, Fe(II) for iron, and according to the homeostatic steady state of the body.

The bile from the gallbladder contains molecules greater than about 375 to 475 in molecular weight. It is instructive to compare the biliary molecular weight thresholds of other species: rat, 275 to 375; and rabbit, 425 to 525. Thus the threshold for humans is nearer the rabbit's than the rat's threshold, so that the rabbit is a better animal model for humans in this regard. Some of these high molecular weight compounds and conjugates can be degraded further enzymatically or by the flora and fauna resident in the intestines to low molecular weight compounds that can be reabsorbed, thus constituting the enterohepatic circulation. Animals with no resident flora in their intestines are called germ-free, and the metabolism and kinetics of xenobiotics in such animals can vary markedly from animals with resident flora and fauna. The symbiotic microorganisms in the intestines and lungs also produce vitamins and essential cofactors for their hosts, in addition to detoxifying xenobiotics. The bile is a major route for expulsion of high molecular weight products of nitrogen degradation related to red blood cell degradation in the nearby spleen (Section 2.11.5). High molecular weight anions acting as digestive detergents are also contained in the bile. Some specific surfactant agents such as bile salts, sodium and potassium salts of fatty acids, and excess lysophospholipids aid in lipid and lipid-soluble vitamin digestion/absorption (Section 2.8.2). Inhibition of cholesterol absorption by ingested resins that bind these detergents (and hence enhance fecal excretion) has resulted in an up to 60% decrease in serum cholesterol concentrations. These resins with bound cholesterol also cannot be attacked efficiently by the symbiotic bacteria to release cholesterol for enterohepatic circulation. Bile salt excretion in the feces is the major mechanism by which excess cholesterol is expelled by the human body (Section 2.8.2).

The digestion and absorption process is regulated by the autonomic nervous system together with many polypeptide hormones. The four best-known gastrointestinal hormones are: gastrin, produced by the gastric mucosa [stimulates gastric secretion of hydrochloric acid and pepsinogen, the inactive precursor (zymogen) of the protease enzyme, pepsin, in response to stomach distension (vagus nerve) and critical concentrations of the degradation products of proteins]; secretin, produced by the upper small intestinal mucosa (stimulates pancreatic secretion of bicarbonate to neutralize gastric hydrochloric acid); cholecystokinin, produced by the cells in the upper small intestine (stimulates the emptying of the gallbladder and the secretion of pancreatic digestive enzymes and bicarbonate, and inhibits gastric emptying in response to high critical concentrations of the products of lipid and protein digestion); and gastric inhibitory peptide, produced by specific cells of the small intestine (inhibits gastric secretions, mobility, and emptying, and stimulates pancreatic insulin release through its response to excess glucose).

Pancreatic insulin and glucagon maintain the blood glucose level. The pancreas also produces serine protease digestive enzymes such as trypsin (cleaves after arginine and lysine amino acid residues in proteins and polypeptides), chymotrypsin (activated by tryptic action), and elastase (also activated by tryptic action) for protein digestion at specific amide links; RNAse

A (hydrolyzes RNA to its component nucleotides at pH 6); α-amylase (hydrolyzes all α-1,4-glucosidic bonds of starches except their outermost bonds and those next to branches) and phospholipase A_2 (Section 2.8.1). α-amylase is the major digestive enzyme of mouth saliva; the pancreatic type causes the production of the disaccharide maltose, the trisaccharide maltotriose, and the dextrin oligosaccharides, which are amenable to further attack by enzymes in the brush border membranes of the intestinal mucosa to produce monosaccharides, which are then absorbable through small and large intestinal membranes. The zymogens (proenzymes) of the pancreatic proteases usually are packaged in the Golgi body–like zymogen granules, and are activated upon release by trypsinogen released initially by a duodenal enteropeptidase (enterokinase) action on the trypsinogen zymogen in an autocatalytic manner. The zymogens have distorted active sites mediated through allosteric binding that prevents substrate binding. Most other zymogens are stored in the Golgi bodies of the specific cells involved in the secretion.

Three important hormones are secreted from the pancreatic islets of Langerhans: insulin from the β cells, glucagon from the α cells, and somatostatin from the δ cells. Insulin stimulates muscles, liver, and adipose cells to store glucose through glycogen (the enzymes uridine diphosphateglucose pyrophosphorylase, glycogen synthase, and glycogen branching enzyme are involved), protein (Sections 2.11.3, 10.1.4, and 10.1.5), and fat (Section 2.7) syntheses. Glucagon has the opposite effects, stimulating glycogenolysis (Section 2.4) and gluconeogenesis (Section 2.4) in the liver and lipolysis in the adipose tissue (Sections 2.5 and 2.6). Somatostatin inhibits release of both insulin and glucagon, and is the master pancreatic paracrine (hormone that acts on nearby cells) hormone controlling insulin and glucagon. Somatostatin is also released by the hypothalamus in an endocrine (acts on cells distant from the point of release) function. Thus ingestion of carbohydrate, lipid, protein, DNA, and RNA-adducted materials may lead to the release of the original xenobiotic or an adducted metabolite of the xenobiotic during the digestive process.

The daily average ingestion of food is about 800 g and 1200 mL of water in male adults. About 1.5 L of saliva, 2 L of acidic gastric secretions, 2 L of pancreatic and biliary secretions, and 1.5 L of intestinal secretions are also produced. Thus 8.5 L of water is absorbed in the gastrointestinal tract above the large intestine, with only 0.5 L reaching the latter.

Undegraded molecules such as cellulose, desquamated cells from the lining of the small intestine, microbes (flora) and invertebrates (fauna), and minerals rejected through homeostatic mechanisms as well as certain excretion products contained in the bile and about 0.5 L of liquid containing the macroions, such as ions of sodium, potassium, magnesium, calcium, phosphate, sulfate, bicarbonate, carbonate, and chloride, reach the large intestine, where water and sodium continue to be absorbed.

The feces contain high molecular weight materials, microorganisms, and excess minerals in addition to products excreted through the bile that have not undergone enterohepatic circulation.

3.2 DERMAL EXPOSURE

Quantitative data on dermal absorption of industrial chemicals for humans are difficult to find, but dermal exposure does occur because toxic effects and production of metabolites or detection of xenobiotics in body fluids have been noted after skin-only exposure.

The skin has approximately 20 ft^2 of surface area for potential contact with foreign substances. A 70-kg man has a skin surface area of 1.8 m^2; a 58-kg female has a skin surface area of 1.6 m^2. The skin protects the body by regulating body heat, receiving sensations, secreting sweat, manufacturing protective pigments, and replenishing itself. The underlying muscles, nerves, and blood vessels are protected from physical and chemical agents. The skin consists of three basic layers: the epidermis (the stratum corneum, 50 μm thick, which consists of horn cells that arise from the basal layer of the epidermal cells and also include melanocytes, which protect against ultraviolet light); the dermis [about 1.25 mm thick, it contains proteins (especially collagen and elastin), sweat ducts and glands, hair follicles that encase hair, and sebaceous (oil) glands that secrete through the hair ducts, as well as nerves and capillaries]; and the hypodermis (connective tissue and fat up to 1.4 mm thick in males and 6.6 mm thick in females). The stratum corneum is a proteinaceous layer that is relatively resistant to mild acids, water, and water-soluble chemicals but is vulnerable to bases, strong detergents, desiccant chemicals, and organic solvents.

Chemicals can penetrate and permeate through the 10-μm-thick outer dead layer of cells of the epidermis into the 40-μm-thick layer of living cells and thence into the dermis, where absorption occurs through the capillaries. The latter absorption is related to blood flow through the capillaries (perfusion), which depends on cardiac output, in turn influenced by environmental and skin temperature, humidity, and physical activity; if the chemical has high affinity for the dermis, then absorption will be slow. The blood perfusion rate in the dermis is about 0.2 L/min, whereas in the hypodermis it is about 0.15 L/min.

Absorption of fat-soluble chemicals, fats, and oils can also occur via the hair follicle, which contains the hair bulb and a portion of the hair shaft; retention of compounds of high K_{ow} will occur in the hypodermis, especially in females.

Uptake through the stratum corneum is called flux (*Fl*), which is defined [5,6,8] as the amount of chemical taken up after direct contact over a defined surface area of skin in square centimeters during unit time. This rate depends on the type of vehicle and the concentration of applied chemical as well as the type of chemical. Other factors such as sweat and oiliness of the skin are important, as well as pH and the extent of ionization of the xenobiotic. Carriers such as acetone dehydrate skin and thus abrade it, so increasing the surface area for absorption. Other carriers such as dimethyl sulfoxide are intrinsically soluble in the stratum corneum, and will promote uptake no matter what the characteristics of the xenobiotic because the carrier is the dominant influence. Water carriers do not promote uptake. Phenol, cresols, and alcohols penetrate quickly, but highly chlorinated phenols do not. 2,3,7,8-Tetrachlorodibenzo-*p*-dioxin is not readily absorbed through the skin unless a solvent carrier such as acetone transports it through.

Any agent causing skin injury increases uptake, for example, sunburn. Inorganic lead salts, which ordinarily will not penetrate the skin like most other inorganic salts, do so in cutting oil because of the dermatitis caused by the latter. Chromates can penetrate, as can organometallic compounds (for example, butyl chromate, tetraalkyl leads, alkyl mercurials, organic tins, and methylcyclopentadienyl manganese tricarbonyl). Skin desiccation with solvents such as acetone also promotes absorption of many other components because skin abrasion occurs.

The regional variation of skin absorption is well known. Thus, dilute aqueous formulations of organophosphate pesticides are 100% absorbed when applied to the scrotum, 32 to 47% when on the head and neck, and 9% when exposed to the forearm. Much of the contradictory nature of the literature may be caused by nonstandardization of the skin sites for dermal exposure investigations.

One simple diffusion model for flux is described by the following equation [6, 8]:

$$Fl = \frac{s}{15}(0.038 + 0.153K_{ow})\mathrm{e}^{-0.016M} \tag{3.13}$$

where:

Fl = flux, $\mathrm{mg\,cm^{-2}\,h^{-1}}$
s = solubility of the xenobiotic in water at skin temperature, mg/mL
K_{ow} = octanol/water coefficient for the xenobiotic
M = molecular weight

Negligible Fl should be shown by compounds of M of 500 or more. As s approaches zero, Fl approaches zero. However K_{ow} increase may counter this effect.

For K_{ow} of less than 0.03:

$$Fl = \frac{0.038s}{15}\mathrm{e}^{-0.016M} \tag{3.14}$$

For K_{ow} of 2 or greater:

$$Fl = \frac{0.153K_{ow}s}{15}\mathrm{e}^{-0.016M} \tag{3.15}$$

Dermal absorption occurs when liquid, solid, or vapor forms contact the skin. Dissolution of impacted aerosols in sweat or sebum can occur to make chemicals available for absorption. Dissolved chemicals are absorbed directly according to their concentration and inversely to their solubility in the carrier.

Prolonged contact with liquids usually causes changes in skin and skin permeability. A familiar example is the softening and crinkling of the skin after prolonged immersion in water. Contaminated clothing or garments can also spread chemicals from their original points of contact over larger skin areas, so enhancing absorption potential. The specific process in the workplace may determine how and where chemicals contact the skin, as well as the work routine and the hygiene and skills of the worker. Such factors often are not corrected for in epidemiological studies. The absorption rate also depends on how saturated the blood is from other routes of exposure.

Very few half-times of dermal exposure have been reported, the extreme variability with skin site and interindividual variability being major delimitations.

3.2.1 Simultaneous Dermal, Gastrointestinal, and Inhalation Exposure

Absorption rates for dermal exposure are related to diffusion of the chemical through any membranes or layers as embodied by equation (3.13). Inhalation absorption and exhalation at blood capillaries have been related to the blood/air partition coefficient K_{ba} of the chemical (Table 3.1) at physiologic conditions, which is defined similarly to the K_{ow}:

$$K_{ba} = \frac{c_{\text{blood}}}{c_{\text{air}}} \tag{3.16}$$

where:

c_{blood} = equilibrium concentration in blood
c_{air} = equilibrium concentration in air

Compounds of high K_{ba} will be absorbed avidly into the blood and will not be readily exhaled. Conversely, compounds of low K_{ba} will tend to be exhaled.

Where fat and blood are in contact, a similar fat/blood partition coefficient, K_{fb} (Table 3.1), can be defined:

$$K_{fb} = \frac{c_{\text{fat}}}{c_{\text{blood}}} \tag{3.17}$$

where c_{fat} is the equilibrium concentration in fat.

Equation (3.17) is applicable for absorption by all routes.

Similarly a fat/air partition coefficient, K_{fa}, is:

$$K_{fa} = \frac{c_{\text{fat}}}{c_{\text{air}}} \tag{3.18}$$

Because there are different kinds of fat and blood, the literature is replete with many contradictory values, all of which may be correct. Individuals may have unique partition coefficients but these vary with age.

Shelley et al. [9] have used a regression equation linking K_{fb} with K_{ow} for chlorinated/brominated hydrocarbons and unsubstituted hydrocarbons:

$$K_{fb} = 70.9 \log K_{ow} - 127 \; r^2 = 0.84 \tag{3.19}$$

Because the literature for K_{ow} is much larger than that for experimentally determined K_{fb}, equation (3.19) is useful for modeling purposes.

An example of the different kinetics of absorption by inhalation (4 h exposure to 100 ppm) and by the skin (30 min immersion of one hand directly in liquid) has been determined in five healthy adult males for trichloroethylene and toluene through analysis of breath alveolar end-tidal volumes for 2 h after exposure [10]. The breath concentrations of trichloroethylene due to inhalation were two times those for skin exposure although uptake through the skin was only about one-third that of inhalation as adjudged by blood trichloroethylene and urinary trichloroacetic acid and trichloroethanol. Toluene was much less absorbed through the skin, the peak blood concentration during inhalation being about four times that during skin exposure. Trichloroethylene caused skin erythema, whereas it was very slight for toluene; this may account for the effects. The disappearance rate constant of blood and breath trichloroethylene for each route of entry is about the same, being $0.187 \pm 0.011\,h^{-1}$, or for a pseudo first-order process (Section 1.8) a half-time of $3.71 \pm 0.22\,h$.

The initial metabolism to chloral hydrate is thus followed by production of trichloroacetate and trichloroethanol in a step so fast that chloral hydrate has not been found in high concentration in human blood. Thus any kinetic differences after skin and inhalation exposure to trichloroethylene are related to uptake processes, not metabolic differences. These data also show that the monitoring of just one route of excretion after exposure, in this case alveolar breath, may not be sufficient for one to interpret results properly. The reason for this is that after absorption from inhalation, any absorbed xenobiotic is carried first to the heart and then distributed to the tissues by the arteries with the unmetabolized xenobiotic coming back to the heart by the venous return for reoxygenation in the lungs, exhalation, and recirculation. For skin or gastrointestinal absorption after an acute or short-duration exposure, the xenobiotic is taken up in the blood capillaries and lymphatics (which eventually empty into the venous system), and is then transported by the venous return to the heart, which forwards the blood to the lungs for reoxygenation and exhalation, and then to the tissues for metabolism and eventual return of unmetabolized xenobiotic.

Alveolar breath concentrations soon after skin absorption and ingestion therefore do not reflect "first pass" tissue metabolism as occurs after inhalation. Thus xenobiotics absorbed through the skin and through the gastrointestinal tract after acute or short-duration exposures have greater opportunity to be exhaled than xenobiotics absorbed after inhalation. Because workplace exposures are generally intermittent rather than continuous (in contrast to the usual conditions utilized in toxicological animal experiments), exhaled breath analysis may not be a good quantitative marker technique for exposure dose under real conditions unless continous exposure can be shown to be occurring. In addition the presence of dermal exposure may cause an overestimation of exposure if inhalation exposure alone is assumed.

The initial penetration of xenobiotics may be quite fast into the skin, but transport away from the area via the blood capillaries depends on many factors, as discussed above. This explains why very high disappearance rates of toluene from the skin ($14–23\,mg\,cm^{-2}\,h^{-1}$) were reported previously in the literature, and yet Sato and Nakajima [10] found blood concentrations to be inconsistent with the same high rate of uptake into the capillaries. Solvents may be confined within the skin layers for a considerable time before being taken up by the circulatory system. For toluene, this was confirmed by maximum blood concentrations being maintained for 15 min after skin exposure ceased. This was not observed for trichloroethylene, which accounts for the higher blood concentrations for that chemical.

Often the washing techniques employed to assess skin contamination may cause penetration. Alternative procedures that have been used to assess skin contamination are fluorescent labels [11] and individual exposure pads [12] at the likely areas of skin exposure. Both techniques have drawbacks. Fluorescent labels may be quenched or enhanced by other chemicals; individual skin patch data are dependent on the initial placement of the patch to reflect representative exposures, a difficult proposition for many situations.

That vapors may also be absorbed through the skin of male human volunteers aged 20 to 35 years wearing supplied air respirators and light pajamas and socks was demonstrated for exposures of 600 ppm of xylene, styrene, toluene, 1,1,1-trichloroethane, and tetrachloroethylene at 25°C at 50% RH for 3.5 h [13]. The estimated dermal exposure compared with inhalation exposure over the same exposure time frame, assuming inhalation and skin to be the only two absorption routes, were 1.4, 1.9, 0.9, 0.08, and 1.1%, respectively. The dermal exposure absorption uptake for xylene was calculated to be 6 nmol $cm^{-2} h^{-1}$, even though liquid xylene can penetrate skin quickly at 1.13 μmol $cm^{-2} h^{-1}$ [14]. This situation can be compared [15] with the percutaneous rate of liquid water or water vapor of high relative humidity of 11 micromole $cm^{-2} h^{-1}$. Permanent gases such as carbon dioxide, oxygen, nitrogen, and helium penetrate the skin at 0.1 to 1.0 micromole $cm^{-2} h^{-1}$ [15].

In a further inhalation study with 20 ppm xylene [15], the uptake from inhalation alone was 57.7%, in agreement with Astrand et al. [1] but with much interindividual variability. Dermally absorbed xylene in the form of urinary methylhippuric acid was excreted 2 to 4 h later than absorbed xylene from inhalation [15]. Styrene inhalation of 10 ppm or dermal exposure at 600 ppm produced equal molar amounts of urinary mandelic acid and phenylglyoxylic acid, with 10 ppm of inhaled styrene being absorbed at an 81% level, as calculated from urinary measurements. Delays of several minutes occurred in the percutaneous absorption of liquid toluene and xylene, but these delays increased to about 1 h for xylene, styrene, and toluene to achieve a steady state.

Methyl chloroform blood concentrations after skin exposure as vapor never attained a steady state, and tetrachloroethylene uptake combined features of both types of kinetics. An individual with atopic dermatitis displayed twice the blood xylene concentrations of volunteers with intact skin, with a threefold increase in urinary methylhippuric acid. When xylene dermal exposure through the skin of one hand was studied for a 1:1 mixture of xylene and isobutyl alcohol, there was a conspicuous delay in, and extent of, *m*-xylene uptake, which was corrected by saturating the mixture with water, so indicating that skin desiccation was involved [16]. It must be remembered that skin absorption through the hand was studied; there is much variability of skin absorption with respect to location.

In contrast with hydrocarbon-type solvents of high vapor pressure, skin absorption predominates as an exposure route for relatively less volatile compounds such as most agricultural pesticides. The pioneering work of Durham and Wolfe [17] in 1962 and that of Wolfe et al. [18–20] have led to much interest on the efficacy of biological monitoring to assess dermal exposure

(Chapter 22), and the comparison of skin patch testing with biological monitoring results [21]. In general, patch testing is not a very representative exposure method, but biological monitoring is, because the latter integrates over all the skin exposed, whereas the patch may or may not be placed in the regions exposed.

A study with malathion as substrate has compared the correlation of a fluorescent tracer (4-methyl-7-diethylaminocoumarin) remaining on the skin and on skin patches, skin patch malathion, and urinary dimethylphosphate and dimethyl dithiophosphate metabolites [22]. The correlation for skin patch deposition to 72-h urinary metabolities [Pearson correlation coefficient (r) between 0.712 to 0.738; nonparametric Spearman rank r between 0.423 to 0.588] was always lower than for the tracer method (Pearson r for all workers, 0.887; nonparametric Spearman r of 0.689 for $n = 19$). The tracer method for the pesticide mixers was less well correlated (Pearson r of 0.733; Spearman rank r of 0.771) than that for the applicators (Pearson r, 0.910; Spearman rank r, 0.709).

The pattern of dermal exposure for mixers of malathion formulations was: hands, 43% (despite the wearing of "protective" gloves); torso and arms, 36%; and head and neck, 20%. For malathion applicators, the pattern was: hands, 12%; torso and arms 64%; and head and neck, 24%. The patch data accounted for about 50% of the total variance, whereas the tracer data accounted for 80%. Urinary excretion represented between 17% and 23% of the estimated exposure. The skin patch technique requires extrapolation from the specific skin patch data to a whole body estimation, involving assumption of uniform coverage. This clearly does not happen for aerosol deposition and for people wearing personal protective equipment of different levels of protection.

Investigation of the influence of protective clothing on skin deposition using the fluorescent tracer technique [11] showed that most of the exposures occurred near sleeve and neck openings in the garments, and that coveralls provided more protection than shirts (reduced exposures from 44% to 77% under these exposure conditions).

Thus biological monitoring is the method of choice to determine skin exposure, but especially to nonvolatile compounds.

3.3 EYE ABSORPTION

The eye is an extraordinary direct sense organ of contact with irritants. Many industrial accidents involve contact of the eyes with chemicals or aerosols. The direct effects can vary from no effect or minor irritation to complete loss of vision. Some mists, vapors, and gases produce varying degrees of eye irritation. Acidic and basic compounds are all potential eye irritants. Lachrymators [such as acetyl chloride, benzoyl chloride, ethyliodoacetate, α-bromobenzylcyanide, and α-chloroacetophenone (Mace) vapors], other chemical irritants (such as acid or alkali mists, photochemical smog, soap, or certain cosmetics), and irritants released by cutting up foods such as onions are well known. All these irritative effects signal that some absorption of the chemical by the eye has occurred.

Sometimes a chemical that causes no overt eye damage can be absorbed in sufficient amounts to cause systemic poisoning. This was discovered for fluoroacetate in rabbits, which caused convulsions and death without affecting the eye itself. Very few references to eye absorption in humans are available. One well-known example is that the efficacy of eye drops requires their absorption. At a time when there were no restrictions on chemical usage in cosmetics in the United States, Lash Lure (major ingredient *p*-phenylenediamine) was reported to have caused a fatality after application to the eyelid. It is good industrial hygiene practice for workers to wear shielded eye goggles if they handle or contact chemicals. Neutral organic solvents contacting the eye directly cause reversible dulling of the eye cornea. Hot solvents may produce irreversible dulling.

Itching of the eyes is a common sign of allergy although this often occurs also in elderly patients who have "dry eye."

Blood is supplied to the visual centers of the brain through the two carotid arteries and the two vertebral arteries. The cavernous sinus drains the eye (via the two ophthalmic veins) and some facial venous blood. Substances absorbed through the eye thus drain to the cavernous sinus and may cause meningitis. The blood supply to the eye itself is through the retinal and ophthalmic arteries.

Superficial punctate keratitis is diffuse edema caused by injury to the eye epithelium, including injury from chemical agents. During slit lamp examination, hazy punctate areas are seen. Grayish-white corneal scars result from burns due to exposure to lye and other bases. Conjunctivitis, the most common eye disease, affects the mucous membranes of the eye, and is characterized by redness and a watery, mucoid, or pus discharge. Chemical exposures may also induce this condition.

Further Reading

Inhalation

Gas Laws: Maron, S. H., and Prutton, C. F. 1967. *Principles of Physical Chemistry*, 4th ed., Macmillan, New York, pp. 5–61.

Lung Physiology and Gas Uptake: Wright, G. W. 1973. The influence of industrial contaminants on the respiratory system. In *The Industrial Environment—Its Evaluation and Control*, NIOSH, pp. 493–498.

Aerosols: Knutson, E. O., and Lioy, P. J. 1989. Measurement and presentation of aerosol size distributions. In *Air Sampling Instruments for Evaluation of Atmospheric Contaminants*, 7th ed., S. V. Hering (ed.), ACGIH, Cincinnati, OH, pp. 59–68.

Hering, S. V. 1989. Inertial and gravitational collectors. In *Air Sampling Instruments for Evaluation of Atmospheric Contaminants*, 7th ed., S. V. Hering (ed.), ACGIH, Cincinnati, OH, pp. 337–341.

Roach, S. A. 1973. Sampling air for particulates. In *The Industrial Environment—Its Evaluation and Control*, NIOSH, pp. 139–140.

Wright, G. W. As for the lung physiology and gas uptake reference, above.

Ingestion

Amdur, M. O. 1973. Industrial toxicology. In *The Industrial Environment—Its Evaluation and Control*, NIOSH, pp. 63–65.

Whittenberger, J. L. 1973. Review of physiology. In *The Industrial Environment—Its Evaluation and Control*, NIOSH, p. 58.

Dermal Absorption

Amdur, M. O. As for ingestion, above.

Birmingham, D. J. 1973. Occupational dermatoses: their recognition, control and prevention. In *The Industrial Environment—Its Evaluation and Control*, NIOSH, pp. 503–509.

Fiserova-Bergerova (Thomas), V., and Pierce, J. T. 1989. Biological monitoring. V: Dermal absorption. *Appl. Ind. Hyg.* **8**: F14–21.

Eye Absorption

Amdur M. O. As in Ingestion.

Leitman, M. W. 1988. *Manual for Eye Examination and Diagnosis*, 3rd ed., Medical Economics Books, Oradell, NJ.

Potts, A. M. 1986. Toxic responses of the eye. In *Casarett and Doull's Toxicology*, 3rd ed., C. D. Klaassen, M. O. Amdur, and J. Doull, (eds.), Macmillan, New York, pp. 478–515.

4

Distribution of Xenobiotics After Absorption

4.0 INITIAL DISTRIBUTION

The various routes of absorption, distribution, and excretion are shown in Figure 4.1.

Absorbed xenobiotics are carried to tissues by the circulatory system, which is comprised of the heart and blood vessels containing the blood. The right side of the heart pumps blood to the lungs for oxygenation and back to the left side, which pumps the aerated blood to the rest of the body. A standard 70-kg man has about 5.5 L of blood; each side of the heart pumps at about 5 L/min and can increase this rate fivefold during heavy work or exercise. The heartbeat is under central nervous system and hormonal regulation. The arterial system, beginning with the aorta, other large arteries, and the peripheral arterioles, contains approximately 15% of total blood volume, with a heart pressure ranging from 70 to 110 mm Hg. The endothelial lining of the arteries has specific receptor sites that recognize foreign molecules, which result in the calling of macrophages (lymphocytes) to the site to deal with the foreign molecule (Chapter 13). The lining also protects against attack of the artery wall by the person's own lymphocytes, and contains vasodilators and constrictors.

The arterioles lead to the capillaries, where blood flow decreases markedly down to 0.07 cm/sec at pressures of about 35 mm Hg. This forces fluid plus its nutrients and xenobiotics out into the tissue spaces; cells in the tissues have pores of about 4 nm diameter and allow molecules passage up to a molecular weight of about 200. At the venous end of the capillary, the pressure is about 15 mm Hg. Also, hemoglobin gives up its oxygen under these conditions and exchanges oxygen for carbon dioxide. The venous system connects the systemic capillary beds to the right side of the heart. It contains about 50% of the blood and is controlled through the central nervous system.

The lymphatic system starts as capillaries in the tissue spaces where the lymph picks up proteins and excess fluid from the blood capillaries as well as

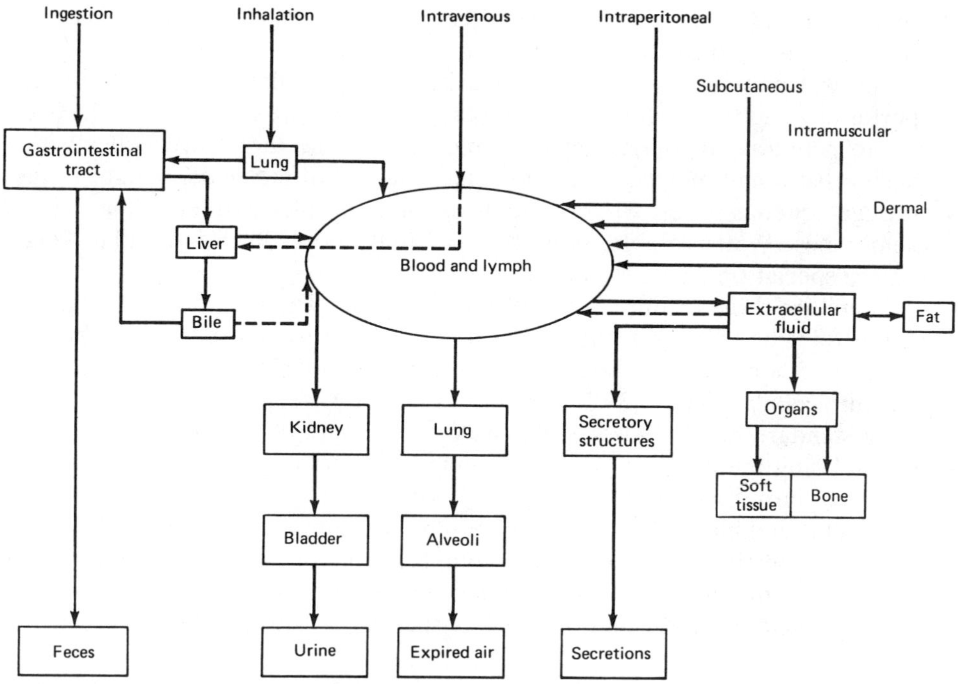

FIGURE 4.1. Routes of absorption, distribution, and excretion of toxicants in the body.

fat droplets absorbed by cells of the intestinal mucosa. Lymph and its contents eventually empty into the veins via trunks in the abdomen and thorax. Lymph nodes filter the lymph en route to the veins.

The distribution of xenobiotics after absorption following an acute exposure (single dose) or an intermittent doses varies according to the route of exposure for relatively low concentrations (ppb to ppm in blood) of absorbed xenobiotic. Inhalation causes direct uptake in the pulmonary artery, which returns blood to the heart, so that the reoxygenated blood plus any xenobiotics are carried out through the aorta and thence to all tissues, with most going to the liver for initial detoxification. The xenobiotics from ingestion and the skin, however, are absorbed first in the venous or lymphatic systems, the latter emptying into the venous system. The venous system returns blood to the heart, which pumps it to the lungs for reoxygenation and then out for distribution to the tissues. Mention has been made already of the fact that xenobiotics taken up through skin absorption and ingestion after an acute dose are more likely to contribute to exhaled air than those absorbed by inhalation because "first pass" metabolism is not important soon after ingestion or skin absorption (Section 3.2.1). The higher the concentration of exposing xenobiotic is, the less important this effect will be because high exposures require multiple passes through the circulatory system and tissues, and low exposures are more easily handled by the "first pass" mechanism.

The time to attain a steady state concentration of xenobiotic in the blood depends on the rates of metabolism and excretion in the tissues, and on whether an individual has enzymes already capable of aiding metabolism that have been induced by previous exposures.

The distribution rate is determined by the blood flow through the organ (perfusion) and the facility of the xenobiotic to cross the arteriole/capillary bed and to penetrate to the target cells and then to the target organelles within those cells. Small molecules and ions less than 50 in molecular weight diffuse through aqueous pores, whereas lipid-soluble molecules permeate lipid bilayer membranes. Water-soluble molecules and ions above 50 in molecular weight require special transport systems to enter cells.

There are three distinct compartments for body water: plasma water (4.5% of the total body weight and 3 L in a male 70-kg standard man), interstitial water (15.5% of the total body weight and 11 L in a male 70-kg standard man), and intracellular water (30.5% of the total body weight and 21 L in a male 70-kg standard man). Extracellular water is the sum of plasma and interstitial water. Using these volumes and assuming that a total of 1 mg of xenobiotic is absorbed into each compartment and without any tissue uptake, biotransformation, and elimination, there would be concentrations in ng/L of 333, 91, and 48, respectively, in these three compartments, assuming distribution with water. Distribution in real life is much more complicated than this because binding and dissolution in storage sites such as fat, liver, or bone are major influences.

If tissues take up the xenobiotic, the xenobiotic's concentration in the blood decreases exponentially with time so that a plot of the logarithm of xenobiotic concentration versus time has linear regions. If only one straight line is observed, this indicates a one-compartment model (equivalent to pseudo first-order kinetics discussed in Section 1.8) defined by a pseudo first-order rate constant with the half-time for disappearance being independent of the initial concentration. When two straight lines are produced from such a plot, a two-compartment model is said to be obeyed, and an *n*-compartment model for *n* straight lines, each compartment defined by its pseudo first-order rate constant. The first straight line nearest the zero time defined for absorption is labeled as alpha (α) or the distributive region; the next is labeled beta (β) or the post-distributive region; and so on with the Greek alphabet. Multicompartment models are obeyed when "deep compartments" such as bone and fat are involved. Such models are strictly empirical and oversimplified because the rate-determining steps of the processes are being reflected by measurements in body fluids. However, the treatment is applied to all biological media as well as whole body data.

The apparent volume of distribution (V_d) is defined as follows:

$$V_d = \frac{\text{mass of xenobiotic in body}}{\text{initial concentration in plasma}} \tag{4.1}$$

To estimate V_d, the plasma concentration versus time curve (plasma disappearance curve) is extrapolated to zero time to find the initial concentration in plasma, a process often fraught with much error because initial rates have the largest intrinsic errors. This extrapolation procedure is accurate only for one-compartment models. The mass of xenobiotic (initial body burden) is obtained from an intravenous dose or from some measure of the total absorbed dose.

A better way of estimating the initial concentration in plasma is to find the area under the curve (AUC) using the trapezoidal rule from time zero to the final time. The usual procedure is to add the area (A) of the trapezoids formed by each two successive plasma concentrations ($A = 0.5[c_1 + c_2][t_2 - t_1]$, where c_1 and c_2 are the plasma concentrations of the xenobiotic at consecutive time intervals and $t_2 - t_1$ is the time interval t_i between the two plasma samples) plus the AUC from the last plasma sample at time t to time infinity. The latter is equal to the final concentration of xenobiotic in plasma divided by the elimination rate constant that is obtained from the slope of a plasma disappearance curve (slope = −elimination rate constant/2.303).

Polar xenobiotics such as formate ion are found mostly in the plasma, as are compounds with high affinities for plasma proteins (such as PCBs); so V_d may approximate the volume of plasma. Ethanol, in contrast, distributes itself evenly in total body water so that V_d approximates body volume. Chemicals that bioaccumulate such as polychlorinated dibenzo-*p*-dioxins (PCDDs) and polychlorinated dibenzofurans (PCDFs) have V_d values much greater than the body volume; so V_d values may have no physiological meaning. Body burden can also be calculated by knowing V_d and the plasma concentration at any time.

When exposures are chronic rather than acute, they may be continuous (exposure to ambient air components), intermittent (exposures in workplace generally, but especially where workers are not always in the same work area; drug taking), or intermittent continuous (when the exposing chemical is regularly encountered at a certain location, for example, cosmetics in bedrooms).

For continuous exposures, any chemical A is eliminated from the target organ or body at a rate directly proportional to body burden at any time t after administration. Thus, from Section 1.8:

$$\left(\frac{dA}{dt}\right)_t = -k_e A_t \tag{4.2}$$

where:

$\left(\frac{dA}{dt}\right)_t$ = rate of elimination of A at time t after administration
k_e = rate constant of elimination assuming pseudo first-order kinetics
A_t = body burden (mass or moles) at time t

The rate of elimination increases as A accumulates until a steady state body burden A_s is reached at which the rate of elimination is equal to the rate of absorption or dose rate (D_r):

$$D_r = k_e A_s \tag{4.3}$$

Thus:

$$A_s = \frac{D_r}{k_e} = \frac{D_r t_{0.5}}{0.693} \tag{4.4}$$

assuming pseudo first-order kinetics.

Using the integrated form of equation (4.2):

$$A_t = A_s[1 - e^{-k_e t}] \tag{4.5}$$

About 97% of the steady state level is reached after five half-times *if* a pseudo first-order process is obeyed. Similarly, 90% of the steady state level is reached after 3.3 half-times. A chemical of short half-time will accumulate little on chronic administration and will reach steady state rapidly. A long half-time means that steady state will take a long time to be attained under continuous-administration conditions.

Body burdens of most xenobiotics reach steady state within a few weeks except those favoring significant fat deposition where gender (females have more fat than males of the same weight on average) and the amount of fat (which varies in an individual manner) influence half-times.

For practical biological monitoring related to recent exposure, half-times of xenobiotics should be less than 12 h for adequate sensitivity and to ensure representative samples of biological media.

When exposure to chemical A is intermittent (the usual case), blood and tissue levels cycle between a maximum, A_{max}, reached early in each exposure interval t_i and a minimum, A_{min}, after the end of each exposure interval:

$$A_{\text{max}} = \frac{D_r}{1 - e^{-k_e t_i}} \tag{4.6}$$

and:

$$A_{\text{min}} = \frac{D_r e^{-k_e t_i}}{1 - e^{-k_e t_i}} = A_{\text{max}} e^{-k_e t_i} \tag{4.7}$$

If the elimination half-time is very short, the body burden after many doses or exposures may only be slightly larger than the body burden following the first dose. In fact, for a number n greater than 3 of equal doses or exposures that are equally spaced at $k_e t_i = 0.6$, the ratio after n doses to that after one is about 2.5. For $k_e t_i$ of 0.1, this ratio for above $n = 3$ decreases by about 0.75.

The intermittent continuous type of exposure can be described by using equation (4.5) in an on–off manner together with equation (4.2) for elimination during the nonexposure intervals. A feature of this treatment is that if A bioaccumulates to any degree, the A_{min} values will show a continuous increase during nonexposure intervals with A_{min} not being equal to preexposure levels. Thus the difference between A_t and the preceding A_{min} is more related to the recent exposure dose than A_t itself, which also contains a component due to past exposure history.

More correctly, the AUC between the two times minus the level at A_{min} multiplied by the t_i between A_{min} and A_t is the quantity directly related to recent exposure dose. Because the time of exposure and the value for A_{min} are usually unknown, it is best to pick an integrative type of marker for biological media (for example, bile excretion over 24 *h*; 24-*h* urines; total hair levels) rather than a differential marker (blood samples; enzyme activities; hair segment levels), and to take preexposure as well as postexposure samples so that the difference between the two results approximates the AUC between the two time points corrected for any preexposure. If the preexposure sample can be shown to be the same as a historical average preexposure sample, the difference between post- and preexposure values is then clearly related to exposure dose. If this is not the case, the kinetics must be defined for one to be able to interpret the results. This matter has plagued the fields of biological monitoring and medical monitoring from the beginning. It applies to the interpretation of data not only for elimination but also for blood and animal pharmacokinetic data where parameters are measured directly.

Needless to say, pseudo first-order kinetics must be demonstrated to occur *before* any of these equations can be applied, a condition often not proven by those who interpret or amass biological monitoring data. The kinetics of elimination from organs and tissues must similarly be known before the above treatment can be applied. It is always tempting to do a "first approximation" or an "order of magnitude" calculation using the above approach.

4.1 REDISTRIBUTION

Often redistribution of the xenobiotic among organs occurs so that distribution changes with time. The initial distribution depends on the blood flow to the area, the permeability of the tissue to the xenobiotic, and the availability of binding sites. Other organs that are less well perfused with blood may have a higher binding potential in terms of type, number, and rate of availability of binding sites, but require many passes of the xenobiotic through the circulatory system for these other factors to become dominant. For example, the skin may contain a high concentration of an absorbed chlorinated organic solvent soon after absorption, but other organs may concentrate the xenobiotic ultimately, particularly the liver which is the chief organ of detoxification. Soon after absorption, lead is localized in the red blood cells, liver, and kidney. Two hours after absorption, about half of it is found in the liver. A month later, 90% of the lead is localized in the bone where it substitutes for calcium in the hydroxyapatite lattice. Another well-known redistribution is that of lipophilic compounds from well-perfused tissues to the adipose tissue over time. Demonstrating steady state to allow representative samples to be taken and interpreted correctly is therefore difficult when half-times and exposure times/durations are not known.

4.2 BIOLOGICALLY EFFECTIVE DOSES

Any adverse toxic effect is related to the biologically effective dose. If a target organ effect is being considered, then the concentration of xenobiotic absorbed by the organ is related to toxic effects for that organ; so only part of the absorbed dose may produce the adverse effect. Moreover, the total dose absorbed by a target organ may not all be the effective biological dose because detoxification, biotransformation, and excretion processes (metabolic pools or turnover) will nullify much of the impact of the organ's absorbed dose. If these systems successfully handle the xenobiotic or its toxic metabolites, then no toxic effects occur. Thus above a critical dosc (threshold), toxic effects (observable adverse effects) may be manifested, a dose that varies from chemical to chemical, organ to organ, animal strain to animal strain, and animal species to animal species. These toxic effects may be reversible or irreversible.

Therefore, although exposure to acetyl chloride may cause involuntary tearing, which is an observable adverse effect, this is a reversible effect because tearing stops after exposure ceases. Pathology in tissues is an example of a generally irreversible toxic effect. Observed effects significantly different from the same tissue in unexposed persons are called lesions. Not all lesions are adverse.

Xenobiotics may be biotransformed into metabolites that are more or less toxic than the xenobiotics. Paraoxon is more toxic than its precursor parathion, an organophosphate insecticide. Generally if metabolites are to be more toxic than the original xenobiotic, they usually occur in the first few activation/Phase I steps. Carbon dioxide, the ultimate oxidation metabolic product of organic compounds, is one of the natural constituents of the air that humans breathe. Elimination products are often nontoxic. There are exceptions for all these statements.

The rate at which biotransformation occurs also is important, as are the rates of clearance and excretion. The faster a chemical can be eliminated from the body, the less hazard it poses to the body. Therefore, any factors that increase residence time of xenobiotics in the body may produce unexpected toxic effects. If the chemical is stored in the fat, it is not readily available for metabolism and is thus eliminated slowly because the slow release from fat is the rate-limiting step of the whole process. However, if fasting occurs, a toxic situation may develop due to the fast depletion of fat stores.

The classic receptor site model used to explain toxicity assumes that a toxicant binds reversibly to the appropriate receptor sites, that toxicant concentration at the receptor sites is an appropriate measure of exposure dose, and that the concentration in blood can be used as a surrogate for concentration at the receptor site. There are also models where total integrated exposure is thought to be the appropriate measure of dose. For example, the total administered dose is the most convenient dose, and absorption is assumed to be 100%. Another case is where lung effects are related to total inhaled xenobiotic mass, rather than absorbed mass, the latter being better related to liver effects. We have already presented the other type of model involving pharmacokinetic measures of effective dose in Section 4.0, namely, the AUC method, and the amount in the blood or tissue at steady state.

Sometimes, the total amount of stable metabolites excreted or eliminated may serve as a surrogate measure (marker) of effective dose for a xenobiotic or its toxic metabolite(s). One example of the former case is the measurement of total trichloro compounds in blood and urine for perchloroethylene and trichloroethylene exposure. An example of the latter case is the greater correlation of hepatotoxicity with metabolite production from perchloroethylene than with perchloroethylene dose itself. More rarely, the rate of metabolism of the administered chemical may serve as a surrogate for the amount of putative intermediate responsible for the toxic effect. This occurs when there is an optimum concentration for the toxic effect caused on the low-concentration side of the maximum by increasing potency due to dose, and on the high-concentration side by factors such as metabolic saturation (capacity-limited processes) or the accelerating destruction of the receptors responsible for the adverse effects. The former situation is the case for rat carcinogenesis (angiosarcoma) elicited by vinyl chloride through the putative carcinogen chloroethylene oxide; the latter explains the toxic effects of acrolein, which gradually denatures the cytochrome P-450 enzyme complex at high concentrations. Such examples in the latter case are obtained from animal data, where the mechanism must be known for one to interpret the data correctly; data for humans of this type are much more difficult to find than animal data.

4.3 STORAGE

Accumulation in target organs may serve as a protective measure. Thus the organ with the highest concentrations or mass of xenobiotic or its metabolites may not necessarily be the target organ associated with toxicity. For example, chlorinated aromatic insecticides often are found in highest concentrations in fat but produce no known toxic effects on this organ. The bloodstream itself may also be a target organ; for example, the hemolysis of red blood cells by absorbed arsine gas and the production of carboxyhemoglobin in red blood cells on exposure to carbon monoxide or methylene chloride. Paraquat accumulates in the lung. Lead is stored in bone, but lead-poisoning symptoms are correlated with soft tissue concentrations. Ceruloplasmin transports most of the copper in serum, but is not associated with a toxic effect.

Binding to plasma proteins usually is determined to be present by equilibrium dialysis or by ultrafiltration. The fraction passing through the dialysis or filter membrane is "free"; the fraction retained after dialysis is "bound." Albumin is the chief binding protein in plasma and can bind xenobiotics at six major sites. Some chemicals that bind to albumin are: acid dyes, adenosine, aspirin, barbiturates, bilirubin, chloramphenicol, dieldrin, digitonin, fatty acids, histamine, penicillin, phenol red, quinocrine, salicylate, streptomycin, sulfonamides, suramin, tetracycline, thyroxine, triiodothyronine, uric acid, vitamin C, and calcium, copper, and zinc ions. If a ligand of greater affinity is present, the first ligand may be displaced from binding sites and then become available to enter the target organ. Because the bound form cannot enter the target organ but the free form can, toxic effects of the first compound may accompany administration of a suitable second compound of higher affinity. An example of this occurs when the drug phenylbutazone is administered to patients who have had prior high workplace exposures; the drug displaces the bound chemicals from their plasma storage forms, and the toxic effects of the free chemicals can be manifested. An interesting example of storage of a drug is the marked increase in plasma binding that is produced on long-term treatment with lidocaine.

Binding to plasma proteins has been analyzed by Scatchard plots [23–26], in which the ratio of bound to free ligand concentration is plotted against the moles of bound ligand where the "affinity constant" can be calculated from the slope (which equals −1/affinity constant), and the maximum number of binding sites is the intercept at a bound/free ligand ratio of zero. A nonlinear Scatchard plot could indicate the presence of more than one type of binding site, each of characteristic affinity constant, or could show that the binding of each successive ligand molecule alters the affinity constant for the next ligand molecule to be bound, or could indicate a mixture of the two possibilities.

Measurements must be made at equilibrium at known concentrations rather than on preparations of unknown composition. Klotz [23] recommended that Scatchard plot data be believed only when a plot of the number of moles bound versus the logarithm of free-ligand concentration shows an asymptote at high free-ligand concentrations and when the binding curve is sigmoidal and symmetric with an inflection point at half the asymptotic concentration. In other words, there should be evidence that the system is near saturation relative to binding. A lively literature discussion has ensued about these points [23–26].

Other target tissues that store specific chemicals include liver (organic anions and acids, azo dye carcinogens, and corticosteroids via Y protein or ligandin); kidney (cadmium via metallothionen); fat (organochlorine alicyclic and aromatic compounds of high K_{ow}); bone and teeth (lead, fluoride, strontium); brain (aluminum and methylmercury in adults, and lead in children); lung (aluminum, asbestos, silica, and inhaled refractory materials) and the fetus (thalidomide, lead).

Further Reading

Klaassen, C. D. 1986. Distribution, excretion and absorption of toxicants. In *Casarett and Doull's Toxicology*, 3rd ed., C. D. Klaassen, M. O. Amdur, and J. Doull (eds.), Macmillan, New York, pp. 33–63.

O'Flaherty, E. J. 1981. *Toxicants and Drugs: Kinetics and Dynamics*, Wiley-Interscience, New York.

Whittenberger, J. L. 1973. Review of physiology. In *The Industrial Environment—Its Evaluation and Control*, NIOSH, p. 58.

5

Metabolism

5.0 GENERAL REMARKS

Section 2.13 outlined the general concepts important to biological monitoring as they relate to general metabolism in humans. One should review the following sections before reading this section: fatty acid degradation (Section 2.5), beta-oxidation (Section 2.6), fatty acid biosynthesis (Section 2.7), other lipids (Section 2.8.2), cytochrome P-450 and hydroxylations (Section 2.9), degradation of nitrogen compounds (Section 2.11.1), glutathione (Section 2.11.4), porphyrins (Section 2.11.5), creatine and creatinine (Section 2.11.6), metabolism regulation (Section 2.12), and especially general body handling of xenobiotics (Section 2.13).

Xenobiotics that are not water-soluble are generally metabolized to more water-soluble, less volatile products (Phase I oxidation products and Phase II conjugates) to enable elimination and excretion (Chapter 6). There are some exceptions. For example, some metals such as selenium and tellurium are methylated and excreted in the breath. These breath markers are more non-polar, less water-soluble, and more volatile than the original xenobiotic. Metabolism may also produce a component of a naturally occurring series of reactions with ultimate oxidation to carbon dioxide, water, bicarbonate ion, and carbonate ion, or with anabolism to a body macromolecule via incorporation in C_2 and C_3 biosynthetic cycles, or transformation to other substrates that can enter general metabolism.

For many compounds, the rate-determining steps of excretion processes are metabolic reactions, but this is not so if the original xenobiotic is the marker. Metabolism often determines how much of the original compound, metabolites, or conjugates are excreted and by what routes. Factors that affect the rate of excretion, the distribution and redistribution of the xenobiotic (Chapter 4), the production of its metabolites and conjugates, and the integrity of any target organs will influence the interpretation of marker concentrations in biological media. Any factor that increases storage of the xenobiotic or its metabolites in tissues such as fat, teeth, or bone will decrease metabolism and excretion, and vice versa.

Certain congeners (same basic family of compounds with different substitutions of common functional groups) of PCBs, polybrominated biphenyls (PBBs), and polychlorinated dibenzo-*p*-dioxins (PCDDs) and dibenzofurans (PCDFs) are more resistant to metabolism than others (the ones with vicinal halogens), and so these accumulate in the liver, breast milk, and blood long after exposure, with the other congeners being more enriched in the blood if the exposure is recent. This means that the compositions of the congeners determined in biological media can change relative to those found in the original exposing mixture. This also occurs in water (enrichment of more soluble congeners), air (enrichment of the congeners with the highest vapor pressures), and soil (enrichment of the congeners resistant to microbiol degradation and those congeners that are least volatile and water-soluble).

This is not really surprising if it is remembered that exposures to multicomponent chemicals can result also in differential accumulation, metabolism, elimination, and excretion of the multicomponents.

If a xenobiotic is not a substrate for a specific enzyme system, its metabolism occurs generally through the nonspecific microsomal enzymes in the cytochrome P-450 complex, which carry out epoxidations, hydroxylations, demethylations, reductions, and hydrolyses, all in the same complex. A hydrocarbon-type xenobiotic will be hydroxylated or a keto group produced at one carbon atom at least, with perhaps further oxidation to aldehydes and carboxylic acids in addition to competing Phase II conjugations. Alkyl side chains on benzene rings will undergo beta-oxidation to produce a benzoic or a phenylacetic acid before amino acid or glucuronic acid conjugation and then excretion. Halogenated compounds and intermediates will form some glutathione (GSH) conjugates, the extent of conjugation depending on the strength of the halogen–carbon bond. The stronger bonds are also partially hydroxylated in the cytochrome P-450 system, this requiring molecular oxygen. Hydroxylated intermediates may also undergo Phase II conjugations. Xenobiotic degradation, like catabolism, consists of several competing, concurrent processes. The choice of a biological monitoring marker for a given xenobiotic must be based on a knowledge of its metabolic fate.

The kinetics of metabolic pathways are not constant in the same person at all times and among individuals, genders, ages, ethnicities, races, or organs. Because a biological monitoring program relies on the rate of appearance of and/or the amount of marker in the bioassay medium, anything that affects this rate or amount will influence the interpretation of biological monitoring data. Composite sampling of biological media over an extended period of time minimizes the effect of a variable excretion rate. This is the fundamental reason why more consistent results are found with 24-h urine samples than with spot urine samples.

5.1 CONJUGATIONS (TYPE II PROCESSES)

This section is a brief summary of comparative conjugations in animals. This is necessary to appreciate why certain animal models for humans are adequate or inadequate.

TABLE 5.1. Phase II major system distribution in male Sprague-Dawley rat tissues.

Tissue	1	2	3	4	5	6
Adrenals			+		+	
Bladder			+			
Blood cells					+	
Brain			+		+	
Gut	+		+	+		+
Kidney	+	+	+	+[a]	+	+
Liver	+	+	+	+	+	+
Lung	+		+	+	+	
Placenta			+			
Skin			+		+	
Spleen	+		+		+	
Thymus			+			

Adapted from references 169 and 170.
[a] Not complete system.
(1) Acetylation; (2) amino acid conjugation; (3) glucuronidation; (4) glutathione; (5) methylation; (6) sulfate formation.

Eight out of ten of the major conjugation reactions (Table 2.2) were discovered between 1842 and 1894, mostly in Prussia and Germany. Knowledge of enzymes, cofactors, and high energy substrates in conjugation (Phase II) reactions mostly has been elucidated since World War II. In the nineteenth century most conjugates were found to be much less toxic and more polar than the original compounds. Instances of the original compound being activated to a more potent compound before conjugation (for example, the paraoxon activated intermediate of parathion) have been reported. Other examples are the conjugation of certain *N*-hydroxy compounds to produce potent carcinogens and the mutagenic glucuronide of the nonmutagenic *N*-hydroxy-4-aminobiphenyl.

Most organisms including humans conjugate in preferred portions of organs and cells. Thus the major amount of metabolism in rats and in humans occurs in the liver, though all organs including skin can metabolize to some extent (Table 5.1). In cells, conjugating systems are concentrated in the membranes, cytosol, mitochondria, lysosomes, and endoplasmic reticulum. Electrophilic and nucleophilic centers (Section 2.13.2) can be conjugated. Each conjugating system except that containing glutathione (GSH) requires the biosynthesis of a high energy nucleotide.

Thus to conjugate with nucleophilic centers (often the lone pair electrons of heteroatoms, anions, or radicals), the following high energy intermediates are available for enzyme-catalyzed conjugation: sulfation—3-phosphoadenosine-5′-phosphosulfate (PAPS) in the cytosol; glucuronidation—uridine diphosphate glucuronic acid (UDPGA) in the endoplasmic reticulum; acetylation—acetyl coenzyme *A* (AcCoA) in the cytosol; methylation—*S*-adenosylmethionine (SAM) in both the cytosol and the endoplasmic reticulum; and amino acid conjugation via activation of xenobiotic with coenzyme A in mitochondria—endoplasmic reticulum and lysosomes.

The sole pathway to detoxify electrophilic centers (cations and protonated activated intermediates) is GSH conjugation, which involves enzymic and nonenzymic reaction between GSH and the foreign compound in the cytosol with eventual conversion to a thioether using AcCoA in the last step in the endoplasmic reticulum. All of these processes occur in specific cellular compartments.

The Phase I products resulting from oxidation/reduction are all amenable to Phase II processes, depending on the target organ (Table 5.1). These conjugations compete with further Phase I processing. This results in many possible biological monitoring markers, the ones produced in the highest yields being the most sensitive ones.

5.5.1 Glucuronidation and Sulfation

Glucuronic acid conjugation (Section 2.11.5 relative to bilirubin) is important because a diverse number of functional groups are conjugated (oxygen atoms in hydroxy- and carboxyl-; nitrogen atoms in amino-, nitro-, nitroso-, and amido-; sulfur atoms in thiols, disulfides, and dithoic acids; and atoms with acidic hydrogens). Also, glycogen, which acts as the ultimate source of β-glucuronic acid, is far more plentiful compared with sulfate and amino acids. Thus the glucuronic acid conjugation pathway is the general last line of defense should the easily saturated pathways, amino acid conjugation and sulfation, be inadequate to detoxify the xenobiotic. There are many glucuronyl transferase isozymes.

The glucuronic acid is bonded at the anomeric carbon with a beta-configuration (below the plane of a Newman structure ring form). β-glucuronidase (β-D-glucuronide-glucuronohydrolase) catalyzes the formation of glucuronides of certain phenols. The enzyme also mediates the transfer of glucuronic acid from aryl and alicyclic glucuronides to aliphatic alcohols and glycols but not to alicyclic alcohols or phenols. The kidney and the bladder can release large amounts of β-glucuronidase so that the enzyme activity in the urine is not just related to the influence of the liver. Metabolites resulting from competing multiple conjugations by different paths are also known. The ultimate end product of the β-glucuronic acid pathway is D-glucaric acid, a urinary marker reflecting the activity of enzymes associated with the endoplasmic reticulum. The D-glucaro-1,4-lactone is the crucial intermediate. Glucuronidation is not important in cats and the "gunn rat." See also Section 9.3.8.

Sulfates ($R{-}O{-}SO_3^-$) are major metabolites of many phenols, alcohols, aromatic amines, and hydroxylamines. Sometimes sulfation occurs to increase the water solubility to the point that cytosolic systems can then conjugate efficiently at the nucleophilic and/or electrophilic centers. Sulfation often serves to introduce a nucleophilic center (the resonance-stabilized oxygens that share a negative charge), which enables elimination or transport between cellular and organ compartments to achieve final conjugation and excretion. Bile elimination is facilitated also. Phenol sulfation requires 3′-phosphoadenosine-5′-phosphosulfate as sulfate group donor and the enzyme arylsulfatase A. There are many types of sulfotransferase enzymes. Many sulfated species have been implicated in DNA, RNA and protein adduct formation (Chapters 10–12). Guanine in DNA and RNA, and Met, Cys, Trp and Tyr in proteins are most estersulfated.

5.1.2 Glutathione Conjugation

It was in the late nineteenth century that the mercapturic acid *S*-(*p*-bromophenyl)acetyl cysteine, was discovered in the urine of animals dosed with bromobenzene. This compound was isolated from urine acidified for preservation purposes. Just after this discovery in the nineteenth century, it was found that dosing other halogenated aromatic and related compounds also caused similar mercapturic acids to be detected in acidified urines. The "premercapturic acid precursors," the true metabolites, were found to be thioethers only in the 1950s. The mercapturic acids were artifacts of the analytical procedures. It was not until the early 1960s that the cysteine moiety in these mercapturic acids was discovered to be derived from GSH. The GSH concentration represents the majority of the available sulfhydryl-containing compounds.

There are four distinct steps to the processing of a xenobiotic by the GSH pathway (Section 2.11.4): enzymic (at least seven isoenzymes of the glutathione-*S*-transferase) and nonenzymic conjugation with glutathione in the cytosol; removal of the glutamyl moiety from the conjugate by γ-glutamyltransferase; hydrolytic removal of the glycine moiety by a dipeptidase to provide the cysteine conjugate; and *N*-acetylation of the latter by an AcCoA-requiring enzyme to yield the thioether. Apart from the initial step in the cytosol, all the other enzymes are membrane-bound. The types of compounds conjugated include *N*-hydroxy compounds, urethanes, sulfides, sulfonamides, aromatic amines, thiophenes, triazines, diphenyl ethers, halogens on aliphatics and aromatics, esters, nitro groups, double bonds, and sulfates.

Thioethers have been found in the urines of many animals, including the rabbit, rat, mouse, dog, cat, hamster, guinea pig, horse, sheep, pig, monkey, cow, lizard, frog, chicken, duck, goldfish, and human. Usually only the thioethers but sometimes also the cysteine conjugates are excreted in the urine. Glutathione-*S*-transferase activity has been found in many tissues, including the lung, liver (about 10% of soluble liver proteins), kidney, and gut. These enzymes have molecular weights of 45,000 to 50,000 and consist of two subunits of approximately equal size.

"Ligandin" and "basic azo-dye binding protein" have been terms used to describe a soluble liver protein that binds many compounds, including bilirubin, some steroids, cholecystographic agents, azo dyes, and carcinogenic hydrocarbons. This substance has been shown to be glutathione-*S*-transferase B. Because most GSH conjugates exceed 300 in molecular weight and are nucleophiles, they are eliminated in the bile. This includes many metal conjugates. The biliary GSH conjugates are further metabolized by the intestine and intestinal flora and fauna to compounds that do not contain the cysteine moiety. The undegraded fraction is excreted in the feces. The degradation products that are less than 300 in molecular weight can be absorbed or reabsorbed, with some being excreted in the urine. The remainder may be metabolized further, may undergo more enterohepatic circulation, or are excreted in the feces.

The thioether content in the urine is not an adequate measure of GSH conjugation because of these many complicating factors. However dose-effect relationships may be obeyed, and specific thioethers may be adequate biological monitoring markers under the appropriate conditions. Urinary total thioethers (Section 9.3.7) is a potential marker that integrates multicomponent exposures in the absence of interactions. GSH conjugation events are usually investigated through bile analysis.

All GSH conjugation substrates have electrophilic centers; that is, the xenobiotic itself, a Phase I product, or an activated intermediate [for example, carbonium ions, episulfonium ions, and protonated oxiranium (epoxide) ions] may possess such a center. Sometimes GSH conjugation leads to a more toxic intermediate, for example, the episulfonium ion with 1,2-dibromoethane which is postulated to form DNA adducts. Most GSH conjugation reactions mechanistically resemble an SN_2 process (Section 1.11) of a sulfur nucleophile with an electrophilic carbon. Many substituted aromatic compounds are conjugated, including simple and complex aromatic systems, furans, pyridines, thiophenes, and triazines.

GSH conjugation of α- and β-unsaturated compounds also occurs by an addition of the nucleophile GS^- to an activated double bond. Some unsaturated bonds are converted to activated protonated epoxide intermediates before GSH conjugation; for example, acetals, aldehydes, esters, ketones, lactones, nitriles, sulfones, and nitro compounds. Alkanes substituted with halogen and nitro-groups, methanesulfonates, and the P and O in the phosphate group of organophosphate pesticides are all conjugated, along with arylalkyl-halides, -alcohols, and -esters (including sulfate esters).

The production of epoxides has been advocated as the most important step to initiate carcinogenesis via electrophilic attack on DNA, RNA, and proteins. This often-heard postulate is contradictory because the epoxides themselves are nucleophiles, not electrophiles. Protonated epoxides (oxiranium ions) and episulfonium ions are electrophiles, which may form before or after epoxide formation. Also all epoxides ought to be carcinogens, but this is not so.

The electrophile has to be stable enough and yet still sufficiently reactive (moderate electrophile) to react with nuclear materials. It cannot be too reactive (strong electrophile) because everything would react around the point of absorption. Concentration thus becomes an important factor, as well as what fraction of the available xenobiotic is converted to an activated epoxide. The types of functional groups on the rest of the molecule are major factors, as, for example, in epichlorhydrin. Electron-donating groups such as alkyl ones will enhance the existence of relatively stable electrophiles if these groups are bonded to the electrophilic atom. Electron-withdrawing groups like nitro- and carboxyl- will cause the reverse events. Conjugated systems tend to have relatively stable electrophiles. Thus the arene oxides, which are relatively stable epoxides and moderate electrophiles, are postulated to be potent carcinogens on a per-molecule basis. Epoxides also can be converted to diols, a reaction that for arene oxides results in formation of catechols and phenols, which are not carcinogenic and which then may be sulfated and glucuronidated to facilitate excretion.

If inefficient metabolism occurs, whether from intrinsic factors or from exposure to other chemicals that may deplete metabolism, the result is to allow the activated and labile intermediates longer life than they should have, a process that may cause attack on the nuclear material or acute toxic effects not noticeable under usual conditions.

5.1.3 Methylation

Experiments in the 1940s and 1950s led to proof that *S*-adenosyl methionine (SAM) is the major source of the methyl group for methylations of xenobiotics. Though it is known that 5-methyltetrahydrofolic acid is the methyl donor in *N*-methylation of biogenic amines in rat and human brain, no methylations of xenobiotics with this donor have been reported. There is a methylation activity associated with the DNA-histone (chromatin) complex.

The enzyme that forms SAM, methionine adenosyltransferase, is widely distributed in animals. The major acceptors are the nitrogen of primary, secondary, or tertiary amines; certain nitrogen-containing heterocycles; the oxygen of phenols and certain *N*-hydroxy compounds; and the sulfur of thiols and certain related compounds.

Methylation of only one hydroxy group catalyzed by catechol-*O*-methyltransferase occurs when there are two or more adjacent hydroxy groups on a benzene ring. Which hydroxy group is methylated depends on the other substitutions on the ring. Demethylation also occurs, this being more facile for *p*-methoxy groups than *m*-methoxy groups so that the ratio of *para*- to *meta*- in the urine is dependent on the balance between methylation and demethylation. For three adjacent hydroxy groups (pyrogallol), the center hydroxy group is methylated in rats and rabbits. If one of the "outer" hydroxy groups is converted to a methoxy, either one of the two remaining hydroxy groups may be methylated but not both. The enzyme has been detected in many tissues, including liver, heart, kidney, spleen, intestines, salivary glands, pituitary, thyroid, pineal body, aorta, central nervous system, and skin. It has been found in many animals, including the rat, cow, pig, mouse, guinea pig, cat, rabbit, and human. It is found mostly in the cytosol, but there is some activity in the microsomes.

Phenol-*O*-methyltransferase catalyzes the *O*-methylation of many alkylphenols, alkoxyphenols, and halophenols in the endoplasmic reticulum. The enzyme has been observed in the liver, lung, and other tissues.

Hydroxy indole-*O*-methyltransferase in the pineal body methylates *N*-acetylserotonin and similar substrates to melatonin.

Nonspecific *N*-methyl transferases *N*-methylate many primary and secondary amines in the cytosol of lung, liver, spleen, adrenals, and brain of chicken, rat, rabbit, mouse, guinea pig, and cat.

Phenylethanolamine *N*-methyl transferase (at least five isoenzymes) catalyzes the SAM-mediated *N*-methylation of noradrenaline to adrenaline, and the *N*-methylation of other aromatic primary and secondary amines. It has been found in the heart, kidney, brain, and adrenals.

A soluble SAM-dependent transferase methylates the *N*-hydroxy group in *N*-hydroxy-2-acetyl aminofluorene and similar compounds to a product more carcinogenic than the parent compound.

Many sulfhydryl groups are methylated by SAM-requiring thiol methyltransferase in the microsomes. There is a distinct cytosolic enzyme that *S*-methylates certain pyrimidines and thiopurines, the products being further metabolized before excretion (Section 9.3.11).

5.1.4 Acetylation

Mammals can acetylate amino, hydroxy, and thiol groups of certain endogenous compounds such as choline, coenzyme A, and amino sugars. The acetylation of xenobiotics appears primarily to occur for primary amino groups. Secondary and tertiary amino groups are not acetylated. Also, diacetyl derivatives are not produced in the urine. In the acetylation of xenobiotics, AcCoA is the acetyl donor. Transaminations occurring during metabolism allow subsequent acetylation.

Aryl amine *N*-transferase (several isoenzymes) in the cytosol catalyzes acetylation of numerous aryl amines and sulfonamides. This enzyme has been detected in the liver, gut, lung, thymus, ovary, spleen, uterus, adrenals, leukocytes, kidney, bone marrow, salivary gland, pancreas, pineal body, red blood cells, brain, and muscle; many animals possess it, including the cat, cow, horse, sheep, goat, monkey, mouse, rabbit, rat, guinea pig, and human. The capacity to acetylate varies with species and strain, and with age. This is so also for humans where it was found that normally therapeutic doses of isoniazid (fast acetylators) were toxic to certain people (slow acetylators). The gut and liver enzyme is thought to make an individual "slow" or "fast." Japanese are "fast" acetylators. Other drugs that are subject to fast or slow acetylation include Hydralazine and Procainamide.

Although acetylation often destroys the biological activity of xenobiotics, the reverse does occur also. *N*-Acetylation appears to be the first step in the conversion of aromatic amines such as 2-aminofluorene, 4-aminobiphenyl, and 2-aminonaphthalene to their ultimate carcinogens.

5.1.5 Amino Acid Conjugation

Xenobiotics that contain a carboxyl group or generate one during metabolism are often excreted as an amino acid conjugate, the most common conjugate being with glycine. Aryl and arylalkyl acids usually are excreted as amino acid conjugates at low concentrations.

In contrast to other types of conjugations, the xenobiotic itself is activated as the high energy donor (–S–CoA) via a synthetase, and the amino acid serves as the acceptor in the transferase reaction. These enzymes appear to be present in the cytosol as well as in mitochondria and in the endoplasmic reticulum. The enzyme for benzoic acid conjugation is in the mitochondria, whereas that for endogenous compounds (for example, cholyl-CoA) is in the cytosol, endoplasmic reticulum, and lysosomes.

Although glycine is the most common acceptor, conjugates with alanine, arginine, glutamic acid, glutamine, glycyltaurine, ornithine, serine, and taurine have been detected. Species variations are pronounced. Glycine conjugation predominates in the human, dog, cat, rat, rabbit, mouse, bovines, goat, sheep, pig, monkey, guinea pig, horse, camel, elephant, and some birds but not in the domestic chicken, geese, duck, and turkey. In humans and certain primates, arginine and glutamine conjugations are common. Birds and some reptiles often use ornithine as the acceptor. Taurine conjugation is common in primates.

TABLE 5.2. **Variation of amino acid conjugation (AAC) and glucuronidation (G) with animal species for some carboxylic acids in male animals.**

	Percentage urinary ^{14}C-acid conjugated					
	Rat		Ferret		Rhesus monkey	
Acid	AAC	G	AAC	G	AAC	G
Phenylacetic	100	0	84	0	91	0
1-Naphthylacetic	23	51	72	19	3	83
Hydratropic	0	64	91	5	0	76
Diphenylacetic	0	94	0	76	0	70

Adapted from reference 171.

5.1.6 Other Conjugations

Phosphate conjugation of aromatic hydroxamic acids has been postulated to produce "ultimate carcinogenic metabolites," for example, for 2-(*N*-hydroxy)-acetamidofluorene and for 2-naphthylamine initiation of bladder cancer. Though phosphate conjugation is not commonly encountered, it may be important in specific processes linked with cancer. N-acetylglucosamine and other UDP-sugars (glucose, galacturonic acid, xylose are the major ones) are known to form glycoside conjugates.

5.1.7 Animal Models as Surrogates for Humans

Tissue distribution of key conjugating systems for acetylation, amino acid conjugation, glucuronidation, glutathione conjugation, methylation, and sulfate formation in male Sprague-Dawley rats (Table 5.1) may be similar to that in humans. The kidney and the liver have all conjugating systems; the lung has all except sulfate formation and amino acid conjugation; glucuronidation is performed by all the 12 organs in Table 5.1 except the blood cells; and methylation is done by all except the bladder, gut, placenta, and thymus. The skin, brain, and adrenals can methylate and glucuronidate. Blood cells can only methylate.

As most organs can glucuronidate and conjugate amino acids, it might be expected that most animals might be uniform in these processes for structurally related carboxylic acids. This is not so for the rat, ferret, and rhesus monkey for phenylacetic, 1-naphthylacetic, hydratropic, and diphenylacetic acids (Table 5.2). If humans are more like the rhesus monkey, then the use of rat data as surrogate for human may not always be justified. The rat liver is generally used as an animal model for human liver; the ferret lung is usually used as an animal model for human lung deposition and physiology. The grossest difference between rat and rhesus monkey data is for 1-naphthylacetic acid where the monkey excretes predominantly (83%) glucuronide and very little amino acid conjugates (3%); in contrast, the rat excretes 23% amino acid conjugates and 51% glucuronides. The rat kidney also has been used as an animal model for the human kidney.

Although the rat is an adequate animal model for microsomal oxidations,

TABLE 5.3. Excretion of ^{14}C-label from trichloroethylene by various excretion routes after an acute dose of 50 mg/kg body weight through intramuscular injection to male (m) and female (f) chimpanzees, baboons, and rhesus monkeys (Rhesus) compared with human data.*

A. Urine and fecal route comparison.

	Percentage Recovery in Animal							
	Chimpanzee		Baboon		Rhesus		Human	
Excretion route	m	f	m	f	m	f	m	f
Urine	56	43	18	9	28	24	38–57	
Feces	3	0.9	6	4	8	5	2–3	
Total urine/feces	59	44	24	13	36	29	40–60	
Unaccounted	41	56	76	87	64	71	40–60	

B. Time course of trichloroacetic acid (TCA) and trichloroethanol (TCE) and their glucuronides (Glu) excretion in urine for chimpanzees.

	Percentage in Urine Relative to Urine Total							
Hours after administration	TCA		TCA–Glu		TCE–Glu		Total TCE/TCA	
	m	f	m	f	m	f	m	f
6	11	14	4	5	85	81	6	4
24	5	4	6	8	89	88	8	7
48	6	7	13	7	82	86	5	6
72	6	3	13	11	81	85	4	6
96	7	6	17	16	76	78	3	4

* Adapted from reference 27.

ascorbic acid is not a vitamin for the rat as it is in humans and guinea pigs, where it is called vitamin C. Thus glucuronidation and production of D-glucaric acid (the end product of the β-glucuronic acid pathway) are not well modelled for humans by the rat because the later products in this pathway can be converted to vitamin C in the rat but not in humans.

The comparative metabolism of ^{14}C-trichloroethylene 50 mg/kg injected intramuscularly in chimpanzees (*Pan troglodytes*), baboons (*Papio paio*), and rhesus monkeys (*Macaca mulatta*) was investigated by Muller et al. [27]. The urinary and fecal excretion routes were compared first, and these results are provided in Table 5.3A. Even among primates there were differences in the urine/fecal ratio, though the urine is always more important than the fecal route. The percent unaccounted for is probably exhaled. In exhalation and fecal excretion, the chimpanzee resembles humans more than the baboon and the rhesus monkey do. The next study involved the investigation of trichloroacetic acid, trichloroethanol, and their glucuronides in chimpanzees because the latter most approached humans (Table 5.3B). The glucuronide of trichloroethanol was the major excretion product and was the only product in feces. When fecal and urinary data were added, the excretion ratio of TCE/TCA was very similar for all three primate species, whereas this was not

TABLE 5.4. Species differences in conjugation products in urine over 24 h after administration for some related aromatic compounds—phenol, 1-naphthol, 2-naphthol, and dopamine.

Substrate	Dose (μmol/kg)	Route	Species	Gender	Percentage recovered				
					1	2	3	4	5
Phenol	266	o	cat	f	59	87	0	—	1[a]
			rat	f	95	54	42	—	2[b]
			pig	f	51	0	100	—	—
1-Naphthol	170	ip	cat	f	91	98	1	—	—
			rat	f	59	51	49	—	—
			pig	f	81	32	66	—	—
2-Naphthol	170	ip	cat	f	73	78	3	—	20[c]
			rat	f	86	43	57	—	—
			pig	f	84	6	94	—	—
Dopamine	64	o	rat	m	88	6	34	17	26[d]
			dog	f	86	71	3	16	2[d]
			rabbit	f	95	1	2	16	78[d]
			mouse	m	70	10	24	9	56[d]

Adapted from references 172 and 173.
o, oral; ip, intraperitoneal; f, female; m, male.
[a]quinol sulfate; [b]quinol conjugates; [c]hydroxynaphthyl sulfate; [d]3,4-dihydroxyphenylacetic acid.
1 signifies % ^{14}C-label recovered in 24-h; columns 2 to 5, % of total ^{14}C-label recovered in 24-h that was sulfated (column 2), glucuronidated (column 3), methylated (column 4), and other metabolites (column 5). Column 1 data for dopamine is for 72 h; column 4 data for dopamine is the sum of free and conjugated homovanillic acid.

so for urine alone. These results show that reliance on one path of excretion may not always provide consistent or interpretable results.

A similar comparison for the cat, rat, mouse, dog, rabbit, and pig for related compounds, phenol, 1-naphthol, 2-naphthol, and dopamine (Table 5.4) showed that whereas sulfation dominated in cats for the phenols and glucuronidation for the pigs, the rat excreted approximately equally through both pathways. There were no similarities for dopamine excretion among the rat, dog, rabbit, and mouse. Phenol metabolite excretion in rats was also dose-dependent. The doses in μmol/kg body weight to produce the indicated percentages of phenyl glucuronide after 2 h (always greater than 90% total recovery) were: 13, 28; 27, 34; 67, 42; 133, 50; and 266, 60. The rest of the ^{14}C-label was excreted as phenylsulfate. This showed that glucuronidation was the overflow pathway for phenol in rats.

The administration of an equal number of moles/kg is probably not the correct biological comparison because each species has a different basal metabolic rate and hence metabolism rate. Interspecies studies should involve normalized doses with respect to metabolic rate because a dose metabolized rapidly in one animal species may be capacity-limiting for another with a lower metabolic rate even if corrected for body weight. Unfortunately, few animal studies have done this. Nevertheless, it is clear that not all animals or animal strains have the same excretion profiles. Analogously, it might be expected that human ethnic groups may also show differences. The latter has been demonstrated for acetylation.

TABLE 5.5. Mono-oxygenase complex contents in several mammal strains and species.*

Species	Gender	Content in nmol/mg Microsomal Protein		
		Cyt P-450	Cyt b_5	Cyt c-reductase
SD rat	m	0.58	0.26	133
	f	0.57	0.35	124
Wistar	m	0.46	0.28	120
Pig—castrated	m	0.38	0.33	117
Mouse	m	0.48	0.20	128
Guinea pig	m	0.75	0.49	136
Rabbit	m	0.67	0.38	115
Monkey	m	0.74	0.45	130
Human, average	m	0.31	0.29	100
age 22	m	0.29	0.42	104
27	m	0.21	0.31	86
35	m	0.37	0.36	84
47	m	0.25	0.15	110
55	m	0.42	0.21	115
Literature	m	0.58	0.40	117

* Adapted from reference 28.
m, male; f, female; Cyt P-450, cytochrome P-450; Cyt b_5, cytochrome b_5; Cyt c-reductase, NADH-cytochrome c reductase; SD rat, Sprague-Dawley rat.
Relative errors in the mean were about 1 to 16%.

Cytochrome P-450 content also varies (Table 5.5) from species to species [28]. The cytochrome P-450 content in human liver microsomes is 20 to 50% lower than for Sprague-Dawley male and female rats, male Wistar rats, male castrated pigs, male mice, male guinea pigs, male rabbits, and male monkeys. There is no significant variation in microsomal cytochrome b_5. The male rabbit and humans have lower NADH–cytochrome c reductase contents compared with the other species. Aminopyrine and benzphetamine *N*-demethylase activities were similar in humans and pigs, as were benzo(a)pyrene hydroxylase activities (also in female Sprague-Dawley rats) but not 7-ethoxycoumarin deethylase and *p*-nitroanisole *O*-demethylase activities (where the rabbit is more similar to humans). For men of different ages, there is much variation in all three cytochromes (Table 5.5). It is known that the rat cannot reduce carbonyl groups to hydroxy ones as readily as can man. This could be so because the ratio between oxidation (cytochrome P-450) and reduction forms (NADH–cytochrome c reductase) is higher for the rat (0.0044) than for humans (0.0031) because the absolute amount of reductase is higher for the rat than for humans.

Generally, tissues from fetuses and very young and very old animals including humans conjugate xenobiotics less efficiently than tissues from adolescent and adult animals. Thus animal age must be carefully considered in the selection of a human model animal. Gender, species, dose, diet, enzyme inducibility (hence pretreatment or acclimation period), disease states, and environmental temperature and strain may influence conjugation. The following sections focus on the factors affecting humans.

5.2 FACTORS AFFECTING METABOLIC AND CONJUGATING RATES IN HUMANS

5.2.1 Variations in Enzymes

If a human is missing an enzyme or has an enzyme with specific activity different from that of most other people, and the enzyme is a critical one in the metabolism and excretion of a marker, the concentrations of such an affected marker will lead to a mistaken interpretation of the individual's exposure. If the elimination half-time is increased, concentrations will indicate less exposure than has happened; also, toxic effects may appear. Even in fraternal twins, the plasma half-time can vary up to one order of magnitude.

Greater variations are expected in the general population. The efficacy of medications is related to this phenomenon. Thus ethnic groups may show differences. Reactions to isoniazid, *p*-pyridinecarboxylic acid hydrazide, were as follows: rapid inactivators in Japanese, Eskimos, American Indians, Latin Americans, U.S./Canadian Caucasians, and U.S. African Americans constituted 87, 95, 77, 67, 45, and 48%, respectively, and slow inactivators were 13, 5, 22, 33, 55, and 53%, respectively. Slow metabolizers have been found for the drug Meperidine. Desipramine is cleared more slowly by Chinese than by other ethnic groups.

5.2.2 Diet

Excessive niacinamide (3–9 g/day) elevates serum glutamatic acid oxalotransaminase (SGOT) and ATPase. A high-protein diet enhances metabolism. Any deficiency in diet relative to vitamins and essential elements may affect the activity of key enzymes, leading to changes in metabolism or metabolic rate and thus a person's ability to cope with a chemical exposure. The presence in the diet of any precursor to a biological marker will affect that marker's concentration, for example, organophosphates and PCBs in food; sodium benzoate food preservative will affect urinary hippuric acid. The urine levels of hippuric acid fluctuated threefold in U.S. subjects, up to 13-fold for Japanese, and almost 40-fold in Finns, mostly because of dietary differences.

Similarly, if a chemical in the diet interacts or competes with the processes producing a marker, then the concentrations of a biological marker may not be interpretable. Analogously, the influence of fully defined diets or undefined chow diets on the toxicology of xenobiotics in animal experiments has been much discussed.

5.2.3 Enzyme Induction and Inhibition

People exposed in the past to chemicals that are metabolized through the nonspecific microsomal enzymes (for example, phenobarbital, spironolactone, alicyclic chlorinated pesticides such as chlordane, heptachlor and dieldrin, DDT, methoxychlor, polynuclear aromatic hydrocarbons, PCBs, and PBBs) may have induced the enzymes necessary to catalyze rate-determining steps of xenobiotic metabolism and hence excretion. Similarly, people may have induced their enzyme systems by exposure to mixtures of chemicals, for example, tobacco smokers, people exposed passively to tobacco smoke, and those exposed to smog. For this case, higher concentrations of urinary marker metabolites would be excreted, leading to the erroneous conclusion that overexposure had occurred. Also, if the analysis is based on unmetabolized xenobiotic, as, for example, with blood, fat, or breath analysis, the estimate of exposure would be low. This problem is especially important in medical monitoring where "normal ranges" are the reference values, as it is often unclear what critical threshold is associated with toxic effects. This same problem exists for exposure concentrations as well. Some drugs whose metabolisms are subject to enzyme induction include diazepam, valproic acid, and antiepileptic drugs.

Inhibition of the nonspecific microsomal enzymes can also occur, leading to lower concentrations of metabolite markers than expected in urine and higher concentrations than usual of xenobiotic in blood and breath. Styrene and benzene epoxidations are hindered by toluene, which successfully competes for the enzyme, allowing styrene and benzene to accumulate more than they would if it were not present. Antabuse (Disulfiram) inhibits oxidation of ethanol to acetaldehyde, causing a nausea used to manage alcoholism. Here biological monitoring markers may be in a "normal" range when in fact toxicity could be occurring. This is the hardest type of situation to interpret.

Some markers of liver microsomal enzyme activity include: plasma and saliva antipyrine (phenazone); urinary D-glucaric acid (end product of the β-glucuronic acid pathway, which is formed from free β-glucuronic acid via D-glucaro-1,4-lactone); and urinary 6-β-hydroxycortisol/17-hydroxycorticosteroids ratio. The antipyrine test is markedly affected by smoking, but the latter two tests are not.

Continued exposure to a chemical can stimulate or inhibit its own metabolism. Pretreatment with trichloroethylene can either stimulate or depress metabolism of subsequently administered trichloroethylene, depending on treatment time and dose. If the dose is high enough or of sufficient duration to destroy key enzymes, then subsequent exposure will result in lower amounts being excreted relative to the amount excreted before the damage. This example illustrates why regular monitoring is necessary for correct interpretation of biological monitoring data. In contrast, pretreatment with perchloroethylene only stimulates the metabolism of subsequent perchloroethylene exposure.

Some drugs whose half-time is increased on prolonged administration include Methotrexate and Verapamil. An example of the reverse is Rifampin.

It takes about 6 months for a new worker to induce the enzymes fully in the glutathione elimination system to produce a stable excretion rate of urinary thioethers on exposure to workplace chlorinated solvents.

5.2.4 Bound and Free Chemical in the Blood

Many chemicals are transported in the bound state as well as free. This is done by physical reversible adsorptive binding, often at several binding sites as opposed to that where covalent bonds are produced to form adducts. Generally there is binding to albumin because this is the dominant plasma protein, or secondary binding to microglobulins. The ratio of the free to the bound form varies from chemical to chemical and with the dose. The total blood concentration (bound plus free) will reflect the absorbed dose. Some of the bound form may be for storage rather than transport.

Clearance into the urine and the breath usually depends on the free concentration, as does toxicity. It is wise always to sample at the same time after exposure to make the bound and free chemical ratio and any circadian rhythms as constant as possible from sampling set to sampling set. This of course is not always possible.

Sometimes some chemicals may have more affinity for the binding sites on blood proteins than others. Some examples are: the drug phenylbutazone prescribed for arthritis and other aches and pains; medications such as aspirin and clofibrate (an anticholesteremic); or the results of massive exposures to chemicals. A genetic defect in the binding capacity of the protein or a disease state (any disease state that lowers plasma protein will increase the ratio of free to bound xenobiotic, as, for example in chronic liver disease, liver cirrhosis, rheumatoid arthritis, diabetes, essential hypertension, nephritis, peptic ulcer, and colitis) may also lower the amount bound. For these cases, the displaced chemical may be excreted faster than expected, thus producing higher concentrations than usual. However, if the key rate-determining steps are also affected, the displaced chemical may also have to wait its turn to be excreted, thus lowering the concentration relative to xenobiotic exposure alone.

5.2.5 Dose of Xenobiotic

According to Waritz, Quick reported in 1931 that high doses of benzoic acid administered to humans caused increasing amounts of urinary benzoic acid glucuronide to be excreted in addition to the hippuric acid observed at low doses. In 1942, von Oettingen et al. determined that 8 h of exposure to 300 ppm toluene caused the additional excretion of the glucuronide of benzoic acid as well as the hippuric acid observed at lower doses. In 1968, Tanada and Ikeda found that trichloroacetic acid excretion in humans after exposure to 150 ppm trichloroethylene became saturated after 8 h of exposure. In 1972, Ikeda et al. showed that trichloroacetic acid formation became saturated after exposure to 50 ppm of tetrachloroethylene for several hours. In the same year, Gotell et al. also reported that urinary concentrations of phenylglyoxylic acid peaked after exposure to styrene at 150 ppm for 8 h, and actually fell above this concentration.

These early data are enough to show that any regression equations linking concentration of biological marker with exposure dose cannot be extrapolated, only interpolated, and that they apply only for the conditions under which they were measured and sampled.

5.2.6 Competition for an Essential Enzyme

If multicomponent exposures occur of chemicals that require the same enzyme(s) for metabolism, the pattern and the rate of metabolism relative to single exposures may be drastically altered. The chemical that is preferentially metabolized will have the pattern and the rate most approaching that of single exposure. The other chemicals not preferentially metabolized have "to wait in line" or be excreted elsewhere. Life-style interactions are considered in Section 5.3.

Relative to markers of adverse effect, anything that decreases the concentration in the target organ of the toxicant molecule (whether it be the xenobiotic, a metabolite, a conjugate, or an activated intermediate) will decrease the hazard; anything that increases it increases toxicity. Interactions, therefore, are among the most important sources of variability in the interpretation of biological monitoring data. Levels deemed to be adverse or safe relative to a single chemical then may not be representative for multicomponent exposures. Thus risk assessment using such single chemical data may not be applicable either.

To facilitate interpretation of their sample results, industrial hygienists and environmental scientists always should send a list of coexposing chemicals along with the samples, a task easier and less expensive for industrial hygienists than for environmental scientists because of the existence of the relevant hazardous materials data sheets. A chemical that interacts may also have to be quantitated at the same time as the xenobiotic. Thus decisions about sampling strategy are best made by the industrial hygienist before any sampling begins, from a knowledge of what variables are important for the specific chemical. Medical personnel cannot interpret these data either without coexposure information. The compilation of a list of coexposing chemicals also helps analytical chemists to perform the analysis, a recommendation of the NIOSH *Manual of Analytical Methods*.

Interactions thus may contribute to the enormous range (at least two- or threefold differences between upper and lower limits in general) in reference ranges observed for many endogenous chemicals, a range already broad because of individual genetic variation, diet, and life-style differences. If a xenobiotic gives rise to an endogenous biological marker (essentially an interaction with an endogenous system), the concentration range expected from a particular exposure level may vary four- to sixfold.

5.2.7 Fraction Metabolized and Excreted

We have already seen how most organic solvents are not fully absorbed through the inhalation route [1], the mass fraction absorbed usually being between 60% and 70% of the mass of xenobiotic inhaled. Inert aerosols are not completely absorbed either because deposition is particle-size-dependent, and clearance depends on aerosol dose and the integrity of the clearance mechanisms. Once absorption occurs, sensitive urinary or blood detection of a marker metabolite is possible only if the fraction metabolized is high and occurs quickly (half-time less than 12 h). This will ensure a steep slope for any marker versus exposure concentration correlations, and will also offset any preexposure levels.

For example [8], methylchloroform metabolites in the urine show a dose-effect relationship up to 50 ppm for 8 h in air, but the relative standard deviation is 40% coupled with a shallow slope (0.073 to 0.28, depending on the metabolite). This makes for a weak biological marker for methyl chloroform.

In another example, styrene is less than 10% converted to hippuric acid at an exposure of 100 ppm. Dose-related hippuric acid was only excreted 24 h after exposure. Compare this with about 70% metabolism of >60 ppm toluene within a day to hippuric acid. Hippuric acid is thus a poor marker for styrene but a good one for toluene even though both may give rise to the same marker.

Metabolic rate also changes with age. Older, healthy people have been found to metabolize some medicinals at half the rate of healthy young subjects with no significant difference in absorption after oral administration. This may have something to do with hormonal (particularly thyroidal) influences although elderly people also have less appetite than young ones, which may cause metabolic rate changes.

Availability for metabolism after absorption varies with gender. The urinary half-time of total trichloro compounds after trichloroethylene or perchloroethylene exposure was almost twice as great in Japanese female workers as in males. Because both of these compounds are extremely fat-soluble, and because females have much more fat than males in general, males have more available xenobiotic in the blood for metabolism. Also, the metabolic rate may have been lower for these females than for males. However, females excreted more daily urinary trichloroacetic acid and much less trichloroethylene than did males, so that the metabolic rate probably is not a factor. This excretion occurred 24 to 36 h after exposure.

Disease and dietary deficiencies also can alter the fraction metabolized, as well as the ratio of xenobiotic bound and free. Kidney damage causing decreased renal clearance causes lower urinary and higher blood levels than those observed in healthy people. Cirrhosis of the liver decreases the efficiency of metabolism.

5.3 LIFE-STYLE FACTORS

There are five major components of life-style: (1) alcoholic beverages—general use, drinking habits, distribution places, Alcoholics Anonymous groups; (2) smoking habits—general use, smoking patterns, passive exposures; (3) life stresses—in the family, in sexual relations, at work, at social events, at play; (4) load stresses—home and material maintenance, education and surveillance of children, care of the aged, compulsory routines including work (ergonomics), traveling to and from work, repeated muscular and psychological stresses, career establishment, and coping with bureaucracies; and (5) dietary stresses. An enormous questionnaire would be required to determine the contributions of all these factors, but good epidemiological studies will attempt the task.

The major chemically related life-style factors are: use of recreational drugs; type of diet; coffee and tea consumption; alcohol drinking habits; smoking tobacco and recreational drugs; and the use of medicines and palliatives. It is recommended that if biological and environmental monitoring markers indicate a possible exposure problem, the influence of these variables for a specific chemical be evaluated by means of a questionnaire. A professional environmental hygienist needs to know about these variables before biological monitoring sampling occurs. Alcohol consumption and tobacco smoking will be considered below.

5.3.1 Alcohol

Alcohol may interact with the metabolism of many workplace chemicals. An example is the competitive excretion of methanol and ethanol [29]. The first step in Phase I metabolism, and the rate-determining step in metabolism and excretion, is oxidation to the corresponding aldehyde catalyzed by liver alcohol dehydrogenase, a zinc-containing enzyme. The enzyme has greater affinity for ethanol than methanol. Therefore, when methanol is also present, only a small amount of the methanol is dehydrogenated, and methanol circulates in the blood as free and bound stored methanol. Blood, urinary, and exhaled breath methanol levels thus are elevated over those for methanol alone. The major acute effect of methanol overexposure is eye damage, which appears to be caused by the Phase I metabolite, formic acid, rather than by methanol itself. Therefore the elevated levels of blood methanol are not biological monitoring markers for eye damage in this situation, but will be for methanol exposure alone. This illustrates how biological monitoring markers of adverse effect depend on the situation.

Another alcohol interaction occurs with trichloroethylene, where urinary trichloroethylene concentration was greater than expected in the absence of ethanol [30]. Ethanol also has been shown to interfere with the metabolism of xylene [31], styrene [32], and toluene [33] in the same manner as for methanol. However, for habitual alcohol consumers, the liver enzymes may exhibit the reverse behavior; liver cirrhosis prolongs the half-time of xeniobiotics in the body and decreases metabolite biological monitoring markers [34].

Perhaps the most famous interaction of alcohol is the one with Antabuse (Disulfiram; tetraethylthiuram disulfide). Antabuse is generally prescribed as a single oral dose of 0.5 g (approx. 7.1 mg/kg) for 1 to 2 weeks followed by 0.25 g/day (approx. 3.6 mg/kg). Rapid pulse, flushing, fall in blood pressure, breathing difficulty, and nausea are produced. At least 13 deaths (mostly from circulatory collapse or cerebral hemorrhage [35]) have occurred. Aldehyde dehydrogenase appears to be inhibited in a competitive manner. The C-to-S double bond and an α-nitrogen are essential for the interaction in the competing molecule. Disulfiram is also used in rubber vulcanization, and exposed workers who drink have also suffered the "Antabuse syndrome." The methyl ester analog is a pesticide, Thiuram. The Thiuram disulfides are components of many fungicides, insecticides, seed disinfectants, larvicides, germicidal soaps, lotions, ointments, rubber goods, and fabric finishes.

Other chemically related substances also may interact with alcohol [34], including pesticidal dithiocarbamates such as pyrazole, Ziram, and Manam; hypoglycemic sulfonylureas, and the explosive nitroglycerol. Industrial chemicals interact: amides such as dimethylformamide, *n*-butyramide, isobutyramidecylamide, cyanamide, and calcium cyanamide; oximes including *N*-butyraldoxime (also inhibits alcohol dehydrogenase), acetaldoxime, acetoxime, isobutyraldoxime, cyclohexanone oxime, and methyl ethyl ketoxime; halogenated hydrocarbons including carbon tetrachloride, trichloroethylene, chloroform, methylene chloride, and 1,2-dibromo- and dichloroethanes; metals such as cobalt (from the era when cobalt was added to beer, 1959 to 1967; the interaction caused enhanced heart disease only if a nutritional deficiency also existed [36]), manganese (ethanol enhances its absorption in rats), and mercury (methyl mercury chloride, methyl mercury acetate in rats). Acute administration of ethanol decreases clearance of pentobarbitone, meprobamate, and warfarin.

Ethanol has been linked as a cofactor in the etiology of cancer, there being more cancers in heavy drinkers than in abstainers or light drinkers. Alcohol and tobacco smoking cancer effects also interact [37]. There are few reports of interactions of alcohol with the carcinogenicity of industrial chemicals. There is a report of an interaction between ingested ethanol and inhaled vinyl chloride in rats, causing enhanced liver angiosarcoma [38].

Little research for alcohol interactions using breath analysis has been reported in spite of the massive use by the authorities of the most used breath test, the Breathalyser. The significance of breath tests will be discussed in Chapter 6.

5.3.2 Tobacco Smoke Exposures

As has been made clear by countless reports of the Surgeon General, tobacco smoke, which consists of thousands of chemicals [39], has been regarded as the chief cause of lung cancer. Suspected and known human carcinogens present in tobacco smoke include in ng/unfiltered cigarette [40]: 4-aminobiphenyl (2.4–4.6), benzene (20,000–50,000), benzo(a)pyrene (10–50), hydrazine (24–43), 2-naphthylamine (4.3–27), nickel (20–3000), particulate matter, polonium-210 (0.03–1 picoCurie), and vinyl chloride (1.3–16). Similarly, animal carcinogens also present include benz(a)anthracene (40–70), benzo(b)-fluoranthene (30), benzo(j)fluoranthene (60), benzo(e)pyrene (5–40), gamma-butyrolactone, chrysene (40–60), dibenz(a,h)acridine (0.1), dibenz(a,j)acridine (3–10), dibenzo(c,g)carbazole (0.7), dibenzo(a,i)pyrene (trace), ethylene oxide, formaldehyde (5000–100,000), indeno(1,2,3-cd)pyrene (4), 5-methyl-chrysene (0.6), 4-(methylnitroamino)-1-(3-pyridyl)-1-butanone (0–950), 2-nitropropane (0–2200), *N*-nitrosodiethanolamine (0–40), *N*-nitrosodiethyl-amine (0.1–28), *N*-nitrosodimethylamine (1–180), *N*-nitroso-ethylmethylamine (1–40), *N*-nitrosopiperidine (0–9), *N*-nitrosopyrrolidine (2–110), *N*′-nitroso-anabasine (40–400), *N*′-nitrosonornicotine (120–3700), chlorinated dibenzo-*p*-dioxins (1.81 pg toxic equivalents of the 2,3,7,8-isomer/m^3 [41]), 2-toluidine (30–160), and urethane (20–38). Unfiltered cigarettes are not much smoked nowadays, but a substantial number of people still roll their own.

The control of and exposure to environmental tobacco smoke is, and will be, the subject of legal strictures. A recent book discussed all biological monitoring aspects and interactions of environmental tobacco smoke [39]. The extent of mainstream and sidestream tobacco smoke exposures has been cofactored out by biological monitoring methods [39] such as the following: blood and urinary nicotine; urinary, serum, and saliva cotinine, the major metabolite of nicotine; blood carboxyhemoglobin and expired carbon mon-oxide; urinary, saliva, sweat, and serum thiocyanate; and urinary mutagenicity. These are the classical biological monitoring markers of exposure to tobacco products. The carboxyhemoglobin, carbon monoxide, and thiocyanate markers are related to exposure to smoke; the nicotine and cotinine markers are related more to nicotine exposure than to smoke, including chewing tobacco and nicotine chewing gum or nicotine transdermal exposures. Newer smoke markers such as hemoglobin adducts of 4-aminobiphenyl and 14 other aromatic amines in cigarette smoke [42] and of hydroxyethylvaline (formed from ethylene oxide in tobacco smoke [43]) are still in the evaluation stage and will be discussed more in Chapters 10 through 12.

Individuals with chronic lung disease such as asthma and vasomotor rhinitis are often more sensitive than healthy people to the acute irritating effects of exposure to tobacco smoke (eye irritation, nasal symptoms, headache, cough, wheezing, sore throat, and nausea) [44]. Dermal effects have also been reported [45].

Smokers metabolize many drugs more rapidly than nonsmokers, for example, theophylline, warfarin (different clearance of S^- and R^+ enantiomers), phenacetin, propanolol, imipramine, pentazocine, caffeine, and antipyrine [46]. Smoking reduced the diuretic effects of furosemide and the suppressive effect of dexamethasone on plasma corticosteroids [46].

Nonsmokers excreted urinary cotinine (the major metabolite of nicotine) more slowly than did smokers; this paralleled the increases in plasma cotinine for nonsmokers relative to smokers [47]. The half-time of cotinine in plasma for chronic smokers was 19 h compared with 50 h in nonsmokers; the corresponding data for the urine were 22 and 33 h, respectively [48]. This shows that the regression equations linking nicotine exposure concentrations to urinary cotinine cannot be used for nonsmokers, and perhaps light smokers and those passively exposed as well. The relative responses of people must be identical, in addition to there being a dose-response relationship, to enable the use of such equations. The same situation pertains in the use of the external standards method to quantitate chemicals in analytical chemistry.

The famous interaction between asbestos and smoking was first announced by Selikoff et al. in 1968 [49] even though it was known in 1935 that asbestos caused lung cancer. Smoking increased the risk of lung cancer eightfold relative to asbestos alone, and caused 92 times the risk relative to nonsmokers. Another interaction is with radon for uranium miners, where the risk of lung cancer was found to be increased fourfold relative to smokers who did not work in the mines [50]. Asbestos and smoking interact also for laryngeal cancer [51]. Rothman and Keller [52] reported a strong interaction between alcohol and smoking, attributing 76% of mouth cancer in males to the interaction; the same interaction was also observed for cancer of the esophagus [53].

Smoking may cause apparent interactions, which arise because the xenobiotic itself or a precursor of a biological monitoring marker may be present in cigarette smoke or tobacco. A famous instance is carbon monoxide in the gas/vapor part of the smoke causing elevated blood carboxyhemoglobin levels a situation that can only be corrected for by taking baseline levels before exposure to the ambient or workplace atmosphere.

5.3.3 Other Life-style Factors

Not much research has been published on the effects of daily stresses and loads on biological monitoring markers, although the influence of physical activity (Table 3.2) has been recognized to require much more research. The major impact of existential stresses and loads is on the nervous, brain, and hormone systems. The secretion and the excretion of adrenaline, noradrenaline, other catecholamines, thyroid hormones, steroids, and adrenocorticoids are related to the stress impacting an individual. This topic will be discussed further in the chapters on medical monitoring.

Further Reading

Fournier, P. E., and Thomas, G. 1988. The impact of life style factors and consumption of pharmacological drugs on toxicokinetics. In *Health Surveillance of Individual Workers exposed to Chemical Agents*, W. R. F. Notten, R. F. M. Herber, W. J. Hunter, A. C. Monster, and R. L. Zielhuis (eds.), Springer-Verlag, New York, pp. 21–30.

Kolmodin-Hedman, B. 1988. Enzyme induction: its relevance for internal exposure and health risks. In *Health Surveillance of Individual Workers exposed to Chemical Agents*, W. R. F. Notten, R. F. M. Herber, W. J. Hunter, A. C. Monster, and R. L. Ziulhuis (eds.), Springer-Verlag, New York, pp. 76–83.

Paulsen, G. D. 1980. Conjugation of foreign chemicals by animals. *Residue Reviews* **76**: 31–72.

Waritz, R. S. 1979. Biological indicators of chemical dosage and burden. In *Patty's Industrial Hygiene and Toxicology*, L. J. Cralley, and L. V. Cralley (eds.), John Wiley and Sons, New York, pp. 257–318.

6

Excretion and the Media for Biological Monitoring

6.0 GENERAL REMARKS

6.0.1 Definitions and Types of Samples

Excretion is a process whereby unwanted substances are expelled to the outside environment; for example, urination, defecation, expectoration, farting, flatulence, blowing the nose, exhalation, burping, or belching. Elimination is a similar process for an organ inside the body, as, for example, the release of bile from the gall bladder or the disappearance of a xenobiotic from blood or an organ; often metabolism and conjugation must occur before elimination of a given xenobiotic is possible. Secretion occurs from a gland whose whole function is this; for example, sebum from sebaceous glands, saliva from the salivary glands, tears from the tear glands, milk from the mammary glands, and hormones from their appropriate glands. Accretion is the accumulation of secretions and eliminations and cellular detritus in a heterogeneous single state of matter, as, for example, when sweat residue, sebum, and sloughed horn cells mix on the skin, and in ear wax. The contents of the lower bowel are an accretion just before expulsion as feces or excrement, as is the content of the urinary bladder. Seminal fluid (semen) ejaculation is not a secretion because muscles are used to effect the process even though secretory processes are involved.

For xenobiotics in all of these media, the pharmacokinetic principles as discussed in Chapter 4 apply. Urine, blood, and exhaled air are the most used specimens for routine biological monitoring. Other biological media have some serious problems: tissue biopsy is very invasive; external contamination limits the interpretation of hair, nails, sputum, saliva, and sebum results; inconvenience hinders obtaining and analyzing feces, tears, sweat, flatulence, teeth, belches, other body involuntary emissions, nasal accretions, milk, and semen.

Matrix effects make analyses difficult for xenobiotics and their metabolites in sebum, teeth, semen, and feces. As a result, dose-effect relationships also are insufficient for many of these media, and they do not necessarily provide results that are consistent with those from blood, urine, or breath.

Nevertheless, if any of these excretion processes are markedly increased, the biological marker under study may also be involved, and concentrations in the media sampled will be influenced because all of these processes are concurrent and competing. Thus monitoring of just one biological medium may not be sufficient to interpret the biological monitoring data. The concentration of a marker in the medium will change with the excretion rate of the medium from the excretory organ because little elimination into the excretory medium usually occurs after the excretory organ. If this rate is intrinsically slow, as is the case with nails, hair, ear wax, teeth, or sebum, negligible dilution effects will occur although accumulation will result in specific parts of these media, as, for example, in the segments of a growing hair shaft and in the growing parts of bone and teeth that are exposed. In breath analyses, the subject usually is sedentary, a condition that does not increase respiratory volume. However, excretion rates of liquids can vary enormously; for example, in sweating, saliva formation, lactation, tearing, and urination. The effect of dilution has to be corrected for in all these fluids. The circulatory system generally has a characteristic constant volume in a healthy person, but the rates of disappearance and appearance of markers in the blood and plasma generally depend on the chemical and the particular kind of homeostasis operating for each person. Cumulative sampling minimizes the dilution effect, such as 24-h urine collections or composite collections of blood relative to spot samples. The situation is analagous to time-weighted average air sampling versus direct reading and grab air sampling in environmental analyses.

As the dosage of the xenobiotic increases, its initial rate of elimination may decrease. This behavior is called saturation or Michaelis–Menton kinetics (see Section 1.10) and usually involves enzymic factors. Biotransformations and active transport processes have finite capacities and can be saturated; so critical threshold concentrations for exposure and internal concentrations exist for every chemical. The transition from pseudo first-order kinetics to saturable (zero-order) kinetics may herald the onset of adverse (toxic) events. Some characteristics of saturable kinetics include: the AUC method (Chapter 4) does not provide results related to absorbed dose; the ratios and identities of metabolites may change from those at lower doses; competitive inhibition effects suddenly appear; the rate of production of metabolites from low doses suddenly becomes constant beyond a critical exposure dose (zero-order kinetics); and the slope increases on dose-response curves.

Some specific examples are as follows: Benzoic acid and toluene at low doses are both metabolized to produce hippuric acid in the urine. At high doses, the glucuronide also is detected. Trichloroethylene similarly is metabolized and excreted as trichloroacetic acid in the urine; the acid concentration plateaus after 150 ppm vapor inhalation for 8 h. The acid concentration decreases after 8 h of exposure at air levels greater than 150 ppm.

It is recommended whenever any biological monitoring is to be used that the donors be educated on the sampling process and on any special behavior expected, as, for example, fasting times and sampling durations, how to sample and store the media, how to cooperate during blood and breath sampling, and why the sampling is being done. The way that the results are to be interpreted should be explained, with assurances given that any unusual concentrations will be reported to the worker with a possible interpretation.

6.0.2 Factors Required to Interpret Biological Monitoring Data

Interpreters of biological monitoring data must know what factors influence their marker, and how and in what time scale these factors affect the marker's excretion rate. Some of these factors have already been discussed, in the sections on absorption (Chapter 3), distribution (Chapter 4), and metabolism (Chapter 5). Important factors include the following: diet (high-protein diets enhance metabolism in humans; the presence of vitamin C in foods will enhance iron absorption and enhance defense mechanisms in the immune system; vegetarians often lack essential elements and vitamins and may be particularly susceptible to the toxic effects of chemicals; children have different nutritional requirements from adults, as have the elderly); induction of rate-limiting enzymes (interactions between ethanol and methanol, trichloroethylene and ethanol, and ethanol and Antabuse); incidence and intensity of cigarette smoking and passive tobacco smoke exposures (the rate-limiting metabolizing enzymes of the liver may be stimulated or inhibited); the taking of drugs (which can inhibit or induce rate-limiting enzymes; for example, penicillamine used to treat Wilson's disease and schizophrenia increases urinary copper, as does Antabuse for alcoholics); home and ambient exposures (blood carboxyhemoglobin may have a high workplace preexposure level because of exposure to carbon monoxide from gas heaters in homes, from automobile exhaust on highways, from the interiors of faulty cars, from exposure to tobacco smoke, or from methylene chloride–based paint strippers used in homes or for hobbies); past history (past exposures can depress or stimulate the xenobiotic's own metabolism; slow release from a storage reservoir such as bone or fat that was filled by previous exposures may increase the apparent concentration of recent exposure, as in blood lead, cadmium, stontium, fluoride, and PCB concentrations); allergies (a small but still substantial fraction of the population is hypersensitive to many chemicals and shows adverse effects at very low exposures compared with most of the population; thus biological monitoring data for these people may not show a dose-response relative to adverse effects, and the dose-response relative to environmental exposure is very different for them); life-style (exposures at discos, hobby sites, recreational facilities, sports venues, and alcohol drinking establishments); specificity [toluene, benzoic acid, quinic acid (the last two are found in coffee, prunes, plums, and cranberries), sodium benzoate (a food preservative), and *n*-propylbenzene all metabolize to hippuric acid]; effects of dilution (as in all spot samples of fluids); absorption differences (Chapter 3); and human factors.

The last element, human factors, can include: genetics, stress, circadian rhythms (need to take samples at the same time of the week to counter this effect), age (children, adults, and the aged may absorb, process, and excrete chemicals with different efficiency), gender (females retain total trichloro compounds from tri- and tetrachloroethylene twice as long as males), disease (presence of HIV-1 and HIV-2 infection, hepatitis, etc.), physical activity during exposure as shown in Table 3.2 (workers in hot, strenuous conditions will show greater uptake of any xenobiotic than under sedentary conditions, and hence greater concentrations than expected might appear in biological monitoring media), and race (sickle cell factor in African Americans; Asians are fast acetylators relative to Caucasians). All of these factors may influence the half-time of chemicals in body fluids. Table 6.1 summarizes half-times for some chemicals and their markers in various biological media.

Personal baseline data also are required before any interpretation of biological monitoring data can be made. That is, at least two and preferably more data points are necessary to determine whether a statistically significant change has occurred or not for samples collected before and during/after exposure. The minimum number of samples for a marker of defined half-time really is three: one before exposure, one near or begun just after the end of exposure, and another 3.3 half-times after exposure and before the next exposure sequence to confirm that the baseline has not changed. This mimics the procedure followed when pumps used to sample workplace air are checked for calibration before and after sample collection but also are monitored during the exposure. If the marker's half-time is not known, it is necessary to define the elimination/excretion curve to be able to interpret what is happening and to estimate a half-time. Practically, this means that each biological sample should be collected, stored, and analyzed separately in a research situation. The inconvenience and the expense of this approach mean that in nonresearch situations some kind of composite sample will be taken, the meaning of its results being difficult to interpret. Unfortunately, when multicomponent chemicals interact at the same receptor sites or saturate enzyme systems prematurely, the "known" half-lives may suddenly become unreliable, and the elimination/excretion curve still needs to be defined in order for one to interpret the data. For workplaces with stable chemical and physical factor/physical stress regimes, it is likely that reproducible and valid results can be obtained on experienced workers. All other situations require greater professional judgment to interpret results.

Initially, therefore, several samples should be collected over equal time durations with the first and last sample analyzed to assess whether the baseline has changed. Practically, this reduces to collecting and analyzing each biological sample. The amount excreted over the entire period can be found by addition of the marker mass of each sample relative to the cumulative volume. The time of urine sampling can be set by selection of a time at which some fraction of the marker, for example, 90% or 50%, is reproducibly excreted by several workers in an exposed group. Often the worker with the highest environmental exposure is the best one to conduct this procedure on, if funds and time are limited. It is much easier to interpret results for the industrial environment, where many of the exposing chemicals are known through labels and hazardous materials data sheets, than in the ambient environment, where the chemicals involved generally are unknown.

A recent study by this author and others showed that the use of biological monitoring "exposure" data without baseline correction for markers that have endogenous levels may lead to spurious results [54]. Some markers for which

TABLE 6.1. Half-times for selected xenobiotics.

Chemical	Fluid	Marker	Half-time (h)
Aniline	urine	total *p*-aminophenol	4.0
Benzene	urine	total phenol	5.7
	breath	benzene	30.0
Cadmium	urine	total cadmium	20 y
	blood	total cadmium	100 d
Carbon disulfide	urine	2-thiothiazolidine-4-carboxylic acid	5.0
Carbon monoxide	blood	carboxyhemoglobin	5.0
	breath	carbon monoxide	5.0
Chromium [VI]	urine	chromium	7, 15–30 d, 3–5 y
Dimethylformamide	urine	*N*-methylformamide	4.0
Ethylbenzene	urine	mandelic acid	4.0
	breath	ethylbenzene	48.0
Fluorides	urine	fluoride	4–7, weeks, years
Furfural	urine	total furoic acid	2.0
n-Hexane	urine	2,5-hexanedione	15.0
	breath	*n*-hexane	0.25
Lead	blood	total lead	900.0
		zinc protoporphyrin	500.0
	urine	total lead	700.0
Methanol	urine	methanol	1.5–2.0
		formic acid	2.5–>5
Methemoglobin inducers	blood	methemoglobin	6–24
Methyl chloroform	breath	methyl chloroform	32.0
	urine	trichloroacetic acid	72.0
		total trichloroethanol	12.0
	blood	total trichloroethanol	12.0
Methyl ethyl ketone	urine	methyl ethyl ketone	4.0
Nitrobenzene	urine	total *p*-nitrophenol	86.0
	blood	methemoglobin	6–24
Organophosphate pesticides	red blood cells	cholinesterase	700.0
Parathion	urine	total *p*-nitrophenol	7.0
	red blood cells	cholinesterase	700.0
Pentachlorophenol	urine	total pentachlorophenol	700.0
	plasma	free pentachlorophenol	700.0
Perchloroethylene	breath	perchloroethylene	96.0
	blood	perchloroethylene	96.0
	urine	trichloroacetic acid	80.0
Phenol	urine	total phenol	3.5
Styrene	urine	mandelic acid	4.0
		phenylglyoxylic acid	7.0
	breath[a]	styrene	0.25, 20
	blood	styrene	0.5, 13
Toluene	urine	hippuric acid	1.5
	venous blood	toluene	0.5
	breath	toluene	0.5
Trichloroethylene	urine	trichloroacetic acid	75.0
	blood	total trichloroethanol	12.0
	breath	trichloroethylene	30.0
Xylenes	urine	methylhippuric acids	3.6

Breath markers were all end-exhaled air except for breath[a], which is mixed-exhaled. The markers are given in the order of reliability. Single half-times are α-phase; a second number in the half-times column signifies β-phase. Half-times are from reference 8.

this procedure is relevant are: red blood cell/serum acetylcholinesterase, metals, enzymes, and red blood cell carboxyhemoglobin; and urinary thioethers, D-glucaric acid, porphyrins, and hippuric acid. Baseline monitoring is also essential when it is necessary to prove that a specific site is causing an exposure. When doing biological monitoring for the very first time on individuals, one must take personal baseline samples to be able to assess if there are other environments that may interfere. For example, phenol is found in many cough lozenges, cleaners, smoked meats, tobacco smokes, mouthwashes, ointments, analgesics, and drugs such as salol, zinc phenylsulfonate, and phenobarbital; and the amount of phenol absorbed from these sources may be mistakenly thought to be of workplace origin from workplace phenol or benzene if a prework sample is not collected and analyzed. Baseline monitoring also is essential to correct for any holdover from past exposures.

In addition, the environments where the biological monitoring sample was taken and where the person was within 3.3 half-times of the marker to be measured should be characterized relative to their physical and chemical makeup, so that the biological monitoring data can be interpreted. Some of these data may be impossible to amass, but much information can be obtained by the design of an appropriate questionnaire to indicate if further information or environmental sampling are necessary.

However, if one is interested in the total absorbed dose from all sources and routes, biological monitoring data do provide that information. Provided that the sample was collected at a representative time in the correct manner and duration, transported properly, and analyzed correctly, one can say that human absorption of a precursor of the marker or of the marker itself, at some time in the past, has occurred. Its further interpretation relies on one's knowing how exposure occurred relative to a potential source, when, under what conditions, and for how long. The influence of the factors discussed above also must be weighed.

6.0.3 Personal versus Group Comparisons

The exposure versus nonexposure group comparison is the basis of epidemiological investigations, a comparison that is dependent on there truly being nonexposure, and on the interindividual variability of both groups being described by the same type of statistical distribution. The amount of variation in the "unexposed" group determines the significance of the marker levels observed for the exposed group.

Taking account of personal baselines involves performing an "exposure versus nonexposure" comparison at the level of each individual, similar to a paired Student's t-test, which is used precisely for those cases where there is much interindividual variability. For such paired data, the distribution of the differences also must be determined for group comparisons. Both uncorrected and baseline-corrected data can be transformed to a known distribution to allow use of parametric statistics. Otherwise, nonparametric statistics must be used, for example, the Kolgomorov–Smirnov statistic.

Industrial and environmental hygienists monitor specific persons first and foremost, whereas epidemiologists study exposed and "nonexposed" groups. The two perspectives do not conflict if negligible marker is excreted in "unexposed" persons, for example, urinary mutagens. However, very different results may be obtained with respect to "exposed" results corrected for the personal baseline if there is a large, variable baseline level in the "unexposed" population [54].

6.0.4 Uses and Disadvantages of Biological Monitoring

Some uses of biological monitoring include: indication of unsuspected exposures, of unexpected routes of exposure, of atypical people, of people with metabolic abnormalities, and of interactions among chemicals for multicomponent exposures as compared with single chemicals; physician guidance on administration of medications when known interactions may occur; documentation of overexposure or acceptable exposure; preemployment screens; validation of personal, grab, or area monitoring; integration of multicomponent exposures for screening markers; accumulation of data to distinguish deviations due to exposure on a personal or a group basis; drug monitoring; and elucidation of predictive markers of adverse effect.

Some of the disadvantages are as follows: the appearance of the marker may occur after organ or tissue damage; the marker may not be specific; there may be a dependence on time for the marker to appear, thus making cause-and-effect difficult to assign; the concentration of the marker may not be related to the absorbed dose; interindividual, gender, ethnic, age, life-style, physical activity, and nutritional differences may make group comparisons difficult; the recommendations to perform biological monitoring, sample collection, sample transport, sample storage, and sample chemical analysis must be done by the appropriate professionals, so making biological monitoring an expensive proposition; and there are legal issues concerning personal rights associated with biological monitoring.

6.0.5 Sampling, Storage, and Transport of Biological Media

Representative biological specimens must be collected and sampled at the correct time and duration with a standardized technique. If the sample is not taken correctly, the analysis, however good, will be for naught. If the sample is not taken at the correct time and for the correct duration, the results may not be interpretable. The sampler also must communicate with the laboratory doing the analysis to determine special precautions, to ascertain the required quality assurance samples (for example, blank containers), to know if the laboratory supplies specialized sampling and shipping containers or if the sampler has to do that, and to note and transmit to the laboratory the names of any other chemicals, processes emitting chemicals, or combustion engine proximity to the sample. The method of cleaning containers also should be ascertained, and blank containers are essential to verify if the cleaning procedure has been adequate.

An important step is to acquire and to read through a laboratory's recommended sampling methodology. If there is time, a sample of the matrix that has a known composition should be sent to the laboratory for analysis to see if the laboratory performs well, or such a sample should be included with the actual samples.

All hand contact with sampling containers should be minimized. The correct kind of gloves (check chemical degradation and permeation characteristics) should be worn, with the hands and the arms cleaned with soap and water. The sampling instructions may require rinsing of the container with the sample fluid, or that the sampled person refrain from eating and drinking for a specified time before the sample is taken. Labeling of sample containers is important: use only unique descriptors that include the time, the date, the sample type, and a unique number that has meaning only to the sampler; and never use water-soluble inks or labels backed with water-soluble glue. Sample containers should not be filled to the top if they are to be frozen because aqueous solutions expand on freezing, so breaking the container. Screw-cap lids (Teflon-lined if possible) should be used in preference to snap-on ones. Seal all caps and labels on. If the bottle is glass, bind it with masking or duct tape to hold it together should breakage occur on transport, storage, or refrigeration. Each sample should be individually wrapped in aluminum foil to negate any photochemical effects. Brown bottles may be recommended for environmental samples.

Transport, storage, and chemical analysis must be characterized by a chain-of-custody documentation. Special containers may be necessary that allow ice (0°C) or dry ice (−70°C) to be used. Coolants may have to be ordered. Always notify the laboratory that a sample is coming, and give it the avenue of shipping and the date shipped. Many samples require special packing or may break if poorly protected from the coolant. One must not assume that a package will not be inverted, even if "This way up" or "Fragile" is written on it; therefore, one must remember to insulate the samples on all sides including the lid side. Shipping may require adherence to Department of Transportation regulations, depending on the size and the toxicity involved. Send the samples for analysis as soon as possible, and know the correct storage conditions pending shipping.

Laboratory personnel must check the received shipment for completeness and sample condition (note broken vials, thawed samples, labels off, etc.), and also must note the date and the time of receipt, and who is making these entries. The sample must be stored in racks without removal of the aluminum foil coverings, and analyzed within the prescribed time (generally within three days of sampling if liquid).

Much biological sample handling now is tied to whether the AIDS or HIV status is known for the source. The minimum safety precautions include: no hand-to-mouth contact, eating, drinking, or smoking in the laboratory; no pipetting by mouth; cleaning and disinfecting work areas and instruments after use; working in a biohazard hood if possible (mandatory for infectious agents); wearing the correct kind of gloves based on chemical degradation and permeation resistance characteristics, as well as laboratory wear such as suitable coats; wearing safety glasses with side-shields and also hair nets; and regularly cleaning all laboratory wear and laboratories. Also, cancer and infectious agent handling may require an air-locked laboratory and glove-box handling. There must be a written safety and chemical disposal program, including storage and transport, labeling, and RCRA testing for all medical and solid waste. Blood and tissues have the greatest hazard potential; serum-derived fluids—for example, urine, sweat, and saliva—are less hazardous because large molecules and cellular elements have been filtered out. However, all chemicals and biological samples should be *handled with care*, as if they were dangerous (Chapter 18).

6.0.6 Analytical Chemistry Methods

Standardized analytical chemistry methods that feature rigorous quality assurance and control must be used. Unless all the sample is used in the analysis, gentle mixing must be done before the sample is taken for analysis because most biological media are suspensions rather than solutions. The calculations for extrapolating from the mass in the volume analyzed assume homogeneity, as they involve multiplying the mass found from a calibration curve by the inverse fraction of the volume analysed relative to the total volume. Thus the duration and the strength of shaking must be optimized initially. The initial volume and mass must be measured. Initially it is best to define a "soluble" fraction (one that passes through a 0.45-μm-pore filter) and a solids fraction (the solid residue after filtration to obtain the soluble fraction), and do analyses on both. Sometimes the sample must be dried to constant weight (for example, tissues to be analyzed for metals).

The analytical chemistry methods used to quantitate markers sensitively are generally complicated, and involve cleanup and chromatography for organics and anions and digestion followed by atomic absorption/emission spectroscopy for metals. The preliminary cleanup and chromatography must be done by skilled personnel.

Chromatography/mass spectrometry is generally essential for confirmation of the identity of organic components. The latter is an expensive technique; so screening with the chromatographic technique in tandem with the appropriate detector should be performed to define which samples require confirmation. This cuts costs markedly. Colorimetric methods and spot tests are generally less specific than those with chromatographic steps.

In comparing the results of different studies, analytical differences may account for any discrepancies as well as the biological variables. It is wise to compare only those studies that utilize the same analytical technique, but this is not always possible.

Problems often arise in analyzing biological monitoring media that contain many compounds, for both "unexposed" and "exposed" samples. This background often has components with the same retention time as the desired marker. In methods development, one needs a baseline sample to be able to optimize cleanup, and resolution on chromatographic columns in addition to recovery experiments over the concentration range of interest [commonly up to ppm (mg/L) concentrations]. The recovery experiments *must* be done with the chemical form of the marker in the medium, not just the free form. If methods of external standards (calibration with known masses of the marker) or of standard additions (addition of at least three known masses similar to the suspected mass of the marker to account for matrix effects; the linear regression line must have the same slope as an external standards slope before extrapolation to zero dependent variable is valid) are not practical, the use of an appropriate internal standard often is recommended. The internal standard must partition and behave exactly like the desired marker does and yet be resolvable. A better procedure is to add the internal standard to the final sample to be analysed.

Gas chromatography (GC) and liquid chromatography (LC) with the appropriate detectors are screening methods that provide maximum concentrations as long as the analytical steps are performed competently along with quality control and assurance. The latter often involves running high and low spikes, simulation samples, controls, and blanks for every ten samples.

Most of the data in the biological monitoring field are of the screening type, especially for organics where no chromatography/mass spectroscopy analysis is usually done because of cost. The detector utilized in these screening techniques depends on the sensitivity desired, such as: electron capture and Hall conductivity GC detectors for halogenated volatiles at picogram (pg) levels; flame GC photometric detectors for S, N, and halogen–containing volatiles; flame ionization GC detectors for volatile hydrocarbons at the nanogram (ng) level; ultraviolet LC detectors at specific wavelengths for compounds of high molar absorptivity for ng levels; fluorescence LC detection for fluorescent compounds at femtogram (fg) levels; electrochemical LC detectors for pg detection of catecholamines; ion chromatography for anions and cations at the ng level; specific ion electrodes for cations and anions; and so on. As most metal determinations involve digestion before analysis, total metal invariably is reported, and the original speciation is lost. This explains why most regulations for metals are written in terms of total metal. An exception occurs if a species is known to be more toxic; for example, chromium (VI) relative to chromium (III) for carcinogenicity.

Cleanup methods before GC/LC/detector quantitation vary, depending on the complexity of the matrix and the sensitivity desired. Biological media with plasma as the ultimate source, such as urine, sweat, saliva, and tears, or breath samples require less cleanup than complex matrices such as blood, plasma, bile, fat, hair, sebum, ear wax, and feces. The greater the sensitivity required, the more likely it is that there will be resolution problems and complex cleanup schemes. Laboratories and glassware must be ultraclean to achieve high sensitivity. A book has been published about all these techniques as they are used in biological monitoring [55], and selected U.S. EPA [56] and NIOSH [57] methods are also available.

6.1 BLOOD

6.1.1 Physiology

Blood consists of a heterogeneous mixture of specific cells (red blood cells, white blood cells or leukocytes, neutrophils, and granulocytes) suspended in an aqueous, straw-colored solution of electrolytes, nonelectrolytes, and macromolecules (including albumin, carrier proteins, and lipids) called the plasma. Turbulent flow in the circulatory system caused by the heartbeat and peristaltic waves in the arterial system and nervous system constriction and dilation for the venous system maintain the suspension. Plasma without fibrinogen (molecular weight 340,000), the clear solution after clotting, is called serum; the cells plus fibrinogen are a clot.

Anticoagulants stop clotting in several ways: the anticoagulant binds calcium (as for oxalates, citrates, or disodium EDTA); it may inactivate thrombin and thromboplastin like heparin; or it may defibrinate (conversion of fibrinogen to fibrin), as for the surfaces of glass beads. Soluble clotting factors (Factors VIIc, VIIIc, and fibrinogen) in the blood itself have been linked to ischemic heart disease [58]. In the laboratory, blood is allowed to stand in its tube or be centrifuged at 1500*g* so that the packed cells separate from the plasma. The ratio of packed cell volume to total blood volume is the hematocrit. Cells occupy 40 to 50% of the blood in males and 37 to 47% in females. When the red blood cells leak or lyse, hemolysis is said to occur. This can be triggered through a change of osmotic strength as with the addition of water; through the addition of detergents; through agitation; through temperature changes; through insufficient anticoagulant; and through radiation treatment. For males, the blood volume is 75 mL/kg body weight; for females, it is 67 mL/kg. More discussion of the medical monitoring characteristics of blood is given in Sections 9.0 and 9.1; the xenobiotic and its interaction with blood are the focus here.

6.1.2 Distribution of Xenobiotics

Chemicals need not be distributed equally between the cellular elements and the plasma. Thus lead is found mostly in the red blood cells and very little in the plasma. Cholinesterases in the two fractions are very different. Hexavalent chromium easily crosses cellular membranes, but trivalent chromium does not. Benzene is equally distributed, but its metabolite phenol is found only in the plasma. PCBs are found mostly in the plasma. The xenobiotic may be present free, bound to proteins, or conjugated. There may be several bound and conjugate forms. Thus phenols and trichloroethanol are conjugated as glucuronides and sulfates. Hemoglobin adducts (Chapters 10 and 12) may be formed in red blood cells, and DNA adducts (Chapter 11) may be present in lymphocytes (but not red cells because they have no nuclei). The concentration units for blood are conventionally given as g/dL where dL is deciliter (that is, 100 mL).

6.1.3 Sampling, Storage, and Transport

Blood monitoring is invasive, painful, and best avoided for regular sample collection in this age of AIDS (always use sterile needles!). Only medical personnel should sample blood.

The skin is usually cleaned with an isopropyl alcohol–soaked swab before blood is taken. Although plastic vessels are good if analysis for metals is desired, these containers cannot be used if organic analysis is required because of the presence of plasticizers, which interfere with GC/HPLC/MS analyses. Thus acid-washed glassware (soaked overnight in 10% nitric acid, rinsed copiously with distilled water, and dried, with anticoagulant added) is essential for both organic and inorganic analyses of blood in glass containers. Sometimes chromic acid cleaning is required.

An anticoagulant such as tetrasodium EDTA or heparin should be used in a container that should not adsorb the xenobiotic; the lid or top should not contain leachable impurities—so include a blank tube with the same volume of distilled water as that of the sample with each batch of samples. To prevent coagulation, the blood must be gently rolled 10 to 20 times to mix the anticoagulant, allowing as little as possible to touch the caps.

Whole blood or serum samples are obtained by venipuncture. Whole blood is collected in a vacuum-collection tube of 15 mL volume containing the anticoagulant; for example a "lavender top" Vacutainer™. Blood for serum samples must be collected in vacuum-collection tubes with no anticoagulants; for example, "red top" Vacutainers™. The blood is allowed to clot for 30 min at room temperature, the tubes are centrifuged at 1500*g* for 15 to 20 min, and the separated serum is transferred with a disposable pipette to a clean container with a screw cap that has a Teflon liner. Samples should be kept at refrigerator temperature for 1 h and then frozen at −20°C until analysis or transport/analysis. Empty vacuum-collection tubes and containers should be analyzed as blanks.

Immediate storage after sampling of whole blood is recommended at 4°C; freezing causes hemolysis. If distribution data between red blood cells and plasma are required, no hemolysis must occur. The blood sample should not be centrifuged, but should be allowed to separate over a period of hours in a sterile, dark environment. Blood samples easily hemolyze if not properly collected, transported (just above the freezing point to inhibit bacterial growth and to retain volatiles), or stored (at 4°C for as short a time as possible for whole blood; freezing can be done once the blood components are separated).

6.1.4 Analytical Chemistry

Often analysis of blood components requires extensive method development because of the presence of interfering or obscuring peaks in samples from "unexposed" people or in baseline samples. Whole blood often is preferred as the analyte when the distribution between plasma and cellular elements is unknown. Thus semivolatile nonpolar organochlorines including pesticides at ppb levels in 3-g blood samples have been extracted with hexane, concentrated, and analyzed by gas chromatography with electron capture and mass spectrometric detection [59]. Backgrounds in "unexposed" people had peaks no greater than 5% of full scale at the retention times of interest, with detection limits arbitrarily defined as peaks greater than 10% of full scale. Recoveries varied from >72% for simple chlorinated hydrocarbons to >36% for the pesticides above 1 ppb. Hexachlorocyclopentadiene reacted or decomposed in blood. The sample storage duration was a major factor in the recoveries of the chlorinated pesticides. All blood and reagent blank samples analyzed contained phthalate ester plasticizers; all blood samples contained butylated hydroxytoluene (a food preservative antioxidant), tris-2-butoxyethylphosphate (from Vacutainers™), cholesterol, and other natural steroids (natural blood constituents). Some "unexposed" bloods also showed dichlorobenzene isomers, hexachlorobenzene, heptachlor epoxide, *trans*-nonachlor, *p,p′*-DDE (major storage metabolite and degradation product of *p,p′*-DDT) and tri- through hexachlorobiphenyls (PCBs).

Although the analysis of nonpolar halogenated and unhalogenated compounds in blood is relatively interference-free because there are few nonpolar naturally occurring low molecular weight compounds and because specific detectors can be utilized for these xenobiotics, analysis for organic acids in plasma is fraught with difficulty. Most human fluids apart from urine have proteins that contain bound smaller molecules including carboxylic acids, the near-ultimate oxidation products of Phase I metabolism (Section 2.13.1). The degradation of proteins unlooses large amounts of polar and nonpolar compounds that may totally obscure any peaks due to small carboxylic acids.

Oleate replacement ultrafiltration was used to replace organic acids bound to plasma albumin with subsequent separation by ultrafiltration and with the formation of oxime derivatives, which were then concentrated by anion exchange chromatography and eluted and trimethylsilylated before capillary GC/MS using tropic acid as an internal standard [60]. The most abundant acids detected were: phosphoric, uric, citric, glucose-oxime, hexuronic, and citric acid and glycolytic cycle acids, in that order. Lactic acid was also a major component but also occurred in blanks. Aspirin users were easily recognized because of their high *o*-hydroxybenzoic acid concentrations.

Polyserositic patients (having a genetic disease of Sephardic Jews and some Arabs and Armenians) exhibited large concentrations of pyruvic acid and lower citric acid than normal. Diabetics showed high concentrations of lactic acid, 3-hydroxybutyric acid, and sugar acids. Only nine people were sampled in this study, so it is difficult to come to general conclusions.

Inorganic species in the blood can be divided into macroelements (greater than 10 ppm) and microelements (Table 6.2). The macroelements are, in mg/L [61]: calcium, 58–78; carbon 250–360, as carbonate/bicarbonate anions; chloride, 2590–3290; iron, 301–530 (mostly in the red blood cells); magnesium, 27–46; phosphorus, 311–510, as dihydrogen phosphate/monohydrogen phosphate anions; potassium, 1450–1920; sodium, 1710–2050; and sulfur, 1680–1930, as sulfate/bisulfite (Schiff bases). These species are present as ions except for iron and sulfur. Microelements, which also include all the toxic elements, usually are chelated or complexed with an organic species, quite often a specific carrier protein or amino acid. Potassium ion prefers singly charged oxygen donors or neutral oxygen ligands; magnesium, calcium, and manganese divalent ions are bound by carboxylate, phosphate, and nitrogen donors, but calcium has less affinity than magnesium for nitrogen donors, phosphate, and other multidentate anions; divalent iron prefers sulfhydryl groups and amino groups and, to a lesser extent, carboxylates; trivalent iron and trivalent cobalt are bound by carboxylates, tyrosine, amino groups, and porphyrins; copper monovalent ions and molybdenum and cadmium divalent ions prefer sulfhydryl groups; copper divalent ions are bound by amines and to a lesser extent carboxylates; zinc divalent ions prefer imadazoyl- and cysteinyl- groups. Under the usual pH 7.4 conditions, the naturally occurring L-α-amino acids can chelate metal ions through coordinate links to produce stable five-membered rings. The elemental contents of whole blood, red blood cells, blood plasma, and blood serum have been compared in Table 6.2 by using many different measurement techniques [61].

Simple peptides without side chains will chelate metal ions less strongly than peptides with side chains. Side chains on peptide and protein backbones dominate any chelation of metals for these species. Trivalent manganese, chromium, and iron ions are transported in the blood by transferrin. Selenium as selenite is bound to plasma albumin (like divalent nickel, cadmium, and zinc

TABLE 6.2. Comparison of the content of elements (E) in whole blood (WB), red blood cells (RBC), blood plasma (BP), blood serum (BS), sweat (SW), tears (T), and saliva (SA).*

	Concentration in μg/L					
E	WB	RBC	BP	BS	SW[c]	SA
Ag	3.4–120	4.3–15	3.6–44	2.9–200	—	—
Al	100–720	64–4600	280–410	110–780	—	—
As	2.5–190	2.7	2.4	20–43	—	—
Au	0.042–0.42	0.8	0.06	0.08	—	—
B	40–740	—	120	—	—	—
Ba	41–95	7	50–66	25–80	—	—
Be	<0.1–3.8	—	<4	—	—	—
Bi	<2–23	—	<0.6	<10	—	—
Br	1.3–8.1[a]	1450	3.1–13[a]	1.04–7.5[a]	0.2–0.5	0.2–2.3[a]
Ca	58–78[a]	0.63–5.2[a]	89–106[a]	92–109[a]	4–206	52–64[a]
Cd	1.1–7.4	—	2.6	2.3–12	—	—
Ce	<2	—	—	—	—	—
Cl	2590–3290[a]	1760–2477[a]	3260–4280[a]	2940–4120[a]	1054–2041	208–1203[a]
Co	0.3–99	0.16–86	0.07–12	0.22–14	—	—
Cr	6.5–107	19–66	26–164	2–20	—	—
Cs	3–4.7	—	3.1	1.3–60	—	—
Cu	640–1280	750–1310	610–1410	970–1640	0.06–1.48	26–320
Dy	<8	—	<2	<100	—	—
Er	<8	—	<6	<30	—	—
Eu	<4	—	<4	<200	—	—
F	1.9–1160	0.45	23–370	19–35	0.2–2.0	80–250[c]
Fe	301–530[a]	985–1140[a]	710–1270	870–1870	0.46–1.5	—
Ga	<80	—	0.21	<40	—	—
Gd	<8	—	<2	<100	—	—
Ge	440–5000	650	<30	<40–290	—	—
Hf	<6	—	<2	<200	—	—
Hg	<5–20	7–50	2–11	12	—	—
Ho	—	—	<2	<200	—	—
I	15–72	—	58–85	45–100	0.01	100–102
In	—	—	<4	<80	—	—
Ir	<4	—	—	—	—	—
K	1450–1920[a]	3030–4230[a]	137–208[a]	160–211[a]	176–350	—
La	—	—	<6	0.44	—	—
Li	3–38	28	30	8–27	—	—
Lu	—	—	<0.6	<50	—	—
Mg	27–46	41–68[a]	13–27[a]	20–28[a]	0.002–48	7.2[a]
Mn	1.6–75	12–66	0.59–68	0.54–61	0.06	2.5–7.0
Mo	0.95–75	18	13	6–27	—	—
N	—	52,250[a]	—	—	—	—
Na	1710–2050[a]	177–360[a]	2990–3330[a]	3130–3370[a]	1017–3370	22–331[a]
Nb	4.7	—	<10	<60	—	—
Nd	<1	—	<2	<30	—	—
Ni	4.8–106	48–106	10–66	7.8–58	0.052–0.163	—
Os	<5	—	<2	<100	—	—
P	311–510[a]	656–978[a]	112–130	115–163[a]	0.24–1.55	—
Pb	88–400	150–610	12–180	16–130	0.05–2.7	—
Pd	<7	—	<10	<40	—	—
Po	0.22[b]	—	—	—	—	—
Pr	—	—	<50	<100	—	—
Pt	<40	—	<40	<50	—	—
Ra	6.6[b]	—	17[b]	—	—	—

TABLE 6.2. *Continued*

	Concentration in μg/L					
E	WB	RBC	BP	BS	SW[c]	SA
Rb	1.17–5.98[a]	4.2–5.3[a]	260–2000	40–580	—	—
Re	<3	—	<2	<100	—	—
Rh	6	—	<4	<60	—	—
Rn	<10	—	—	<90	—	—
Ru	—	—	<4	—	—	—
S	1680–1930[a]	—	330	1120–1270[a]	—	—
Sb	1.2–4.7	4.6	3.2–54	2.5–3.2	—	—
Sc	7.6	—	<30	0.15	—	—
Se	57–320	71–340	<30–590	98–327	—	—
Si	1.2–8.9[a]	4.1[a]	430	2.5–10[a]	—	3.5[a]
Sm	8	—	<2	<70	—	—
Sn	8.5–290	250–510	<4–105	30	—	—
Sr	16–95	7.2	28–44	<20–46	—	11–22
Ta	—	—	<6	<100	—	—
Tb	—	—	—	<90	—	—
Te	<6	—	<30	<40	—	—
Th	<0.2–2.4	0.16	<0.04	<40	—	—
Ti	28–100	50–180	<40–110	<10–120	—	—
Tl	0.47–0.48	—	<2.5	<30	—	—
Tm	<2	—	<0.6	<100	—	—
U	0.1–0.8	0.24	<0.13–59	<20	—	—
V	7.9–58	17–89	<10–56	4.6	—	—
W	1	—	<700	0.4	—	—
Y	4.7	—	<10	<100	—	—
Yb	<6	—	<2	<100	—	—
Zn	4.8–9.3[a]	7.6–16[a]	790–1700	670–1830	0.50–1.58	51
Zr	6.3–19	12	1.7	100	—	

* Adapted from reference 61.
[a] mg/L. [b] fg/L. [c] μg/g. —, no data. A 24-h collection of sweat contained, in μg: Al, 6130; Ba, 85; Br, 200; Co, 17; Cr, 59; Cu, 1590; F, 650; Fe, 130–500; Hg, 1; I, 24; Mn, 97; Mo, 61; Nb, 3; Ni, 83; Rb, 50; Sb, 11.

ions) and to α^2 and β^1 globulins. Selenium in selenomethionine can replace sulfur where methionine is utilized. Metallothionen transports cadmium and zinc in the red blood cells.

In the analysis for metals, blood and tissues usually are digested in nitric acid and then subjected to atomic absorption, emission or inductively coupled plasma so that all speciation is lost, an artifact masking the great complexity of metal speciation.

6.1.5 Interpretation of Blood Data

Blood measurements are differential in that they reflect the absolute concentrations of substrates at a given time and location of the circulatory system and are analogous to grab air samples. Blood data are a function of circulatory system volume and perfusion, and whether a steady state of xenobiotic distribution has been attained (as was discussed in Chapter 4). Blood concentrations, however, can be related to recent exposures (Section 4.0), but they may also reflect storage (Section 4.3), elimination from tissues (for example, blood urea nitrogen—BUN), secretion (hormones), and reabsorption (enterohepatic circulation, as for many glutathione conjugates eliminated in the bile). Redistribution (Section 4.1) after distribution often is marked by a transient increase in concentration of the xenobiotic in blood; sampling during this phase leads to difficult-to-interpret data. If the concentrations of the xenobiotic are not in a steady state, blood concentrations will differ from one blood vessel to another. Xenobiotics that are not efficiently metabolized and are not too fat- or bone-soluble are often good candidates for blood monitoring. The sampling technique is uncomplicated (fingerstick, vacuum-collection tubes), and the marker often is highly specific.

Uptake by the excretory organs is favored when there is a large concentration gradient caused by active excretion and metabolism. The same is true for concentrations in blood relative to those in the tissues it serves, if the compound is diffusible. Sometimes the membranes are selective barriers that compartmentalize chemical species within or outside of organelles and cells. We have already discussed this phenomenon in Section 2.6, where β-oxidation of fatty acids is organelle-specific. Thus different organs may have their own threshold whereby elimination occurs instead of uptake.

Generally, the more quickly a sample is taken up after exposure, the higher the blood concentration. If hand dermal exposure is involved, for example, the concentration in arm blood will reach a peak much sooner than that in the rest of the circulatory system. Concentrations increase if the elimination half-time is greater than 5 h. Physical activity increases the absorption rate, and this factor remains one of the most important unrecorded variables in most studies (see Table 3.2 for the effect of work activity on some physiological parameters).

The elimination of most hydrocarbon solvents from blood follows exponential curves. Thus one hour after cessation of exposure, blood concentrations drop by about 50% of the initial concentrations. This holds at least for white spirit, toluene, xylenes, styrene, trichloroethanol, and *n*-butanol. In contrast, acetone and isopropanol are cleared very slowly from blood. Macroelement concentrations are under homeostatic control; much of the control is exerted at the level of absorption. The toxic elements generally are efficiently absorbed and may have very long body half-times with short blood half-times, as, for example, lead and cadmium. They may also have short body half-times and short blood half-times, as, for example, chromium and mercury.

Medical monitoring parameters of blood such as enzyme activities and cellular elements are considered in Sections 9.0 and 9.1.

6.2 URINE

6.2.1 Physiology

The urine is the product of a complex set of processes in the kidneys that includes ultrafiltration of blood to remove low molecular weight, polar, water-soluble molecules without loss of proteins or cellular elements, as well as the controlled reabsorption and elimination of electrolytes, water, some hormones, and some vasoactive substances. This strict regulation is required for the proper functioning of cells in mammals because they require near constancy of the internal environment relative to temperature, oxygen supply, nutrient supply, hydrogen ion concentration, water, sodium, potassium, calcium, magnesium, vitamins, carbon, sulfur, nitrogen, phosphorus, and trace element compounds. Much of this is achieved through redistribution from storage reservoirs and movement among compartments. The balance for water, for example, involves a daily intake of about 2.5 L for a 70-kg male: 1 L from food, 0.3 L from metabolic conversions, and 1.2 L from drinking water or beverages. An equal amount is lost each day through urination (1.5 L), evaporation from the skin, and exhaled breath (0.9 L), and the remainder in the sweat or feces.

The kidneys are only 1% of total body weight but receive one quarter of the output of the heart. The kidney achieves its control through three processes: each fundamental unit of the kidney (the nephron) includes a capillary tuft (the glomerulus) that filters the blood at the end of an afferent arteriole so that plasma ultrafiltrate enters the surrounding space (Bowman's capsule), which is the beginning of a tubule. The tubule allows reabsorption, secretion of specific compounds, and elimination before joining other tubules that eventually lead to the bladder, where more processing and enzymic reactions continue before the urine issues through the urethra in females and also through the ureter in the penis in males.

The kidney glomeruli and the blood capillaries have pores of about 70 nm that allow molecules smaller than albumin (molecular weight 60,000) to pass through. Many xenobiotics have special transport forms, some being large proteins. Unless there is an exchange mechanism, most protein-bound xenobiotics are not filtered. The glomerular filtrate is large (about 180 L per day from a perfusion rate of 1.2 L blood/min, and a plasma flow of 600 mL/min via an afferent arteriole to the glomerulus). About 20% of plasma flow is filtered and delivered to the tubule. All compounds above 5000 in molecular weight are absent in the ultrafiltrate. The entire plasma volume passes through the kidneys some 60 times in one day with reabsorption being 99% for water, 99.5% for sodium ion, 100% for glucose, and 50% for urea, a waste product of nitrogenous compounds.

Reabsorption in the tubule is both passive and active. Sodium ion is reabsorbed by an energy-consuming process triggered by aldosterone, a hormone secreted by the adrenal cortex. Water reabsorption occurs along with that of sodium, but is regulated also by the antidiuretic hormone (ADH) produced by the hypothalamus, as well as by such diuretics as alcohol and caffeine. Reabsorbed glucose normally is returned to the peritubular capillaries, but is not if blood glucose reaches a critical limit. Then the excess escapes into the urine, as occurs in diabetes. Ions and polar compounds generally are reabsorbed. The pH of the urine ranges from 4.6 to 8.0.

A third mechanism involves secretion from tubular cells, a process often encountered for xenobiotics or their metabolites, which is both active and passive. Very few of the molecules secreted are normally found in the body (some of the exceptions are potassium and hydrogen ions and hippuric acid). This secretion appears to be a defense mechanism designed to eliminate xenobiotics and their metabolites. Sometimes xenobiotics also are stored in the kidneys; for example, cadmium, which is excreted when the metallothionein sites in the renal cortex become saturated. The appearance of a usually stored element or compound in the urine generally signifies some kind of kidney damage, and the marker then becomes one of adverse effect. Markers of adverse effect often are indicated when normal ranges of reference markers are not obeyed; for example, creatinine clearance decreases in the urine, and creatinine concentrations increase in the plasma, or proteinuria (protein in the urine). Medical monitoring markers for urine are discussed in Section 9.2.

6.2.2 Urine Composition and Normalization of Concentrations

Urine is 90 to 98% water. The variability of the urine daily volume (usually 600 to 2500 mL/day) is related to water intake and loss, which depend on temperature, ventilation conditions, humidity, and physical activity in the absence of genetic factors. Dilution differences among the urines from different people make comparisons difficult if the mg/L concentration type of reporting is used. It has become customary to normalize concentrations to urine properties, which fluctuate less than water volume. Some such components are specific gravity, creatinine clearance, and the less often used sulfate concentration, and osmolarity. When any of the normalization parameters lie outside their upper and lower normal ranges, the parameters cannot be used for normalization purposes. Another often used method is to report in terms of the amount collected over a specific time period.

The solids in urine are thousands of organic and inorganic compounds. Dissolved solids output varies markedly from individual to individual, varying between 30 and 70 g/day, but is relatively constant for each individual. The specific gravity is mostly related to solids content and varies between 1.003 and 1.030. It must be measured on fresh urine with a urinometer before the solids precipitate because the latter cannot easily be resolubilized. NIOSH uses 1.024 as its reference specific gravity, and the corrected specific gravity is obtained by use of the following equation:

$$\text{Corrected specific gravity} = \frac{\text{Observed value} \times 24}{\text{Last two digits of observed specific gravity}} \tag{6.1}$$

Renal clearance measures the excretion efficiency of substances. For non-reabsorbed compounds below a molecular weight of 5000, the concentration in the plasma (c_p) equals the concentration in the urine (c_u); then for the clearance Cl (volume of plasma cleared per unit time) relative to urine output V_u (volume of urine per unit time):

$$Cl \times c_p = V_u \times c_u \tag{6.2}$$

where V_u is the clearance and is an imaginary volume assuming 100% ultrafiltration efficiency.

Substances reabsorbed in the tubules have small clearances, whereas those that are secreted there have large ones. Weak electrolyte excretion is very dependent on urinary pH. Excretion of weak acids in alkaline urine is greater than in acid urine, and vice versa for weak bases. Some volatile chemicals such as toluene, styrene, methanol, and nitrous oxide are eliminated in the kidney by diffusion, which is driven by the urine/blood distribution coefficient.

Creatinine, as shown in Section 2.11.6, is a metabolic product of the energy processes in skeletal muscle. The clearance rate through the glomeruli is related to the lean body mass [62], that is, minus fat. A 70-kg man has about 28 kg of total muscle, and because 20% is protein and 80% is water, there is 4 to 6 kg protein in muscle or about 50% of the body protein. The creatinine equivalence is 17 to 22 kg muscle mass/g urinary creatinine. Its daily excretion ranges from 1.0 g to 1.6 g, and its concentration in urine varies between 0.3 and 3.4 g/L, with lower values being found for women (0.0–2 g/day with the mode between 1 and 1.5 g/day) than men (0.5–3.5 g/day with the mode being between 1.5 and 2 g/day). The creatinine concentration usually remains constant for urine flows greater than 1 mL/min; below this, it is proportional to urine flow. This makes it a good normalization parameter.

Creatinine clearance increases under physical stress but not by more than 10%. For healthy persons, the clearance rate is not much affected by diet, dehydration, and diuresis, and commonly varies only 4 to 8% for each individual. The exception occurs when the diet contains creatine, creatinine, and proteins containing amino acid precursors of creatinine. The average raw meat contains 700 mg creatine and 37 mg creatinine; cooked meat contains 570 mg and 160 mg, respectively. Vegetarians therefore have lower creatinine levels than meat eaters. There is thought to be no circadian rhythm (biological clock) to complicate matters, though this has been challenged [63]. Creatinine clearance decreases with age for an individual. Creatinine is measured, usually in an automated manner, by a colorimetric technique based on the production of an intense red color by reaction with alkaline picrate. Creatinine normalization accounts for individualized rates of uptake, metabolism, and elimination.

Normalization to creatinine is the major such procedure in urinary biological monitoring. It is not justified if the excretion mechanism of the marker to be normalized is not the same as for creatinine, if the urine is more concentrated than the upper normal range or more dilute than the lower normal range, or if elimination of the marker increases with urine flow. Thus methanol, nitrous oxide, and other compounds excreted by tubular diffusion should not be normalized to creatinine.

An average specific gravity value of 1.02, a mean urine output of 50 mL/h, and an average creatinine concentration of 1 g/L are used for interconversion purposes. For benzene, the ACGIH's biological exposure index (BEI) for phenol metabolite is 50 mg/L. This is equivalent to 50 mg/g creatinine or an excretion rate of 2.5 mg/h.

6.2.3 Sampling, Storage, and Transport

The concentrations of compounds found in the urine usually reflect the time weighted average concentrations in the plasma during collection and storage in the bladder. Sometimes this is not so if the kidney also stores the marker (as for cadmium and chromium). Spot samples that reflect urine collection in the bladder over the last 2 to 4 h are convenient and small enough to be stored without difficulty, yet the volume is large enough for adequate analysis. The link to exposure is tenuous for spot samples because the biological half-times determine whether spot sampling is effective. For example, the best time to collect a spot sample is that of the void with peak concentration. This cannot be known a priori without knowledge of the exposure pattern, which depends on the person's work or activity schedule, exposure process involved, and physical activity level. Direct-reading instrumental investigation of both the atmosphere and the urine may be necessary to decide when a spot sample should be taken for a marker of given half-time, assuming no interactions. Intermittent exposures commonly encountered in the workplace are not well correlated to spot sampling because a very complex exposure pattern may result in a spot urine sample that is not representative.

The only way to ensure complete collection in an 8-h time frame characteristic of shift work is to collect all voids in one container (analogous to "composite" sampling of environmental media except that all the biological medium is collected, not just a portion) or in separate containers, the latter contents all being analyzed along with any normalization parameters.

Thus 12- or 24-h sampling (that is, all voids are combined in the one container) is more representative than spot sampling, and usually correlates better with exposure. Any variations in excretion time, assuming half-times less than 12 h, are evened out. However, the bulky containers and their transport are awkward, and the collection of all voids for some people often is impossible, though it has been achieved in some studies. This may be a less sensitive technique for markers of short half-time because dilution relative to spot samples will occur for half-times of less than 2 h. This can be compensated for by analytical techniques with concentrative steps. Twelve-hour sampling will allow 75% collection of a compound with a half-time of 6 h and 62.5% collection for a half-time of 8 h. Similarly, 24-h sampling allows 75% collection of a compound with a half-time of 12 h and 87.5% collection for a half-time of 8 h.

To decide the time at which to sample, not only must the half-time of the exposure chemical be known, but also worst-case exposure scenarios have to be allowed for. For example, most of the exposure could occur in the last 5 min of a shift or an activity (some direct-reading instrument sleuthing is recommended to assure oneself of the exposure pattern if airborne exposures are suspected, and the chemicals are known). Taking a spot sample at the shift's end under these exposure conditions will be futile no matter what the half-time; if the half-time is less than 2 h, an extra 4 h of sampling will enable 75% of the compound to be collected. However, if the half-time is 12 h, another 24 h of sampling must be done. Clearly, any universal prescription for urine sampling can fail to achieve representative samples. Generally for the workplace, spot samples are taken at the end of a shift (for short half-times), at the end of a shift for the last working day of the week (for longer half-times that cause bioaccumulation), or on the morning after the exposure day (for markers that are Phase I oxidation products of long half-time). See Chapter 21 on BEIs.

One of the great advantages of urine collection is its noninvasive mode in contrast to blood. The ease of collection and the privacy generally involved during sample collection make tampering with (spiking or diluting) samples easy, however. The sampling containers used must be acid-washed in the same manner as for blood. The timing of sample collection must be precise, with the initial void and the final void noted. If volatiles are to be measured, the urine must fill the entire container, and the latter must be sealed immediately. Headspace analysis must be done with containers strong enough to withstand overpressure caused by temperature changes during transport or storage after sealing of the freshly collected sample. Only spot samples will give valid headspace samples owing to gas/vapor loss necessarily incurred for integrated sampling. However, the results of a number of spot samples in a given sampling period can be combined mathematically using a total mass of marker approach.

Some investigators have used preservatives such as thymol, boric acid, and nitric acid. These often interfere with extractions or other tests (for example, thymol with the Coomassie Blue protein method), and any chemical speciation may be destroyed (for example, glucuronides are hydrolyzed by nitric acid and sulfuric acid). The use of preservatives is not recommended if conjugates are also to be analyzed. Misinterpretation of analytical artifacts from the use of preservatives also can result; for example, it may be thought that certain compounds could be excreted "free" when in fact they are conjugated. Another famous artifact was the postulate that mercapturic acids were the ultimate products of the glutathione detoxification pathway in acidified urines (acid used as preservative and as part of the analytical workup), when in fact the ultimate products were thioethers (Section 5.1.2).

If the urinary half-time is not known, each void should be collected separately over 24 h, stored, and transported frozen, and then stored frozen in the laboratory, thawed just before analysis (if volatiles are required, sample the headspace while thawing is occurring), mixed well, and analyzed separately by much the same general methods as those used for blood in Section 6.1.4. Time-integrated data then can be generated mathematically from the void data. If it is known how much urine is to be used in subsequent analysis, the fresh urine should be dispensed into a suitable container in the field for freezing before transport, storage, and analysis. The larger volume then can serve as a backup if more sensitivity is required, if the smaller sample is lost, or if mishaps occur. The larger sample also can remain frozen at the sampling site until the results are received and interpreted. Failure to freeze urine causes microbiological growth, creatinine decomposition, loss of enzyme activities, and enhanced oxidation.

6.2.4 Chemical Analysis and Urine Chemical Composition

Fewer cleanup problems during sample analysis are generally found for urine in comparison to blood or plasma. Although digestion or extraction of urine is required for metals if atomic absorption analysis is the analytical technique, dilution with acid is all that is required for inductively coupled plasma atomic emission spectrometric analysis [64]. For the elements below the least quantifiable limit, digestion and concentration are still necessary. Extraction of nonpolar organics with nonpolar organic solvents is easier for urine than for blood because urine is more aqueous than blood and contains salts that promote a "salting-out" effect. Blood also has much more affinity for nonpolar organics than urine has. Nevertheless, the urine should be saturated with a salt such as sodium chloride to ensure uniform aqueous ionic strength for organic solvent extractions. The use of a buffer may be necessary to control the effects of pH and the buffering capacity of the urine.

Urinary elimination of the unchanged parent compound has been investigated for xylene, styrene, acetone, methyl ethyl ketone, ethanol, methanol, isopropanol, butanol, and oxitol, and it amounts to less than 1% of the amount absorbed. More polar xenobiotics such as amines or carboxylic acids may be excreted to a greater extent.

The influence of atmospheric concentration, respiratory uptake, and work load have been studied on parent compounds in urine by Pezzagno et al. [65] for acetone, styrene, toluene, xylenes, methyl chloroform, and perchloroethylene. Work load influences pulmonary ventilation, which governs uptake and thus the absorbed dose (Table 3.2). Five volunteers were exposed as follows: a 2-h exposure at rest (also another group of 15 subjects); a 4-h exposure at rest (also another group of 15 subjects); a 2-h exposure alternating between light physical exercise (20 min at a work load of 50 W on a bicycle ergometer followed by 20 min at rest repeated three times during exposure) (also another group of 15 subjects); a 1-h exposure at 50 W; and a 30-min exposure at 100 W.

Another workplace study, involving 528 participants, examined the relationship between weighted environmental and biological concentrations. Spot urine samples were taken before and after exposure using a specific gravity correction. Urinary analyses for xenobiotic were done by headspace analysis. Mixed air breath samples also were analyzed. Exposure concentrations in the air were obtained by passive sampling. The regression equations relating uptake, air concentration, and urinary concentration corrected for specific gravity are given in Table 6.3. The results showed that acetone, styrene, and xylenes depend only on pulmonary ventilation for the volunteers at rest and doing light work because there was no dependence on compound retention (Table 6.3), whereas toluene was lung-ventilation-dependent only at rest. The excretion of chlorinated solvents depends also on retention. For retention-independent solvents, the ratio of urine concentrations after effort relative to those at rest varied between 3.1 and 3.6, whereas for those solvent vapors also dependent on retention this ratio was less than 3.

The uptake of methyl chloroform, however, is greater during light than heavy exercise because the retention is not constant. Thus any standards should be set on at-rest data, as they provide the lowest C_u, which is the most conservative case, provided that no interactions are occurring. Many workers are sedentary for substantial portions of their work routines. However, because the urine concentrations increase with physical effort, a safe exposing concentration could be mistaken as overexposure if urine data were used alone under conditions of various degrees of physical activity. Thus exposure information still is necessary for one to be able to interpret this situation.

Urinary protein is restricted to proteins of molecular weight of less than 5000. The recommended method for detecting proteinuria presently is the Coomassie Brilliant Blue dye-binding technique [66] for albumin, but the Biuret method was the least dependent on γ-globulin content. Amino acid content in urine and serum has been determined [67] at femtomole levels with good resolution by *o*-phthalaldehyde/2-mercaptoethanol derivatization followed by reverse phase high performance liquid chromatography (HPLC) using a fluorescence detector (excitation wavelength 230 nm; emission at 418 nm). The half-times of the fluorescent derivatives were all greater than 2.3 min after dilution in 72 : 20 : 8 water/sodium propionate/acetonitrile. The amino acid content varied markedly from person to person, aspartic acid and ornithine being the most consistent. Serum and urine levels agreed for

TABLE 6.3. Regression equations linking uptake (U) at different physical activities, urinary concentration obtained from headspace analysis corrected for specific gravity, (C_a), and air concentrations (C_a).

A. Controlled 2–4 h exposures with 15 volunteers.

Solvent	U versus C_u		C_u versus UC_a
Acetone	$U = 47.5C_u + 23.2$	$[r = 0.82]$	$C_u = 0.021UC_a - 0.49$
Styrene	$U = 4.2C_u - 14.1$	$[r = 0.83]$	$C_u = 0.24UC_a + 3.36$
Toluene	$U = 1.3C_u - 0.2$	$[r = 0.85]$	$C_u = 0.77UC_a + 0.15$
Perchloroethylene	$U = 3.2C_u + 14$	$[r = 0.82]$	$C_u = 0.31UC_a - 4.37$
Methyl chloroform	$U = 2.0C_u - 50$	$[r = 0.88]$	$C_u = 0.50UC_a + 25$
Xylenes	$U = 2.4C_u + 6.1$	$[r = 0.83]$	$C_u = 0.42UC_a - 2.54$

B. Field study for 4 hours of exposure.

Solvent	C_u versus C_a	
Acetone[a]	$C_u = 33.61C_a - 0.33$	$r = 0.87; n = 104$
Styrene	$C_u = 0.33C_a + 18.90$	$r = 0.88; n = 200$
Toluene	$C_u = 0.60C_a - 1.40$	$r = 0.88; n = 80$
Perchloroethylene	$C_u = 0.33C_a + 11.90$	$r = 0.87; n = 40$
Methyl chloroform	$C_u = 0.45C_a + 12.60$	$r = 0.95; n = 60$
Xylenes	$C_u = 0.38C_a + 1.77$	$r = 0.94; n = 44$

C. Data for tetrachloroethylene and methyl chloroform for varying physical activities for 4-h exposures.

Solvent	Work (W)	C_u versus C_aV_p
Perchloroethylene	0	$C_u = 4.22 \times 10^{-2}C_aV_p - 4.37$
	50	$C_u = 3.98 \times 10^{-2}C_aV_p - 4.37$
	100	$C_u = 3.59 \times 10^{-2}C_aV_p - 4.37$
Methyl chloroform	0	$C_u = 3.69 \times 10^{-2}C_aV_p + 25$
	50	$C_u = 3.15 \times 10^{-2}C_aV_p + 25$
	100	$C_u = 1.86 \times 10^{-2}C_aV_p + 25$

Adapted from reference 65

[a] The equation for acetone does not correct for preexposure levels; when these are subtracted, the following equation results:

$$C_u = 0.019C_a + 236$$

Each environmental breathing zone measurement C_a in mg/m^3 corresponds to a range; each biological measurement C_u in µg/L (except mg/L for acetone) corresponds to a range of UC_a; U in mg was calculated by $K \times V_p \times R_e \times t$, where K is a constant depending on the units used, here 0.06; V_p is the pulmonary ventilation, defined here as the inspired minute pulmonary ventilation for the compound, which is also equal to the expired minute pulmonary ventilation; t is the time of exposure in minutes; R_e is the compound retention in the body measured by $[C_a - C_m]/C_a$ where C_m is the concentration in mixed exhaled air. R_e values are: acetone, 0.53 ± 0.06; styrene, 0.65 ± 0.016; xylenes, 0.64 ± 0.07 (mean and standard deviation) at rest and for light work. The value for toluene at rest is 0.50 ± 0.015, but at 50 W work it is 0.40 ± 0.21; the chlorinated solvent vapors induced decreasing R with increasing V_p.

cysteine, serine, glutamine, arginine, alanine, taurine (interfered with probably by β-aminoisobutyric acid), phenylalanine, and leucine. Urinary noradrenaline, adrenaline, and dopamine were separated and analyzed by HPLC-electrochemical cell detection or by fluorometry [68]. In 80 nonhypertense controls the daily excretion was: noradrenaline, 11 to 58 μg; adrenaline, 1.2 to 29.2 μg; and dopamine, 34 to 294 μg. Natural amines in urine included methylamine, dimethylamine, ethylamine, piperidine, and pyrrolidine [69].

Urinary α-, β-unsaturated, aromatic and α-carboxylic organic acids in the urine of infants have been separated by cation exchange/reverse phase HPLC using ultraviolet (200/280 nm) and electrochemical detection in series in a screening method [70]. For example, excess orotic acid was found in an infant with citrullinemia. Other genetic diseases and their associated biological acid marker include: propionic acidemia—methylcitrate; oxalosis—oxalic; Lesch–Nyhan syndrome—uric; urea cycle enzymopathies—orotic; lactic acidoses—pyruvic; branched chain ketoaciduria—α-ketoisocaproic, α-ketomethylvaleric, and α-ketoisovaleric; phenylketonuria—phenylpyruvic; tyrosinemia—*p*-hydroxyphenylacetic; alkaptonuria—homogentisic; β-methylcrotonyl CoA carboxylase deficiency—β-methylcrotonic. Inborn genetic errors in infants usually announce their presence by the accumulation of these specific acids at over 20 times their usual concentration. This screening analytical method resolves all of these carboxylic acids. Such techniques are valuable in medical monitoring or health surveillance.

Analysis for oxalic acid is important because it acts as a marker for kidney stones, hypercalcinuria, and poisonings from oxalate and ethylene glycol. Dietary deficiency in calcium or vitamin D reduces oxalate absorption and decreases excretion. Hyperglycinuria also decreases urinary oxalate. As early as the eighteenth century, there were reports identifying urinary calculi as calcium oxalate.

The analysis of ultraviolet-absorbing compounds in urine has been related to exposure of carcinogens. Ion exchange and reverse phase HPLC after filtration of urine through a 0.45-μm filter revealed [71] that the major ultraviolet-absorbing compounds at 254 nm were uric, hippuric, 3-methoxymandelic, uracil, mandelic, and 2-hydroxy-phenylacetic (quinaldic acid and 4-hydroxybenzylglycine have the same retention times) acids. This particular method of analysis favored detection of carboxylic acids.

The elemental composition of 24-h urines in mg for the blood macroelements is [61]: calcium, 145–460; chloride, 4400–6530; iron, 0.131–1.2; magnesium, 60–154; phosphorus, 538–1160; potassium, 1833–3000; sodium, 2944–4620; and sulfur, 800–1320. Other elements with daily masses greater than 1 mg include: bromine, 3.7–7.0; fluorine, 1.6; rubidium, 1.1–2.4; and zinc, 0.042–1.25. Trace elements include, in μg/day: Ag, 0.55–9.5; Al, 100–1000; As, 6.5–195 (depending on seafood diet); Au, 0.011–0.032; B, 570–1075; Ba, 14–420; Be, 130; Bi, 1.6; Cd, 2.1–88; Ce, 36; Co, 0.73–235; Cr, 0.6–150; Cs, 9.9–50; Cu, 11–325; Ga, 42; Ge, 1400; Hg, 1–17; I, 50–376; La, 0.28–0.71; Li, 690–800; Mn, 0.22–1570; Mo, 49–150; Nb, 360; Ni, 2.4–931; Pb, 11–120; Sb, 1.5–3.5; Sc, 0.073–0.57; Se, 20–187; Sm, 2.1–2.8; Sn, 17–95; Sr, 110–390; Te, 530; Ti, 330–480; U, 0.34; V, <6–27; and W, 11–32.

Spot urines show [61] the following elemental concentrations in μg/L (except as noted): Ag, 10; Al, 60; As, 15–120; B, 709–919; Ba, 89; Bi, 20; Br, 1300–5300; Ca, 55–164 mg/L; Cd, 0.64–8.9; Co, 98; Cr, 0.7–12; Cs, 80; Cu, 17–300; F, 430–3800; Fe, 180; Ge, 1300; Hg, 4.3–114; I, 66–388; K, 1415–1910 mg/L; Mg, 48–200 mg/L; Mn, 30–300; Mo, 10–100; Nb, 260; Ni, 2.3–85; P, 24–621 mg/L; Pb, 6.3–110; Rb, 154–1520; S, 1650 mg/L; Se, 4.8–46; Si, 4700–5200; Sn, 13; Sr, 100; Te, 630; Th, 1.3–100 ng/L; Ti, 10; Tl, 0.3–0.4 ng/L; U, 0.015–7; V, 2.2–22; and Zn, 193–2040.

The U.S. Department of Commerce published a specific set of analytical methods to identify priority pollutants in urine [72]. Normal safety precautions were used then because hepatitis A and B were shown not to be transmitted in urine. Since the advent of AIDS, all biological fluids have been handled routinely in a biohazard hood if the patient's AIDS or HIV status is unknown. (See also Chapter 18.)

Many workplace, environmental, and pharmacological compounds and/or their metabolites have been sampled in urine. The discussions of the BEIs (Chapter 21), medical monitoring (Section 9.2), and special topics (Chapters 22 and 23) should be consulted for specific compounds.

6.3 EXHALED BREATH

6.3.1 General Remarks

In Section 3.0 we saw that most volatile organic solvents were between 60 and 70% absorbed on inhalation in sedentary individuals, leaving 30 to 40% exhaled in the breath [1]. As the vapor pressure decreases, exhalation will become less important after absorption. Volatile, water-insoluble substances absorbed through the skin or by ingestion have also been detected in exhaled breath. For the latter, increased physical activity will increase the amount exhaled. The situation relative to exhalation and increased physical activity for inhaled gases and vapors is more complex. We have also seen (Sections 3.0.2 and 3.0.3) that particles between 0.5 and 10 μm and <0.1 μm in aerodynamic diameter deposit in the alveoli, whereas those between 0.1 and 0.5 μm do not completely deposit and may also be breathed out.

Breath analysis has been used in clinical diagnosis to detect diabetes (fruity odor), uremia (fetid odor), hydrogen for gastric disorders, and alkanes from overactive lipid peroxidation [73], as well as for alcohol exposure of motorists. It is used to identify and quantify xenobiotics in exhaled breath after ambient and occupational exposures, and to complement environmental and other biological monitoring. Along with urine sampling, breath sampling is noninvasive.

Specimens collected from subjects with abnormal pulmonary function—for example, bronchospasm, bronchitis, asthma, emphysema, endobronchial lesions, heart failure, pulmonary emboli, atelectasis, pneumoconiosis, fibrosis, alveolitis, pulmonary edema, vasculitis, and hypertension—are not suitable for analysis. Higher concentrations than expected may be an indicator of skin absorption or ingestion. The kinetics of exhalation also depends on how much and which part of the body is exposed to a xenobiotic via skin absorption, whole hand absorption differing markedly from thumb absorption.

6.3.2 Physiological Aspects

Exhalation serves to discharge waste gases and vapors, especially carbon dioxide from its hemoglobin complex in venous blood to produce oxyhemoglobin on inhalation and to transport oxygen to the tissues and brain by the arteries. Inhalation and exhalation of xenobiotics thus is adventitious. Gas/vapor exchanges depend on the existence of a concentration gradient to favor exhalation, on the air/blood partition coefficient (the inverse quantities are provided in Table 3.1), on the solubility in blood (increasing solubility lessens concentration in alveolar air for expiration), on the vapor pressure of the substance (increasing vapor pressure increases volatilization) into alveoli from the blood, on cardiac output (because this affects the amount of blood per unit time coursing through the alveolar veins), on the duration of lung exposure, and, if this is intermittent, on the diffusion of the fraction of xenobiotic that can cross the blood/air barrier into alveolar air. Blood composition does affect partition coefficients, meals increasing partition coefficients of halothane, methylene chloride, benzene, toluene, and trichloroethylene by about 60% [74]. If the blood/air partition coefficient is below 5, alveolar air does not reflect mixed venous blood composition [75].

The total volume expired in 15 breaths/minute (tidal volume) is about 500 mL in sedentary healthy humans. Only 350 mL is used for active gas exchange, and the other 150 mL is dead space volume. Available alveolar air mixed with inspired air has a volume of about 2 L, and average alveolar ventilation is about 5 L/min with an average blood flow of 6 L/min. The ventilation/perfusion ratio varies throughout the lung.

Body build, gender, physical activity, pulmonary ventilation, and metabolism (partition coefficients, elimination, metabolic rate) differences, along with the mode of exposure (fluctuating concentrations, time intervals between exposure, type and route of exposure), often cause large interindividual differences that are difficult to interpret or to correct for, especially if group comparisons are desired [76].

6.3.3 Sampling

Breath is a difficult fluid to sample with good reproducibility. Expired air under normal breathing conditions (mixed exhaled air) is a heterogeneous unmixed mixture of unused prior inspired breath (dead space volume), which is sampled first, and gases and vapors exchanged with blood (alveolar air), which is sampled last. Different results are obtained, depending on what part of the exhaled breath is sampled. The dead space volume has the same composition as the prior inhaled breath. The latter needs to be analyzed also so that one can interpret the significance of the expired air sample—that is, whether dilution due to the absence of the marker or higher-than-true values due to inspired breath contamination are occurring.

The gases and vapors from venous blood exchange are in higher concentrations in end-tidal air (end-exhaled air), but are even more concentrated in forced expiration air if the compounds are not water-soluble or reactive. Single breaths reflect free (unbound) venous concentrations just before exhalation for inert, water-insoluble organics, and constitute differential measurements.

Inhaling by nose and exhaling by mouth is preferred over the use of a two-way valve and mouthpiece.

Breath-holding is used to obtain a steady, representative concentration of alveolar air. Breath-holding with the lung full or partially emptied gives different results [77]; more reproducible results occur with the lung full than partially empty.

Rebreathing consists of exhaling several times into a closed system, usually with removal of carbon dioxide, to obtain a large volume of homogeneous breath. As many breaths as are necessary to at least half-fill gas bags or fill glass containers should be collected.

The gradient in concentration of components through the pulmonary tree is analogous to the dilution effect for spot urines. Thus normalization to carbon dioxide concentration (as a marker of venous system contribution) is being increasingly performed [78], and is recommended.

It is important that subjects who are donating breath samples not "tense up"; otherwise, nonrepresentative samples will be obtained. This can cause hyperventilation (increased volume exhaled without need for more oxygen) or hypoventilation (decreased exhaled volume).

During breath sampling and analysis, volumes and concentrations usually are recorded at the temperature and pressure of the recording instruments, often assuming that equation (3.2) applies. Volumes have to be corrected to 25°C and 760 mm Hg conditions (ATP) for reporting purposes. The converted volumes are themselves converted to body temperature pressure saturated (BTPS) conditions (equation 6.3) or, less frequently, standard temperature pressure dry (STPD) conditions (equation 6.4):

$$V_{BTPS} = V_{ATP} \times [237 + 37]/[237 + t_C] \times [p_B - P_w]/[p_B - P_w(37)] \quad (6.3)$$

$$V_{STPD} = V_{ATP} \times 273/[273 + t_C] \times [p_B - P_w]/p_B(0) \quad (6.4)$$

where t_C is the temperature of measurement in degrees C, p_B is the barometric pressure, and P_w is the vapor pressure of water at t_C.

Workshift breath sampling or analysis are convenient and enforceable by management but reflect instantaneous exposures. Breath concentrations do not correlate with average exposure or dose during intermittent and variable exposures. Thus, this sampling time cannot be used for routine evaluation of time-weighted average exposures.

Sampling and analyzing just after a work shift (5–30 min) have the advantage that the concentrations still will be elevated, but have the disadvantage that they will be decreasing fast, causing much variability. This also assumes that no exposure is still occurring, which is sometimes untrue, or that a large exposure did not occur just before work ended, so biasing the results. It is best to detect environmental concentrations with a direct-reading instrument that can also detect breath concentrations so that the kinetics can be followed, and to verify that no exposures are still occurring.

Performing the sampling or analysis the morning after exposure but before the next shift is convenient, and any concentrations that are detected should not change rapidly, assuming no further exposure to the marker being monitored. However, some compounds will be below the detection limit of the technique, especially rapidly metabolized ones. For inert volatile organics, the concentration 16 h after exposure is about 100 times lower than the last substantial exposure concentration. Redistribution processes for certain compounds also may complicate the interpretation of the measurements, especially for high-fat individuals and for women relative to men. This sampling time had less interday variability for the compounds that could be detected compared with the other two methods.

The factors that most bias sampling 30 min and 15 h after an exposure for aromatics are metabolism and physical activity. Another factor that is extremely important for sampling 30 min after an exposure is variation in exposure concentrations during the day, whereas repeatability and interday variations must be considered for sampling at 15 h [76]. Personal baseline samples are again recommended, as for urine and blood samples.

Different types of gas bags have been used for breath sampling. Teflon, Tedlar, and aluminum bags are most used, the first two showing adsorption/resorption cycling phenomena; this is not so important with aluminum bags once the large initial adsorption process has occurred. Sampling occurs by breathing into the bag. Analysis is done by a gas sampling valve on a gas chromatograph connected by Teflon tubing to the bag, or by injecting a known volume into a gas chromatograph by a gas-tight syringe.

Glass pipettes, burettes, or bulbs also have been used but are easily broken. Sampling is done by breathing through the tube and then sealing the open ends with Teflon- or aluminum-lined seals. Analysis is performed by a gas-tight syringe transferring a defined volume to a gas chromatograph. Volumes for expired breath should be sufficiently large; end-exhaled breath containers should accommodate the last 30 to 50 mL.

Solid sorbent sampling with a backup section (Tenax GC, charcoal, XAD types, silica gel, molecular sieves, and precolumns for gas chromatographs) has the disadvantages of a high pressure drop and of breakthough in charcoal, silica gel, and molecular sieves caused by high humidity in the breath. Tenax GC and XAD type resins allow water vapor to break through yet retain aromatics and chlorinated compounds but not very volatile compounds; they are useful for subsequent thermal desorption/GC. After sampling they must be capped and preferably stored and transported at refrigeration temperatures. They have the advantage over the gas bag and glass vessel containers of being small, transportable, and light. Migration of adsorbed compounds occurs at room temperature, or if samples are stored too long. Desorption, done by solvents or thermally, has the same difficulties associated with these processes for air samples.

6.3.4 Analysis of Breath Samples

Breath has a simple matrix for analysis compared with blood (proteins, fats, and cellular elements) and urine (salts). Gas chromatography with the appropriate column material followed by mass spectral analysis is the best single technique for volatile organics. Screening techniques using the various GC detectors have also been widely used. Adequate sensitivity appears to be the major problem rather than resolution or interfering background compounds.

Direct reading instruments give real-time results. Detector tubes are inexpensive, simple, and rapid but rather imprecise (about 25% error) and nonspecific. Carbon monoxide and carbon dioxide have been sampled in gas bags and analyzed from there with the appropriate detector tubes/pumps. The alcohol Breathalyzer test for motorists is based on the decolorization reaction of alcohol with potassium permanganate crystals [79]. Infrared and gas chromatographic methods have also been used [79]. All alcohol tests are extremely variable during the alcohol absorption phase but are reliable after this stage. Electrochemical-type detectors, which operate by oxidizing a compound, for example, carbon monoxide to carbon dioxide, are used in tandem with a sampling valve. Infrared detectors are often utilized for carbon dioxide.

Gas chromatographs equipped with gas sampling valves or cryogenic retention have been used. The advent of portable gas chromatographs equipped with gas sampling valves has made field measurements accessible. The availability of small quadrupole mass spectrometers has made field breath samples a distinct possibility, albeit an expensive one.

Air that has reached the lung and participated in the blood–gas exchange in the alveoli contains about 5% carbon dioxide, 6.5% water (equivalent to the vapor pressure of water at body temperature), and 14% oxygen. The air that is exhaled is more like ambient air than alveolar air. Humans not exposed overtly to chemicals breathe out over 100 compounds, mostly at ppb levels [80, 81], whereas people exposed overtly to chemicals breathe the latter out in the ppm range.

Compounds and their concentrations expressed in μg/h and detected in at least seven out of ten assays on eight subjects not overtly exposed to chemical emissions included [80]: acetone, 1.3–2000; butane, 0.24–9.4; 1-butene, 1.3–510; dichlorobenzene, 0.001–26; dimethyldifluorosilane, 1.2–140; dimethyl sulfide, 0.54–53; ethanol, 11–440; furan, 0.25–98; indene, 0.14–83; isoprene, 15–390; and isopropyl alcohol, 2.0–160. The breath of an individual who was assayed three times varied greatly in composition and concentration. Of these compounds, dichlorobenzene may have reflected chemical exposures. Isoprene was suggested to arise from psychological stress. Dimethyldifluorosilane was thought to be a metabolite of dietary silicones. Dimethyl sulfide is probably a result of microbial processes. The only compounds to exceed 1 ppm in the breath were acetone (2 ppm) and *n*-propyl alcohol (1.4 ppm). Smokers generally had higher concentrations of chemicals in their breaths, especially aromatic compounds. Hydrocarbons such as butane, 1-butene, 2-butene (*cis* and *trans*), ethyl acetylene, ethylene, 1-hexane, 2-hexene, methyl acetylene, methyl cyclohexane, methyl cyclopentane, octyne, 1-pentene, and propane were detected variably, as well as compounds such as acetaldehyde, *n*-butyl alcohol, capryl alcohol, cyclohexyl alcohol, dimethyl disulfide, ethyl acetate, isobutyl alcohol, methanol, methyl ethyl ketone, methyl isobutyl ketone, propyl acetate, and refrigerant Freons.

Particulate matter also is emitted, up to 4 particles/cm^3 during breathing, fewer while sedentary, and the most during severe physical activity [82]. The particle size was usually below 0.3 micrometer. Fewer than 2% had diameters above 1 micrometer.

6.3.5 Field Studies

Two breath tests, based on aminopyrine and caffeine, are in general use to determine the induction or the inhibition of enzymes located in the endoplasmic reticulum of liver cells [137]. These tests complement the antipyrine test used on saliva, plasma, or urine.

The aminopyrine breath test involves oral administration of ^{14}C-aminopyrine (about 2 Curie) labeled in the methyl group. The latter is oxidized by the cytochrome P-450 enzyme complex, and eventually is excreted as $^{14}CO_2$ in the breath at a rate assumed to reflect the rate of liver demethylation. The label is collected for 2 h after administration (the patient must be sedentary during this period) by blowing through a trapping agent for carbon dioxide, and the radioactivity is determined by liquid scintillation. The cumulated exhalation from administration to sampling then is calculated by multiplying the sample activity with the endogenous CO_2 output for a sedentary person of 9 mmol $\times$ kg body weight $\times$ h^{-1}. The correlation coefficient with unlabeled aminopyrine in plasma or saliva is about 0.8. The test has been used to assess the prognosis of patients with cirrhotic liver disease, but potent inducing agents such as glutethimide are also detected. The marker has not been used much in the workplace, probably because of the requirement that the subject be sedentary for 2 h after administration of the drug, an inconvenience for management and the worker.

Aminopyrine was introduced in the late nineteenth century as an analgesic, antipyretic, and anti-inflammatory agent, but its use in the United States was curtailed in 1938 when frequent reports were made of fatal agranulocytosis. However, it is still widely available in other countries, in some as an over-the-counter preparation. Hence baseline breath samples must be taken for this technique, as the metabolite 4-aminoantipyrine or 4-aminophenazone has been detected even in the United States (in Mexican workers), where its use has been officially ended [139]. The half-time for aminopyrine is 1.4 to 3.2 h [139], and it is 95% metabolized.

The caffeine breath test is similar [137] to the aminopyrine test in that it uses ^{14}C-caffeine with the label in one or all three methyl groups in a similar 2-h cumulative collection for breath $^{14}CO_2$. This measures the activity of animal hepatic enzymes induced by 3-methylcholanthrene but not phenobarbital, which induces the enzymes of the cytochrome P-450 complex. Vinyl chloride and polycyclic aromatic hydrocarbons are activated by 3-methylcholanthrene-inducible enzymes. The same advantages and disadvantages of the aminopyrine breath test apply here. It is an advantage that caffeine is much less toxic than aminopyrine. However, again baseline measurements are necessary to account for the influence of coffee, tea, and other caffeinated drinks.

Other substances that have been used in similar breath tests include diazepam and phenacetin, but they have no advantages relative to the two breath tests above. They have not been widely used [137].

Most of the breath analysis studies in the workplace have involved volunteers rather than workers in the field, as difficulties are much greater in the field than in a laboratory setting. Alveolar air concentrations in volunteers are related to increasing exposure time under continuous exposure conditions only for vapors and gases that are poorly soluble and/or poorly metabolized. Thus, concentrations of toluene, xylene, styrene, and trichloroethylene are constant [83] in alveolar air after 15 min of continuous exposure for the next 8 h of continuous exposure, but methyl chloroform, tetrachloroethylene, and dichloromethane under the same conditions gradually increase during continuous exposure [84]. This behavior is interesting, but when intermittent exposures characteristic of workplace exposures are considered, one must know the time intervals between exposures to be able to interpret the data; for once exposure ceases, rapid decreases in concentration in alveolar air occur.

Benzene [85], cyclohexane [86, 87], dichloromethane [88, 89], Freons [90], halothanes [91], *n*-hexane [92], isopropanol [93], methanol [94], methyl chloroform [95], pentanes [96], perchloroethylene [97], styrene [98–101], toluene [102–104], trichloroethylene [105], and xylene [106] derivatives have been breath-sampled in the workplace. About half of the studies utilized end tidal air, one used forced end tidal air [102], one used breath-holding [100], two did not indicate what type of sample was collected [99, 103], and the rest [85, 89, 94, 95, 101, 106] sampled expired air. Most breath analysis was performed on the xenobiotic except for methylene chloride, where breath carbon monoxide was quantified along with blood carboxyhemoglobin [89].

Although acetone can arise from endogenous biochemical processes (Section 2.6) as well as from the workplace [92], it can be produced in the breath of rats from the metabolism of halogenated C_1 and C_2 compounds [107], including vapors of carbon tetrachloride, chloroform, *cis*- and *trans*-dichloroethylene, methylene chloride, 1,1,2-trichloroethane, trichloroethylene, vinyl bromide, vinyl chloride, vinyl fluoride, and vinylidene fluoride, and after administration of fluoroacetate and chloroacetate but not after exposure to vapors of methyl chloroform or *n*-hexane. Similar metabolism probably will occur in humans; so if acetone is being measured, exposure to other compounds that may give rise to it should be quantitated also.

6.3.6 Predictive Models for Volatile Organic Solvents

Caperos et al. [108] have discussed a model for methyl chloroform based on one developed to simulate absorption, distribution, metabolism, and excretion for trichloroethylene by the same group [109] involving urine and breath. Earlier work by Stewart et al. in the 1960s and 1970s [110–112] was the inspiration behind the model. In the Caperos et al. approach [108], tissue volumes, blood volumes, blood perfusion, and partition coefficients for four compartments (vessel-rich, muscle, fat, and lung) were considered (Table 6.4), along with the experimental rate constants of elimination for the principal metabolites and for the xenobiotic in urine, breath, and other excretion routes, as well as the rate constants for each principal metabolic step leading to the biological monitoring markers. The liver is included in the vessel-rich compartment.

The volume of alveolar air was the functional residual capacity (2.43 L) plus half of the tidal volume (0.25 L). The lung-tissue/gas partition coefficient was assumed to be the same as the blood/gas partition coefficient. A fixed flux of blood was considered to be cleared of the xenobiotic (0.025 L/min for methyl chloroform from experimental observations). The cardiac output was assumed to be 6.791 L/min with a cardiac index of 3.501 L/min/m^2 and a surface area of 1.24 m^2. The alveolar ventilation was the one at rest (5.45 L/min). Physical activity was accounted for by varying the cardiac output and alveolar ventilation (Table 3.2). A urinary output of 1 mL/min was assumed, and that the bladder was emptied at 7 A.M., 12 noon, 5 P.M., and 10 P.M. with exposure

TABLE 6.4. Four-compartment model parameters for methyl chloroform.*

Parameter	Compartment			
	Vessel-rich	Muscle-rich	Fat-rich	Lung
Tissue volume (L)	8.8	36.3	11.5	1.0
Blood volume (L)	3.19	0.63	0.18	1.4
Blood perfusion (%)	79.9	15.7	15.7	—
Partition coefficient	9.1	6.1	373.0	4.35

* Adapted from reference 108.

The relevant pseudo first-order rate constants used were:

Total trichloroethanol/trichloroethanol glucuronide: urine, $0.026\,h^{-1}$; other excretion/metabolism, $0.0082\,h^{-1}$.

Trichloroacetate: urine, $0.00685\,h^{-1}$; other excretion/metabolism, $0.00685\,h^{-1}$.

Conversion of trichloroethanol to trichloroacetate: $0.01919\,h^{-1}$

The model was:

methyl chloroform → trichloroethanol → trichloroacetate → other
→ trichloroethanol-glucuronide
→ other metabolites/excretion

These variables are valid also for trichloroethylene because the latter has the same metabolic products.

occurring between 8 A.M. and 12 noon and between 1 P.M. and 5 P.M. for workplace exposures.

Based on their model, Caperos et al. [108] showed that total trichloroethanol in urine corrected for preexposure baseline and, collected just before the next work shift after exposure began, was the best biological monitoring marker for methyl chloroform. The breath methyl chloroform marker was too dependent on intermittent concentrations, the latter not affecting urinary trichloroacetate and trichloroethanol concentrations, however. Urinary trichloroacetate had the disadvantage of a lower correlation coefficient at lower exposure air concentrations of methyl chloroform than had total urinary trichloroethanol. Alveolar samples were recommended to be most representative 6 h after exposure ended. The model assumed that only inhalation occurred as a route of exposure.

A similar model [113] for unchlorinated solvents also uses four compartments (vessel-rich, muscle-rich, fat-rich, and vessel-poor), the major parameters for it being summarized in Table 6.5. The sharp-eyed reader will immediately note that the values for the same-name compartments in Table 6.4 and 6.5 for the same physiological parameters do not generally agree. Each research group tends to use the values it has found to work for it; hence the proliferation of different "standard values." A concentration 90% of steady state occurs in 3.3 half-times, and 99% in 5 half-times. All other things being equal (in spite of disagreement over the actual values), the half-time for residence in each compartment for different compounds is influenced primarily by the tissue/blood partition coefficient. For many unchlorinated organics, the half-time in the vessel-rich tissues varies between 0.8 and 3.2 min; or, 3 to 10 min is the time required to reach 90% of steady state. Within this time frame, 75% of the venous blood has the same concentration of xenobiotic as

TABLE 6.5. Data for methyl ethyl ketone (MEK), toluene (TOL), and *n*-hexane (HEX) to fit a four-compartment model to account for the elimination of the xenobiotic from the body of a male, 70-kg person.*

		Compartment			
Parameter	Solvent	Vessel-rich	Muscle-rich	Fat-rich	Vessel-poor
Volume (L)		6.0	33.0	14.5	12.5
Perfusion (L/min)		5.25	1.27	0.38	0.1
Cardiac output (%)		75.0	18.1	5.4	1.5
Tissue/blood distribution coefficient	MEK	1.0	1.2	0.88	—
	TOL	2.3	1.6	82.0	1.9
	HEX	4.0	5.0	130.0	—
Distribution volume (L)	MEK	6.0	39.6	12.8	—
	TOL	13.8	52.8	1189.0	23.7
	HEX	24.0	165.0	1885.0	—
Half-time (min)	MEK	0.8	21.8	23.3	—
	TOL	1.8	28.8	36.1 h	2.7
	HEX	3.2	90.0	57.4 h	—

* Adapted from reference 113.

has arterial blood, assuming cardiac output to the vessel-rich compartment to be 75%. Blood at the extremities tends to have lower concentrations than venous blood [113]. Thus the fingerstick samples often used in studies of children may not be representative of venous blood samples, which are more closely related to exposure than fingerstick samples.

No generalized models for inorganics have appeared apart for specific elements such as lead. Clearly, it would be highly worthwhile to develop a predictive model for chemicals where complete information is not available. A variant of these models [108, 113] will be discussed in Chapter 21. Models also indicate that monitoring for one marker may be insufficient for an investigator to interpret the situation correctly.

Few models exist that take into account the metabolic pools and turnover in other biological monitoring media such as hair, nails, teeth, fat, milk, saliva, sebum, tears, ear wax, sweat, semen, sputum, feces, or gaseous emissions of the body.

6.4 KERATINIZED BIOLOGICAL MONITORING MEDIA

6.4.1 Hair

Hair has good storage qualities, and some spectacular discoveries have been made with hair analysis of long-dead people. For example, arsenic was found in the hair of Napoleon Bonaparte; and mercury was discovered in the hair of physicist Isaac Newton, and was related to his experiments in alchemy.

Hair is plentiful and is easily collected, transported, stored, and analyzed for metals. It can be analyzed segmentally to obtain an exposure history since the last cutting, or analyzed whole to provide a total exposure since the last cutting. Hair metal measurements have been performed since the early 1900s.

Clinically, Menkes' steely-hair syndrome, caused by a rare genetic defect in copper transport and storage, not only is recognizable by kinky or steely hair but also by depigmentation of the skin and hair, hypothermia, seizures, cerebral degeneration, and vascular defects. Low serum, hepatic, and cerebral copper levels, low ceruloplasmin, and little or no cytochrome oxidase activity in nerve tissue accompany the other symptoms, which are fully manifested in infants by age 3 months.

Hair analysis has been used mostly to detect metals, which are excreted into the hair shaft in the same concentration as in the nearby plasma and are not known to have any functional role in hair protein although Menkes' syndrome points to a role for copper. Each segment of hair reflects plasma concentrations from all sources at the time of hair shaft synthesis; thus the analysis of one whole hair is a cumulative measure of exposure from the last time of cutting to the time of sampling, assuming no external contamination.

This last caveat is the single biggest obstacle to the acceptance of hair as a biological monitoring medium. Surface contamination from the external environment, shampoos, cosmetics, sweat, sebum, water during showers, hair oil, greases, and combing are still major obstacles in spite of many methods of washing. The interferences may be inhaled, absorbed through the skin, or ingested to add to the absorbed dose, and are indistinguishable from true exposure from a known source. Hair generally has also a natural oily coating, which can trap external sweat or external dust. The frequency of hair washing will affect cleanliness of the hair also. Because any adsorbed material is not related to the absorbed dose, such material must be removed. The old question "How clean is clean?" still is unsolved. Where does cleaning merge with leaching out of hair material?

The simplest washing technique employs distilled deionized water rinses and oven drying. Some investigators have used acetone, nitric acid, ether, and trisodium ethylenediamine tetraacetic acid; and others have tried detergent, followed by distilled water and then organic solvent washes, or have done this in reverse order. A method often mentioned is the one recommended [114] by the International Atomic Energy Agency, involving successive triplicate washings in acetone, deionized water, and acetone again. Some procedures such as nitric acid treatment have also removed internal hair metals as well as adsorbed species. Ionic detergents solubilized ionic species but essentially left intact any oils, natural or otherwise, whereas neutral detergents also removed the natural oily coating of the hair.

External contamination might be minimized if pubic, armpit, or breast hair were used instead of scalp hair. However, sweat becomes a greater problem here, as do the material and the cleanliness of clothes worn over the skin surface. Hair from different areas may grow at different rates. Axillary hair grows at about two-thirds the rate of scalp hair, and pubic hair at about half the rate. Body hair grows at the same rate as scalp hair. If clothes are tight-fitting, that is doubtless a factor, since prolonged friction against the legs is well known for producing naked patches of skin devoid of hair.

Nevertheless, many metals have been detected in hair, as documented in innumerable reviews [115–121]. The difficulty is not that metals can be detected; the problem lies in the interpretation of the concentrations.

Some diseases or pathological conditions have been associated with altered trace elements in hair [117]. Chromium is decreased by parity and juvenile diabetes mellitus [122, 123]; severe thermal burns decrease zinc [124]; manganese is decreased in the hair of infants with congenital malformations [125]; cadmium and lead increases in the hair of children have been associated with learning disabilities [126]. Hair mercury on samples cut in 1973 indicated a massive poisoning incident that occurred in Iraq in 1971–72 due to the consumption of homemade bread contaminated with a methylmercury fungicide [127]. Dose–response neurologic effects were observed in 82 infant–mother pairs with a threshold effect about 10 to 20 μg/g hair. Epidemiological studies on fish-eating populations in Canada [128] and New Zealand [129] appeared to confirm this threshold. In an experiment in which volunteers consumed fish containing methylmercury [130], 8-mm hair segment levels cut close to the scalp paralleled blood levels with a lag of about 20 days. The data for methylmercury are the strongest illustration of a dose-effect for hair analysis. Recently, hair root analysis has been performed to assess the most recent exposures.

A number of laboratories in the United States analyze hair and provide their clients information on nutritional deficiencies and overburdens [121]. There has been at least one case of misinterpretation through commercial laboratory testing [131].

Hair grows at a rate of about 1 cm in 30 days; so analysis of hair clippings provides data related to plasma content, depending on the shaft length and the length of the remaining proximal shaft since the last cutting.

Interpretation of hair concentrations would be difficult even if the external-contamination washing problem were to be solved. Many metals are transported in the blood in the bound form (for example, iron in ferritin) or are stored in the body (for example, lead and strontium in bone). Anything that causes release of the free ion could result in a short- or long-term "overexposure," which may have nothing to do with exposure since the last time of hair cutting. The converse is also true for "underexposure."

Chemicals such as xenobiotics or medicinals may also displace metals bound to transport proteins, peptides, and amino acids. Wasting diseases like AIDS may release stored metals. Certain absorbed complexes from ingested green plants may chelate metals. Meats also constitute a more highly absorbable form of many metals; for example, heme iron is more efficiently absorbed than inorganic divalent iron. High-fiber diets lower metal absorption in the intestine. Cosmetics and hair dyes may not only be adsorbed to hair directly, but they may be absorbed by the skin and thus contribute to any absorbed dose reflected in the blood, and hence the hair shaft. Many metals are found [117] in hair dyes, dye formulations, and cosmetics, including aluminum, arsenic, barium, boron, calcium, chromium (III), cobalt, copper, fluorine, iron, lead, magnesium, selenium, silicon, sodium, tin, titanium, zinc, and zirconium. Thus a complete medical history as well as knowledge about prior exposures, medicines, cosmetics and hair dye use, and diet is required for one to be able to interpret hair analyses.

The effects of age and gender are contradictory. A concentration of 30 to 40 mg lead/kg hair has been advocated as the upper normal concentration, and this has been found to correspond to about 90 μg lead/100 g blood. Other correlations, notably with copper, cadmium, and zinc, are contradictory.

Hair is generally collected from the back of the head at the nape, using stainless steel scissors to cut as close as possible to the scalp. Collected hair should be no longer than 1 to 2 inches, measuring from the scalp outward. The ends of hairs that exceed this length usually are cut and discarded. About 0.5 to 1 g (1–2 tablespoons) is collected, and if metals analysis is to be done, the hair is placed in labeled plastic bags.

The chief methods for hair metal analysis are digestion in nitric acid followed by atomic absorption or inductively coupled plasma; other types of metal analyses that have been used include neutron activation analysis, anodic stripping voltammetry, proton induced X-ray emission, spectrophotometry, spark source mass spectrometry, and X-ray fluorescence [132].

The elemental composition of normal hair is given by Iyengar et al. in ppm [61]: Ag, 2–766; Al, 2–66; As, 0.13–3.71; Au, 0.0017–1.25; B, 5; Ba, 0.55–4.2; Be, 0.0063–0.021; Bi, 2; Br, 0.65–53.3; Ca, 146–3190; Cd, 0.24–2.7; Cl, 950–4805; Co, 0.2–1.05; Cr, 0.13–3.65; Cs, 0.37–1.1; Cu, 11–34; Fe, 5–44.7; Ga, 0.07–25; Ge, 2.3; Hg, 1.25–7.6; I, 2–750; K, 2–282; La, 2–718; Mg, 19–163; Mn, 0.25–5.7; Mo, 2–282; N, 140–157; Na, 18–1720; Nb, 2.2; Ni, 0.6–6.5; P, 83–165; Pb, 3–70; Po, 18.5–72; Ra, 19; Rb, 0.21–0.5; S, 42,200–47,700; Sb, 0.09–3.0; Se, 0.64–2.53; Si, 20–1950; Sn, 1; Sr, 0.046–0.92; Ti, 0.048–14; Tl, 0.016; U, 0.00013; V, 20–90; W, 66; Zn, 99–450; and Zr, 1.15–1.6.

Some organics that have been found in hair include PCBs and *o*-dichlorobenzene [132].

6.4.2 Nails

These media (fingernails, toenails) are very like hair in that they are keratinized tissues and have been used to detect metals. Human fingernails grow about 100 μm/day, whereas human toenails grow about 25 μm/day [119].

All of the same physiological factors discussed for hair analysis apply here. Varnishes, shoe interiors, socks, sweat, skin, and microbes (for example, athlete's foot) may have to be considered as sources of other metals. Hygiene and the frequency of cleaning also must be factored in.

Iyengar et al. give the elemental composition of nails in ppm as [61]: Ag, 0.0003–1.4; Al, 132–927; As, 0.2–3.3; Au, 0.03–0.78; B, 33; Ba, 7.5; Be, <0.01; Bi, 1.35; Br, 9–10; Ca, 368–3400; Cd, 0.08–3.4; Ce, 0.6; Cl, 1090–3570; Co, <0.2; Cr, 6.2; Cs, 6.6; Cu, 11.2–53; Fe, 27–347; Ge, 1.2; Hg, <0.07–7.27; K, 357–2800; La, 0.31; Mg, 16.2–125; Mn, 0.04–2.1; Mo, <0.15–5.6; N, 146–148; Na, 332–3010; Ni, 0.033–11.9; P, 180–990; Pb, 13.8–39; Rb, 3.1; S, 4780–36,600; Sb, <0.03–0.75; Se, 1.14–8; Si, 310–3550; Sn, 12; Sr, 0.017–0.65; Ti, 0.28; Tl, 0.0022–1.6; V, <0.15; Zn, 73–304; and Zr, 0.96.

Like hair, nails can concentrate mercury after methylmercury exposure [127].

The sampling, washing, and analytical methods for nails are the same as for hair. Nails are less convenient to sample than hair because of the pain involved in removing them. The parts that people habitually cut are the oldest, and their concentrations will be related to long-past exposures. The nail nearest the quick is the youngest, and it is not practical to sample it from living persons. Nails have an advantage over hair in that they do not have an oily covering to adsorb chemicals from the external environment.

6.5 AQUEOUS MEDIA DERIVED FROM BLOOD PLASMA

Saliva, tears, and sweat contain chemicals transferred from blood plasma as well as the urine. The concentrations in the first three fluids appear to reflect free levels in plasma. Because dilution effects occur, any xenobiotic concentrations should be normalized to a reference compound in these fluids. Such reference compounds, however, still have not been agreed upon. Collection of sweat and tears is not convenient, nor is it very practical for routine sampling, though saliva is easy to sample. The degree of contamination from the last meal varies with mouth hygiene and eating habits. The elemental contents of blood, red blood cells, blood plasma, blood serum, saliva, and sweat are compared in Table 6.2.

These fluids should be collected in plastic, acid-washed glass, or stainless steel containers if inorganic analysis is to be performed; the acid- and organic solvent–washed glass containers are recommended for samples to be analyzed for organics. Control containers containing the same volume of distilled deionized water as the sample should be analyzed also. All the containers should be wrapped in aluminum foil to decrease the likelihood of photodecomposition. If possible, if the samples have to be stored or transported, they should be frozen.

6.5.1 Sweat

Sweat tests were reported in 1953 when it was found that children with cystic fibrosis of the pancreas (probably the most serious genetic disease among Caucasians) secreted abnormally high concentrations of electrolytes in sweat [133]. In early studies, sweat was stimulated by hyperthermia, which caused some deaths. There were also many false positives and negatives. In 1959, Gibson and Cooke reported a technique called quantitative pilocarpine iontophoresis that induced localized sweating pharmacologically. Sweat was collected efficiently with absorbent pads, which then were analyzed for metals or chloride. This is still the reference method for sweat analysis. Alternative methods were developed in the 1960s and 1970s, including chloride ion electrodes that measured chloride directly on the skin and plastic cup collection as an alternative sampling method. The cup's cleanliness and potential to adsorb created problems. The chloride electrode had to be skillfully used, was easily contaminated, was hard to decontaminate, and was easy to break. In 1984, another device, the Macroduct™, was introduced [134]. A disposable collection device combined the fluid output from several hundred sweat microducts into a single macroduct in the form of coiled plastic tubing. This minimized evaporation and external condensation of water, and allowed the sweat sample to be visible so that the volume could be determined. Localized sweating is induced by pilocarpine from battery-operated Pilogel™ reservoirs for ionotophoresis. The conductivity of the sample can be read with as little as 6 μL, and other analytical techniques for elements, anions, cations, conductivity, and osmalality can be applied.

Organics have also been found in sweat, including benzoic acid, ethanol, phenol, salicyclic acid, and urea. Arsenate appears very quickly in sweat after its administration. Rapid skin absorption in humans of finely powdered lead metal (20 mg; 100 mesh) or 0.5 M lead nitrate solution (60 μL) has been observed [135], with the absorbed lead appearing in sweat induced by pilocarpine-induced iontophoresis within 2 days after a 24-h exposure (from 15–25 μg Pb/L to >300 μg/L) and in saliva (2.5–15 μg Pb/L), but not in the blood or the urine. The absorption rate increased with increased skin sweating. Nine battery plant workers exposed occupationally showed high sweat lead (71–17,700 μg/L sweat) in spite of only moderately high blood lead concentrations (19–95 μg/dL). The sweat concentrations may be more related to dermal exposure than to inhalation exposure, for which a well-studied link to blood lead has been determined. The roles of skin contamination and the dependence of skin absorption on sweaty conditions are not clear.

Osmone 1 is a steroid found in human sweat that is chemically similar to animal musks [136]. It is secreted by the sebaceous glands and reportedly has possible tranquilizing effects when sniffed. It is a possible precursor of 5-α-androsterone. The odoriferous component of sweat is postulated to be 3-methyl-2-hexonic acid.

6.5.2 Saliva

Saliva is very available and convenient to sample, the sampling being noninvasive. Generally, the individual to be sampled rinses out his or her mouth with water and then chews on an inert material such as rubber or wax from 30 sec to several minutes. The first mouthful of saliva is discarded, and thereafter the saliva is collected into an acid-washed glass bottle. However, saliva is still prone to contamination by food residues, and to contamination if the teeth, mouth, tongue, and gums are not clean and healthy. Tooth fillings may contribute metals. Microbial products may accumulate in the mouth saliva produced from teeth with many caries.

Saliva secretion usually is initiated by reflex parasympathetic stimulation of the acinar cells [137]. Mechanical stimulation also is well-known, for example, while brushing the teeth. An increase of intracellular calcium ion has been shown to be the primary trigger for saliva secretion and also is correlated with the loss of intracellular chloride and potassium ions [138].

Saliva concentrations of the antiepileptic phenytoin show a good correspondence with blood concentrations. Salicylic acid has been detected in the saliva.

The major use of saliva as a biological monitoring medium has been for antipyrine clearance determinations to monitor the activity of the hepatic endoplasmic reticulum enzymes [139]. The technique has been used since 1978. Laypersons themselves can take the samples. Four to seven samples can be taken 24 to 48 h after administration of the drug (usually 1 g). This has now been simplified to taking one sample at least 18 h after drug administration, along with computing the volume of distribution with regard to age, gender, body weight, and height. Saliva, urine, or plasma can be used. Personal baseline sampling also is necessary to minimize the coefficient of variation of the volume of distribution. People exposed to xenobiotics that require processing by cytochrome P-450 complex enzymes for detoxification can be sampled to assess whether induction or inhibition of the liver enzymes occurs relative to concentrations before exposure. If the baseline requires measurement in already exposed people, they should not be exposed for at least one week before the baseline measurement is taken (for example, after a vacation). The two samples must be collected at the same time on the same day of the week because the hepatic enzymes have an intrinsic circadian rhythm. This means that drug administration must be strictly timed in this regard also. A sensitive liquid chromatographic method is available for the analysis [140].

Antipyrine is rapidly and completely absorbed from the gastrointestinal tract and distributed with less than 10% bound to plasma and tissue proteins and with less than 5% eliminated unchanged in the urine [139]. Antipyrine has a negligible first-pass metabolism, and the metabolism is virtually independent of changes in liver–blood perfusion. There are three major Phase I metabolites out of five known ones, and Phase II conjugation allows excretion. Its elimination obeys pseudo first-order kinetics with a half-time of about 10 h in healthy people. The distribution volume is equal to total body water (Chapter 4), implying equal distribution.

Antipyrine clearance is enhanced [141] by organochlorine alicyclic pesticides such as chlordecone and lindane, chlorinated aromatic pesticides such as DDT and the chlorinated phenoxy herbicides, halothane above 20 ppm in air, PCBs, tobacco smoke, alcohol, caffeine, and gasoline vapors. No change occurs for styrene or toluene, or for halothane vapors in air at less than 20 ppm. Lead and spray-painting chemicals inhibit it.

Clinically, saliva is used to test for secretory IgA in infant hypogammaglobulinemia, for β^2-microglobulin in Sjogren's syndrome, for steroids, and for zinc for gustin decrease during taste impairment. The difference in pH of saliva and serum is such that ratios of bound/free drugs are not the same; so saliva measurements are not surrogates for serum ones.

6.5.3 Tears

Tears are very inconvenient to sample on a routine basis. Urea has been detected in this medium.

Chemicals such as acids and alkalis stimulate lachrymation, as do compounds that hydrolyze in water to irritants such as acids and bases, as, for example, acetyl chloride, α-chloroacetophenone, α-bromobenzyl cyanide, benzoyl chloride, and ethyl iodoacetate. Photochemical smog and onion aerosol are other agents that elicit tears, in addition to tear gas.

The tears drain through the lacrimal puncta at the inner nasal margins of the upper and lower eyelids. The flow enters the lacrimal canaliculi in the lid margins and flows through the common caniculus, lacrimal sac, and nasolacrimal duct into the nasopharynx. Tears running down the cheek (epiphora) is the alternative route. The drug furfuryl trimethyl ammonium iodide (Furmethide) blocks lacrimation by inflaming the walls of the entire drainage system.

6.6 BREATH TESTS AS RELATED TO INTESTINAL GAS

These tests have not been used in a workplace setting because of the inconvenience, but clinicians have used them to diagnose malabsorption, for example, of lactose, of other carbohydrates, and even of fats [142]. The chief marker used in such cases is hydrogen concentration. Some ^{13}C-labeled organics have been used to investigate fat malabsorption with analysis of ^{13}C-labeled carbon dioxide or methane.

Oxygen, nitrogen, carbon dioxide, hydrogen, and methane comprise 99% of all intestinal gases, whether they be emitted as flatus, burps, coughs, belches, or farts. Swallowing of food and mouth breathing carry oxygen and nitrogen into the stomach. Hydrogen, carbon dioxide, and methane are all produced, primarily within the colon by microbes that metabolize undigested food. Gluttony is a prime cause of malabsorption. Certain foods also contain carbohydrates not metabolized by pancreatic digestive enzymes or in the mucosal brush border of the small intestine, for example, stachyose and raffinose found in beans. Thus the test is useful as a biological marker for lactose intolerance, secondary lactose intolerance from injury to the intestinal mucosa (confirm with the D-xylose absorption test), bacterial overgrowth caused by partial obstruction, a blind loop, or dysmotility, or for infants with rotavirus or without a known pathogen.

The bacterial flora release predominantly hydrogen and carbon dioxide, but a third of people have bacterial flora that produce methane predominantly. This appears to be related to diet. The concentration of hydrogen at sea level is 0.02 mmol/L. Because hydrogen is not a product of any known metabolic process in humans, any increase in hydrogen concentration above this level reflects the activity of bacterial flora and hence the available undigestible hydrogen sources [143]. About 79% of hydrogen produced is excreted as flatulence, and 21% is absorbed into the blood and is excreted by the lungs. For obvious reasons flatulence and other bodily gaseous emissions are impossible to monitor routinely; so the breath test for hydrogen, though relying on the minor route of excretion, is accessible routinely and conveniently.

A typical methodology is to fast overnight (4–6 h for infants) so that a baseline sample can be collected. Then 2 g/kg body weight (maximum dose 50 g) of lactose or sucrose in a 20% solution is taken orally, and breath sampling is repeated every 30 min for 3 h. If the samples cannot be stored immediately, they are stored at −20°C [144]. A rise of hydrogen greater than 10 ppm within 2 h is regarded as abnormal, and can be accompanied by such clinical symptoms as diarrhea, flatulence, abdominal distention, or pain. The latter become important symptoms for the 2% of patients who do not produce hydrogen, and can be identified through ingestion of lactulose, which will not produce hydrogen in atypical individuals. If there is also bacterial overgrowth, maximum levels of hydrogen are attained by the first 30-min sample.

Susceptible infants more than 2 months of age can be detected by this test in response to a normal lactose load. Assessment of the stool for a reducing substance is not as sensitive as this test. The infant colon of less than age 2 months converts lactose to volatile fatty acids, which act as important sources of energy. Thus the lactose breath hydrogen test is itself unreliable in this situation. Atypical infants usually exhibit watery diarrhea after breast or lactose-formula feeding, often around the time of weaning. This varies with ethnicity, but lactase activity in the small bowel drops to about 10% of the values at birth in Caucasians by 6 years of age [145]. The diagnosis needs to be confirmed by a small bowel biopsy to document normal morphology with absent lactase activity. An abnormal lactose test in Caucasians under five years of age, or an African-American or Asian child under 3 years, often indicates mucosal injury. Celiac disease will not be signaled by a positive lactose test.

This test has not been used in the workplace but could be to indicate the contribution of the intestinal and lung flora and fauna to xenobiotic metabolism, using correlations with hydrogen or methane as appropriate. It could also be used to assess microbial overgrowth during AIDS or HIV infection.

6.7 FATTY MEDIA

6.7.1 Adipose Tissue

Body fat is estimated primarily from skinfold measurements. The assumption here is that one-half of total body fat is deposited as subcutaneous tissue loosely attached to underlying muscles. The skin and the fat are lifted up with the fingers into a fold, and the thickness is measured with a caliper. The triceps and subscapular skinfolds are usually summed. Such a technique is invalid with patients who have edema. Other research methods for body fat have utilized ultrasound, computed tomography, prompt γ neutron activation, and underwater weighing.

The sampling of adipose tissue for xenobiotics is invasive and is not a good routine technique. Females of the same weight have more fat than males. Orientals have more adipose than Caucasians and African peoples of the same weight. Naturally, exceptions will abound, individual diet and physical activity routines being important variables. Neutral fats of an obese male may constitute between 20 and 60% of body weight relative to 20% for a lean, athletic person. The chemical analysis of fats has been well summarized [146].

The toxicity of compounds with high K_{ow} may be lower in obese relative to lean individuals. Fasting or starvation may release any stored toxicants in the fat. Disease states also may mobilize the fat depots. Adipose accumulation is specific for xenobiotics that do not metabolize readily and are not breathed out, and which bioaccumulate (log K_{ow} values >5). Such chemicals are specific polyhalogenated congeners of biphenyls, dibenzofurans, dibenzo-*p*-dioxins, diphenyl ethers, biphenylenes, and similar compounds substituted in the vicinal ring positions, as well as polyhalogenated and polynitro aromatic systems.

Table 6.6 compares chlorinated pesticides found in adipose tissue collected between 1979 and 1981 for two Canadian cities [147]. Most adipose tissues did not contain consistent residues until after age 25 years. These data are probably representative of the huge range of residue concentrations that generally are nonnormally distributed.

Table 6.7 compares 2,3,7,8-tetrachlorodibenzo-*p*-dioxin (2,3,7,8-TCDD) concentrations in people in Times Beach, Missouri, sampled for 20 g of their adipose from the anterior abdominal wall in 1985, with "unexposed" populations [148]. People with greater than 20 pg/g are evidently beyond the "non-

TABLE 6.6. Organochlorine residue ranges in ng/g wet weight in the adipose tissues of male and female persons autopsied at two Canadian cities.*

Chemical	Kingston, Ontario		Ottawa, Ontario	
	Male (51)	Female (40)	Male (53)	Female (31)
α-Chlordane	nd–80	nd–50	10–30	10–20
p,p'-DDD	nd–80	nd–50	nd–30	nd–60
p,p'-DDE	10–17,100	180–7,590	280–10,200	80–8,190
p,p'-DDT	nd–740	10–710	nd–350	30–740
Dieldrin	nd–100	nd–120	nd–130	nd–90
Heptachlor epoxide	10–110	10–90	nd–130	10–130
Hexa CBz	10–402	32–458	17–315	21–280
β-HCH	nd–210	10–3,430	10–680	10–370
Mirex	nd–190	nd–70	nd–120	nd–70
Oxychlordane	10–120	10–80	20–110	10–80
PCB	90–28,300	600–7,350	790–4,760	450–3,570
PCP	nd–277	nd–247	nd–66	5–168
Penta CBz	nd–8	nd–16	nd–44	nd
Photomirex	nd–60	nd–20	nd–30	nd
1,2,3,5/1,2,4,5-Tetra CBz	nd–8	nd–16	nd	nd–3
2,3,4,6/2,3,5,6-Tetra CBz	nd–133	nd–92	nd–31	nd–44
2,3,4,5-Tetra CP	nd–22	nd–22	nd–22	nd–17
1,3,5-Tri CBz	nd–14	nd–22	nd–13	nd–61
1,2,4-Tri CBz	nd–653	nd–122	nd–39	nd–156
1,2,3-Tri CBz	nd–1,320	nd–54	nd	nd–8

*Adapted from reference 147.
nd = not detected. The age ranges were: Kingston, 7–87 for males and 14–88 for females; Ottawa, 16–91 for males and 20–91 for females. DDD and DDE are impurities and metabolites of DDT. Other chemicals are: CBz, chlorobenzene; β-HCH, β-hexachlorocyclohexane; PCB, polychlorinated biphenyls; PCP, pentachlorophenol; CP, chlorophenol.

TABLE 6.7. Comparison of Times Beach, Missouri, 2,3,7,8-TCDD concentration ranges in pg/g in the adipose tissue of exposed and "nonexposed" groups.*

Group	Categories			
	Recreational	Residential	Occupational	Total
Exposed	5.0–577	2.8–59.1	3.5–750	2.8–750
Number	8	16	15	39
Men	3	7	14	24
	Place	Source	Number	Concentration
Unexposed	Missouri	surgical	57	1.4–20.2
	Ohio	autopsy	6	5–12
	Missouri, Canada	autopsy veterans	61	1–15
	Georgia, Utah	autopsy	35	2.7–19

*Modified from reference 148.

exposed" range. The whole-body half-time for 2,3,7,8-TCDD was calculated to be between 5 and 8 years.

Polyhalogenated phenols, plasticizers such as the phthalate esters, polynuclear aromatic hydrocarbons, aromatic organophosphate pesticides, aromatic nitrosamines, aromatic acids, and highly halogenated aliphatics also have been detected. A bioconcentration factor in 20 humans (aged 16–87 years) for pentachlorophenol relative to dietary intake was calculated for their organs, based on wet weight calculations, to be [149]: liver, 5.7; brain, 3.3; blood, 1.4; spleen, 1.4; and adipose tissue, 1.0. The half-time was about 20 days. The log K_{ow} is 2.50. Pentachlorophenol thus is not a large bioaccumulator in the adipose tissue, but the chemical still can be detected. The bioconcentration factors for pentachlorophenol for several countries relative to their diet were: Federal Republic of Germany, 1.0; United States, 2.7–3.0; Canada, 2.2; and Japan, 2.2.

The U.S. EPA has sponsored a broad-scan analysis of xenobiotics in human adipose tissue from people in the general population [150]. Purge and trappable organics were detected. The compounds with an upper range greater than 100 ng/g wet weight were: xylene (1400), methyl chloroform (830), chloroform (580), 1,4-dichlorobenzene (500), ethylphenol (400), styrene (350), ethylbenzene (280), and toluene (250). Similarly, the major semivolatile organics were: *p,p'*-DDE (6800), dieldrin (4100), PCBs (1700), butylbenzyl phthalate (1700), di-*n*-butylphthalate (1700), hexachlorobenzene (1300), diethyl phthalate (970), triphenyl phosphate (850), dioctyl phthalate (850), β-BHC (570), *p,p'*-DDT (540), *trans*-nonachlor (520), heptachlor epoxide (310), *tris*-(2-chloroethyl) phosphate (210), and tributyl phosphate (120). Toxaphene was present in most samples but was not quantified. PCDDs and PCDFs were also detected in pg/g: 2,3,7,8-TCDD, 1.3–14; 1,2,3,7,8-PeCDD, 1.3–5000; all HxCDD, 13–620; 1,2,3,4,7,8,9-HpCDD, 26–1300; OCDD, 19–3700; 2,3,7,8-TCDF, 1.3–660; 2,3,4,7,8-PeCDF, 1.3–90; all HxCDF, 3.0–60; 1,2,3,4,6,7,8-HpCDF, 3.5–79; and OCDF, 1.2–890.

Metals such as Ag, As, Cd, Cr, Cu, Mn, Pd, V, and Zn also have been detected after exposure in the workplace. The U.S. EPA broad-scan study for constituents of adipose tissue in the general population detected the following elements in μg/g wet weight [150]: Ag, 0.12–0.38; Al, 0.6–8.3; Au, 0.0025–0.0030; B, <0.32; Br, 0.33–2.4; Ca, 15–41; Cl, 240–1500; Co, 0.035–0.078; Fe, 3.0–36 by ICP-AES and 3.5–40 by neutron activation analysis; I, 1.4–13; K, 52–270; Mg, 6.5–25; Na, 150–640 by ICP-AES and 240–1200 by neutron activation analysis; P, 130–220; Rb, 0.18–0.27; Se, 0.030–0.056; Sn, 8.7–15; Zn, 1.1–6.0 by ICP-AES and 1.4–4.5 by neutron activation analysis.

Adipose tissue commonly is sampled from the buttocks by a needle biopsy (about a 200-mg sample) or by a surgical procedure for larger amounts. In the latter, fat sometimes is taken from the peritoneal cavity. Tissue samples should not be wrapped in plastic if organics are to be analyzed but in aluminum foil with the shiny side outside (this contains chlorinated organics). Preservatives, saline, or fixatives must not be added. The wrapped-up sample should be placed in an acid-washed glass container and frozen at −20°C within 30 min after sampling.

The analytical chemistry laboratory then saponifies [146] the sample with potassium hydroxide/ethanol to form ethers and carboxylates. The neutral xenobiotics then are removed by multiple extractions in an appropriate organic solvent such as hexane or methylene chloride after removal of the ethanol. The salts remain in the aqueous phase, and can be removed as free acids after acidification by diethyl ether extraction. The free acids then can be esterified by standard techniques for GC/MS quantitation.

The U.S. EPA in its broad-scan study of constituents of adipose tissue [150] classified "volatile organics" by their ability to be amenable to the heated purge-and-trap technique; "semivolatile organics" separation was based on further gel permeation chromatography and Florisil fractionation; PCDDs and PCDFs were separated from PCBs by column chromatography. Organics were confirmed to be present by gas chromatography/high resolution mass spectrometry.

6.7.2 Breast Milk

There are few lactating women in the workplace, but there are many women exposed to chemicals in the general environment and to those in food. Because nursed infants have body weights as small as one-twentieth the body weight of the mother, concentrations that do not affect the mother may affect the child, whether exposure occurs by breast milk or in the womb, where the potential hazard is even greater but often is mitigated by the placental barrier. In addition, the neonatal enzyme system for metabolism often is incomplete, leading to bioaccumulation of xenobiotics. Such bioaccumulation is seen for lead, which causes greater neurobehavioral problems in children than adults.

Milk has an aqueous and a lipid phase. The concentrations in the aqueous phase might be expected to be related to unbound blood concentrations, as for the aqueous biological fluids in Section 6.5. All the chemicals that accumulate in adipose tissue also accumulate in breast milk in the lipid phase.

A risk assessment approach for nursing infants exposed to volatile organics through the mother's occupational inhalation exposure has appeared [9]. Compounds with low blood/air and octanol/water coefficients present low risks, and high partition coefficients give high risks. For intermediate blood/air coefficients between 2 and 25 and octanol/water coefficients between 100 and 1500, the dose to the child is never greater than 35% that of the mother. A seven-parameter model for the mother and eight parameters for the child were assumed. A three-compartment model was assumed: central, fat, and mammary/milk. The mother's parameters were: cardiac output, 214 L/h; pulmonary ventilation, 171 L/h; fat tissue perfusion, 19 L/h; mammary tissue perfusion, 42 L/h; central compartment volume, 48 L; fat volume, 5 L; and mammary tissue volume, 1 L. The child's parameters were: cardiac output, 38 L/h; pulmonary ventilation, 30 L/h; fat perfusion, 0.85 L/min; fat volume, 0.4 L; central compartment volume, 4.1 L; uptake per milk feeding, 0.3 L; feeding duration, 5 min; and feeding frequency, 3.5 times/h. The efficiency of absorption of milk by the child is assumed to be 100%. Thus, assuming a Michaelis–Menten type of metabolism (Section 1.10):

$$dA_i/dt = Q_i[CBM - CV_i] - V_{max}CV_i/[K_m + CV_i] \tag{6.5}$$

where:

A_i = amount of xenobiotic in tissue$_i$ at time t
Q_i = blood flow to tissue$_i$

$CV_i = A_i/[V_iP_i]$
V_i = the volume of tissue_i
P_i = tissue/blood partition coefficient for tissue_i
V_{max} and K_m = Michaelis–Menten parameters (equation 1.22)

If xenobiotics themselves are being considered in the milk, the second Michaelis–Menten term is unnecessary. However, if metabolites are being measured, this term must be included to account for the metabolic rate. For the xenobiotic itself, as discussed in Section 4.0, an effective dose at a given point in time is given by the area under the curve for blood (AUCB). The relative effective dose for the child (REDC) can be calculated as follows:

$$\text{REDC} = \text{AUCB[child]/AUCB[mother]} \tag{6.6}$$

The AUCB[child] is a function of the metabolism of the chemical in the mother and in the child, and of excretion by the mother and the child as well as transfer in the milk, placental transfer to the child before birth, and the bioaccumulatory potential of the chemical. Except for the bone-seeking species lead (II), strontium (II), and fluoride, most stored xenobiotics in the child are excreted soon after birth so that placental transfer for organics is often a negligible factor on a suckling child's exposure except for soon after birth.

The milk/blood partition coefficient ($K_{\text{milk/blood}}$) is calculated by equation (6.7), in which a 4% fat content is assumed:

$$K_{\text{milk/blood}} = c_{\text{milk}}/c_{\text{blood}} = 0.04\ K_{\text{fat/blood}} + 0.96[1.0] \tag{6.7}$$

where c_{blood} is the equilibrium concentration in blood, and c_{milk} is the equilibrium concentration in milk.

Equation (3.19) connects the partition coefficients for fat/blood and octanol/water. Thus, REDC can be calculated for many workplace chemicals (Table 6.8). The highest REDC values are for toluene (0.1658), 1,2-dichloroethane (0.0931), trichloroethylene (0.0861), and benzene (0.0810).

After one exposure, the REDC continues to rise for days afterward, according to this model. For multiple 9-h workshifts it can be shown that the REDC approaches an asymptotic value, 90% of this being achieved by two months of exposure using the assumptions of the model. According to the constraints of the model, the following empirical predictive equation has been derived for REDC:

$$\text{REDC} = 0.0011\ K_{\text{blood/air}}\ K_{\text{octanol/water}}^{0.35} \tag{6.8}$$

for these intermediate partition coefficients.

Because the mechanism of transport between mammary tissue and bulk milk is not known precisely, two separate models have been advocated. Model 1 has milk concentration controlled by continual equilibration with mammary blood flow; model 2 has xenobiotic accumulation in the milk based on mammary tissue concentration at the time of milk production.

Model 1 assumes the xenobiotic diffuses between the mammary tissue and milk (indicated by subscript *m*) so that, applying equation (6.5):

TABLE 6.8. **Relative child-to-mother blood concentrations (REDC) and partition coefficients for blood/air ($K_{blood/air}$) and for fat/blood ($K_{fat/blood}$) for various chemicals, calculated by using equations (3.19) and (6.6) and assuming 2 months' exposure of 9 h/day work exposure of the mother and 7 days/week exposure of the child to the mother's milk.***

Chemical	$K_{blood/air}$	$K_{fat/blood}$	REDC
Benzene	8.2	60.9	0.0810
Chloroethane	2.7	14.3	0.0123
Chloroform	6.9	29.6	0.0430
1-Chloropropane	2.9	41.4	0.0224
1,1-Dichloroethane	4.9	33.2	0.0329
1,2-Dichloroethane	19.5	17.6	0.0931
1,1-Dichloroethylene	5.0	13.7	0.0221
cis-1,2-Dichloroethylene	9.9	23.0	0.0537
trans-1,2-Dichloroethylene	6.0	24.5	0.0340
Dichloromethane	8.9	13.4	0.0385
1,2-Dichloropropane	8.8	57.0	0.0823
Diethyl ether	12.2	3.9	0.0395
Halothane	5.3	34.6	0.0364
n-Hexane	2.3	69.4	0.0254
Isopropyl bromide	2.6	61.5	0.0262
Methyl chloroform	2.5	104.0	0.0374
n-Propyl bromide	7.1	33.3	0.0474
Toluene	18.0	56.7	0.1658
Trichloroethylene	7.9	70.2	0.0861
Vinyl bromide	2.3	21.7	0.0124

* Adapted from reference 9.

$$dA_m/dt = Q_m[CBM - CV_m] - QO[CV_m]K_m \tag{6.9}$$

where QO is the suckling rate of the child, and K_m is the milk/blood partition coefficient of the chemical considered (Table 6.8).

Thus:

$$CM = \text{concentration of chemical in milk} = CV_mK_m \tag{6.10}$$

Model 2 treats mammary tissue and milk as two separate compartments with irreversible transport of the xenobiotic to the milk, with the application again of equation (6.5):

$$dA_{mt}/dt = Q_{mt}[CBM - CV_m] - QP[CV_m]K_m \tag{6.11}$$

$$dA_{mk}/dt = QP[CV_m]K_m - QO[CM] \tag{6.12}$$

$$CM = A_{mk}/V_{mk} \tag{6.13}$$

where:

A_{mt} = mass in mammary tissue at time t
A_{mk} = mass in milk at time t
QP = rate of milk production
V_{mk} = volume of milk

TABLE 6.9. Concentrations in ng/g milk fat of lindane isomers (HCHs), 1,1,1-trichloro-2,2-*bis*-(p-chlorophenyl) ethane compounds (DDTs), and polychlorinated biphenyls (PCBs) in mother's milk in India.*

				Concentrations in ng/g milk fat		
1	2	3	4	HCHs	DDTs	PCBs
5	19–28	3–420	0.26–3.4	8773[7623] 3400–26,000	1022[706] 100–2400	180[275] 21–770
6	22–33	90–510	1.3–15	2120[1195] 1100–4000	1652[2527] 110–6100	59[75] 7.0–190
7	22–29	90–360	0.95–4.3	2850[822] 1900–3800	758[381] 230–1300	108[174] 7.0–190
8	21–26	60–150	1.8–5.1	10,300[7692] 1900–17,000	2347[1963] 140–3900	21.1[15.4] 3.3–31
9	19–33	3–510	0.26–15	6204[6398] 1100–26,000	1244[1376] 100–6100	120[206] 7.0–770

*Modified from reference 153.
(1) Sampling location in India; (2) mother's age in years; (3) age of nursed child in days; (4) fat content in %; (5) Chidambaram, 250 km south of Madras City (11 persons sampled Aug. 7–14, 1988); (6) Chinnoor Parangipettai, a fishing village 30 km north of Chidambaram (5 persons sampled Sept. 1, 1988); (7) Madras, a city located on the southwest coast (6 persons sampled Sept. 6, 1988); (8) Nattarasankottai, a rural area 250 km south of Chidambaram (3 persons sampled Dec. 28–31, 1988). The numbers under HCHs, DDTs, and PCBs are arithmetic mean/standard deviation on the first line, with the range underneath.

Model 2 is an accumulatory model rather than a blood equilibrium one like Model 1. The time span for accumulation is not known; so which model is correct has not been demonstrated.

Many compounds have been detected in milk, and some specific instances follow. Canadian data on the major organochlorine compounds in breast milk and milkfat similar to fat data have been reported. Unfortunately, the use of arithmetic means instead of ranges for these data, which undoubtedly are distributed nonnormally, precludes their quotation here [151]. The same applies for some 1988 Norwegian data [152], and most of the data reported by investigators worldwide [153].

Some Indian data are quoted [153] in Table 6.9 to illustrate the extreme nonnormality of most residue data. Clearly, the use of arithmetic means is not representative of any of the data in Table 6.9 except for total HCHs for Madras. The major HCH isomer was the β, followed by the alpha among α, β, γ, and δ isomers, *p,p′*-DDE predominated among the DDTs (*p,p′*-DDD and *p,p′*-DDT in addition). DDT and lindane are still being used in India and account for more than 50% of the insecticides applied there. Most underdeveloped countries use these pesticides heavily (including Latin America, where breast milk concentrations are also very high) even though their use in the United States has ceased.

Congener patterns of polychlorinated dibenzo-*p*-dioxins (PCDDs) and dibenzofurans (PCDFs) in milk and the adipose tissue are identical (Table 6.10). All the major components are 2,3,7,8-substituted. This means that the congener and isomer patterns relative to the exposing mixture change so that the original isomer/congener pattern is not helpful in identifying sources of these chlorinated compounds [154]. These congeners are also the ones that

TABLE 6.10. Comparison of concentrations of PCDDs and PCDFs in adipose tissue from 31 people and breast milk from 4 mothers in Sweden.*

Compound class	Congener	Mean Concentrations [range] in pg/g	
		Adipose tissue	Breast milk
PCDDS	2,3,7,8-	3[nd–9]	0.6
	1,2,3,7,8-	10[3–24]	6.5[3.5–13.8]
	1,2,3,4,7,8-	nd	nd
	1,2,3,6,7,8-	15[3–55]	nd
	1,2,3,7,8,9-	4[3–5]	nd
	1,2,3,4,6,7,8-	97[12–380]	59.5[28–86]
	OCDD	414[90–763]	302[197–484]
PCDFs	2,3,7,8-	4[0.3–11]	4.2[2.2–8]
	2,3,4,7,8-	54[9–84]	21.3[7–53]
	1,2,3,4,7,8-	6[1–15]	nd
	1,2,3,6,7,8-	5[1–13]	nd
	2,3,4,6,7,8-	2[1–7]	nd
	1,2,3,4,6,7,8-	11[1–49]	7.4[4.4–12]
	OCDF	4	3.2[nd–11]

* Modified from reference 154.
nd, not detected; PCDD, polychlorinated dibenzo-*p*-dioxin; PCDF, polychlorinated dibenzofuran; OCDD, the octachlorinated isomer of PCDDs; OCDF, the octachlorinated isomer of PCDFs.

TABLE 6.11. Comparison of PCB isomer and congener pattern in human breast milk and exposing Aroclor 1260.*

Ratio in Milk/Aroclor	Ballschmiter PCB number [156]
O (not detected in milk but detected in Aroclor)	018, 017, 024, 016, 029, 026, 021, 053, 045, 043, 042, 040, 100, 095, 091, 134, 131, 176, 129, 178, 175, 173, 200, 084, 083, 097, 085, 136, 154, 082, 149, 199, 207
<0.1 but >0	185, 174, 196, 195
>10 but <100	033, 022, 046, 049, 118, 099
>100	028, 037, 074
Infinity (not detected in Aroclor but detected in milk)	114, 130, 119, 157

* Modified from reference 155.

accumulate in human liver, but especially those above the tetrachlorinated isomers. These are also the most toxic congeners (except for the fully chlorinated congener), and many investigators are now using "TCDD toxic equivalents" (concentration weighted by the biological potency of the congener) to aid in risk assessment. When it is remembered that there are 135 PCDFs and 75 PCDDS, this approach simplifies their analysis even if there is no relation to the original isomer pattern in the exposing mixtures.

The vicinally substituted isomers again predominate [154] for PCBs (Table 6.11). As there are 217 PCBs [155], this again simplifies analysis. Blood PCB patterns well after exposure are also different from that of the exposing PCB; blood patterns soon after exposure are very similar to the exposing PCB [155].

The tasks of identifying and quantifying mixtures such as PCBs, PCDDs, PCDFs, toxaphene, Stoddard Solvent, and chlordane are much greater than for single compounds in biological media as well as in the environment, where enrichment also occurs.

Metals are also found in breast milk [61]. Concentrations for some elements in mature transitional colostrum are, in μg/L (except as noted): Al, 330 ± 42; As, 36; Ba, 20; Br, 1520 ± 200; Ca, 150–481 mg/L; Cl, 375–910 mg/L; Cd, 2.19; Co, 1–8.6; Cr, 10–29; Cs, nd; Cu, 197–500; F, 0.5; Fe, 130–3150; Hg, 1–6; I, 120; K, 336–745 mg/L; Mg, 28–42 mg/L; Mn, 7–120; Mo, nd; N, 1920–3800 mg/L; Na, 136–635 mg/L; Ni, 20–83; P, 90–198 mg/L; Pb, 12–30; Rb, nd; S, 140–230 mg/L; Sb, nd; Sc, nd; Se, 13–128; Si, 292–392; Sn, 20; Sr, 20; Ti, 20; and Zn, 316–8250 (where nd = no data).

Milk concentrations usually are reported either in whole milk or in milk fat. Whole milk can be diluted with water to negate salt effects for elemental analysis by ICP-AES [64]. Metals can be analyzed by standard techniques such as digestion followed by atomic absorption.

Probably the most used method to extract chlorinated derivatives from milk fat is the Association of Official Analytical Chemists (AOAC) technique [153]. This involves extraction by mixed solvents of ethyl alcohol, diethyl ether, and hexane, concentration, and further concentration of chlorinated derivatives on a Florisil column, another hexane extraction with concentration, another fractionation on a silica gel column, and then GC/MS.

6.7.3 Feces

Feces are not a convenient medium to sample in the workplace. Fecal analyses for calcium (reduced with improper nutrition), chymotrypsin (reduced in pancreatic disease), hemoglobin [increased with internal bleeding (occult blood) as for ulcers], porphyrins (occasionally for porphyria diagnosis), protein (analysis for α^1-antitrypsin), trypsin (decreased in pancreatic disease although compromised by the presence of bacterial flora), lipids (to diagnose malabsorption due to intestinal or pancreatic disorders; steatorrhea; lipid balance studies), and urobilinogen (stool that loses color due to biliary obstruction as an index of liver disease) are routine in clinical practice.

The most important fecal clinical test, and one that has been included in many health examinations, is that for occult blood. It should be performed on discrete stools and not on the small amount of feces present on surgical gloves after a physician does a rectal examination. The tryptic test is done especially for cystic fibrosis in children. For metabolic studies, stool collections are generally made over 72 h using a controlled and defined diet for at least 3 days before the sampling begins.

No preservative should be added to the fecal sample (containers are wide-mouthed polyethylene for metals and wide-mouthed acid-washed glass vessels for organics and metals). The vessel should be preweighed so that on completion of sampling the weight of feces can be easily calculated. The sample usually is homogenized ("pureed") before analysis. Some investigators have ground up the feces with sodium sulfate into a fine, dry powder for analysis by the usual techniques.

Because feces contain a large component of fat, fat analysis is an important part of fecal analysis [157]. This also implies that compounds with high K_{ow} values can be candidates for fecal analysis, especially those known to be eliminated in the bile. Such a compound is 2,3,7,8-TCDD [158]. Fecal isotope dilution measurements imply that TCDD at 0.25 pg/g in a 0.5-g sample from a 20-g original stool is about 50% metabolized in humans. Though not confirmed by human measurements as yet, animal metabolism studies on TCDD have resulted in the formation of hydroxylated tri- and tetra-CDDs, chlorinated diphenyl ethers, and dichlorocatechols.

Elemental analysis of feces reflects the diet and the biliary excretion route balanced by gastrointestinal absorption, symbiotic bacterial uptake/excretion, and enterohepatic circulation. Human studies have determined that Si, Ti, and Al may be dietary marker elements [64].

6.7.4 Skin Lipids

Whereas the skin can be the site of absorption of xenobiotics (Section 3.2), it can also be the site of excretion from such processes as sweat secretion from the sweat glands and sebum (skin oil) secretion from the sebaceous glands. Excretion of excessive sebum also occurs in cases of dermatological pathogenesis. Skin oil from the forehead had been proposed as a noninvasive source of sampling skin lipids for chlorinated xenobiotics [159]. This is not an advantageous site because sebum accumulation here is slow, accumulation being much faster on fleshy parts near the lymph nodes, for example, on the neck or on the scrotum.

Skin oil was sampled [159] by gauze backed by two absorbent papers held in place by an elastic headband. Sampling was performed for 10 min (discarded), followed by another 10-min sample, a 30-min sample, and then a 180-min sample. The papers were stored in clean glass vials and maintained at −20°C until analysis. The workup involved ether/hexane extraction and concentration; half the sample was then subjected to Florisil column workup and final concentration before GC/MS analysis for xenobiotics, and the other half was analyzed for lipids.

Lipid excretion was 1 to 2 $\mu g\, cm^{-2}\, min^{-1}$, with excretion higher in males than in females. Samples taken over 30 min or more had greater than 0.5 mg weight of lipids. PCBs, *trans*-nonachlor, and *p,p'*-DDE were detected at ng/mg lipid concentrations. The corresponding range of serum concentrations were: *p,p'*-DDE, 1 to 75 ng/mL with excellent correlation with skin lipids; and *trans*-nonachlor, PCBs, and hexachlorobenzene, 1 ng/mL with correlation that was not good except among individuals highly exposed to PCBs. These preliminary studies implied that at least 3 h may be the necessary sampling time for low serum concentrations. Thus skin oil analysis for xenobiotics is a qualitative technique rather than one related to body burden for low doses.

6.7.5 Semen

Semen consists [160] of secretions from apocrine cells (portions of the cytoplasm, membrane fragments, and parts of the apical cytoplasmic matrix are discharged along with soluble secretory products) and merocrine cells (secretory cells that remain intact on secretion).

The apocrine sources also account for the many enzymes in semen, especially those of glycolysis. The testis contributes a clear, watery, and protein-poor fluid that is conveyed by the cauda epididymis; the prostate and the seminal vesicle also secrete particulate matter and cellular detritus (debris) into the vas deferens. The contents of the cauda epididymis and the vas deferens meet to form the semen.

Xenobiotics enter the semen by blood, lymph, and the skin, especially as scrotum skin has a large surface area for absorption and has high blood perfusion (Section 3.2). Inhalation of the nematocide dibromochloropropane in the workplace, the skin absorption of *tris*-(2,3-dibromopropyl) phosphate (Tris-BP) from underwear, and excessive administration of Antabuse for management of alcoholism have caused testicular atrophy. Many of these changes are reversible.

The blood/testis barrier of animals does not prevent such xenobiotics as barbiturates, α-chlorohydrin, dimethylnitrosamine, ethanol, glycerol, iodoantipyrine, methanesulfonate, and sulfonamides from appearing in the testicular plasma, which is composed of secretions from the seminiferous tubules, tubuli recti, rete testis, and ductuli efferentes. This plasma also contains immotile and infertile spermatozoa at the point of their entry into the caput epididymis.

The plasma may also receive metabolites from the testis itself. For example, the testis has high glutathione and glutathione-*S*-transferase contents so that Phase II conjugation products of glutathione and others that are cytosolic may be present in the testicular plasma.

The succeeding parts of the epididymis (the corpus and the cauda) also are sites of further secretion. α-Chlorohydrin is secreted in animals by both the testis and the epididymis. The main site of accumulation of carnitine (Sections 2.6 and 2.7) in many animals is the cauda epididymis, even though very little of it is manufactured in that organ. Carnitine is secreted into the semen at this point.

The major means of elimination in the reproductive system of ethyl alcohol, of some antibiotics that are weak bases such as erythromycin, and of sulfonamides is via the prostatic fluid. Even proteins very similar to blood proteins are eliminated, a phenomenon that is suggestive of blood plasma as the source. Zinc in the semen comes mostly from the prostate, probably in the form of a polypeptide.

The seminal vesicles also contribute weak basic xenobiotics such as ergothioneine. Many of the mechanisms of secretion are unknown.

Whole ejaculates obviously are much easier to procure than the individual accessory fluids. They can be collected repeatedly and noninvasively over long periods of time so that the elucidation of a time course is possible. The semen can be separated by centrifugation or filtration into spermatozoa and seminal plasma. The possibility that xenobiotics originally in either portion could partition into each other after ejaculation should be remembered; it is the source of a potential systematic error common to all subcellular separations.

The spermatozoa consist of the following organelles: plasmalemma, acrosome, mitochondria of the middle piece, and the axoneme. The ejaculate also may contain urinary components because it travels along the ureter. Xenobiotics may be present in semen and yet not affect the motility or fecundity of spermatozoa; for example, ethyl alcohol, sulfonamides, and salicylic acids. The last decrease biosynthesis of prostaglandins and hence their content in semen, however. Some xenobiotics do affect spermatozoa: thalidomide is absorbed avidly, binds irreversibly in the spermatozoa, and affects pregnancy outcome. Ions of zinc and calcium, steroid hormones, retinyl acetate, tetracycline, and the antigens and antibodies of the seminal plasma are all absorbed and firmly bound inside human spermatozoa.

Sometimes drug concentrations in semen are equal to, or greater than, those in blood plasma; for example, for trimethoprim, sulfamethoxazole, and methadone (diphenylhydantoin). Phenytoin and valproic acid (dipropylacetic acid) are found in lower concentrations in semen than in blood. Chlorinated compounds of high K_{ow} such as hexachlorobenzene, DDT metabolites, *tris*(dichloropropyl) phosphate, and polychloronaphthalenes also have been detected in human semen.

Through the appropiate masturbation techniques, at least three separate fractions (split ejaculates) can be sampled: pre-sperm or "pre-cum," chiefly derived from the bulbourethral and urethral glands; sperm-rich, which comprises spermatozoa and prostatic secretion; and post-sperm, which is mostly seminal vesicle secretion. There is some overlap in these ejaculates. Chemical markers are used to assign the secretion source in human ejaculates. Thus, fructose is the marker secreted by the seminal vesicles and ampullae; citric acid and acid phosphatase derive mostly from the prostate. The order of these fractions can be upset by drugs that affect the nerves controlling the ejaculation process. It is recommended that these markers be used for normalization purposes.

6.8 OTHER BIOLOGICAL MONITORING MEDIA

6.8.1 Ear Wax

Another medium that could be used for biological monitoring is ear wax. It is produced by the sebaceous glands (apocrine) and sweat glands, with the plasma in the carotid artery being the ultimate source of compounds. Because the ear is a relatively protected environment, external contamination would not be so important there as for hair, sebum, sweat, or nails. Most of the secretion is organic waxes (at least 98%), but this author has shown that metals are also present [167]. Bioaccumulatory pesticides such as lindane and DDT have also been detected in ear wax [168].

6.8.2 Sputum

Sputum has been used to detect hemoglobin as a marker of internal bleeding in the respiratory tract because it does not usually contain blood. However, it has not been used for the workplace relative to xenobiotics contained in it. Sputum cytology has been utilized in clinical situations to detect the presence or absence of malignant cells shed from the bronchial epithelium [161]. Such tests have been used for smokers and those with chronic shortness of breath and coughing. Approximately 14% of persons with moderate dysplasia of the bronchial epithelium developed lung cancer, 83% with severe dysplasia developed squamous carcinoma, and 46% of the latter exhibited underlying squamous carcinoma at bronchoscopy. Many of these phenomena in smokers can be reversed by cessation of smoking, and sputum cytology confirms this effect. The major components found in the sputa of nonsmokers are, in order of frequency: macrophages, neutrophils, pigmented macrophages, mucus, columnar cells, metaplastic cells, and mucous spirals. For smokers, the macrophages, pigmented macrophages, and neutrophils are about equal and increase over 50% relative to nonsmokers; the mucus and columnar cells are approximately equal, and increase about twofold relative to nonsmokers; metaplastic cells also increase about twofold. Mucous spirals increase over 30-fold, and dysplastic cells appear in smokers. Increased neutrophils in sputum have been correlated with emphysema although AIDS patients with *Pneumocystis carinii* infection of the lung also show this effect.

6.8.3 Teeth

Shed teeth have been used in infants to test for chronic body burden of lead. Lead is not distributed evenly throughout the various parts of each tooth, and different teeth have varying amounts of lead. Other bone-seeking species such as strontium and fluoride could also be sampled in the same manner. The technique has no promise in adults except at autopsy or after tooth extraction.

6.8.4 Organs

Organs are accessible only at autopsy for analysis. The book by Iyengar et al. gives the metal content of the various organs [61], and Table 6.6 provides an example of the chlorinated residues found in the adipose tissues of some Canadian corpses.

6.8.5 The Menses

The menses is shed 14 or 15 days after the luteinizing hormone and body temperature surge about midway in the fertility cycle of females. No one has yet reported if the menses contains xenobiotics, though it is expected that it should. Its irregularity is its chief disadvantage, but its analysis is a noninvasive technique.

6.9 DIRECT-READING METHODS OF BIOLOGICAL MONITORING

Noninvasive techniques have been used for *in vivo* measurement of chemical elements for humans since the early 1960s [162]. The technique requires no sampling, sample preservation, storage, and transport. However, the results often cannot be easily interpreted. Sensitivity, specificity, radiation scattering, and geometry considerations are always problems with these techniques.

Nevertheless, the advantages of direct-reading instruments are so numerous that much more research must be done with them. Time studies thus are possible, which would be too expensive by conventional techniques. In these measurements, no chemical reactions are used; rather, atomic luminescence, atomic absorption, or some other physical property specific for the atom using various energy sources are measured. Most of the reported research has concerned metals. The majority of the current direct-reading instruments for biological monitoring [162] use ionizing radiation (ionizes air molecules).

Whole-body counting of naturally occurring ^{40}K in the body, X-ray and X-ray fluorescence analysis of bones and organs, and neutron activation analysis for body elements are probably the best-known techniques. Most of these methods have detection limits of about 1 to 100 μg/g. X-rays and gamma rays, unlike alpha and beta particles, are not appreciably absorbed by the skin; hence their use for these techniques. However, exposure to this radiation does pose a hazard to the subject for extended analysis times and strong sources. These energy sources require shielding to safeguard against radiation poisoning.

Cadmium has been detected by prompt gamma neutron activation analysis in kidney and liver and by X-ray fluorescence in kidney and liver. Lead has been quantified in teeth, finger, and leg by X-ray fluorescence. Mercury has been found in brain, kidney, and liver by prompt gamma neutron activation analysis, and in head, wrist, and kidney by X-ray fluorescence. Silicon has been monitored in the lung by neutron activation analysis. Aluminum in the whole body and in the hand has been detected by total body neutron activation analysis using the delayed component.

Other techniques have been utilized: NMR specific organ and whole body techniques are of great interest [163–166]; infrared thermosensing has been used to detect vasodilators and vasoconstrictors [163]. Neither technique has been used to trace xenobiotics. Fluorescent dye used as a tracer has indicated the sites of skin exposure of pesticides [22] on illumination with ultraviolet light.

Further Reading

BEI Committee, ACGIH. 1989. *Documentation of the Biological Exposure Indices*, ACGIH, Cincinnati, OH, BEI-vii to xxii [88].

Brugnone, F.; Perbellini, L.; Apostoli, P.; and Gaffuri, E. 1987. Monitoring of industrial exposure to organic volatile compounds by analysis of alveolar air and blood. In *Biological Monitoring of Exposure to Chemicals*: Organic Compounds, M. H. Ho and H. K. Dillon (eds.), John Wiley and Sons, New York, pp. 59–71.

Hill, R. H., Jr.; Guillemin, M.; and Droz, P. O. 1988. Sample Collection. In *Methods for Biological Monitoring: A Manual for Assessing Human Exposure to Hazardous Substances*, T. J. Kneip and J. V. Crable (eds.), American Public Health Association, Washington, DC, pp. 37–63.

Potts, A. M. 1986. Toxic responses of the eye. In *Casarett and Doull's Toxicology The Basic Science of Poisons*, 3rd ed., C. D. Klaassen, M. O. Amdur, and J. Doull (eds.), MacMillan New York, pp. 478–515.

Tietz, N. W. 1986. *Textbook of Clinical Chemistry*, W. B. Saunders, Philadelphia, PA.

Waritz, R. S. 1979. Biological indicators of chemical dosage and burden. In *Patty's Industrial Hygiene and Toxicology*, L. J. Cralley and L. V. Cralley (eds.), John Wiley and Sons, New York, pp. 257–318.

References for Part 2 (Chapters 3–6)

1. Astrand, I.; Engstrom, J.; and Ovrum, P. 1978. Exposure to xylene and ethylbenzene. I: Uptake, distribution and elimination in man. *Scand. J. Work Environ. Health* **4**: 185–194.

2. Petrofsky, J. S., and Lind, A. R. 1978. Comparison of metabolic and ventilatory responses of various lifting tasks and bicycle ergometry. *J. Appl. Physiol.* **45**: 60–63.
3. Khalil, T. M.; Genaidy, A. M.; Asfour, S. S.; and Vinciguerra, T. 1985. Physiological limits in lifting. *Am. Ind. Hyg. Assoc. J.* **46**: 220–224.
4. Sato, A.; Fujiwara, Y.; and Hirosawa, K. 1972. Solubility of benzene, toluene and *m*-xylene in blood. *Jap. J. Ind. Health* **14**: 1–8.
5. Berner, G., and Cooper, E. R. 1987. Models of skin permeability. In *Transdermal Delivery of Drugs*, Vol. II, A. F. Kydonieus and B. Berner (eds.), CRC Press, Boca Raton, FL, pp. 41–55.
6. Fiserova-Bergerova (Thomas), V., and Pierce, J. T. 1989. Biological monitoring. V: Dermal absorption. *Appl. Ind. Hyg.* **8**: F14–21.
7. Verschueren, K. 1983. *Handbook of Environmental Data on Organic Chemicals*, 2nd ed., Van Nostrand Reinhold, New York.
8. ACGIH. 1991. *Documentation of the Biological Exposure Indices*, 6th ed., American Conference of Governmental Industrial Hygienists, Cincinnati, OH.
9. Shelley, M. L.; Andersen, M. E.; and Fisher, J. W. 1989. A risk assessment approach for nursing infants exposed to volatile organics through the mother's occupational inhalation exposure. *Appl. Ind. Hyg.* **4**: 21–26.
10. Sato, A., and Nakajima, T. 1978. Differences following skin or inhalation exposure in the absorption and excretion kinetics of trichloroethylene and toluene. *Br. J. Ind. Med.* **35**: 43–49.
11. Fenske, R. A. 1988. Comparative assessment of protective clothing performance by measurement of dermal exposure during pesticide applications. *Appl. Ind. Hyg.* **3**: 207–213.
12. Jongeneelen, F. J.; Scheepers, P. T. J.; Groenendijk, A.; van Aerts, L. A. G. J. M.; Anzion, R. B. M.; Bos, R. P.; and Veenstra, S. J. 1988. Airborne concentrations, skin contamination, and urinary metabolite excretion of polycyclic aromatic hydrocarbons among paving workers exposed to coal tar derived road tars. *Am. Ind. Hyg. Assoc. J.* **49**: 600–607.
13. Riihimaki, V., and Pfaffli, P. 1978. Percutaneous absorption of solvent vapors in man. *Scand. J. Work Environ. Health* **4**: 73–85.
14. Engstrom, K.; Husman, K.; and Riihimaki, V. 1977. Percutaneous absorption of *m*-xylene in man. *Int. Arch. Occup. Environ. Health* **39**: 181–189.
15. Scheuplein, R. J., and Blank, I. H. 1971. Permeability of the skin. *Physiol. Rev.* **51**: 702–747.
16. Riihimaki, V. 1979. Percutaneous absorption of *m*-xylene from a mixture of *m*-xylene and isobutyl alcohol in man. *Scand. J. Work Environ. Health* **5**: 143–150.
17. Durham, W. F., and Wolfe, H. R. 1962. Measurement of the exposure of workers to pesticides. *Bull. WHO* **29**: 279–281.
18. Wolfe H. R.; Durham, W. F.; and Armstrong, J. F. 1967. Exposures of workers to pesticides. *Arch. Environ. Health* **14**: 622–633.
19. Wolfe, H. R.; Armstrong, J. F.; Staiff, D. C.; and Comer, S. W. 1972. Exposure of spraymen to pesticides. *Arch. Environ. Health* **25**: 29–31.
20. Durham, W. F.; Wolfe, H. R.; and Elliott, J. W. 1972. Absorption and excretion of parathion by spraymen. *Arch. Environ. Health* **24**: 381–387.
21. van Heemstra-Lequin, E. A. H. and van Sittert, N. J. 1986. Biological monitoring of workers manufacturing, formulating and applying pesticides, *Toxicol. Lett.* **33**, Elsevier, Amsterdam.
22. Fenske, R. A. 1988. Correlation of fluorescent tracer measurements of dermal exposure and urinary metabolite excretion during occupational exposure to malathion. *Am. Ind. Hyg. Assoc. J.* **49**: 438–444.

23. Klotz, I. M. 1982. Numbers of receptor sites from Scatchard graphs: facts and fantasies. *Science* **217**: 1247–1249.
24. Scheinberg, I. H. 1982. Scatchard plots. Lett. Ed. Science **215**: 312–313. Reply by Weisiger, R. A.; Gollan, J. L.; and Ockner, R. K., p. 313.
25. Munson, P. J., and Rodbard, D. 1983. Number of receptor sites from Scatchard and Klotz graphs: a constructive critique. Lett. Ed. Science **220**: 979–981. Reply by Klotz, I. M., p. 981.
26. Light, K. E. 1984. Analyzing nonlinear Scatchard plots. Lett. Ed. Science **223**: 76–77. Reply by Paul, S. M.; Hauger, R. L.; Hulihan-Giblin, B. A.; and Skolnick, P., p. 77–78.
27. Muller, W. F.; Coulston, F.; and Korte, F. 1982. Comparative metabolism of ^{14}C-trichloroethylene in chimpanzees, baboons and rhesus monkeys. *Chemosphere* **11**: 215–218.
28. Souhaili-El Amri, H.; Batt, A. M.; and Siest, G. 1986. Comparison of cytochrome P_{450} content and activities in liver microsomes of seven animal species including man. *Xenobiotica* **16**: 351–358.
29. Leaf, G., and Zatman, L. J. 1952. A study of the conditions under which methanol may exert a toxic hazard in industry. *Br. J. Ind. Med.* **9**: 19–25.
30. Muller, G.; Spassowski, M.; and Henschler, P. 1975. Metabolism of trichloroethylene in man. III. Interaction of trichloroethylene and ethanol. *Arch. Toxicol.* **33**: 173–189.
31. Savolainen, H.; Vainio, H.; Helojoki, M.; and Elovaara, E. 1978. Biochemical and toxicological effects of short-term intermittent xylene inhalation exposure and combined ethanol intake. *Arch. Toxicol.* **41**: 195–205.
32. Wilson, H. K.; Robertson, S. M.; Waldron, H. A.; and Gompertz, D. 1983. Effects of alcohol on the kinetics of mandelic acid excretion in volunteers exposed to styrene vapor. *Br. J. Ind. Med.* **40**: 75–80.
33. Waldron, H. A.; Cherry, N.; and Johnston, J. D. 1983. Effects of ethanol on blood toluene concentration. *Int. Arch. Occup. Environ. Health* **51**: 365–369.
34. Hills, B. W., and Venable, H. L. 1982. The interaction of ethyl alcohol and industrial chemicals. *Am. J. Ind. Med.* **3**: 321–333.
35. Alha, A. R.; Hjelt, E.; and Tamminen, V. 1957. Disulfiram–alcohol intoxication: investigation of five fatal cases and the chemical determination of disulfiram and blood acetaldehyde. *Acta Pharmacol. Toxicol.* (Copenhagen) **13**: 277–278.
36. Kesteloot, H.; Roelandt, J.; Willems, J.; Claes, J. H.; and Joossen, J. V. 1968. An enquiry into the role of cobalt in the heart disease of chronic beer drinkers. *Circulation* **37**: 854–864.
37. Schottenfeld, D. 1979. Alcohol as a co-factor in the etiology of cancer. *Cancer* **43**: 1962–1966.
38. Radike, M. J.; Stemmer, K. L.; Brown, P. G.; Larson, E.; and Bingham, E. 1977. Effect of ethanol and vinyl chloride on the induction of liver tumors: preliminary report. *Environ. Health Perspect.* **21**: 153–155.
39. National Research Council 1986. *Environmental Tobacco Smoke: Measuring Exposures and Assessing Health Effects*, National Academy Press, Washington DC.
40. Hoffman, D., and Wynder, E. L. 1986. Chemical constituents and bioactivity of tobacco smoke. In *Tobacco: A Major International Health Hazard*, D. G. Zaridze and R. Peto (eds.), International Agency for Research on Cancer, Lyon, France, 1986, pp. 145–193.
41. Muto, H., and Takizawa, Y. 1989. Dioxins in cigarette smoke. *Arch. Environ. Health* **44**: 171–174.
42. Bryant, M. S.; Vineis, P.; Skipper, P. L.; and Tannenbaum, S. R. 1988. Hemoglobin adducts of aromatic amines: associations with smoking status and type of tobacco. *Proc. Nat. Acad. Sci. USA* **85**: 9788–9791.

43. Bailey, E.; Brooks, A. G. F.; Dollery, C. T.; Farmer, P. B.; Passingham, B. J.; Sleightholm, M. A.; and Yates, D. W. 1988. Hydroxyethylvaline adduct formation in hemoglobin as a biological monitor of cigarette smoke intake. *Arch. Toxicol* **62**: 247–253.
44. Speer, F. 1968. Tobacco and the nonsmoker. *Arch. Environ. Health* **16**: 443–446.
45. Zussman, B. M. 1974. Tobacco sensitivity in the allergic population. *J. Asthma Res.* **11**: 159–167.
46. Surgeon General. 1979. *Smoking and Health: A Report of the Surgeon General*, U.S. Dept. Health, Education, and Welfare, Washington, DC, pp. 12-28–12-58.
47. Jarvis, M. J., and Russell, M. A. H. 1984. Measurement and estimation of smoke dosage to non-smokers from environmental tobacco smoke. *Eur. J. Respir. Dis.* **65**(Suppl. 133): 68–75.
48. Sepkovic, D. W.; Haley, N. J.; and Hoffman, D. 1986. Elimination from the body of tobacco products by smokers and passive smokers. *J. Am. Med. Assoc.* **256**: 863 (letter).
49. Selikoff, I. J.; Hammond, E. C.; and Churg, J. 1968. Asbestos, smoking, and neoplasia. *Am. J. Med.* **204**: 104–110.
50. Archer, V. W.; Wagoner, J. K.; and Lundin, F. E. 1973. Uranium mining and cigarette smoking effects on man. *J. Occup. Med.* **153**: 204–211.
51. Morgan, R. G. H., and Shettigara, P. T. 1976. Occupational asbestos exposure, smoking and laryngeal carcinoma. *Ann. N.Y. Acad. Sci.* **271**: 308–310.
52. Rothman, K., and Keller, A. 1972. The effect of joint exposure to alcohol and tobacco on risk of cancer of the mouth and pharynx. *J. Chron. Dis.* **25**: 711–716.
53. Kaminonkowski, M. D., and Fleshler, B. 1965. The role of alcoholic intake in esophageal carcinoma. *Am. J. Med. Sci.* **249**: 696–700.
54. Newman, M. A.; Que Hee, S. S.; Schoeny, R.; and Lowry, L. 1990. Biological monitoring screening of patients provided antineoplastic drugs including adriamycin, cyclophosphamide, 5-fluorouracil, methotrexate, and vincristine. *Cancer Res.* **50**: 3351–3366.
55. Kneip, T. J., and Crable, J. V. (eds.). 1988. *Methods for Biological Monitoring: A Manual for Assessing Human Exposure to Hazardous Substances*, American Public Health Association, Washington, DC.
56. U.S. EPA. 1982. Direct measurement of volatile organic compounds in breathing-zone air, drinking water, breath, blood and urine, EPA 600/4-82-015, NTIS, U.S. Department of Commerce, Springfield, VA.
57. NIOSH. 1984. *NIOSH Manual of Analytical Methods*, 3rd ed., Cincinnati, OH.
58. Hoyt, D. W. 1987. Drug testing in the work place. *J. Am. Med. Assoc.* **258**: 504–509.
59. Bristol, D. W.; Crist, H. L.; Lewis, R. G.; MacLeod, K. E.; and Sovocool, G. W. 1982. Chemical analysis of human blood for assessment of environmental exposure to semivolatile organochlorine chemical contaminants. *J. Anal. Toxicol* **6**: 269–275.
60. Issachar, D.; Holland, J. F.; and Sweeley, C. C. 1982. Metabolic profiles of organic acids from human plasma. *Anal. Chem.* **54**: 29–32.
61. Iyengar, G. V.; Kollmer, W. E.; and Bowen, H. J. M. 1978. *The Elemental Composition of Human Tissues and Body Fluids: A Compilation of Values for Adults*, Verlag Chemie, New York.
62. Heymsfield, S. B.; Arteaga, C.; McManus, C.; Smith, J.; and Moffitt, S. 1983. Measurement of muscle mass in humans: Validity of the 24-hour urinary creatinine method. *Am. J. Clin. Nutrit.* **37**: 478–494.
63. Ransil, B. 1977. Evidence of systematic temporal variation in 24-hour urinary creatinine excretion. *J. Clin. Pharmacol.* **17**: 108–119.

64. Que Hee, S. S., and Boyle, J. R. 1988. Simultaneous multielemental analysis of some environmental and biological samples by inductively coupled plasma–atomic emission spectrometry (ICP-AES). *Anal. Chem.* **60**: 1033–1042.
65. Pezzagno, G.; Imbriani, M.; Ghittori, S.; and Capodaglio, E. 1988. Urinary concentration, environmental concentration, and respiratory uptake of some solvents: effect of work load. *Am. Ind. Hyg. Assoc. J.* **49**: 546–552.
66. McElderry, L. A.; Tarbit, I. F.; and Cassells-Smith, A. J. 1982. Six methods for urinary protein compared. *Clin. Chem.* **28**: 356–360.
67. Turnell, D. C., and Cooper, J. D. H. 1982. Rapid assay for amino acids in serum or urine by pre-column derivatization and reversed-phase liquid chromatography. *Clin. Chem.* **28**: 527–531.
68. Oka, K.; Sekiya, M.; Osada, H.; Fujita, K.; Kato, T.; and Nagatsu, T. 1982. Simultaneous fluorometry of urinary dopamine, norepinephrine and epinephrine compared with liquid chromatography with electrochemical detection. *Clin. Chem.* **28**: 646–649.
69. Audunsson, G. 1988. Determination of low parts per billion levels of amines in urine by liquid membrane sample cleanup directly coupled to a gas–liquid chromatograph. *Anal. Chem.* **60**: 1340–1347.
70. Buchanan, D. N., and Thoene, J. G. 1981. HPLC urinary organic acid profiling: role of the ultraviolet and amperometric detectors. *J. Liq. Chromatog.* **4**: 1587–1600.
71. Hanai, T., and Hubert, J. 1981. Analysis of urine by liquid chromatography in the ion-exchange or hydrophobic mode. *J. High Resol. Chromatog. and Chromatog. Commun.* **4**: 500–507.
72. U.S. Department of Commerce. 1983. Priority toxic pollutants in human urine: their occurrence and analysis, NBSIR 83–2690, Washington, DC.
73. Manolis, A. 1983. The diagnostic potential of breath analysis. *Clin. Chem.* **29**: 5–15.
74. Fiserova-Bergerova, V.; Vlach, J.; and Cassady, J. C. 1980. Predictable "individual differences" in uptake and excretion of gases and liquid soluble vapours simulation study. *Br. J. Ind. Med.* **37**: 42–49.
75. Kelman, G. R. 1982. Theoretical basis of alveolar sampling. *Br. J. Ind. Med.* **39**: 259–264.
76. Droz, P. O.; and Guillemin, M. 1986. Occupational exposure monitoring using breath analysis. *J. Occup. Med.* **28**: 593–602.
77. Filser, J. G.; Bolt, H. M.; Maliawan, H.; and Kapus, H. 1983. Quantitative evaluation of ethane and *n*-pentane as indicators of lipid peroxidation *in-vivo*. *Arch. Toxicol.* **52**: 135–147.
78. Nire, H. C.; Scholler, D. A.; and Klein, P. D. 1979. Improved gas chromatographic quantitation of breath hydrogen by normalization to respiratory carbon dioxide. *J. Lab. Clin. Med.* **94**: 755–763.
79. Mason, M. F.; and Dubowski, K. M. 1975. Breath-alcohol analysis: uses, methods, and some forensic problems. Review and opinion. *J. Forensic Sci.* **4**: 9–41.
80. Conkle, J. P.; Camp, B. J.; and Welch, B. E. 1975. Trace composition of human respiratory gas. *Arch. Environ. Health* **30**: 290–295.
81. Krotioszynski, B.; Gabriel, G.; and O'Neil, H. 1977. Characterization of human expired air: a promising investigation and diagnostic technique. *J. Chromatogr. Sci.* **15**: 239–244.
82. Fairchild, C. I.; and Stampfer, J. F. 1987. Particle concentration in exhaled breath. *Am. Ind. Hyg. Assoc. J.* **48**: 948–949.
83. Sato, A.; and Nakajima, T. 1979. Partition coeficients of some aromatic hydrocarbons and ketones in water, blood and oil. *Br. J. Ind. Med.* **36**: 231–234.

84. Sato, A., and Nakajima, T. 1979. A structure–activity relationship of some chlorinated hydrocarbons. *Arch. Environ. Health* **34**: 69–75.
85. Berlin, M.; Gage, J. C.; Gullberg, B.; Holm, S.; Knuttson, P.; and Tunek, A. 1980. Breath concentrations as an index of health risk from benzene. *Scand. J. Work Environ. Health* **6**: 104–111.
86. Perbellini, L., and Brignone, F. 1980. Lung uptake and metabolism of cyclohexane in shoe factory workers. *Int. Arch. Occup. Environ. Health* **45**: 261–269.
87. Mutti, A.; Falzio, M.; Lucertini, S.; Cavartorta, A.; Franchini, I.; and Pedroni, C. 1981. Absorption and alveolar excretion of cyclohexane in workers in a shoe factory. *J. Appl. Toxicol.* **1**: 220–223.
88. Perbellini, L.; Brugnone, F.; Grigolini, L.; Gunegatti, P.; and Tacconi, A. 1977. Alveolar air and blood concentration in shoe sole factory workers. *Int. Arch. Occup. Environ. Health* **40**: 241–247.
89. Fleeger, A. K., and Lee, J. S. 1988. Characterization of worker exposures to methylene chloride resulting from application of aerosol glue in the asbestos abatement industry. *Appl. Ind. Hyg.* **3**: 245–250.
90. Brugnone, F.; Nordelotto, O.; and Guidice, S. 1981. Monitoraggio dell' esposizione professionale a fluorocarburi mediants l'analisi dell' aria alveolare e del sangue. *Med. Lavoro* **6**: 480–487.
91. Goethe, C. J.; Oevrum, P.; and Borje, H. 1976. Exposure to anesthetic gases and ethanol during work in operating rooms. *Scand. J. Work Environ. Health* **2**: 96–106.
92. Brugnone, F.; Perbellini, L.; Grigolini, L.; and Apostoli, P. 1978. Solvent exposure in a shoe upper factory I. *n*-Hexane and acetone concentration in alveolar and environmental air and in blood. *Int. Arch. Occup. Environ. Health* **42**: 51–62.
93. Brugnone, F.; Perbellini, L.; Apostoli, P.; Bellomi, P.; and Caretta, D. 1983. Isopropanol exposure: environmental and biological monitoring in a printing workshop. *Br. J. Ind. Med.* **40**: 160–168.
94. Angerer, J., and Lehnert, G. 1977. Occupational exposure to methanol. *Acta Pharmacol. Toxicol.* **41**(Suppl.): 551–556.
95. Prost, G. H.; Maniller, D.; and Girard, R. 1972. Analyse toxicologique de l'air expire chez des sujets utilisant du 1,1,1,-trichloroethane. *Arch. Mal. Prof.* **33**: 197–198.
96. Brugnone, F.; Perbellini, L.; Grigolini, L.; and Apostoli, P. 1979. Solvent exposure in a shoe upper factory. II. Methylcyclopentanes, 2-methylpentane, and 3-methylpentane concentration in alveolar air and in environmental air and in blood. *Int. Arch. Occup. Environ. Health* **42**: 355–363.
97. Lauwerys, R.; Herbrand, J.; Buchet, J. P.; Bernard, A.; and Gaussin, J. 1983. Health surveillance of workers exposed to tetrachloroethylene in dry cleaning shops. *Int. Arch. Occup. Environ. Health* **52**: 69–77.
98. Teramoto, K. 1978. Studies on styrene poisoning from the standpoint of occupational health. I. Surveys of the actual conditions of plastics factories using styrene. *J. Osaka City Med. Cent.* **27**: 249–262.
99. Engstrom, J.; Astrand, I.; and Wigaeus, E. 1978. Exposure to styrene in a polymerisation plant. Uptake in the organism and concentration in subcutaneous adipose tissue. *Scand. J. Work Environ. Health* **4**: 324–329.
100. Fields, R. L.; and Horstman, S. W. 1979. Biomonitoring of industrial styrene exposure. *Am. J. Ind. Hyg.* **40**: 451–459.
101. Brooks, S. M.; Anderson, L. J.; Emmett, E. A.; Carson, A.; Tsay, J. Y.; Elia, V. J.; Buncher, R.; and Karbowsky, R. 1980. The effects of protective equipment on styrene exposure in workers in the reinforced plastic industry. *Arch. Environ. Health* **35**: 287–294.

102. Brugnone, F.; Perbellini, L.; Grigolini, L.; Cazzadori, A.; and Gaffuri, L. 1976. Alveolar air and blood toluene concentration in rotogravure workers. *Int. Arch. Occup. Environ. Health* **38**: 45–50.
103. Ovrum, P.; Hultengren, M.; and Lindqvist, T. 1978. Exposure to toluene in a photogravure printing plant. Concentration in ambient air and uptake in the body. *Scand. J. Work Environ. Health* **4**: 237–245.
104. Apostoli, P.; Brugnone, F.; Perbellini, L.; Cocheo, V.; Beelomo, M. L.; and Silvestri, R. 1982. Biomonitoring of occupational toluene exposure. *Int. Arch. Occup. Environ. Health* **50**: 153–168.
105. Pfaffli, P., and Backman, A. L. 1972. Trichloroethylene concentrations in blood and expired air as indicators of occupational exposure. A preliminary report. *Work Environ. Health* **9**: 140–144.
106. Engstrom, K.; Husman, K.; Pfaffli, R.; and Riihimaki, V. 1978. Evaluation of occupational exposure to xylene by blood, exhaled air and urine analysis. *Scand. J. Work Environ. Health* **4**: 114–121.
107. Filser, J. G.; Jung, P.; and Bolt, H. M. 1982. Increased acetone exhalation induced by metabolites of halogenated C_1 and C_2 compounds. *Arch. Toxicol.* **49**: 107–116.
108. Caperos, J. R.; Droz, P. O.; Hake, C. L.; Humbert, B. E.; and Jacot-Guillarmod, A. 1982. 1,1,1-Trichloroethane exposure, biologic monitoring by breath and urine analyses. *Int. Arch. Occup. Environ. Health* **49**: 293–303.
109. Fernandez, J. G.; Droz, P. O.; Humbert, B. E.; and Caperos, J. R. 1977. Trichloroethylene exposure. Simulation of uptake, excretion, and metabolism using a mathematical model. *Br. J. Ind. Med.* **34**: 43–55.
110. Stewart, R. D.; Gay, H. H.; Erley, D. S.; Hake, C. L.; and Schaffer, A. W. 1961. Human exposure to 1,1,1-trichloroethane vapor: relationship of expired air and blood concentration to exposure and toxicity. *Am. Ind. Hyg. Assoc. J.* **22**: 252–262.
111. Stewart, R. D.; Gay, H. H.; Schaffer, A. W.; Erley, D. S.; and Rowe, V. K. 1969. Experimental human exposure to methyl chloroform vapor. *Arch. Environ. Health* **19**: 467–472.
112. Stewart, R. D.; Hake, C. L.; Wu, A.; Graff, S. A.; Forster, H. V.; Lebrun, A. J.; Newton, P. E.; and Soto, R. J. 1975. 1,1,1-trichloroethane: Development of a Biologic Standard for the Industrial Worker by Breath Analysis, Report No. NIOSH-MCOW-ENVM-111-T-75-4, Milwaukee, WI.
113. Brugnone, F.; Perbellini, L.; Apostoli, P.; and Gaffuri, E. 1987. Monitoring of industrial exposure to organic volatile compounds by analysis of alveolar air and blood. In *Biological Monitoring of Exposure to Chemicals: Organic Chemicals*, M. H. Ho and H. K. Dillon (eds.), John Wiley and Sons, New York, pp. 59–71.
114. Obrusnik, I. 1986. Activation analysis of human hair as a tool for environmental pollution monitoring. *J. Hyg. Epidem. Microbiol. Immunol.* **30**: 11–25.
115. Schroeder, H. A., and Nason, A. P. 1969. Trace metals in human hair. *J. Invest. Dermatol.* **53**: 71–78.
116. Klevay, L. M. 1978. Hair as a biopsy material. Progress and prospects. *Arch. Intern. Med.* **138**: 1127–1128.
117. Klevey, L. M.; Bistrian, B. R.; Fleming, C. R.; and Neumann, C. G. 1987. Hair analysis in clinical and experimental medicine. *Am. J. Clin. Nutrit.* **46**: 233–236.
118. Chittleborough, G. 1980. A chemist's view of the analysis of human hair for trace elements. *Sci. Tot. Environ.* **14**: 53–75.
119. Hopps, H. C. 1977. The biological bases for using hair and nail for analyses of trace elements. *Sci. Tot. Environ.* **7**: 71–89.
120. Gibson, R. S. 1980. Hair as a biopsy material for the assessment of trace element status in infancy. A review. *J. Hum. Nutrit.* **34**: 405–416.

121. Barrett, S. 1985. Commercial hair analysis. Science or scam? *J. Am. Med. Assoc.* **254**: 1041–1045.
122. Hambridge, K. M.; Rodgerson, D. O.; and O'Brien, D. 1968. Concentrations of chromium in the hair of normal children and children with juvenile diabetes mellitus. *Diabetes* **17**: 517–519.
123. Hambridge, K. M., and Rodgerson, D. O. 1969. Comparison of hair chromium levels of nulliparous and parous women. *Am. J. Obstet. Gynecol.* **103**: 320–321.
124. Henzel, J. H.; De Weese, M. S.; and Pories, W. J. 1967. Significance of magnesium and zinc metabolism in the surgical patient: Part II. Zinc. *Arch. Surg.* **95**: 991–999.
125. Saner, G.; Dagoglu, T.; and Ozden, T. 1985. Hair manganese concentrations in newborns and their mothers. *Am. J. Clin. Nutrit.* **41**: 1042–1044.
126. Phil, R. O., and Parkes, M. 1977. Hair element content in learning disabled children. *Science* **198**: 204–206.
127. Clarkson, T. W. 1987. The role of biomarkers in reproductive and developmental toxicology. *Environ. Health Perspect.* **74**: 103–107.
128. McKeown-Eyssen, G. E.; Reudy, J.; and Neims, A. 1983. Methylmercury exposure in northern Quebec. II. Neurological findings in children. *Am. J. Epidemiol.* **118**: 470–479.
129. Kjellstrom, T.; Kennedy, P.; Wallis, S.; and Mantell, C. 1986. Physical and mental development of children with pre-natal exposure to mercury from fish. Nat. Swed. Environ. Protect. Board, Solna, Sweden.
130. Hislop, J. S.; Collier, T. R.; White, G. F.; Khathing, T.; and French, E. 1983. The use of keratinized tissues to monitor the detailed exposure of man to methylmercury from fish. In *Chemical Toxicity and Clinical Chemistry of Metals*, S. S. Brown and J. Savory (eds.), Academic Press, New York, pp. 145–148.
131. Guidotti, T. L. 1983. Unjustified employee concern aroused by a direct-service toxicologic testing laboratory. *J. Occup. Med.* **25**: 693.
132. Sheldon, L.; Umana, M.; Bursey, J.; Gutknecht, W.; Handy, R.; Hyldberg, P.; Michael, L.; Moseley, A.; Raymer, J.; Smith, D.; Sparacino, C.; and Warner, M. 1986. *Biological Monitoring Techniques for Human Exposure to Industrial Chemicals: Analyses of Human Fat, Skin, Nails, Hair, Blood, Urine and Breath*, Noyes Publications, Park Ridge, NJ.
133. Gibson, L. E. 1983. The sweat abnormality of cystic fibrosis. In *Textbook of Cystic Fibrosis*, J. D. Lloyd-Still (ed.), John Wright–PSG Boston, INA, p. 37.
134. Barlow, W. K. 1989. The sweat test—recent advances. *Am. Clin. Lab.*, June, p. 6.
135. Lilley, S. G.; Florence, T. M.; and Stauber, J. L. 1988. The use of sweat to monitor lead absorption through the skin. *Sci. Tot. Environ.* **76**: 267–278.
136. Anonymous. 1990. Compound in sweat said to act as tranquilizer. *Chem. Eng. News*, Sept., p. 56.
137. Young, J. A.; Cook, D. I.; van Lennap, E. W.; and Roberts, M. 1987. In *Physiology of the Digestive Tract*, L. R. Johnson (ed.), Raven Press, New York, pp. 773–815.
138. Foskett, J. K., and Melvin, J. E. 1989. Activation of salivary secretion: coupling of cell volume and $[Ca^{2+}]_i$ in single cells. *Science* (U.S.A.) **244**: 1582–1584.
139. Dossing, M. 1984. Noninvasive assessment of microsomal enzyme activity in occupational medicine: present state of knowledge and future perspectives. *Int. Arch. Occup. Environ. Health* **53**: 205–218.
140. Danhof, M.; DeGroot-van der vis, E.; and Breimer, D. D. 1979. Assay of antipyrine and its primary metabolites in plasma, saliva, and urine by HPLC, and some preliminary results in man. *Pharmacology* **18**: 210–223.
141. Bailey, D. N. 1983. The unusual occurrence of 4-aminoantipyrine (4-aminophenazone) in human biological fluids. *J. Anal. Toxicol.* **7**: 76–78.

142. Winter, H. S. 1987. Breath tests as a diagnostic technique for malabsorption. *Pediat. Ann.* **16**: 258–262.
143. Levitt, M. D. 1969. Production and excretion of hydrogen gas in man. *N. Engl. J. Med.* **281**: 122–127.
144. Ostrander, C. R.; Cohen, R. S.; and Hopper, A. O. 1985. Breath hydrogen analysis: a review of the methodology and the clinical application. *J. Pediatr. Gastroenterol. Nutrit.* **2**: 525–533.
145. Simoons, F. J. 1978. The geographic hypothesis and lactose malabsorption. A weighing of the evidence. *Dig. Dis. Sci.* **23**: 963–980.
146. Kates, M. 1975. *Techniques of Lipidology: Isolation, Analysis and Identification of Lipids*, American Elsevier, New York.
147. Williams, D. T.; LeBel, G. L.; and Junkins, E. 1984. A comparison of organochlorine residues in human adipose tissue autopsy samples from two Ontario municipalities. *J. Toxicol. Environ. Health* **13**: 19–29.
148. Patterson D. G., Jr.; Hoffman, R. E.; Needham, L. L.; Roberts, D. W.; Bagby, J. R.; Pirkle, J. L.; Falk, H.; Sampson, E. J.; and Houk, V. N. 1986. 2,3,7,8-Tetrachlorodibenzo-*p*-dioxin levels in adipose tissue of exposed and control persons in Missouri: an interim report. *J. Am. Med. Assoc.* **256**: 2683–2686.
149. Geyer, H. J.; Scheunert, I.; and Korte, F. 1987. Distribution and bioconcentration potential of the environmental chemical pentachlorophenol (PCP) in different tissues of humans. *Chemosphere* **16**: 887–899.
150. Stanley, J. S. 1986. Broad scan analysis of the FY82 national human adipose tissue survey specimens. EPA 560/5-86-035/036/037/038/039.
151. Davies, D., and Mes, J. 1987. Comparison of the residue levels of some organochlorine compounds in breast milk of the general and indigenous Canadian populations. *Bull. Environ. Contam. Toxicol.* **39**: 743–749.
152. Skaare, J. U.; Tuveng, J. M.; and Sande, H. A. 1988. Organochlorine pesticides and polychlorinated biphenyls in maternal adipose tissue, blood, milk, and cord blood from mothers and their infants living in Norway. *Arch. Environ. Contam. Toxicol.* **17**: 55–63.
153. Tanabe. S.; Gondaira, F.; Subramanian, A.; Ramesh, A.; Mohan, D.; Kumaran, P.; Venugopalan, V. K.; and Tatsukawa, R. 1990. Specific pattern of persistent organochlorine residues in human breast milk from South India. *J. Agric. Food Chem.* **38**: 899–903.
154. U.S. EPA. 1988. Health assessment document for polychlorinated dibenzofurans, EPA 600/8-86/018F, Washington DC.
155. U.S. EPA. 1987. Drinking water criteria document for polychlorinated biphenyls, ECAO-CIN-414, Cincinnati, OH.
156. Ballschmiter, K., and Zell, M. 1980. Analysis of polychlorinated biphenyls (PCB) by glass capillary gas chromatography. Composition of technical Aroclor– and Clophen–PCB mixtures. *Fresenius Z. Anal. Chem.* **302**: 20–31.
157. Esteves, W.; Soares, L. A. S.; Hartman, L.; and Pereira, A. S. 1982. Determination of lipids, including medium-chain fatty acids, in human feces. *Clin. Chem.* **28**: 603–605.
158. Wendling, J. M.; Orth, R. G.; and Poiger, H. 1990. Determination of (^{3}H)-2,3,7,8-tetrachlorodibenzo-*p*-dioxin in human feces to ascertain its relative metabolism in man. *Anal. Chem.* **62**: 796–800.
159. Wolff, M. S. 1984. Analysis of skin lipids for halogenated hydrocarbons. *Anal. Chem.* **56**: 1492–1496.
160. Mann, T., and Lutwak-Mann, C. 1985. Passage of chemicals into human and animal semen: mechanisms and significance. *CRC Crit. Rev. Toxicol.* **11**: 1–14.
161. Tandon, M. 1989. Review of quantitative sputum analysis. *Am. Clin. Lab.* **8**(9): 26–29.
162. Ellis, K. J. 1988. *In-vivo* monitoring techniques. In *Methods for Biological*

Monitoring: A Manual for Assessing Human Exposure to Hazardous Substances, T. J. Kneip and J. V. Crable (eds.), Am. Public Health Assoc., Washington, DC, pp. 65–80.

163. UCLA Symposia Colloquium. 1990. *Frontiers of NMR in Molecular Biology*, D. Live, I. N. Armitage, and D. Patel (eds.), Wiley-Liss, New York.
164. Int. Soc. Optical Engineering. 1990. *International Conference on Thermal Infrared Sensing for Diagnostics and Control* (*Thermosense XII*), S. A. Semanovich (eds.), Int. Soc. Optical Engineering, Bellingham, WA.
165. Moonen, C. T. W.; van Zijl, P. C. M.; Frank, J. A.; Bihan, D. L.; and Becker, E. D. 1990. Functional magnetic resonance imaging in medicine and physiology. *Science* (U.S.A.) **250**: 53–61.
166. Smith, I. C. P., and Chmurny, G. N. 1990. NMR spectroscopy and cancer research: the present and the future. *Anal. Chem.* **62**: 853A–859A.
167. Krishnan, U., and Que Hee, S. S. 1992. Ear wax: a new biological monitoring medium for metals? *Bull. Environ. Contam. Toxicol* **48**: 481–486.
168. Wang, X. Q.; Gao, P. Y.; Lin, Y. Z.; and Chen, C. M. 1988. Studies on hexachlorocyclohexane and DDT contents in human cerumen and their relationships to cancer mortality. *Biomed. Environ. Sci.* **1**: 130–151.
169. Vainio, H., and Heitanen, E. 1980. Role of extrahepatic metabolism. In *Concepts in Drug Metabolism*, Part A, P. Jenner and B. Testa (eds.), Marcel Dekker, New York, NY, pp. 256–257.
170. Lake, B. G. and Gangolli, S. D. 1980. Toxification and detoxification as a result of xenobiotic metabolism, In *Concepts in Drug Metabolism*, Part B, P. Jenner and B. Testa (eds.), Marcel Dekker, New York, NY, p. 173.
171. Caldwell, J. 1982. Conjugation of xenobiotic carboxylic acids. In *Metabolic Basis of Detoxification: Metabolism of Functional Groups*, W. B. Jakoby, J. R. Bend, and J. Caldwell, Academic Press, San Diego, CA, p. 277.
172. Testa, B. and Jenner, P. 1980. A structural approach to selectivity in drug metabolism and disposition. In *Concepts in Drug Metabolism*, Part A, P. Jenner and B. Testa (eds.), Marcel Dekker, New York, NY, p. 97.
173. Mulder, G. J. 1982. Conjugation of Phenols. In *Metabolic Basis of Detoxification: Metabolism of Functional Groups*, W. B. Jakoby, J. R. Bend, and J. Caldwell (eds.), Academic Press, San Diego, CA, p. 257.

PART 3

Medical/Health Surveillance, Medical Screening, and Medical Monitoring

Medical screening involves a physical examination, questions on personal past history, or laboratory tests on apparently healthy people to diagnose atypical symptoms or pathology. The major biological markers are the standard medical blood, urine, and physical tests used to confirm apparent health.

Medical monitoring involves discovering early symptoms of disease and following their time course through progression and/or regression. This implies that the biological markers monitored are of adverse effect and appear once damage or the adverse effect have started.

Medical surveillance is a part of a bigger program integrating health and safety training, environmental monitoring, engineering controls, administrative controls, personal protective equipment use, and interactions with the community. The surveillance takes the form of measuring potential biological markers of good health, of adverse health, and of health maintenance. Medical surveillance is part of hazardous waste identification, handling, transport, and disposal programs, as well as an adequate occupational safety and health program in the workplace. The issuance of an advance notice of proposed rulemaking by OSHA for a generic standard for medical surveillance of workplace hazards will drive the future scientific investigation of medical markers.

Another type of monitoring is a medical program, one that includes diagnosis, treatment, and monitoring the time course of adverse effects. This is a purely clinical program, once a definite organic malfunction has been located in a person.

Another type of clinical monitoring is called health surveillance, where predictive markers are identified before adverse effects occur so that prophylactic treatment can prevent the effects—especially for disorders that have no physical signs to warn of impending adverse effect (for example, serum potassium for hyperkalemia or hypokalemia before cardiac arrest). It is most often a research endeavor.

All of these entities may overlap or succeed one another, depending on the circumstances. All may include application of medical, occupational, home, environmental, family, personal, and social history, as well as physical examinations and laboratory tests, so that the contributions of the suspected sources of adverse effects can be distinguished. All require the skills and judgments of physicians and pharmacists, and sometimes nurses and dentists.

The general process of a medical examination involves answering the following questions: (1) Is there a recognizable disease or injury? (2) Is there a disease or an injury in an apparently healthy person (medical screening)? (3) What is the disease process (pathophysiology)? (4) How is the tentative diagnosis to be verified (confirmation)? (5) How severe is the disease process (prognosis)? (6) Has a change occurred since the last examination (medical surveillance for nonsevere diagnoses and medical monitoring for definite adverse effects)? (7) How can the disease or injury be cured (treatment including medications, surgery, or physiotherapy)?

Obtaining a medical history, considering any symptoms described by the patient, giving a physical examination, and keeping accurate records are the minimum requirements at an initial medical examination.

One of the major advantages of medical or health surveillance markers is that an atypical result should trigger further investigation. Once a discrete cause is found, treatment or preventive action can be pursued. Medical screening also becomes important in monitoring the effectiveness of treatment or preventive action.

In addition to the patient, the people who prescribe drugs (physicians and dentists) and their helpers (nurses, pharmacists, anesthesiologists, clinical laboratory workers, operating room staff, and the waste disposal personnel for these occupations) are all exposed to many common drugs.

This section, comprising Chapters 7 through 9, considers the medical monitoring, medical screening, and health/medical surveillance monitoring of people exposed to physical and chemical agents; the factors influencing the common markers; and descriptions of the usual medical markers themselves.

The section references are located at the end of Chapter 9.

7

Medical Surveillance

7.0 OCCUPATIONAL PROGRAMS

There are over 6 million workplace establishments in the United States and over 120 million civilian workers, of whom about a third have a periodic medical examination. To serve these numbers, there are fewer than 1000 board-certified occupational health physicians plus about 1000 other full-time physicians and many part-time ones. The need for more occupational physicians is clear and pressing.

There are presently over 70,000 chemicals in use in industry, with only a fraction being regulated, usually through environmental sampling evaluations. The Occupational Safety and Health Administration (OSHA), which is in charge of workplace regulation in the federal sphere in the United States, has promulgated only one medical or biological monitoring standard—the one that drives the lead standard through blood lead. OSHA has medical screening recommendations for 24 compounds. The National Institute for Occupational Safety and Health (NIOSH), which is in charge of health research pertaining to the workplace in the federal arena in the United States, has recommended some form of medical screening in over 100 of its Criteria Documents. OSHA and NIOSH have issued joint recommendations for 386 chemicals.

The American Conference of Governmental Industrial Hygienists (ACGIH) issues yearly recommendations for Biological Exposure Indices (BEIs) for biological monitoring of workplace chemicals (Chapter 21). This volunteer body has played an important role in recommending safe levels of exposure of physical and chemical agents for the typical healthy worker since 1940.

The American Industrial Hygiene Association (AIHA), also established in 1940, is a non-profit, professional society for practising industrial hygienists. The important roles of licensing laboratories that analyze workplace samples, and also of certifying industrial hygienists are facilitated through the American

Board of Industrial Hygiene. The laboratories participate in an interlaboratory collaboratory program to ensure the quality of analytical results. The industrial hygienist, nurse practitioner, engineer, or physician, ("occupational professionals") must provide the analytical laboratory with a representative sample, which is collected and shipped in an approved manner as set out in the current NIOSH *Manual of Analytical Methods* or its equivalent. The ACGIH and AIHA jointly cosponsor an annual conference at which training and research topics are presented, in addition to a trade show.

Physicians often have no training in the fundamentals and unit processes of the workplace, nor are they taught how to separate occupational diseases from nonoccupational ones. Generally physicians are not familiar with risk assessment, nor are they exposed to how regulations are drafted and implemented. They often are ill-equipped to liaise with industrial hygienists and engineers on the technical aspects of control and environmental measurement. Industrial hygienists and engineers also find it difficult to communicate with physicians on medical matters. The nurse practitioner is somewhere between a doctor and an industrial hygienist in expertise with emphasis on the medical. Because of their less "hard science" training, they often find it difficult to communicate with engineers and industrial hygienists. Clearly a purpose of this book is to foster better communication among these professions. Another aspect of the problem is that the few occupational physicians and nurse practitioners often are perceived to be management-oriented.

Prevention is better than cure, but managements, especially in small businesses, often regard preventive measures as a waste of money. Many small businesses "share" clinics and occupational physicians or nurse practitioners. A wise occupational professional keeps abreast of the latest regulations and recommendations (and incorporates them into the existing file of hazardous materials data sheets!); can identify and justify the appropriate substitutes of "bad actor" chemicals; knows when to ask for engineering controls, personal protective equipment (PPE), and administrative rotation or removal of workers; and knows when physical examinations and biological and/or medical monitoring need to be done.

Industrial hygienists are in charge of environmental monitoring, worker training, monitoring the safety and exposures associated with the industrial process, recommending source control measures, recognizing when hazardous conditions prevail relative to regulations and recommendations, managing the PPE program, and keeping records for all of the above. The links between environmental exposure dose, absorbed dose, and adverse effects can be elucidated by cooperation between industrial hygienists and physicians. Both together must decide on a worker's fitness for a respirator program and how effective that program is.

Engineers particularly safety ones, often are asked to do industrial hygiene and safety as well as design and build unit processes and any safeguards like ventilation systems and guarding. Their lack of training in biology handicaps their communication with physicians.

When worker health is at stake, management must be educated by the occupational professional on how to improve working conditions, to provide adequate staffing, funding, and support, and to stop traditional procedures that are unsafe. In addition, worker confidentiality and confidence must be maintained, as well as management confidentiality and confidence. An occupational professional expert must be able to distinguish between the work-place as the cause of adverse effects, as a contributor to adverse effects, and as a aggravator of an established disease. These possibilities have to be evaluated through time on both personal and group levels.

The occupational physician must have a plan to care for workers who show atypical symptoms or results, those who think they are atypical, or those who exhibit stress. The physician must weigh when to contact local poison centers, hospitals, ambulances, fire stations, and specialists; and must be able to justify any recommendation scientifically, fiscally, and with respect to workplace harmony and production, and to communicate well with both management and workers. The need for worker counseling before and after "bad news" must be evaluated. The scientific, medical, ethical, and legal standing of the medical monitoring program also must be reviewed at least once a year. In the absence of physicians or of nurse practitioners, the onus falls on industrial/environmental hygienists to do the best they can.

7.1 HAZARDOUS WASTE SITE MEDICAL PROGRAMS

NIOSH, OSHA, U.S. EPA, and U.S. CG (U.S. Coast Guard) have issued a comprehensive criteria document detailing guidelines for medical programs at hazardous waste sites. The four major considerations for the medical program are: whether site hazards pose immediate dangers to life or health; whether the hazards are obvious and identifiable; whether the hazards vary according to the site location, the task performed, or the person doing the task; and whether any of these factors change as site activities and seasons change. All of these factors are important as well in the medical programs of the workplace. Many of the following procedures also are implemented in good occupational health workplace programs.

Consulting off-site physicians must become familiar with the types of materials on-site and the potential for worker exposures, and must recommend a specific medical program appropriate for the site to the hazardous waste site project team leader. Medical personnel at local hospitals and clinics must be able to provide adequate emergency treatment and decontamination procedures, and to obtain special drugs, equipment, or supplies necessary for successful treatment. Off-site ambulance personnel must be organized to provide instant and adequate emergency treatment procedures. The phone and fax machine numbers of these off-site personnel, plus fire station, police station, government (local, state, federal), and poison-center numbers, should be publicly posted in the appropriate areas of the work site, including the decontamination area.

On-site, the site safety and health officer (site safety officer), who often is an occupational physician, advises the project team leader on all aspects of health and safety on-site, and recommends stopping work if any operation or condition threatens worker or public health and safety. The specific responsibilities include: selecting PPE, inspecting PPE regularly, and ensuring that PPE is properly stored and maintained; controlling access and exit at the site access control points; coordinating the safety and health program with the scientific advisor; confirming each team member's suitability for work based on a physician's recommendation; monitoring work parties for physical stress (cold, heat, or sunstroke) and fatigue; monitoring on-site hazards and conditions; participating in preparation of the site safety plan and implementing it; conducting regular inspections to ensure compliance with the site safety plan; enforcing the "buddy" system (no team member ever should be alone); knowing and posting emergency procedures, evacuation routes, and telephone and fax numbers of the ambulance, local hospital, poison control center, fire department, local government agencies (federal, state, city, and county), and police department; notifying local public emergency officials when necessary; and coordinating emergency medical care. The site safety officer liaises with the field team leader to determine the level of PPE required; with the project team leader to recommend the site safety plan and to enforce health and safety requirements; with the command post supervisor in rescues; with the decontamination station officer(s) on decontamination procedures, equipment, and supplies; with the work party when unsafe conditions occur; and with the record-keeper who maintains the official records of site activities. Telephones, two-way radios, and fax machines should be available for emergency use.

Health and safety staff must be trained in all relevant areas, and this is also the responsibility of the site safety officer. Each health and safety staff member must have a record of training in his or her personnel file to confirm the adequacy of the training and that it is up-to-date.

Workers at hazardous waste sites may be exposed to toxic chemicals, physical agents, biologic hazards, and safety hazards. They also may develop heat or cold stress, and may face explosions and fires. The medical program must assess and monitor workers' health and fitness both prior to and during employment, and sometimes postemployment; must provide viable emergency and other treatment as needed; and must maintain accurate records and keep them for 30 years after the worker leaves the employment. OSHA requires a medical evaluation for employees who are to wear respirators, and other specific medical requirements must be observed (29 CFR Part 1910.95 and 29 CFR Parts 1910.1001 through 1910.1045). Accurate record-keeping is necessary for use in retrospective epidemiology studies, to adjudicate claims, to support evidence in litigation, and to report workers' medical conditions to federal, state, and local agencies. Medical surveillance complements other protective procedures at the site, such as administrative and engineering controls, use of PPE, and decontamination procedures.

The director of the site medical program should be an occupational physician or a physician with great experience in occupational matters. Often a local physician aided by an occupational physician consultant performs these duties. Sometimes a qualified registered or occupational health nurse or a certified state-licenced physician's assistant performs the day-to-day duties under the direction of a physician, who has legal responsibility for the program.

All medical test analyses must be performed by a laboratory of demonstrated satisfactory performance in an established interlaboratory testing program to meet the requirements of the Clinical Laboratories Improvement Act of 1967 [42 CFR Part 74 Subpart M Section 263 (a)] and Medicare.

7.1.1 The Medical Program

The essential elements of a medical program are: surveillance in preemployment screening, periodic and follow-up medical examinations, and termination examinations; treatment on an emergency and an individual-case nonemergency basis; record-keeping; and program review. Worker involvement must be active and self-interested. Management should urge prospective employees to provide complete and detailed occupational and medical histories, should assure confidentiality, and should ask for reporting of all suspected exposures, and also of atypical physical, psychological, and subjective disturbances and complaints.

The necessary preemployment screening data include the medical history, the occupational history, physical examination results, a determination of fitness to wear respirators and other protective equipment, and baseline urine and blood monitoring for specific exposures (or, better, freezing the preemployment serum specimen for later testing). Periodic medical examinations should update the medical and occupational histories, including the results of a yearly physical examination and of testing based on examination results, exposures, and job class and rank. Testing frequency should reflect the importance of the specific exposures.

Emergency treatment includes: provision of emergency first aid on-site; prearranged procedures for transport of victims to hospitals and to the first aid center; developed and working links with local hospitals and medical specialists; training for all emergency treatment team members; and up-to-date record-keeping on incidents and of the medical history so that medical records can be transferred to the appropriate physician.

Nonemergency treatment must involve an ongoing system of nonemergency health evaluation and care. Record-keeping and review personnel must maintain and provide access to medical records so that OSHA, state, and local regulations are obeyed. These personnel also must make accessible details of on-site occupational injuries and illnesses, review the site safety plan regularly in writing, test its adequacy for specific situations, and review the performance of record-keeping at least annually (focusing on current hazards, exposures, and industrial hygiene standards and recommendations).

The advent of right-to-know laws also means that the appropriate hazardous material data sheets, records of workers' compensation, and any management formal plans on health and safety and emission inventories must be available for worker scrutiny.

There is general agreement that not all xenobiotics, potential hazards, and medical markers can, or should, be monitored, for reasons of cost and practicality. The interagency document on hazardous waste recommends that certain chemical groups and compounds should have priority—the known "bad actors." These chemicals include: aromatic hydrocarbons (benzene, ethyl benzene, toluene, and xylenes); asbestos (asbestiform particles); halogenated aliphatic hydrocarbons [carbon tetrachloride, chloroform, ethyl bromide, ethyl chloride, ethylene dibromide (1,2-dibromoethane), ethylene dichloride, methyl chloride, methyl chloroform, methylene chloride, perchloroethylene, tetrachloroethane, trichloroethylene, and vinyl chloride]; heavy metals (arsenic, beryllium, cadmium, chromium, lead, and mercury); herbicides and related compounds (chlorophenoxy herbicides such as 2,4-dichlorophenoxyacetic acid, 2,4,5-trichlorophenoxyacetic acid, and PCDDs such as 2,3,7,8-tetrachlorodibenzo-*p*-dioxin and other toxic congeners); organochlorine insecticides (DDT and related compounds, chlorinated cyclodienes such as aldrin, chlordane, dieldrin, endrin, and heptachlor, together with chlorocyclohexanes such as lindane); organophosphate and carbamate insecticides (organophosphates such as diazinon, dichlorovos, dimethoate, malathion, methyl parathion, parathion, and trichlorfon, and carbamates such as aldicarb, baygon, and zectran); and PCBs. This listing largely reflects the U.S. EPA's Priority Pollutant list of chemicals or those on the Toxic Substances list.

To account for other chemical factors, direct-reading instruments should be used as much as possible to detect potential situations involving explosion, fire, oxygen deficiency, and radioactivity. Most of these measurements are for air rather than water although headspace and purge-and-trap techniques are utilized to detect volatile organics in liquid samples. A major unexplored area is nonvolatiles in liquid samples because simple screening techniques based on ultraviolet, visible, infrared, or fluorescence spectrophotometry are nonspecific and difficult to interpret. The present screening technique of choice is inductively coupled plasma emission spectroscopy because it is multielemental and also capable of detecting high concentrations of organic and chlorinated compounds. Analyses, which are relatively expensive, are laboratory-based. Samples may change character before analysis although the total elemental content of nonvolatiles will not be changed.

Aromatic hydrocarbons and halogenated aliphatic hydrocarbons cause central nervous system effects such as depression, decreased alertness, headache, sleepiness, and loss of consciousness. In addition, the halogenated group may induce kidney changes (decreased urine flow), eye swelling, and anemia, as well as liver changes leading to fatigue, malaise, dark urine, enlargement of the liver, and jaundice. The aromatic hydrocarbons may produce defatting dermatitis. The chlorophenoxy herbicides, PCB, and polychlorinated-*p*-dioxin (PCDD) groups can cause chloracne, weakness and numbness of the arms and legs, and long-term nerve damage. The organochlorine insecticide group may produce acute symptoms of apprehension, irritability, dizziness, disturbed equilibrium, tremor, and convulsions, as well as liver toxicity and permanent kidney damage. PCBs may elicit many skin ailments, including chloracne from the PCDF contaminants, and liver toxicity. Organophosphate and carbamate insecticides may produce neuromuscular blockage, headaches, fatigue, dizziness, increased salivation and tearing, sweating, nausea, vomiting, cramps, diarrhea, tightness in the chest, muscle twitches, slower heartbeat, unconsciousness, seizures, and delayed effects such as weakness and numbness in the feet and hands and nerve damage. Asbestos can cause lung cancer (especially in smokers and miners), mesotheliomas, asbestosis, and stomach disturbances. All classes have specific carcinogens.

The medical end points recommended for markers of possible adverse effects of all these chemical groups include: taking an occupational/environmental and general medical history, emphasizing prior exposure to the suspected agents; and performing medical examinations focusing on the lungs, liver, kidney, blood, urinalysis, nervous system, and skin, and supported by the appropriate laboratory testing. Complete blood counts are applicable for aromatic hydrocarbons, heavy metals, and organochlorine insecticides (lindane). Platelet counts differentiate aromatic hydrocarbon effects. Chest X-rays and pulmonary function testing are necessary for ascertaining exposure to certain heavy metals and asbestos. Asbestos causes gastrointestinal problems, and a stool test confirms any suspected gastrointestinal malignancy. Metals in blood (all metals) and urine (not beryllium) are specific. Red blood cell and plasma cholinesterase levels differentiate recent exposures to organophosphate and carbamate insecticides, in addition to measuring delayed neurotoxicity. Serum PCB, serum triglycerides, and blood liver function tests are applicable for PCBs.

Naturally, any specific biological monitoring markers of exposure for specific chemicals in any biological medium (Chapters 5, 6 and 21) should be measured as part of preemployment screening or before a person actually begins work. Their measurement during work at the site must take into account the effect, of multicomponent and intermittent exposures, and that any recommended levels based on single exposures may be inapplicable, with the need for establishment of the kinetics of excretion before the data can be interpreted (Section 1.8 and Chapter 4). As Chapters 3 through 6 also have emphasized, age, gender, weight, stress, diet, susceptibility to allergic-type reactions, medications taken, life-style factors, and off-site exposures may also have to be known for an investigator to be able to pinpoint a waste site as the source of any problems.

7.1.2 Preemployment Screening

As part of the hiring process, the worker should fill out an appropriate occupational and medical history questionnaire. The physician should review this information before the first medical examination (whether during preemployment screening or before the worker actually begins work). The information should be discussed with the worker, and more information should be noted if necessary relative to prior exposures to chemical and physical hazards. Past illnesses and chronic diseases (especially asthma, skin, lung, and heart) should be discussed. Shortness of breath and labored breathing on exertion, chest pain, high blood pressure, and heat intolerance should be inquired about. Life-style–type information (smoking, alcohol and drug use, hobbies and entertainment venues) should be as complete as possible.

7.1.3 First Medical Examination

At the first medical examination, a physical examination must be conducted on all body organs, especially lung, heart, skin, ear (do audiometric tests at 500, 1000, 2000, 3000, 4000, and 6000 Hz pure tone in an approved audiometric booth; confirm the integrity of the eardrum because perforated eardrums can lead to internal exposure to vapors and gases), eyes (do vision tests that assess refraction, depth perception, and color), nose, throat, nervous system, bone, genitourinary, reproductive, gastrointestinal, abdomen and rectum (examine for hernia), and musculoskeletal systems. Factors that may contribute to heat stroke such as obesity and lack of exercise should be noted. Factors mitigating respirator use should be detailed, including missing or arthritic fingers, facial scars, dentures, poor eyesight, poor hearing, color blindness, claustrophobia, or poor reaction time. People who wear contact lenses cannot wear full-facepiece respirators. Standard measurements such as height, weight, temperature, pulse, blood pressure, respiration, and eye responses also should be obtained. People who have severe lung disease, heart disease, or back and leg/arm problems must be disqualified.

Baseline conditions must be characterized as much as possible for each individual worker, based on questionnaire material. The physician may then perform the following and compare with prior data: chest and lung X-rays, pulmonary function testing (measure forced expiratory volume in one second, forced vital capacity, and their ratio, and compare these to normal values—in addition to measuring forced expiratory flow, maximal expiratory flow rate, maximal voluntary ventilation, functional residual capacity, residual volume, and total lung capacity), electrocardiograms (at least one standard 12-lead resting EKG and one stress test, especially if heat stress is probable), blood and urine medical monitoring markers (Chapters 8 and 21), and any other relevant testing. Freeze a serum and a urine sample from the worker for future testing if possible.

A written, dated review and summary of the major baseline parameters of each individual should be placed in the worker's file. This should be reviewed, signed, and dated by the Site Safety Officer and project team leader.

7.1.4 Periodic Medical Examinations

Comparison of periodic medical monitoring data with baseline prescreening data is essential to detect trends that may mark the onset of adverse health effects and so be suggestive of the need for protective measures. At the least there should be annual examinations, with greater frequency necessary for specific situations.

Periodic screening examinations should include at the very least: an interval medical history with a focus on changes in health status, illnesses, and possible work-related symptoms, based on the physician's knowledge of personal and area monitoring data for the worker or for other industrial sites, and supplemented by a worker-reported exposure history for the interval; a physical examination; and medical monitoring tests, if appropriate, such as pulmonary function tests, audiometric tests, vision tests, and blood and urine medical marker measurements.

The periodic medical examination is the same as the preemployment screening modified for current conditions relative to the worker's symptoms, site hazards, or exposures. Ongoing written summaries focusing on differences between sequential and baseline results should be prepared. This is facilitated if physicians are computer-literate.

7.1.5 Termination Examination

At the end of employment, all personnel should have a medical examination along the same lines as the prescreening medical examination (that is, medical history, physical examination, and laboratory tests). This could be a periodic medical examination devoted to an interval medical history since the last full medical examination if the latter was performed within the last 6 months, if no exposures occurred since the last examination, or if no symptoms associated with specific exposures occurred since the last examination.

7.1.6 Emergency Treatment

Preplanning is absolutely essential for successful emergency treatment. The range of actual and potential hazards must be considered, including chemical, physical (heat, cold, injuries, burns, sunburn, and eye injuries), and biological (animal bites, plant poisonings, medical wastes, and other biological wastes) hazards. Site workers, contractors, visitors, firefighters, ambulance personnel, and administrators must be covered in these plans. Emergency medical treatment should be part of the overall site emergency response program.

The medical part of planning involves:

- Training an on-site team (include an emergency medical technician if possible) in emergency first aid (Red Cross or equivalent certified courses in resuscitation, treatment for explosion and burn injuries, heat and cold stress, and acute chemical toxicity).
- Training in emergency decontamination procedures (development of standard operating procedures for prevention, measuring, removing, and remeasuring contamination plus associated worker, instrument, and tool protection, encasement, dress codes, water and steam jets, air jets, detergent types, brushes, scrapers, sponges, waste disposal and transport, incineration, chemical neutralization by acids and bases, heat sources, halogen stripping, chemical disinfectants, irradiation, protective clothing, and encasing-material recycling, and other decontamination concerns).
- Predesignating roles and responsibilities by writing a responsibilities chart for emergencies, and practising by organizing simulated emergencies.
- Establishing and stocking an emergency or first aid station on-site to be able to provide a safe environment for victims, and to be able to respond to general first aid to injuries, sprains, cuts, burns, and appendage breakages. The station should be located next to the decontamination area. There must be a first aid kit plus additional items such as emergency or deluge showers, stretchers, portable water, ice, eyewashes, decontamination solutions, fire-extinguishing blankets, and ordinary blankets to isolate contaminated personnel from others. Supplies, equipment, and solutions must be restocked after use and checked regularly.
- Arranging for a physician who can be paged directly 24 h every day.
- Setting up a team of medical specialists to criticize the emergency plans (for example, toxicologist, dermatologist, hematologist, allergist, opthalmologist, cardiologist, and neurologist).
- Establishing protocols for measuring heat and cold stress and their remediation.
- Planning and simulating emergency transportation, treatment, contamination control, decontamination procedures, and transportation to a pre-identified nearby medical facility.

  For this, local emergency transport and hospital personnel have to be educated about: possible medical problems they may have to be prepared for on-site; hazard types and their consequences; exposure potentials; and what the site program will do, and what outside help is supposed to do. The hospital also has to know how to protect its patients and personnel, and how to minimize delays due to concerns about hospital safety or contamination. Each on-site medical record for each worker sent to a hospital in an emergency must be provided at a moment's notice (and must be up-to-date; fax machines are useful here) to aid in treatment.

- Posting conspicuously with duplicates near telephones the names, phone or beeper numbers, fax numbers, and addresses of and procedures for contacting on-call physicians, medical specialists, ambulances, and medical facilities, as well as emergency, fire, police, and civil defense services and poison control centers.
- Making up maps and directions to be provided in an emergency.
- Ensuring that all managers and all medical response personnel have all contact data, maps, and directions.
- Establishing a radiocommunication system for emergency use.
- Reviewing emergency procedures daily with all site personnel at formal safety meetings before beginning the work shift.

7.1.7 Nonemergency Treatment

Workers suffering health effects from site exposures need off-site care as well as on-site care, through medical surveillance. Off-site medical care workers should have the worker's on-site medical record because any interactions due to work exposures may influence the effectiveness of any treatment. Off-site medical care providers must diagnose, measure, and treat non-job-related illnesses that may put the worker at risk because of task requirements, for example, a bad cold that may interfere with fitness to wear a respirator. The non-job-site medical record also should be placed in the medical record file on-site.

7.1.8 Medical Records

Accurate and up-to-date information about past and present chemical exposures, medical history and treatment regimens, work routines, allergies, and medical surveillance information must be included in the medical record so that personnel can respond quickly to emergencies, can prescribe safe treatments by avoiding any interactions, and can consult with physicians familiar with the patient.

OSHA has mandated that in general employers must:

- Maintain and preserve medical records on exposed workers for 30 years after they leave employment (29 CFR Part 1910.20).
- Make available to workers, their authorized representatives, and authorized OSHA representatives the results of medical testing, full medical records, and analyses (29 CFR Part 1910.20).
- Maintain records of occupational injuries, illnesses, and worker's compensation, and post a yearly summary report (29 CFR Part 1904).

7.1.9 Program Review

Regular evaluation of the effectiveness of the medical program is important; so record-keeping and review of the records are essential. The site safety officer, a medical consultant, and/or a management representative should, at least annually:

- Ascertain the promptness of treatment of each accident and illness, its cause, and whether changes in procedures are necessary.
- Evaluate the effectiveness and the expense of specific medical marker measurements in the context of potential site exposures.
- Add or delete medical tests as suggested by current industrial and environmental measurements.
- Review potential exposures and site safety plans at all sites to determine if additional medical and environmental testing are required.
- Review emergency treatment procedures, review any emergency responses for defects, and update lists of emergency contacts.

7.2 NURSING

Legally registered physicians have the legal responsibility to diagnose, prescribe drugs, enter patients into the hospital, operate on them, make recommendations regarding their convalescence, discharge them from the hospital, and treat them in and out of hospitals. Nurses assist registered doctors during diagnosis, operations, treatment, and convalescence. Also nurses often prepare, mix, and administer medicines. They package medical wastes in the approved manner for disposal. Therefore they contact chemical, physical, and biological media associated with the patient and his/her treatment. They keep precise records of treatments and patient health; they bathe and feed patients, and serve their needs.

Nurses also must prepare a patient before diagnosis, evaluation, treatment, and surgery by a physician. The nurse often must explain the purpose of the above, who will perform what procedure, any restrictions on food and drink, sedation procedures, sampling methods and any likely pain, type of specific positioning for sampling and the rationale, how the patient should act during nonoperative procedures, what injections are to be injected and where and why, what vital signs are to be monitored and why, what signs should be reported immediately to the nurse after surgery or to the physician after nonoperative treatment, and whether any special site care is necessary. Nurses have to encourage questions and the verbalization of any concerns by the patient. They must ensure that any informed consent is understood and signed.

Nurses also have to make physical preparations for specific treatments—for example, sterilizing and cleaning syringes and the area to be treated or occupied by the patient administering enemas; doing biopsies and injections if so ordered by the physician; providing the utensils for operations and injections; administering medications; taking and recording vital signs and comparing them with baseline values; helping the patient to undress, urinate, defecate, spit, drink, exercise, or eat; caring for the patient after operations and treatments; making observations and interpreting the appearance of samples; loading samples into automatic analyzers; and performing medical monitoring tests such as blood typing if so ordered by a physician.

Nurses often are more exposed to many of the medicines and biological media of the patient (after vomiting, breathing, drooling, defecation, urination, and diarrhea) than are many physicians. A good physician will ensure that members of the nursing staff are protected appropriately, especially against specific hazards such as antineoplastic drugs, HIV-containing samples, or contagions. Often, the health and safety aspects of nursing are the responsibility of a head nurse or an administrator.

Medical and biological monitoring of nurses should be carried out in the same manner as for exposed workers at hazardous waste sites. Because of their long hours and often inadequate diet, interactions with these factors must be allowed for, as well as the generally multicomponent exposures through all absorption routes that most nurses are subjected to in the course of their duties. To cope with job stress, many nurses smoke and take recreational drugs; so these factors are important in considering potential interactions and for prescribing effective medications in case of ill health.

The intelligent application of closed systems employing transparent plastic bags can minimize many potential exposures, as in, for example, mixing concentrates and sampling the resultant solutions for subsequent patient injection. Such systems are already in wide use for the handling of antineoplastic drugs. Appropriate gloves must be worn that are protective for the specific chemical relative to glove degradation and permeation. Control of hazards at the time of patient injection is particularly difficult, and training in hygienic matters as well as nursing technique are essential to minimize nurse exposure and to attain optimum efficiency. The demand for occupational nurses, like that for occupational physicians, is not being met.

Nurses should observe the guidelines for handling biological media as set forth in Chapter 18.

7.3 PHARMACISTS

Pharmacists weigh, mix, and prepare medicines prescribed by physicians and dentists, and are subjected by all exposure routes to many drugs and solvents, all in their most concentrated forms so maximizing exposures. Often weighing or liquid transfer are not done in a laminar-flow hood—most weighings occurring in a small, confined-space with inadequate ventilation, with many spills and cross-contaminations in the general area. Pharmacists usually wear a white laboratory coat, whose material is not necessarily protective against the specific chemicals handled. Pharmacists also generally do not wear respirators or gloves, or handle very toxic chemicals in glove boxes or glove bags.

Although 99% of all prescriptions in 1983 were for precompounded drugs, the 1% remaining represented some 140 million prescriptions. This percentage is probably not very different now. Skin exposure is especially important for unprecompounded prescription formulating because pharmacists produce many mixtures using various solvents [for example, elixirs (alcoholic solutions), syrups (concentrated aqueous sugar solutions), and aromatic waters (saturated aqueous solutions in contact with such natural oils as peppermint and orange)], which are easily spilled and may facilitate skin penetration of the drug.

Ointments may easily be spread inadvertently over exposed skin or may contaminate surfaces where contact may occur.

Particulates exposure also is encountered because of the many solids weighed. The application of closed systems in transparent plastic bags to dispense and mix drugs still needs greater application in pharmacies.

The top ten drugs prescribed in 1985 according to the National Prescription Audit of 1986, were, in descending order: Dyazide, consisting of triamterene (potassium-sparing diuretic) and hydrochlorothiazide (diuretic and antihypertensive); Lanoxin or Digoxin (cardiac glycoside); Amoxil or Amoxicillin (antibiotic); Tylenol/codeine, consisting of acetaminophen and codeine (nonopioid analgesic); Tagamet or cimetidine (hydrogen antagonist for ulcers); Xanax or Alprazolam (antianxiety agent); Imodium or Loperamide (antidiarrhea agent); Lasix or Furosemide (antidiuretic or antihypertensive); Motrin or Ibuprofen (analgesic); and Tenormin or Atenolol (beta adrenergic blocker). The situation probably has not much changed now except for the advent of anti-AIDS drugs, which are extremely toxic.

7.4 DENTISTS AND THEIR PATIENTS

Dentists and their patients are exposed to many chemicals (contact anesthetics, tooth filling ingredients, pain-killers, psychotherapeutics, drugs, anticonvulsants, hormones, diuretics, antimicrobials, and antivirals, to name some), biological media (blood, breath, saliva and sputum), and physical factors such as noise, vibration, trauma, and stress. Dentists also prescribe drugs, as do doctors.

Patients who are undergoing extensive dental care and dentists themselves should have at least yearly medical examinations. Since the advent of AIDS, dental personnel have to wear gloves and face masks and utilize disposable PPE. Heat sterilization is recommended for dental utensils/tools in contact with biological media. Chapter 18 should be consulted for guidelines for handling biological media.

7.5 LABORATORY TECHNOLOGISTS

Laboratory technologists or laboratory technicans handle many types of chemicals and in clinical laboratories many kinds of biological media also. The guidelines in Chapter 18 also apply here for the latter. Generally a laboratory coat and latex gloves are worn as the sole PPE. Latex gloves, however, are known to have a definite shelf life and to allow permeation of many chemicals. Whenever possible, the type of chemical handled should determine the type of glove worn. The correct pairing should be chosen from the chemical degradation and chemical permeation data now supplied by many glove manufacturers.

Surprisingly little information has been published on the biological monitoring of laboratory technologists or of students doing research on often unknown materials. This situation accords with the small amount that has also been published on the biological monitoring and occupational exposures of physicians, nurses, pharmacists, and dentists and their patients. It is time for an annual medical monitoring examination with the appropriate endpoints selected according to potential hazard to be officially introduced for all these workers as a part of their benefits, and for them to have explicit training on health and safety. It is recommended that all concerned about HIV status should utilize the facilities of HIV anonymous testing sites.

Further Reading

Cella, J. H., and Watson, J. 1989. *Nurse's Manual of Laboratory Tests*, F. A. Davis Company, Philadelphia, PA.

Clark Cooper, W. 1979. Health surveillance programs in industry. In *Patty's Hygiene and Toxicology*, Vol. III, L. L. Cralley and L. V. Cralley (eds.), John Wiley and Sons, New York, pp. 595–609.

Swinyard, E. A. 1985. Principles of prescription order writing and patient compliance instruction. In *Goodman and Gilman's The Pharmacological Basis of Therapeutics*, 7th ed., A. G. Gilman, L. S. Goodman, T. W. Rall, and F. Murad (eds.), Macmillan New York, pp. 1651–1662.

U.S. Department of Health and Human Services. 1985. *Ocupational Safety and Health Guidance Manual for Hazardous Waste Site Activities*, NIOSH/OSHA/USCG/EPA, DHHS (NIOSH) Pub. No. 85–115, pp. 3.1–3.7, 5.1–5.10, 10.1–10.7, and 12.1–12.12.

U.S. Department of Transportation. 1990. *1990 Emergency Response Guidebook*, DOT P 5800.5.

8

Medical Markers and Factors that Affect Them

8.0 INTRODUCTION

Medical markers often used by occupational physicians are provided in Table 8.1. Most of the markers have characteristic reference values ("normal values") in individuals that may change with age and diet; so personal baseline monitoring is essential for the investigator to be able to interpret any change in the marker. Many of the marker levels are related to damage to target organs, whatever the doses and chemicals involved. Such markers thus are related to the net effect on target organs rather than dose alone, unlike biological monitoring for exposure. The markers are nonspecific as to ultimate cause; they are related to the biological effect. However, dose may be important if there is a dominant exposure. In the presence of exposures to many chemicals, interactions among the chemicals often occur, with the target organ responding to the cumulative effect of interactions that may have no relation to the dose of any specific chemical. Reversible changes in medical markers imply that no permanent damage has been inflicted. Slow increase or decrease over time imply a perturbing process. Sharp increases or declines require immediate attention as to cause.

Some general considerations on medical markers follow.

8.1 NORMAL VALUES VERSUS REFERENCE VALUES

The concentration of a medical marker in a biological medium is related to the extent of damage. The concept of "normal values," now obsolete, was used to describe "commonly found" values in humans. It was used to mean variously the range of values observed or the range that contained over 95% of the concentrations of those measured. Such was the proliferation of such values

TABLE 8.1. Medical markers often required by occupational physicians.

Organ	Injury	Medium	Examples
Liver	General	Serum	Albumin, bilirubin (total and direct), globulin, total protein
	Obstruction	Serum	Alkaline phosphatase activity
	Cell injury	Serum	Activities of γ-glutamyltranspeptidase (GGTP), serum glutamic-oxaloacetic transaminase (SGOT), serum glutamic pyruvic transaminase (SGPT), lactate dehydrogenase (LDH)
Kidney	General	Blood	Blood urea nitrogen (BUN), creatinine, uric acid
Many	General	Urine	Acetone, appearance, bile, color, microscopic examination of centrifuged sediment, occult blood, pH, qualitative glucose, specific gravity
Blood forming	General	Blood	Complete blood count (CBC) with differential and platelet evaluation with white cell count (WBC), red cell count (RBC), hemoglobin (Hb), hematocrit, and other indices; reticulocyte count if hemolytic chemicals are involved

that much confusion resulted about their interpretation and the significance of the differences in them. For example, what was "normal" for one group often, on later data acquisition from the same and other experimental groups, appeared to be unique. Nowadays the term has been supplanted by "reference values of apparently healthy individuals" commonly shortened to "reference values."

By definition, a reference value is a value obtained by observation or measurement of a particular type of quantity on an individual selected for comparison using defined criteria (a "reference individual"). Such reference values can be subject- or population-based. Most of the literature data usually are population-based.

Comparison to population reference values has been utilized to imply health of individuals, a practice that flies against probability theory which cannot predict a certain outcome for an individual based on the behavior of the group. "Health" is itself relative and has been characterized by Gräsbeck "by a minimum of subjective feelings and of objective signs of disease, assessed in relation to the social situation of the subject and the purpose of the medical activity." It is in the absolute sense an unattainable ideal state.

The definition of criteria factors for reference individuals has led to culture-dependent criteria even for such apparently nondiverse groups as Caucasians. Thus, the Scandinavian Committee on Reference Values has recommended the use of national age, gender, and height-specific mean weight ±20% as the upper limit for inclusion in reference measurements. A male of 180 cm height and 55 years old is considered overweight at 89 kg in Norway, at 97 kg in Finland, at 104 kg in Denmark, and at 111 kg in Sweden.

Some causes for exclusion by this Committee are: disease; high risk factors such as obesity (greater than 20% of the national mean weight); hypertension (for ages 16–39, diastolic pressure in mm Hg >95 and systolic pressure 150; for age >39, diastolic pressure >100 and systolic pressure 160); occupational and environmental exposures; genetic factors; intake of pharmacologically active agents such as drugs, oral contraceptives, alcohol, and tobacco-related chemicals, through usage or exposure; and specific physiological states such as pregnancy, stress, and excessive exercise. Obviously it might be exceedingly difficult to obtain reference individuals who meet all the criteria!

The same Committee also has recommended exclusion criteria based on laboratory examinations: urinary albumin, above detection limit; urinary glucose, above detection limit; red blood cell sedimentation rate in 1 h for venous blood: <50 years, >21 mm for females and >14 mm for males; >50 years, >28 mm for females and >20 mm for males; venous blood hematocrit, <31% for females and <36% for males; fasting serum cholesterol, >9.1 mmol/L or >350 mg/dL; and fasting serum triglycerides, >2.4 mmol/L or >195 mg/dL.

The Scandinavian Committee on Reference Values has recommended that the following subgroups be the smallest number of subgroups in epidemiological and personal examination studies relative to medical analysis: age; gender; genetic factors [race/ethnic origin, blood groups (groups A,B,O), and histocompatability antigens (HLA)]; physiological factors (stage in menstrual cycle, stage in pregnancy, and physical condition); and other factors (socioeconomic, environmental, and chronobiological).

8.2 SAMPLING AND ANALYSIS CONSIDERATIONS

8.2.1 Standardized Presampling and Sampling Factors

The Scandinavian Committee of Reference Values has recommended that apparently healthy people eat ordinary diets with the last meal before 2200 h; that there be a maximum of one small bottle of beer or an equivalent other beverage taken with a meal; and that the subject abstain from solid food and food and tobacco with a maximum of one glass of water after 2200 h. Unprescribed medications or drugs must be avoided for at least 2 days before the sampling.

For ambulatory subjects where the sample is to be collected in the morning, the person should awake 1 to 3 h before collection (record time); transport by car or public transport should not take longer than 45 min; the subject should not walk more than 500 m at moderate speed; the subject should sit for at least 15 min with no arm muscle work before sampling; and the sample should be collected between 0800 and 1000 h (record time) with the subject in a sitting position with the arm approximately 45 degrees below the horizontal position for blood sampling. The person should have sat in this position at least 20 min before sampling. An arm with an inserted venous line, one with extensive scarring, or one with a hematoma should not be chosen for sampling. Arm veins on the side of the body where an operation or mastectomy has been performed should not be used.

For ambulatory subjects where the sample is to be collected in the afternoon, there should be a light meal in the morning (310 kcal or 1300 kJ) composed of milk, coffee, or tea (a maximum of two cups), two open sandwiches with butter, and slices of lunch meat or cheese or marmalade; there should be no exercising or heavy work; the subject should sit for at least 15 min with no arm muscle work; the sample should be collected between 1300 and 1500 h (record time) a minimum of 4 h after breakfast with the arm positioned as for the morning collection.

For subjects lying in bed with sample collection in the morning, there should be bed rest from 2200 h until collection, with a short visit allowed to the toilet but at a minimum of 1 h before collection; the sample should be collected between 0700 and 0900 h (record the time) with the subject in the supine position with the arm approximately in the horizontal plane.

8.2.2 Blood Sampling

Venipuncture should be in the cleaned (with 70% isopropanol saturated gauze), dry cubital fold with no torniquet [the latter causes changes of up to 10% in serum values for aspartate aminotransferase, bilirubin, cholesterol, iron, lipids (total), potassium, and protein (total) after 3 min occlusion], with finger pressure allowed proximal to the site. If blood ethyl alcohol is being sampled, the skin should be cleaned with a benzalkonium chloride solution free of any alcohol. If the first sampling attempt is a failure, a new attempt can be done on the opposite arm after 15 min rest. Stress associated with blood collection may increase cortisol, growth hormones, glucose, and enzymes originating in skeletal muscle, especially in frightened or hyperactive children.

Skin puncture often is used in tests not requiring much blood for such substrates as glucose and lead in children, though peripheral blood often is not representative of venous blood. A fingerstick or an earlobe pierce is satisfactory for blood typing. In an infant less than one year old, the lateral or medial plantar surface of the foot should be used for skin puncture; in older children, the plantar surface of the big toe is a favorite sampling site.

Arterial punctures require much skill and should be performed only by physicians, specially trained technicians, or nurses. The preferred sites of arterial puncture are, in order, the radial artery at the wrist, the brachial artery in the elbow, and the femoral artery in the groin. The latter is not recommended in the elderly. Firm pressure over the puncture site must be applied for at least 5 min. Arterialized capillary blood may be sampled in young children or in adults where the usual routes are not possible. The earlobe or the heel is the preferred site of sampling, with the skin first warmed with a hot moist towel.

Sampling may have to be modified, depending on local conditions, needs, and the intended use of the data. Discussion of anticoagulants and vacuum container tubes was presented in Section 6.1.3.

Blood samples obtained from different sites differ in composition. Thus glucose and potassium are higher in capillary blood relative to venous blood, with no differences for phosphorus and urea. Lower values are found in capillary blood for bilirubin, calcium, chloride, protein (total), and sodium. Blood obtained by skin puncture is contaminated with interstitial and intracellular fluids. Interstitial fluid has as much as 0.3 mM less potassium than venous serum, and one-third the total protein of plasma. Tissue debris also may contaminate the venous blood samples, and this may cause higher potassium levels than those of capillary blood.

Arterial and central venous and peripheral venous bloods also may differ for certain substituents; but those markers that are not affected include: albumin aspartate aminotransferase, calcium, chloride, creatinine, γ-glutamyltransferase, potassium, sodium, and uric acid. Arterial and central venous bloods also agree for alanine aminotransferase, alkaline phosphatase, amylase, protein (total), and urea nitrogen. The peripheral venous blood is higher than the central venous blood for alanine aminotransferase, amylase, creatine kinase, and protein (total), but lower for alkaline phosphatase and urea nitrogen.

8.2.3 Urine Sampling

Section 6.2.3 details the major principles and sampling and analysis considerations for urinary biological monitoring, all of which apply to medical surveillance. We focus only on clinical medical monitoring applications here.

A clean early morning fasting specimen generally is the most concentrated one and usually is preferred for microscopic examination and analysis of low-concentration substrates. Clean timed specimens obtained after the first void usually are partitioned: the first 10 mL is used to detect urethritis via bacterial detection (also nitrite ion concentration), whereas the midstream has been found best to detect bladder disorders. The double-voided urine specimen is the specimen excreted during a timed period after complete emptying of the bladder; it is used to assess glucose excretion during a glucose tolerance test. The collection time must be known in relation to glucose ingestion. Catheter and suprapubic tap specimens often are used for microbiological examination in critically ill patients or those with urinary tract obstruction.

Patients should be given written instructions relative to fasting, collection of samples and their storage, and dietary or drug intake restrictions. For example, if 5-hydroxyindoleacetic acid is being collected, the patient must avoid avocados, bananas, plums, dates, walnuts, pineapples, eggplant, acetaminophen, and cough syrups containing glyceryl guaiacolate (guaifenesin). The dietary items are sources of 5-hydroxytryptamine, and the other compounds may be chromatographic interferences.

8.2.4 Other Biological Media Sampling

Samples other than blood and urine for biological monitoring media are considered in Sections 6.3 through 6.8. Clinicians also may sample spinal, synovial, pleural, pericardial, ascitic, and amniocentesis fluids, as well as biopses. We will not be concerned with these samples to any great extent because they are invasive, and primarily of clinical import.

8.2.5 Analytical Chemistry and Quality Control

The pertinent sections in Chapter 6 should be read for analytical chemistry applications relative to specific biological monitoring media. Valid comparisons can be done when the same analytical chemistry method and the same analytical laboratory are used to produce comparison data. This minimizes the effect of systematic errors between analytical chemistry methods and laboratories. In lieu of meeting this rather stringent condition, the laboratory should be accredited for the marker in question and/or participate successfully in a recognized interlaboratory collaborative testing program for the marker. Any analytical method should be a standard one of known precision and accuracy or its demonstrated equivalent. Reference values for the marker used by the laboratory should be requested. The sample sender should send a sample of known concentration to the laboratory to test the laboratory's accuracy.

Quality control should be practised, with controls, blanks, known concentrations, simulated samples, and reference samples from reference individuals analyzed every ten samples. The associated intrarun, interrun, and interlaboratory precisions and inaccuracies should be no more than 10%, so that the use of two significant figures is required to report results. There is no point in measuring markers with greater precision than their personal variation allows. To define this variation, at least 3 samples taken at the same time on three consecutive days should be collected, analysed, and the arithmetic mean and standard deviation calculated. The biological markers under strict personal homeostatic control (calcium, chloride, osmolality, and sodium) should be measured to an accuracy of at least 1.4% (use three significant figures), preferably by automated procedures. Albumin, alkaline phosphatase, cholesterol, creatinine, glucose (fasting), phosphate phosphorus, protein (total), thyroxine, and uric acid should be measured with a precision of better than 4%.

The College of American Pathologists employs a total error concept based on the sum of bias and imprecision to certify participating clinical chemistry laboratories. For example, values for potassium deviating by more than 0.5 mM from the mean of all participating laboratories, for calcium by more than 1 mg/dL, for sodium by 4 mM, or for chloride by 5 mM are rejected.

Confirmation by a different technique may be necessary if concentrations associated with adverse effects are detected. Many markers are not specific, and the suspected adverse concentrations or activities need to be confirmed, usually by taking another sample for analysis.

The mindsets for monitoring and diagnosis differ. For monitoring, day-to-day variation and inter- and intrarun precisions are all-important because changes since the last measurement are the key observations. Subtraction of two large values has an associated error that is approximately the sum of the individual absolute errors (standard deviations for a Gaussian distributed data set; geometric standard deviations for a lognormally distributed data set).

For diagnosis, on the other hand, comparison with an established reference interval is most important, the quality of the data usually being questioned initially when the measurement lies out of the reference interval (assess with a Q-test or an outlier test (199)). Also, the result should be confirmed by measuring another sample, validating with a different technique, or both. In emergencies, time may be so important that a somewhat lower standard of performance is acceptable, and direct-reading screening tests become all-important. For example, a high or a low result for blood glucose in a comatose, insulin-dependent, diabetic patient would enable the physician to treat hypoglycemic coma or ketoacidosis.

Incidence is the number of cases in a specified period of time, whereas prevalence is the frequency of cases at a specified point in time. Diagnostic sensitivity is a measure of the frequency of a positive test when a particular disease is known to be present; diagnostic specificity is a measure of frequency of a negative test in the absence of a particular disease. The predictive value of a positive (negative) result is the percentage of all positive (negative) results that are true positives (negatives), or, alternatively, the frequency of the disease in question in all cases with positive results (vice versa for predictive value of a negative result). The efficiency of a test is the percentage of patients who are correctly classified by the test result. Commonly in medical monitoring, the predictive value of a positive result is most often required:

$$\text{Predictive value} = \left[1 + \frac{(1 - \text{prevalence})(1 - \text{specificity})}{\text{prevalence} \times \text{sensitivity}}\right]^{-1} \tag{8.1}$$

If the laboratory test is useful, the predictive value of a positive test should be greater than the disease prevalence.

If two tests are used to make decisions, there are three general approaches: test 1 positives are subjected to test 2 (series approach); test 2 positives are subjected to test 1 (series approach); positives for test 1 and for test 2, and for both tests 1 and 2, are all positives (parallel approach). The series approach provides the highest specificity and lowest cost, whereas the parallel approach has the greatest sensitivity and highest cost. The optimal sequence has to be determined by using the predictive value model. The appropriate application of the predictive value model depends on the correct classification, on matching reference criteria factors in both populations, and on the disease itself. A guesstimate of prevalence is required because it is rarely known in the early stages of a new epidemic.

Biochemical profiles or batteries of laboratory tests (such as the standard 20 marker medical blood screen) have very high sensitivity but low specificity characteristic of the parallel approach. Their high negative predictive value often is used to exclude diagnoses with high certainty. The taking of just one sample rather than multiple samples causes a minimum of inconvenience to the patient, is less expensive than sampling and processing multiple samples, and has less associated paperwork. Also, characterization at a single time point is potentially more useful for several connected markers than characterization at different time points for each marker. The obvious problem with a one-sample regime is that it may be nonrepresentative or clinically misleading.

There are many aspects to selecting a new analytical method. The stoichiometry of any reaction or principles of the assay must be known; and the composition and purity of reagents and standards, the quantity required for the number of desired tests, and storage requirements (space, temperature, light, humidity, compatibilities, corrosiveness) as well as disposal must be considered. Also needed is knowledge of: the stability of reagents and standards (shelf life at room and refrigerator temperatures); possible hazards, safety precautions, and which protective equipment to wear; specimen requirements such as conditions for collection, specimen volume, anticoagulants, preservatives, and storage conditions; anticipated analytical performance (accuracy, precision, analytical range, linear range, specificity, recoveries, reaction efficiencies, interferences, confirmations, matrix effects, reference analytical chemistry methods, and regression analysis) relative to the laboratory's own results; reference range relative to health and disease plus its bases, and whether an in-house referent range will be necessary; the complete and detailed protocol for performing the analysis; instrumental requirements and limitations; and the availability of technical support, supplies, and service. There must be written quality control and assurance procedures for the method.

8.3 SUBJECT AND POPULATION REFERENCE VALUES

Assuming that the data results for both reference individuals and subjects obey the same parametric statistical distribution (Gaussian, lognormal, binomial, rectangular, Poisson, square root, reciprocal, etc.), standard tests such as the Student's t-test, F-tests, and the various analysis of variance (ANOVA) techniques can be utilized with the appropriate means and standard deviations. Otherwise nonparametric statistics or subsectioning of data sets to allow application of parametric statistics must be used. The reader should consult statistics books for more information on nonparametric statistics [1].

Most of the reported medical and biological monitoring data are univariate; that is, the result was elicited with just one analytical chemistry method or independent variable. Multivariate data are obtained when the same sample is analyzed by several different analytical techniques, or the results are dependent on more than one independent variable.

A recent review of the results of a 20-test chemistry profile yielded the following: 68% of the subjects had at least one test result outside univariate reference 95% confidence intervals; only 5% of the patients were outside the 95% multivariate reference level; transformation to Gaussian distribution for univariate data was necessary; the univariate data were sensitive to outliers, whereas multivariate data were not very sensitive; sensitivity to sample differences was increased by defining multivariate reference regions related to physiologically related tests (for example, for liver function).

Similar remarks apply for personal baseline values. Tests of homogeneity for personal versus population values may fail even if the same statistical distribution is obeyed, as the population mean may not be representative of an individual's personal mean. The personal mean may lie outside the 95% confidence interval of the other distribution, suggestive of an individual being in a hyper- or a hypo- group. Nevertheless, this individual may be in good health. The square root of the ratio of the personal-to-population variances (R) is a criterion of usefulness of the population-based reference interval. For $R > 1.4$, the population-based reference interval is reliable for homogeneous variances. At $R < 0.6$, the interval does not have enough sensitivity. Adverse effects may not occur even if atypical values are obtained relative to both personal and population reference intervals. There may be a critical level that corresponds to adverse effects that is well above the upper limit of the reference range. This is a major criticism of the interpretation of reference interval data to imply health, and data not in this range to imply adverse effects. Conversely, hypersensitive individuals may show adverse effects even when values of the marker fall within the reference interval.

Serum proteins and enzymes require personal reference ranges, whereas a homeostatically controlled variable such as sodium or electrolyte concentration is adequately evaluated by using population-based reference intervals. It is clearly advisable to know which markers are controlled homeostatically and which are not. Most medical care ignores these issues, mainly because of cost.

An error analysis often is necessary to locate the major sources of error in medical monitoring data. Thus, the error due to analytical method, laboratory interrun precision, laboratory intrarun precision, interlaboratory precision, homogeneity of the population sampled, sampling biases, or other sources should be defined to determine where the problem resides. If population homogeneity is the problem, dividing the data into subgroups may help. This procedure may be necessary for a relative standard deviation >30%, if a transformation fails to reduce the relative standard deviation.

Time-dependent phenomena can be detected only by regular measurements to assess whether personal baseline values are changing. Thus, any ongoing monitoring program must have the capability to visualize the data as well as to accept and transform them. Because life is a dynamic process, most processes are expected to vary with age and with stress, physical or chemical.

8.4 CONTROLLABLE PHYSIOLOGICAL FACTORS AFFECTING THE COMPOSITION OF BIOLOGICAL AND MEDICAL MONITORING MEDIA

Standardization of presampling conditions, sampling times, sampling techniques, storage conditions, transport conditions, analytical chemistry conditions, quality assurance, and quality control are essential controllable variables. Some of the physiological variables are often subtle.

8.4.1 Position of the Sampled Body

The volume of blood in a body in an upright condition compared with the supine position is 600 to 700 mL less, or about 10% of the total volume, and the reduction in plasma volume is larger than this. Thus values of markers measured in plasma (for example, alanine aminotransferase, albumin, alkaline phosphatase, amylase, aspartate aminotransferase, calcium, cholesterol, IgA, IgG, IgM, thyroxine, and triglycerides) increase up to 11% relative to the recumbent position within 30 min. To compensate, the heart rate and systolic and diastolic blood pressures increase to keep the oxygen supply adequate. Secretions of catecholamines, aldosterone, angiotensin II, renin, and antidiuretic hormone also are enhanced. Increases also occur when a person changes from a lying to a sitting position.

Standing also reduces renal blood flow within 1 h, thus reducing the glomerular filtration rate and urine production. Urinary sodium, potassium, lithium, pH, bicarbonate, and protein also are reduced. All these changes are greater in hypertensive people and in the elderly relative to the young.

During hospitalization and immobilization the blood hematocrit may increase by 10% within 4 days. With prolonged bed rest, serum protein and albumin decrease by an average of 0.5 g/dL and 0.3 g/dL, respectively. Enhanced calcium mobilization from bones keeps serum calcium less affected than this. When skeletal muscle begins to waste, there is a lowering of serum creatine kinase, aspartate aminotransferase, lactate dehydrogenase and aldolase activities, and potassium. Urinary nitrogen, calcium, phosphate, potassium, sodium, pH, and sulfate excretions are increased; reductions are seen for catecholamines (up to one-third) and vanillyl-mandelic acid (one-fourth after 2–3 weeks abed). Recovery after prolonged bed rest is a long process: 3 weeks for calcium excretion, another 3 weeks for positive calcium balance, and several weeks for positive nitrogen balance.

8.4.2 Physical Activity

The duration and the intensity of physical activity also affect the composition of body fluids. Moderate activity increases blood glucose and insulin, plasma pyruvate and lactate, serum creatinine, urate, and enzymes originating from skeletal mudscle. Arterial pH and partial pressure of carbon dioxide are reduced, as are serum cholesterol and triglycerides.

Strenuous physical activity exaggerates the above effects for moderate activity. Plasma lactate increases twofold after moderate activity but may increase tenfold after strenuous activity. Heavy physical activity for 10 min can increase renin activity fourfold.

Some representative serum increases 15 min after a 20-min activity interval, in %, included: acid phosphatase, 11; alanine transferase, 41; aspartate aminotransferase, 31; creatinine, 17; and phosphorus, 12. Decreases, in %, were shown by: iron, 11; potassium, 8; and total lipids, 12. Plasma proteins, creatine kinase activity, aldosterone, growth hormone, prolactin, and catecholamines, and urinary free cortisol and catecholamines, are also increased. Blood pH, oxygen saturation, and venous bicarbonate decrease.

People who habitually experience strenuous physical activity at work or in sports have higher resting serum activities of enzymes of skeletal muscle origin but are less inducible on physical activity than less active people. Their resting serum urea, urate, creatinine, and thyroxine are also higher. Their total resting serum lipids, LDL-cholesterol, and triglycerides (up to 20 mg/dL) are decreased, but their HDL-cholesterol and free fatty acids are increased.

8.4.3 Circadian Rhythms

Cyclical variations of many constituents of body fluids occur through the day. For example, serum iron and cortisol concentrations change by as much as 50% at 1400 h relative to 0800 h. Serum potassium declines from 5.4 mM to 4.3 mM over the same time interval. Constitutents that vary by more than 10%, corrected for analytical variation and measured at 0800, 1100 and 1400 h in males aged 21 to 27 years are, in %: urea nitrogen, 20; cholesterol, 33; total lipids, 21; aspartate aminotransferase, 19; alanine aminotransferase, 39; and alkaline phosphatase, 17. Hormone concentrations are difficult to interpret because of biological cycling. These changes are often greater in females than in males.

Many circadian rhythm effects are also influenced by body position, physical activity, light, food ingestion, sleep, wakefulness, darkness, and stress. Disentangling the independent variables often is extremely difficult.

For example, blindness reduces the cyclic light stimulation of the hypothalamic–pituitary axis. This reduces urinary excretion of 17-ketosteroids, 17-hydroxycorticosteroids, and urate; plasma sodium, chloride, glucose, insulin tolerance, and protein can be reduced also. Increases are seen for serum bilirubin and cholesterol. The circadian rhythm for serum iron often is lost.

Sleep and wakefulness are important variables. Corticotropin is increased three- to fivefold from its minimum between afternoon and midnight, to a maximum around wakening for morning risers. Cortisol concentrations also are greatest around 0600 to 0800 h. Maximum renin activity usually occurs early in the morning during sleep, with its minimum late in the afternoon, and this affects glomerular filtration in an inverse manner. Prolactin concentration is greatest during sleep. Growth hormone secretion is greatest shortly after sleep begins, whereas plasma insulin is highest after wakening.

The excretions of 17-ketosteroids and 17-hydroxycorticosteroids are low at night with a maximum around midafternoon. Plasma testosterone is 20 to 40% increased at night. Serum thyroid stimulating hormone is greatest between 0200 and 0400 h and is at a minimum between 1800 and 2200 h with 50% variation. Peak urinary excretion of sodium and potassium occurs around noon, but that of calcium and magnesium occurs during the night. Serum phosphate is 30% higher at night than during the day, and urinary phosphate is correspondingly lower. Urinary volume and creatinine excretion (by up to 10%) are low at night, but urine is enhanced in ammonium ion and hydrogen ions.

Prolonged immobilization reduces the amplitude of the circadian rhythm for cortisol.

Five days are required to establish a new diurnal rhythm after travel across ten time zones. The changes are thought to be caused by altered pituitary and adrenal functions. Urinary excretion of catecholamines is increased generally for 2 days, and serum cortisol is reduced. Urine excretion rate and sodium excretion are decreased, reverting after 2 days.

8.4.4 Life-style Factors: Acute Effects of Diet

The concentrations of glucose, iron, total lipids, and alkaline phosphatase increase after recent meals. The alkaline phosphatase concentration (mainly intestinal isoenzyme) is greatest for a high-fat meal, with the increase influenced by the blood group of the individual. Lipidemia may interfere with analyses of fatlike constituents.

Ingestion of a protein-rich meal will cause increases in serum urea nitrogen, phosphorus, and urate concentrations that are still apparent 12 h later. Serum cholesterol and growth hormone concentrations increase for at least 1 h after a meal, and glucagon and insulin secretions also are stimulated. Insulin also is increased by carbohydrate meals.

Because the stomach secretes hydrochloric acid in response to a meal, plasma chloride concentrations decrease. Venous bicarbonate and the partial pressure of venous carbon dioxide increase because of stomach activity, and these changes cause a reduction in serum calcium ion. The liver increases its release of enzymes and retention of xenobiotics.

The ingestion of a standard 700 kcal (2.93 MJ) meal in 200 apparently healthy individuals caused less than a 5% change 2 h after a meal relative to before the meal for serum albumin, alkaline phosphatase, calcium, cholesterol, lactate dehydrogenase, protein (total), sodium, urea nitrogen, and uric acid; greater than 10% increases were observed for aspartate aminotransferase (27%), bilirubin (14%), glucose (13%), and phosphorus (16%); and between 5 and 10% increases were observed for alanine aminotransferase and potassium. Glucose increases more than this, and phosphorus decreases after high-carbohydrate meals. The type of meal affects the values also. Drinking one glass of water alters many of these variables.

8.4.5 Life-style Factors: Long-term Effects of Diet

Day-to-day changes in the amount of dietary protein are reflected in the plasma and the urine (end products of protein metabolism) within a few days of the change. Four days after the change from a normal diet to a high-protein diet, up to a doubling of plasma urea and urate may be observed, with increases also in the urine. Serum cholesterol and phosphate also increase. High-fat diets deplete the nitrogen pool because ammonium ions must be excreted to maintain an acid–base homeostasis. Thus serum urate also is reduced. Reduction of the fat intake reduces serum lactate dehydrogenase activity. Ingestion of cholesterol does not appear to affect serum cholesterol, unlike the ingestion of unsaturated fats.

If dietary carbohydrate is mostly starch or sucrose, serum activities of alkaline phosphatase and lactate dehydrogenase are increased. Aspartate aminotransferase activity may be increased by certain sugars. Plasma triglyceride is decreased when the sucrose intake is reduced. More consistent glucose tolerance curves are obtained with a bread diet than for a high-sucrose diet. A high-carbohydrate diet decreases serum very-low-density (VLD) lipoprotein, triglycerides, cholesterol, and protein.

8.4.6 Life-style Factors: Vegetarians

In long-standing vegetarians, the concentrations of VLD and low-density lipoproteins are low. Total lipid and phospholipid are reduced, as are plasma cholesterol (15%) and triglycerides (by as much as one-third). Plasma calcium and blood hemoglobin are lower by about 3%. Blood glucose, blood urea nitrogen, and plasma urea decrease between 9 and 15%. However, vegetarians' serum albumin and plasma high-density lipoprotein and cholesterol do not differ compared to individuals eating mixed diets. Lipid concentrations are also less for those who eat only a vegetable diet, compared to those who also consume eggs and milk.

These effects for long-term vegetarians are much less marked for people who have been vegetarians for a short time. Serum albumins may fall by 10% and serum urea by 50% in a week, but most other parameters do not change for some months, depending on the fat stores. The urinary pH is generally higher for vegetarians relative to meat-eaters because of vegetarians' reduced intake of precursors of acid metabolites. Plasma vitamin B_{12} and iron may be enough reduced that deficiencies develop. Higher serum bilirubin also is often observed in vegetarians.

Habitual ingestion of bran hinders gastrointestinal absorption of calcium, cholesterol, and triglycerides. Pectin and high-fiber diets reduce serum apolipoprotein-B and cholesterol. Many fruits such as bananas and vegetables that contain 5-hydroxytryptamine (serotonin) increase urinary 5-hydroxyindoleacetic acid. Avacados affect insulin secretion and impair glucose tolerance. Onions reduce plasma glucose and the insulin response to glucose.

8.4.7 Life-style Factors: Malnutrition

In cases of malnutrition, total serum protein, albumin, and β-globulin are drastically reduced, as are complement C_3, retinol-binding globulin, transferrin, and prealbumin. These are the accepted biological monitoring markers for the state of malnutrition. Plasma lipoprotein, serum cholesterol, and triglycerides may be reduced by 50%, but glucose is not much affected. However, serum urea, serum creatinine, plasma total triiodothyronine (T_3), thyroxine, thyroid stimulating hormone, blood hemoglobin, and serum enzyme activities related to skeletal muscle are greatly reduced, as is creatinine clearance. Plasma cortisol is increased because of decreased metabolic clearance. Red cell and plasma folate are reduced in protein–calorie malnutrition, but serum vitamin B_{12} is not; plasma vitamin A and vitamin E are much decreased.

Malnutrition produces an added stress that may cause exposures to xenobiotics at "safe" concentrations to elicit toxic responses. Often animal experiments involve pair-feeding when dietary intake is not optimal for the animal exposed to a toxicant. The pair-fed control is appropriate only if there are no interactions—usually a matter of faith rather than of science.

8.4.8 Life-style Factors: Fasting and Starvation

Fasting causes the body to conserve protein at the expense of such other energy sources as fat. Blood glucose decreases by as much as 18 mg/dL within the first 3 days of food withdrawal. Insulin secretion is markedly reduced, but glucagon secretion may double in an attempt to achieve glucose homeostasis (Section 2.12). Lipolysis and liver ketogenesis are stimulated. Ketoacids and fatty acids become the major energy sources for muscle. The ketone bodies, fatty acids, and glycerol in serum rise greatly (Sections 2.4–2.6, 2.8.2, and 2.12). Serum triglycerides increase by about 20% after 2 days of food lack and decline thereafter. Serum cholesterol (Section 2.8.2) decreases, and amino acids (Sections 2.11.2 and 2.11.3) are released from skeletal muscle, with plasma branched-chain amino acids increasing by up to 100% within one day. The breakdown of fat leads to a transient increase in body water, which, however, soon decreases because of osmotic diuresis in spite of an impairment of glomerular filtration signaled by increased serum creatinine (Section 2.11.6) and reduced urinary creatinine clearance. The blood supply to the liver may be reduced. Serum bilirubin (Section 2.11.5) rises, with the unconjugated form more than doubling within 2 days. Increased serum activities of aspartate and alanine aminotransferases and of lactate dehydrogenase occur. The catabolism of nucleoproteins produces increased serum urate (Sections 2.11.1 and 2.11.7), which is exacerbated by the reduced glomerular filtration rate and competition for clearance from lactate and ketoacids. Metabolic acidosis is common with reduced blood pH and reduced partial pressure of carbon dioxide. Often the blood partial pressure of oxygen is reduced.

The plasma growth hormone concentration can rise up to 15 times at the start of the fast but may return to normal after 3 days. The free and the total triiodothyronine decrease by up to 50% within 3 days, but free thyroxine is less affected than triidothyronine. Total thyroxine is not much affected, however. The urinary free cortisol decreases, with plasma free and total cortisol increasing a little with loss of the normal diurnal circadian rhythm.

The onset of starvation is signaled by an increase of aldosterone secretion, and by increased urinary excretion and decreased plasma potassium. Magnesium, calcium, and phosphate also increase in the urine, but phosphate excretion declines gradually.

Early on refeeding, sodium retention is marked, but potassium retention takes longer than sodium. This is so because aldosterone secretion is even greater on refeeding than during fasting. Most markers rapidly return to their typical values. The nitrogen balance soon becomes positive, especially if the nonprotein calories come mainly from carbohydrates.

Pregnancy under fasting and starvation conditions may cause the signs of malnutrition in both mother and fetus.

8.4.9 Life-style Factors: Caffeine

Caffeine, found in coffee, tea, and colas, stimulates the adrenal medulla to increase the excretion of catecholamines and their metabolites and to increase plasma glucose with impairment of glucose tolerance. The adrenal cortex also secretes cortisol, with increased excretion of free cortisol, 11-hydroxycorticoids, and 5-hydroxyindoleacetic acid. The diurnal circadian rhythm of plasma cortisol may be eliminated. Caffeine stimulates gastric juice, pepsin, and hydrochloric acid secretion. Two cups of coffee may increase plasma free fatty acids by as much as 30%, with lesser increases for glycerol, total lipids, and lipoproteins. Chronic coffee ingestion causes a small reduction in serum cholesterol but increases serum triglycerides. Three cups of coffee may increase serum gastrin concentration fivefold. Coffee causes diuresis and allows the kidney to excrete an increased amount of red blood cells and renal tubular cells into the urine.

8.4.10 Life-style Factors: Smoking

The extent of the effects of smoking is related to the number of cigarettes smoked, smoking duration, and to the amount and type of smoke inhaled. Nicotine in tobacco and smoke stimulates the adrenal medulla, increasing plasma adrenaline and urinary catecholamines and their metabolites. Plasma glucose concentration is enhanced 10 min after the start of smoking, often persisting for 1 h after smoking ceases. Plasma lactate is increased, but plasma pyruvate is reduced. Plasma insulin rises 1 h after smoking. Plasma growth hormone concentrations may increase tenfold within 30 min after the smoking of one cigarette.

Smokers have higher plasma β-lipoprotein, cholesterol, and triglyceride concentrations than nonsmokers. Inhalation during smoking causes an increase of about 30% of free fatty acids immediately. Serum albumin, cholesterol, and phospholipids increase less than 5%, but glucose and urea nitrogen typically increase 10%, and triglycerides are enhanced 20% in smokers relative to nonsmokers. Serum vitamin B_{12} often is markedly reduced, in inverse proportion to the serum thiocyanate concentration. Creatinine and albumin decrease also.

Smoking also stimulates the adrenal cortex. Plasma 11-hydroxycorticosteroids may be increased 75% by heavy smoking; plasma cortisol increases by as much as 40% within 5 min of the start of smoking. Unlike the case of caffeine, the diurnal circadian rhythm for cortisol is unaffected in smokers. Smokers also excrete more 5-hydroxyindoleacetic acid than nonsmokers.

Smoking increases total red blood cells, carboxyhemoglobin (may exceed 10%), and leukocytes (as much as 30%), but decreases blood partial pressure of oxygen by 5 mm Hg in habitual smokers and decreases leukocyte ascorbic acid concentration. There is a decrease in plasma protein, plasma urate, serum urea, and serum creatinine. The hematocrit is increased.

Because nicotine stimulates gastric juice secretion, both the gastric juice volume and acid secretion are increased within 1 h of smoking several cigarettes; the bicarbonate concentration and the volume of pancreatic juice are reduced.

Smoking affects the immune response, lowering serum IgA, IgG, and IgM but raising IgE. The presence of antinuclear antibodies and weak positive tests for carcinoembryonic antigen (CEA) may also be shown. Hansen et al. [2] in 1974 detected serum CEA above 2.6 ng/mL in 7.8% of smokers (118/1512), and in 1.7% it was above 5 ng/mL. The corresponding figures for nonsmokers were 3.0% (27/892) and 0.22%, respectively. Similarly, for former smokers the figures were 6.8% (16/235) and 1.7%, respectively, and for pregnant females, 3.8% (14/369) and 0.81%, respectively. The reference cutoff value for CEA appears to be 5 ng/mL because this corresponds to the same percentage for smokers and former smokers. Stevens and MacKay [3] in 1973 measured serum CEA in 955 people aged 60 years and older. Three months after smoking cessation, CEA concentrations in former smokers became the same as for nonsmokers. Among the 903 current smokers, ex-smokers, and nonsmokers who had no detectable cancer, 13.6% of the 110 smokers and 1.8% of the 433 nonsmokers had CEA concentrations above 5 ng/mL. Similar serum CEA results were reported by Alexander et al. [4] in 1976 for 154 smokers and 122 nonsmokers, and by Meeker et al. [5] in 1973 for 176 individuals.

As pointed out in Section 5.3.2, the classical biological monitoring markers for exposure to tobacco are blood and urinary nicotine; urinary, serum, and saliva cotinine, the major metabolite of nicotine; blood carboxyhemoglobin and expired carbon monoxide; urinary, saliva, sweat, and serum thiocyanate; and urinary mutagenicity [6, 7]. The carboxyhemoglobin, expired carbon monoxide, and thiocyanate markers are markers for tobacco smoke, whereas the nicotine and cotinine markers are for both smoked and smokeless tobacco.

8.4.11 Life-style Factors: Alcohol

A single moderate dose of alcohol does not affect many medical markers. Mildly inebriated drinkers show increased blood glucose (20–50%), which is more marked in diabetics. Alcohol ingestion inhibits gluconeogenesis (Section 2.4), culminating in hypoglycemia and ketonemia. In hypoglycemia, lactate accumulates and competes with urate in the kidneys so that serum urate is also increased. The massive increase in serum triglycerides after alcohol ingestion is due to increased triglyceride formation in the liver and the impaired removal of chylomicra and very-low-density lipoprotein from the circulation (Section 2.8.2). Fatty meals show the biggest effect. The elevation may last longer than 12 h. Serum γ-glutamyltransferase, isocitrate dehydrogenase, and ornithine carbamoyl transferase are increased.

Moderate amounts of alcohol ingested for one week cause serum triglyceride concentration to increase by more than 20 mg/dL. Alcohol intoxication results in cortisol secretion, elevated plasma catecholamines, increased luteinizing hormone, but sharply reduced plasma testosterone.

Chronic alcohol ingestion affects the activities of many serum enzymes, and is associated with abnormal pituitary, adrenal cortical, and medullary function. Serum γ-glutamyltransferase activity is used as a marker for persistent drinking.

8.5 UNCONTROLLABLE FACTORS INFLUENCING THE COMPOSITION OF BIOLOGICAL MONITORING MEDIA

Many factors are beyond the control of the biological monitoring subject and often any physician. Such factors are medications, medical conditions, injuries, and such long-term influences as age, gender, and race.

8.5.1 Medications

Most patients are given more than one drug; and healthy people often take many drugs simultaneously, for example, vitamins, oral contraceptives, sleeping tablets, and aspirin-type derivatives. Also many people take medications to be able to function. Reference 8 discusses the effects of such drugs on common laboratory procedures.

Medications are effective only in a blood concentration range called the therapeutic range (Appendix B), analagous to the reference range but for therapeutic effect. Below this range, medications are generally ineffective. Above the upper range toxic side-effects are to be expected. As for reference ranges, an individual's response cannot be predicted, and side-effects may still be observed if concentrations are in the therapeutic range. Thus the remarks in Section 8.3 can be applied to therapeutic ranges too. Toxic side-effects will render any biological monitoring marker measurements uninterpretable. The same remarks apply to recreational drugs also.

Drugs administered intramuscularly, for example, penicillin derivatives, may cause enough muscle irritation to increase creatine kinase, aldolase, and the skeletal muscle component of lactate dehydrogenase activities in the serum, often for several days. Creatine kinase activity is increased by intramuscular injection of ampicillin, analgesics, antibiotics, barbiturates, carbeicillin, chlorpromazine, clindamycin, digoxin, diuretics, lidocaine, meperidine, morphine, penicillin, phenothiazines, and tubocurarine.

Liver and pancreatic enzymes are increased by opiates such as morphine or meperidine, which cause the sphincter of Oddi to have spasms. The latter transmit pressure to the liver and pancreas, stimulating serum enzymes from these organs. Also, massive increases in aspartate aminotransferase activity may be mistaken for the occurrence of a myocardial infarction.

Diuretics often cause a moderate reduction of plasma potassium; hyponatremia may be observed. Hypercalcemia may occur with hemoconcentration (also the calcium ion fraction sometimes). Thiazides cause hyperglycemia, as well as reduced glucose tolerance, and sometimes also prerenal azotemia and hyperuricemia, leading to a decreased glomerular filtration rate. In such situations, normalization to creatinine for urinary biological monitoring is not applicable.

Epileptics receiving anticonvulsants excrete elevated urinary copper and zinc and show increased serum ceruloplasmin and copper as well; reduced T-cell function and decreased high-density lipoprotein-cholesterol, uric acid, and urea occur. Low serum IgA and IgG are seen in 25%, systemic lupus erythematosus in about 10%, and antinuclear antibodies in 55%. In 20 to 30% of epileptic children receiving anticonvulsant therapy, red blood cell aspartate aminotransferase activity is low, indicative of a vitamin B_6 nonutilization.

8.5.2 Common Medical Conditions: Fever

People who are being medically monitored may be suffering from fever, shock, trauma, injury, and mental states. These factors will also affect the composition of biological monitoring media.

Fever induces early hyperglycemia, insulin secretion, and increased serum growth hormone, glucagon, creatinine, uric acid, aldosterone, sodium, chloride, antidiuretic hormone, and copper; serum iron, hydrogen ion, and zinc decrease. Thyroxine secretion is reduced, but corticotropin is increased. Serum concentrations of cholesterol, nonesterified fatty acids and other lipids can decrease initially at onset, but after a few days the free fatty acid concentration increases markedly. Some representative range changes relative to individual baseline values at 18, 48, 72, and 96 h after fever onset are: calcium, −6 to −13%; chloride, −5 to −10%; creatinine, −1 to −10%; magnesium, −4 to −12%; phosphate, −30 to +12%; potassium, 0 to −17%; sodium, −4 to −8%; urea nitrogen, +4 to +38%; and uric acid, +10 to +24%. Many of the decreases are due to increased blood volume and hence dilution.

Plasma shows increased acute-phase reactants, cortisol (diurnal rhythm may be abolished), and glycoproteins, and decreased phosphate. Urinary excretions of free cortisol, 17-hydroxycorticosteroids, 17-ketosteroids, phosphate, and electrolytes are enhanced.

Glycogenolysis and a negative nitrogen balance are prompted by decreased food intake and wastage of skeletal muscle; the bigger the wastage is, the higher the serum uric acid and creatinine.

8.5.3 Common Medical Conditions: Depression, Profound Shock, and Schizophrenia

Experiments in mammals have shown that the brain neurotransmitter dopamine is essential for movement [9]. Dopamine metabolism in the caudate nucleus accumbens of the rat brain was most strongly correlated to speed (energy expended) and direction of movement, whereas both dopamine and its metabolite 3,4-dihydroxyphenylacetic acid were affected most by posture and direction. Loss of dopaminergic neurons in patients with Parkinson's Disease drastically reduces voluntary movements, a state treatable by the administration of L-dopa. Cocaine and amphetamine interfere with the neuronal uptake of dopamine from the surrounding fluid [10]. Antipsychotic drugs bind more avidly to these neuronal receptors than does dopamine itself [10]. Carbon fiber electrodes implanted in the surrounding fluid have detected voltammetric activity related to ascorbic acid, dopamine, and 3,4-dihydroxyphenylacetic acid [10]. The same technique applied to the neuron has shown that dopamine is the major neurotransmitter.

It has been proposed [11, 12] that "some, if not all, depressions are associated with an absolute or relative deficiency of catecholamines, particularly norepinephrine (noradrenaline), at functionally important adrenergic receptor sites in the brain [11, 12]." Noradrenaline and normetanephrine cannot cross the blood–brain barrier but the major metabolite of noradrenaline, 3-methoxy-4-hydroxyphenylglycol, can. The concentration of the latter metabolite in urine was found to be lower in depressed than in nondepressed subjects, but higher when these subjects also suffered from mania. The excretion is subject to a diurnal circadian rhythm as well as to the diet. Subjects with low 3-methoxy-4-hydroxyphenylglycol or 5-hydroxyindoleacetic acid responded to the antidepressants imipramine, maprotiline, dextroamphetamine, and desipramine, which enhance the effects of noradrenaline. The subjects with high concentrations of the urinary metabolite responded favorably to amitriptyline, with those at intermediate concentrations not responding to the high- and low-metabolite treatments. Low urinary concentrations of normetanephrine, noradrenaline, and vanillyl-mandelic acid are also correlated with low 3-methoxy-4-hydroxyphenylglycol. The concentration of blood 3,4-dihydroxyphenylglycol, another metabolite of noradrenaline, also responds to amitriptyline and phenelzine (an inhibitor of monoamine oxidase).

The red blood cells of patients with manic depression concentrate lithium more than normal patients do relative to the plasma, probably because of low membrane lecithin. Such lithium-sensitive patients with paranoid schizophrenia respond to physostigmine like manic patients. In such cases, choline therapy may have a chance of being effective. The dexamethasone suppression challenge test identifies depressed patients with elevated blood cortisol and lacking feedback inhibition on challenge with dexamethasone.

The β-phenethylamine (2-phenylethylamine) excretion rate in the urine is markedly enhanced (2.5–5.4 times over 24 h post-event relative to pre-event) after profound physical stress [13]—in this case, an initial parachuting experience for three males and three females, 18 to 28 years of age. Physical stress was defined here as a significant reversible elevation of heart rate. In an extra three subjects studied for 34 h post-jump, the factors were 3.0, 8.6, and 15.8

relative to pre-jump values. β-phenethylamine is the decarboxylation product of phenylalanine, and is metabolized further to phenylacetic acid by monoamine oxidase B, perhaps in the hypothalamus. In unstressed humans, the excretion of β-phenethylamine is not affected by foods containing this base, and is not tied to the circadian rhythm for urinary pH.

β-phenethylamine has been found also to be excreted at high levels by patients diagnosed with paranoid schizophrenia. Physical stress may precipitate psychotic episodes, and the excretion of β-phenethylamine may be more related to this than to the psychosis itself. The compound also may trigger the psychosis. A theory [14] has been enunciated that the amine is a neuromodulator responsible for triggering or sustaining wakefulness, alertness, and excitement. The 24-h urinary excretion of its metabolite, phenyl acetate, with the aid of the monoamine oxidase B enzyme system is inversely related to how much the enzyme is inhibited during depression [14]. Thus the difference between baseline levels and those found when the patient is depressed is related to the degree of inhibition of the enzyme.

Schizophrenics excrete low concentrations of phenylacetic acid but also have high concentrations of it in plasma. Effective treatment for depression also causes the phenylacetic acid concentration to increase in urine. Another explanation is that the β-phenethylamine concentration itself is lowered during depression, but this is the opposite of what actually happens. Other possibilities to explain the decreased urinary excretion could include dietary and microbial transformation of phenylalanine by the flora and fauna of the gut. Other work showed that fasting and oral phenylalanine administration did not affect the excretion of phenylacetic acid, nor did the killing of gut flora. Antibiotics known to kill off gut flora and fauna reduced the excretion [15], but it was unclear whether the reduction was truly by gut flora reduction or by a direct biological effect of the antibiotic.

Plasma homovanillic acid also has been found to correlate with the severity of schizophrenia in drug-free humans, but the marker is not responsive to treatment with haloperidol [16]. Fifty percent of this marker reflects brain turnover of dopamine in rodents and nonhuman primates. The plasma marker was thought to be better than the cerebrospinal fluid marker.

Yet another possible marker for schizophrenia is cerebrospinal fluid dopamine β-hydroxylase activity, which was much lower in schizophrenic patients who had successful neuroleptic treatment than those who remained psychotic [17]. This enzyme catalyzes the synthesis of noradrenaline from dopamine. The hydroxylase has been localized in the brain noradrenergic neurons, the peripheral sympathetic nerves, and the chromaffin granules of the adrenal medulla. The enzyme is bound to storage vesicles and is released along with catecholamines by exocytosis. Human blood serum activity arises from sympathetic nerve endings, whereas the cerebrospinal activity is thought to arise from brain noradrenergic neurons. The latter activity for each individual is rather constant.

8.5.4 Common Medical Conditions: Shock, Trauma, and Oxygen Lack

People who are in trauma or have experienced shock, common occurrences in emergencies and emotion crises, show three- to fivefold increases in serum cortisol with enhanced urinary 17-hydroxycorticosteroids. Aldosterone, glucagon, insulin, and growth hormone secretions as well as plasma renin activity invariably are increased. Anxiety and stress increase the excretion of catecholamines. Trauma causes plasma fibrinogen to increase up to twofold in 2 to 8 days after surgery. Shock causes mobilization of lipids (not triglycerides), an increase in plasma glucose, and reduced glucose tolerance. The protein-rich fluid lost from the intravascular space following trauma is replaced by protein-poor fluid from the interstitial spaces. This is subsequently succeeded by a fluid similar in composition to plasma. Serum iron and potassium concentrations are reduced immediately following an injury.

Surgery stress reduces serum T_3 by 50%. When surgery involves destruction of muscle, serum enzymes emanating from muscle depots are increased [up to 76% for creatine kinase; 50% for aspartate aminotransferase; 28% for α-hydroxybutyrate dehydrogenase; 18% for lactate dehydrogenase (LDH)-1 isoenzyme, with LDH-1 > LDH-2 by 10%, and 20% for LDH-5 isoenzyme]. Increased tissue catabolism requires increased oxygen consumption and leads to the production of acid metabolites. Thus blood lactate may also increase up to threefold. With tissue anoxia and impairment of renal and respiratory function, a metabolic acidosis can develop.

Irregular sleep hours often are encountered in hazardous waste cleanup, nursing, or emergency and maintenance operations. Swedish railroad workers [18] who worked during a light, warm summer and during a dark, cold winter showed stable circadian rhythms for urinary excretion of potassium (though not for sodium, chloride, and noradrenaline), body temperature, and blood cortisol with a daylight pattern. Decrease in sleep during work at night may have been responsible for marker perturbations and the occurrence of ulcers and gastritis.

Firemen not only are potentially exposed to many chemicals; they also suffer much physical strain and stress in their work. The impact of stress at a Finnish fire alarm center where a 24-h work cycle was followed [19] by 48 h off for three teams doing firefighting and rescue, ambulance, and alarm center work. A preliminary questionnaire revealed that work in the alarm center and the ambulance was more burdensome than actual firefighting and rescue. Urinary 17-ketogenic steroids, adrenaline, and noradrenaline were measured for selected women and men at the alarm center. Stress, especially during rush periods, obliterated the diurnal circadian rhythm for 17-ketogenic steroids but not for adrenaline or noradrenaline, even though the concentrations for the last two markers were higher than on nonworking days. Women excreted much lower concentrations of adrenaline and noradrenaline than did men for the morning shift postulated to be because they did not feel as stressed as men.

People who drive tractors in the workplace, in agriculture, and at hazardous waste sites also are subject to much physical activity and stress. Noise, vibration, physical effort, an unfavorable microclimate, heat, an atypical sleeping cycle, and exhaust fumes all contribute. Total urinary 17-ketosteroids, total 17-oxycorticosteroids, and catecholamines were all elevated in tractor drivers [20]. The work routine reduced the circadian rhythm variations for noradrenaline and adrenaline, and also decreased the amplitudes for 17-ketosteroids and 11-oxycorticosteroids.

Anoxia (oxygen lack) particularly affects the brain, and this is an important effect in confined spaces such as tanks and sewers. During cardiac arrest, the electroencephalograph becomes isoelectric within 15 to 20 sec [21]. This period is followed by a massive efflux of potassium ions from neurons with an influx of sodium ions because of the failure of membrane ion pumps (when regional blood flow is about 10% of typical). When the potassium ion concentration in the extracellular fluid drops to about 12 to 13 mM, changes in membrane potential activate or open voltage-dependent calcium ion channels to allow calcium ions to flood in. This activates phospholipases, thus increasing the production of lysophosphatidyl lipids and free fatty acids, which culmulate in membrane phospholipid hydrolysis and consequent disruption of cell and mitochondrial membranes. Diacylglycerol and inositol triphosphate accumulate in hypoxia-sensitive tissues. However, when oxygen is scarce, the brain undergoes these reactions only slowly. Tissue anoxia may produce an eventual metabolic acidosis.

Hypothermia (cold) disrupts the metabolic rate, regulated metabolism, and ion gradients across membranes [21]. A breakdown of glucose homeostasis ensues, with loss of potassium ion from cells, the eventual opening of the voltage-dependent calcium channels, and the influx of calcium ions. A drop in cell temperature lowers the ion dissociation constant of imidazole groups in proteins. The influx of calcium ions activates phospholipases as for hypoxia, together with sequelae.

8.5.5 Common Medical Conditions: Tissue Injury

When tissue is injured, a loss of fluid occurs to extravascular tissues, decreasing the plasma volume. If the decrease is great enough, the glomerular filtration rate is diminished, causing urea, creatinine, and uric acid and the end products of metabolism to accumulate in the blood. In burn victims, the serum total protein concentration can fall by as much as 0.8 g/dL through fluid loss to extravascular spaces and protein catabolism. Even though concentrations of serum α-1, α-2, and γ globulin increase, the increase is not enough to offset the reduced albumin concentration. When tissues are destroyed in injuries, urinary excretion of the major components of skeletal muscle increases, especially enzymes such as creatine kinase produced from this tissue. Surgery also causes this effect, and it would be expected that the effects of minor injuries often experienced in the workplace would not be as great as for surgery relative to serum enzymes.

8.5.6 Long-Term Influences: Age

Intraindividual variability is much less than interindividual variability. Because most reference value ranges are broad, the values found for one individual may be statistically different from those in another or for a group of similar people, even if they fall within a predetermined reference range. Whether there is a biological difference is quite another question. Even when specimens are obtained from individuals under standardized conditions, as recommended in Section 8.2.1, interindividual differences still are present.

Genetic and life-style factors probably are responsible for these differences. There is better agreement between serum concentrations or activities for

TABLE 8.2. Effect of gender and age on selected serum constituents of Caucasians.*

	Change for Age									
	<29 y		30–39 y		40–49 y		50–59 y		60–69 y	
Marker	R	B	A	B	A	B	A	B	A	B
Albumin (g/dL)	4.6	0.1	−0.1	0.1	−0.3	0	−0.4	0	−0.6	−0.1
Alkaline phosphatase (U/L)	51	14	−3	12	−1	−8	1	2	4	−1
Aspartate aminotransferase (U/L)	41	5	3	8	3	8	1	1	1	−1
Bilirubin	0.4	0.1	0.1	0.1	0	0.1	0	1	0	−1
Calcium	9.8	0.1	−0.1	0.1	−0.2	0.1	0	−0.1	−0.3	−0.2
Cholesterol	211	−14	29	2	43	6	48	−16	36	−34
Creatinine	1.1	0.2	0	0.2	0.1	0.2	0.1	0.2	0	0.1
Glucose	108	5	1	3	6	6	2	0	9	6
Phosphorus	4.0	0.1	−0.1	0.1	−0.3	0	−0.2	−0.1	−0.2	−0.2
Protein (g/dL)	7.6	−0.1	−0.1	−0.1	−0.2	−0.1	−0.2	−0.1	−0.2	−0.2
Urea N	15	3	1	3	1	3	2	2	3	0
Uric acid	5.9	1.5	0	1.7	0.2	1.7	−0.1	1.0	−0.2	0.5

*Modified from reference 22.
R, reference value for a <29-year-old adult male.
A, change for males compared with adult male <29 y value.
B, change for females compared with males of same age.
Values are in mg/dL except as noted.
U are International Activity Units.

monozygotic twins than for dizygotic twins, which shows that genetic factors are important. Genetics influence the concentration of uric acid, α-1 antitrypsin, cholesterol, and alkaline phosphatase.

Gender and age [22] are very important variables affecting the concentration of serum constituents (Table 8.2). The degree of sexual maturity and the amount of skeletal muscle are also independent variables reflected in gender, race, and age. Four age groups usually are considered: the newborn, the older child to puberty, the sexually mature adult, and the elderly adult.

The body fluids of a newborn infant reflect the trauma of birth and the changes related to adaptation to independent functioning. In a mature newborn 9 months in the womb, most of the hemoglobin is in the adult form (hemoglobin A). A premature newborn or one suffering from δ β-thalassemia minor may have much hemoglobin F (the cyanmethemoglobin is resistant to alkali denaturation and subsequent precipitation by ammonium sulfate, unlike hemoglobin A).

The arterial blood oxygen saturation is very low initially in all infants. In the first 24 h after birth, newborns develop a metabolic acidosis resulting from the accumulation of organic acids, particularly lactic acid. A few minutes after birth fluid passes from the blood vessels into the extravascular spaces; the composition of this fluid is similar to that of plasma. Blood glucose and lipid are low in newborns; the latter reaches 80% of adult values after 2 weeks. Initial values of plasma urea nitrogen and amino acid concentration are low, and only rise when tissue catabolism predominates.

Serum activities of serum enzymes of creatine kinase, γ-glutamyl-transferase, and aspartate aminotransferase are high at birth relative to adult values, with only a moderate increase for alanine aminotransferase activity. The concentration of bilirubin rises to a peak on the third to fifth day but hardly ever exceeds 5 mg/dL. Plasma sodium and chloride initially are slightly higher, and decrease at 12 h to below the adult value before increasing to a value slightly greater than in the adult. These changes reflect the finishing touches on the capillary system for an independent existence. The plasma potassium may be as high as 7 mM at birth but falls rapidly. Similarly, plasma calcium also is enhanced, and its concentration can fall by as much as 1.4 mg/dL on the first day of life. The urinary excretion of amino acids may be quite high in infants with immature absorption mechanisms of the renal tubules. Plasma urate initially is increased but declines quickly because of high clearance, eventually to be below the adult value.

Serum thyroxine is very high, and it increases as more thyroid stimulating hormone is secreted. The values reach adult concentrations in about one year of life.

Most of the changes from infancy to puberty are gradual. Plasma protein increases to adult levels in 10 years, with serum IgG increasing more than α-2 globulins. Most serum enzymes attain their adult levels by puberty or earlier. The activity of alanine aminotransferase may continue to rise, especially in men, until middle age. Serum alkaline phosphatase decreases during childhood and rises again in the prepuberty growth spurt correlating with skeletal growth and sexual maturity. The activity decreases rapidly after puberty, especially in girls. Serum creatinine increases steadily to puberty, paralleling development of skeletal muscle. Serum uric acid concentration decreases until age 7 to 10 years and then increases to a peak at about age 16, but especially in boys.

The concentrations of most test markers remain quite constant between puberty and menopause in women, and between puberty and middle age ("male menopause") in men, accounting for the low intraindividual variation characteristic of this group, which is taken as reference.

During midlife, serum protein and albumin decrease slightly, as may calcium. Serum phosphorus in men decreases markedly after age 20; a decrease also occurs in women until menopause, when a sharp increase follows. Serum alkaline phosphatase increases also after menopause, so much so that elderly women may show activities higher than those of men. Serum uric acid peaks in men in their twenties, and in women during middle age. Urea increases in both genders in middle age. Age does not affect serum creatinine in men, but increases it in women. Serum cholesterol and triglyceride concentrations increase in both genders at a rate of about 2 mg/dL per year to a maximum between ages 50 and 60 years. The activities of most serum enzymes decrease relative to adolescence, reflecting lessened physical activity.

Very striking changes occur in many serum parameters after menopause in women. The following increases are observed: alkaline phosphatase, 25%; alanine aminotransferase, aspartate aminotransferase, phosphorus, cholesterol, and uric acid, 10 to 12%; phospholipids, 8%; apolipoprotein AI, 4%; albumin and glucose, 2%; sodium, 1.5%; and protein, 0.7%. Blood urea increases with age, as does urinary excretion of protein.

In elderly adults, the renal concentrating ability is reduced. The tubular maximum capacity for glucose is reduced. Creatinine clearance may decline as much as 50% between the thirties and the nineties. This is related to loss of lean body mass. The secretion of most hormones is reduced: triiodothyronine (T_3) decreases by up to 40% past 40 years of age, but total thyroxine is unchanged because its degradation is also reduced. This also occurs for cortisol. Other decreases include those of plasma parathyroid hormone, aldosterone (halved), testosterone in males in excess of 50 years, urinary 17-hydroxycorticosteroids, and 17-ketosteroid (halved).

Women show increased pituitary gonadotropins such as follicle stimulating hormone in blood and urine. Estrogen secretion in women decreases before menopause, and gonadotropins increase correspondingly. Serum concentrations decrease by 70% or more, with urinary excretion depressed comparably. Men show an age-related decline. Serum cholesterol increases up to age 60 years in women.

8.5.7 Long-Term Influences: Gender

Before puberty, there are few differences between Caucasian boys and girls relative to serum and urinary medical markers. After puberty, serum activities are greater in males than in females for alkaline phosphatase, the aminotransferases, creatine kinase, and aldolase. The total lactate is similar for both; but LDH-1 and LDH-3 are higher and LDH-2 is lower in women than in men, with no differences after the menopause. The older the woman is, the greater is the alkaline phosphatase activity. Albumin, calcium, magnesium, iron, hemoglobin, cholesterol, serum bilirubin, plasma amino acids, creatinine, urea, and uric acid are higher in men than in women; γ-globulin, and α-lipoprotein concentrations are less. Serum iron is low during a woman's fertile years, and women's plasma ferritin may be only one-third the concentration in males because of menstrual blood loss. The effect of age on serum constituents in men and women is provided in Table 8.2.

8.5.8 Long-Term Influences: Race

Differentiation of the effects of race from socioeconomic conditions is often a problem, especially in epidemiological studies. Diet is another factor that is also difficult to account for.

Total serum protein in Blacks is higher than in Whites because of a much higher γ-globulin; the α_1- and β-globulins are also increased in Blacks but not as much as γ-globulin. Albumin concentrations are less in Blacks than in Whites. Serum IgG is also 40% higher in Blacks, and serum IgA can be more than 20% greater in Black males relative to White men. Other markers that are higher in Blacks than in Whites include creatine kinase and lactate dehydrogenase (paralleling more skeletal muscle). Because Black children have greater skeletal development at puberty than Whites, they have greater activities of serum alkaline phosphatase.

Whites show less glucose tolerance than Blacks, Polynesians, American Indians, and Eskimos, relative to comparable age- and gender-matched Whites. After age 40 years, serum cholesterol and triglyceride levels are higher in whites relative to Blacks. This difference could be a dietary effect because plasma levels differ among the same racial group over the world. Blood hemoglobin can be more than 1 g/dL higher in Whites than in Blacks. The Maori of New Zealand have higher urate concentrations than Caucasians.

8.5.9 Long-Term Influences: Blood Groups and Disease

The links between blood groups and disease have been explored [23]. The ABO blood groups were proposed in 1900 by Landsteiner about the same time that Mendel's work on genetics was rediscovered. At about the same time, Ehrlich and Morgenroth also found the existence of blood group antigens and antibodies in goats. The ABO blood group system was the only one used between 1900 and 1927. Landsteiner and Levine in 1927–28 discovered the M, N, and P blood groups, and in 1940 Landsteiner and Wiener reported the rhesus or Rh blood groups.

Blood group frequencies are known now to be stable features of different populations. The ABO antigens of red blood cells are glycolipids soluble in alcohol but not in water. Very few data are available for the AB system because of its rare occurrence.

The first disease-blood group association proved was shown in 1941 between Rh antibodies and hemolytic disease of the newborn, with the next one in 1953 between group A and carcinoma of the stomach. The advent of gel electrophoresis in 1955, together with the older agglutination tests, enabled the field to grow markedly after that. A major extension of the latter technique is the voluminous research on histocompatibility antigens, especially in regard to transplants, disease and in immunology (Chapter 13).

Research on plasma protein and red-cell–enzyme polymorphisms now constitutes the major ongoing effort in the field. Pauling, in 1949, first found that people suffering from hereditary sickle-cell anemia have a hemoglobin (hemoglobin S) different from that in most adults (hemoglobin A). This incidence is more common in Black than in Caucasian women. Most infants with this abnormality usually die quickly. The incidence of hemoglobin S appears to be related also to resistance to malaria.

Some other examples of red blood cell markers under genetic control include: glucose-6-phosphate dehydrogenase deficiency (for hemolytic anemia caused by consumption of the broad bean *Vicia faba* and by administration of the antimalarial primaquine to some Black American soldiers during World War II; and for jaundice among newborn Chinese), which is controlled by three genes, two abnormal types being known in African populations; and acid phosphatase deficiency, for which three genes are known, plus a rare fourth one in the Khoisan of Africa.

Some examples of protein markers under genetic control are as follows: Weak and inactive variants of plasma-protease inhibitor predispose humans to emphysema and hepatic cirrhosis. There is an association between disorders of calcium metabolism and the concentration of proteins that carry vitamin D in the plasma. The relative proportions of plasma alkaline phosphatase from the liver, bone, and intestine are correlated with the ABO group and the secretor status of individuals. Activities of plasma cholinesterases (Section 22.2) and pseudocholinesterases are genetically controlled, and a small percentage (0.3 to 0.5 in Europeans) have abnormally low activities, a trait that is generally hereditary. This may influence susceptibility to organophosphate and carbamate pesticide poisoning (Chapter 22), and may decide the appropriateness of using succinyl choline as an anesthetic.

Various cancers are more associated with various blood groups than others.

There are more cancers for Types A and B than for Type O (there is an association for the latter with cancers of the skin and Hodgkin's disease). Carcinomas of the stomach (very marked), lip, salivary glands, large intestine, gallbladder, bile duct, pancreas, breast, female reproductive organs, nervous system, prostate, and bladder correlate best with Group A. Other infectious diseases associated with Group A are syphilis, meningitis, tapeworm anemia, and ascariasis. Group A individuals also show enhanced allergic dermatosis, rheumatic fever, rheumatic heart disease, diabetes mellitus, thrombosis, anemias, and tropical eosinophilia. Peptic ulcers are associated with Group O, as are bleeding, multiple sclerosis, autoimmune diseases, and influenza infection. Group B associations include cancers of the tonsils, oropharynx and hypopharnyx, gallbladder, pancreas, bile duct, nervous system, and bone; and incidence of syphilis, rheumatic heart disease, thrombosis, tropical eosinophilia, epilepsy, and dermatosis.

8.5.10 Long-Term Influences: Environmental Factors

Dietary and hence cultural influences, which may be related to area agricultural and societal traditions, are important. Thus, endemic goiter has been associated with a cabbage diet since 1928, and less so with turnips. This condition is associated with thioureas and cyanogens, but especially the former. The thioureas inhibit peroxidase action in the thyroid. This discovery led to the use of the phenylthiocarbamide tasting test.

Individuals living at high altitudes relative to sea level show marked increases in blood hemoglobin, red blood cell 2,3-diphosphoglycerate, turnover of red cell nucleoproteins, fasting basal concentration of growth hormone, and urinary excretion of urate.

Heat causes the plasma volume to expand by influx of interstitial fluid into the intravascular space and by reducing the glomerular filtration rate. The plasma protein may decrease up to 10%. Salt and water are lost by sweating, but usually there are no changes in plasma sodium and chloride concentrations. Plasma potassium may decrease by as much as 10% because of tissue uptake. In very extensive sweating, hemoconcentration occurs.

Geographical and geological factors may be important. Serum cholesterol, triglycerides, and magnesium increase in people living in areas with hard water compared to areas with soft water. Relatively water-soluble natural ore deposits, for example, of selenium and mercury, may cause relatively high concentrations in area waters, and in foods grown in area soils. Lead poisoning in acidic water supplies that are conveyed by lead-pipe redistribution systems is well known, as is lead poisoning in acidic natural waters.

8.5.11 Long-Term Cyclical Changes: Seasonal Influences

Generally seasonal changes do not affect medical marker values substantially relative to changes in posture and the use of a tourniquet, but seasonal changes in diet and physical activity may be important . The greater the temperature change between seasons is, the more the effects expected. Day-to-day variability is greater in summer than in winter, but this variability is only a little higher than analytical variability.

In Northern Hemisphere summers, the γ-globulin concentration may increase by as much as 50% relative to winters. Similar increases include: serum urate, 5 to 7%; serum triglycerides, 10%; serum cholesterol, up 50 mg/dL in men and 30 mg/dL in women; and activities of serum enzymes from skeletal muscle, with the increase for lactate dehydrogenase being as high as 20%. Changes for summer relative to winter for some serum components are: alanine aminotransferase, −5%; creatinine, +5%; lactate dehydrogenase, +2%; urea nitrogen, −3%; and uric acid, +4%. Some serum components have their maxima–minima in spring–fall rather than summer–winter, for example: aspartate aminotransferase, +12%; glucose, −2%; and triglycerides, +5%. Maxima–minima in summer–fall include: albumin, −1%; and urea nitrogen, −3%.

Calcium has its maximum in fall and its minimum in winter (−1%). Calcium metabolism is affected by how much sunlight a person is exposed to. Dehydrocholecalciferol in the skin is changed by the ultraviolet component to cholecalciferol, which is further metabolized in liver and kidney to 1,25-dihydroxycholecalciferol. This increases serum and urinary calcium. Exposure to the sun for one weekend during summer may cause enough photodegradation of bilirubin to reduce its serum concentration by 20%.

Serum concentrations of thyroid hormones are not affected by the seasons, but the urinary excretion of triiodothyronine is increased in summer, as is that of metabolites of adrenal hormones.

8.5.12 Long-Term Cyclical Changes: Menstrual Cycle Variations

Plasma corticosterone is 50% higher in the luteal phase than in the follicular phase. Plasma androstenedione and plasma aldosterone increase in the reverse manner. On a preovulatory day, the aldosterone and the renin activity may be twice the concentration in the early follicular cycle, especially for women who retain fluid. Plasma cholesterol is least at ovulation and rises immediately prior to menstruation, after which it remains high for one week. Ovulation marks the lowest concentrations for serum total protein, serum albumin, serum calcium, plasma ascorbate, and serum creatine kinase. Minima at menstruation occur for plasma fibrinogen, serum phosphate, plasma iron, and plasma magnesium. Maxima at menstruation are exhibited for serum creatinine and urate, both being lowest toward the end of the intermenstrual period. Plasma sodium and chloride increase to the onset of menstruation but fall by as much as 2 mM during postmenstrual diuresis.

Urinary excretion of 17-hydroxycorticosteroids peaks at midcycle. Urinary catecholamines increase at midcycle and stay high thereafter through the luteal phase.

Further Reading

Tietz, N. W. 1986. *Textbook of Clinical Chemistry*, W. B. Saunders, Philadelphia, PA, pp. 356–409, and 478–518.

9

Significance of Selected Medical Monitoring and Medical/Health Surveillance Markers

9.0 BLOOD SERUM MARKERS

Many books treat the significance of medical markers from the perspective of physicians [24–28], nurses [29], and dentists [30]. It is too great a task here to cover all these perspectives and all markers; instead we focus on the interpretative aspects of the medical markers shown in Table 8.1, as well as some nonspecific markers used in health surveillance. Appendix A gives the reference ranges for most medical markers. Appendix B contains the therapeutic ranges (Section 8.5.1) for some common drugs. Textbooks contain different ranges; so due allowance for this fact must be made in evaluating the significance of medical monitoring tests.

9.0.1 Albumin

For the adult the reference range is 3.3 to 5.0 g/dL blood; for the newborn, 2.5–5.0; at three months, 3.0–4.2; at one year, 2.7–5.0; and at 15 years, 3.2–5.0.

Albumin, a protein, is formed in the liver. It helps maintain normal distribution of water in the body; it also transports ions, pigments, bilirubin, hormones, fatty acids, enzymes, certain drugs, and certain xenobiotics. Albumin can be taken into cells and catabolized and so can act as an amino acid reserve.

Albumin has a molecular weight of 68,000 and has 575 amino acid residues and no carbohydrate residues. Its circulation half-time is about 21 days, decreasing to 7 days during increased catabolism.

Albumin is increased above the reference range in dehydration together with total protein, but the albumin/globulin ratio (usually greater than 1) is unaffected. Albumin is increased by the administration of bromsulfalein.

Albumin is decreased below the reference range during inadequate food intake (e.g., malnutrition, inadequate iron intake); decreased absorption (e.g., malabsorption syndromes); increased need (e.g., hyperthyroidism; pregnancy); impaired synthesis (liver diseases, chronic infections including those of the skin, congenital analbuminemia); increased breakdown (e.g., cancers, infection, trauma, shock); increased loss (e.g., edema, ascites, burns, diarrhea; hemorrhage, kidney damage, skin loss, protein-losing enteropathy); decreased transport function (e.g., hypocalcemia); excessive administration of IV glucose; and administration of medications (e.g., Cytoxan, Dextran, Enovid, Estinyl, Heroin, Imuran, Niacin, Premarin, Roniacol, Tylenol).

9.0.2 Globulin

For the adult the reference range is 2.0–4.2 g/dL blood; for the newborn, 1.2–4.0; at three months, 1.0–3.3; at one year, 2.0–3.8; at 15 years, 2.0–4.0.

Between 3.9 and 4.2 g/dL, 45% of adults had diagnoses not associated with this elevation; 9.1% had myeloma, sarcoidosis, or collagen disease; 17% had carcinoma; and 21% had acute and chronic inflammation. Between 4.21 and 4.99 g/dL, 28% had diagnoses not associated with elevation; 8.9% had myeloma, sarcoidosis, or collagen disease, with the most common diagnoses being liver disease (20%), metastatic carcinoma (20.2%), and acute and chronic inflammation (22%). Above 5.0 g/dL, 8.4% had diagnoses not associated with the elevation; 43% had myeloma, sarcoidosis, or collagen disease; 18% had liver disease; and 20% had acute and chronic inflammation. The blood sample must have minimum hemolysis. The lipoproteins (Section 2.8) in globulin keep the lipids in solution.

Globulins are divided into α-1, α-2, β, and γ globulins, so named from their electrophoretic band patterns. They are produced mostly by the liver. Dehydration, fever, and malnutrition increase all globulins.

α_1-globulin (reference range 2.4–5.3% of adult total protein) is elevated in pregnancy, malignancies, acute infections, renal disease, and tissue necrosis, but decreased in genetic deficiency of α_1-antitrypsin, liver necrosis, and nephrosis. The major components are: α_1-lipoprotein, which transports lipids, fat-soluble vitamins, and hormones; α_1-antitrypsin (reference range 159–400 mg/dL), which inhibits trypsin and chymotrypsin and is elevated by strenuous exercise, stress, persistent inflammatory disorders, and oral contraceptives, and decreased by genetic factors, early onset of emphysema in nonsmokers, and unexplained cirrhosis and jaundice, especially in the under-20 age group; α-acid glycoprotein (inactivates progesterone and is an acute phase reactant); and thyroxine-binding globulin, to bind thyroxine.

α_2-globulin (reference range 6.6–13.5% of adult total protein but elevated at birth) is increased in acute infections, trauma, burns, advanced malignancies, rheumatic fever, rheumatoid arthritis, acute myocardial infarction, tissue necrosis, collagen diseases, liver disease, sarcoidosis, Cushing's syndrome, and nephrotic syndrome, but decreased by hemolytic anemia and severe liver disease. The major components are: α_2-macroglobulin, which inhibits plasmin and trypsin, has growth factor activity, and binds insulin; α_2-lipoprotein, which transports lipids, especially triglycerides; haptoglobin (referencc range 0–10 mg/dL in the newborn and 30–160 mg/dL in adults), which binds hemoglobin and prevents iron loss, is elevated by some steroids, diffuse inflammatory processes, and tissue destruction, and is decreased by excessive red cell hemolysis, chronic liver disease, and congenital ahaptoglobinemia; ceruloplasmin (reference range 2–13 mg/dL in the newborn and 23–50 mg/dL in the adult), which transports copper and has oxidase activity, is increased by acute infections, hepatitis, Hodgkin's disease, hyperthyroidism, pregnancy, cancer of the bone, lung, and stomach, myocardial infarction, rheumatoid arthritis, and drugs such as oral contraceptives, estrogens, methadone, and dilantin, but is decreased in Wilson's disease (because of hepatolenticular degeneration), hyperalimentation, malabsorption, Menkes' kinky hair syndrome, nephrosis, and severe liver disease and in early infancy; cholinesterase, which hydrolyzes acetycholine; prothrombin, which is essential to blood coagulation; and α-HS glycoprotein, zinc–α_2 glycoprotein, and G-globulin (multiple molecular forms), which are of unknown function.

β-globulins (reference range 8.5–14.5% of adult total protein) are elevated by hypothyroidism, biliary cirrhosis, nephrotic syndrome, diabetes mellitus, Cushing's disease, viral hepatitis, lipid disorders, myeloma, polyarteritis nodosa, and malignant hypertension, but decreased by hypocholesterolemia and severe hepatic necrosis. The major components are: β-lipoprotein, which transports lipids, lipid-soluble vitamins, and hormones; transferrin (reference range 60–170 mg/dL in the newborn and 250–450 mg/dL in adults, with 65% saturation in the newborn and 20–55% saturation in adults), which transports iron and defends against certain infectious agents, is increased with low serum iron by iron-deficiency anemia, hemachromatosis (serum iron 200–300 μg/dL), lead poisoning, multiple blood transfusions, severe hemolytic disorders, pregnancy, menstruation, and oral contraceptives, but is decreased with increased serum iron by diminished protein synthesis, low iron absorption, iron malnutrition, malabsorption, infection states, and nephrotic syndrome; hemopexin, which binds heme; plasminogen, which lyses fibrin in blood clots; complement, which has phagocytic activity; β_2-glycoprotein of unknown function; and fibrinogen, which is essential to blood coagulation.

γ-globulins (reference range 10.7–21% of adult total protein) are elevated by connective tissue diseases such as systemic lupus erythematosus and rheumatoid arthritis, but decreased by nephrotic syndrome, lymphocytic leukemia, lymphosarcoma, and some drugs such as BCG vaccine and the anticancer drug methotrexate. The major components are: immunoglobulin G (IgG), of four subcomponents, which defend against attacks of viruses, bacterial toxins, Rh antibodies, nuclear antibodies, anti-insulin, and ragweed pollen antibodies; immunoglobulin A (IgA), which includes antibodies such as antibacterial agglutinins and antinuclear and anti-insulin antibodies, and constitutes the predominant antibody in body fluids and secretions; immunoglobulin M (IgM), which includes antibodies such as the blood group ABO isoagglutinins, cold agglutinins, antibodies to gram-negative bacteria, Wasserman antibody, antithyroglobulin, and others; immunoglobulin E (IgE), which sensitizes mast cells through binding to their surface so that combination with antigen triggers mediator release independent of the alternative or classical complement pathways (Sections 13.0 and 13.1); and immunoglobulin D (IgD), of unknown function.

The reference ranges for adult antibodies are: IgG, 565–1765 mg/dL; IgA, 90–450 mg/dL; and IgM, 60–280 mg/dL; there are very small amounts of IgD and IgE. All of these values are age-dependent, and personal values in a year may fluctuate by 20%. Synthesis begins at 3 months of age with adult levels attained by 3 years. The immunoglobulins are produced by plasma B-lymphocytes, which are 10 to 20% of circulating lymphocytes. The major analytical techniques used are serum protein electrophoresis, radial immunodiffusion, radioimmunoassay, and immunoelectrophoresis.

For known clinical implications, decreased α_1-antitrypsin is associated with juvenile pulmonary emphysema; increased α_1-acid glycoprotein occurs with chronic inflammatory, degenerative, and some malignant diseases; increased α_2-globulins are associated with altered vascular permeability (e.g., nephrotic syndrome and acute inflammatory diseases), with most other increases involving haptoglobin, α_2-macroglobulin, or both.

Changes in β-globulins are related generally to disorders in γ-globulin function. Increases of γ-globulins are associated with antibodies in which one or more of the immunoglobulins are elevated, and decreases in γ-globulins occur in genetic deficiencies of immunoglobulin production or immunosuppression.

9.0.3 Total Protein

Total protein is the sum of the albumin and the globulin components of serum. The reference range in adults is 6.6–7.9 g/dL. In newborns it is 4.0–7.1; at 3 months, 4.7–7.4; at one year, 5.0–7.5; and at 15 years, 6.5–8.6. The albumin/globulin ratio in adults is 1.5–2.5. Albumin in adults is 52 to 68% of total protein. High serum lipid levels may interfere with the analysis.

Increased total proteins occur in kala-azar, dehydration, macroglobulinemias, and sarcoidosis, and by administration of some drugs such as ACTH, corticosteroids, BSP, clofibrate, dextran, growth hormone, heparin, insulin, X-ray contrast media, thyroid preparations, and tolbutamide, as well as by prolonged stasis with a tourniquet before sampling.

Decreases are caused by renal disease, ulcerative colitis, water intoxication, intravenous infusion, cirrhosis, severe burns, scleroderma, malnutrition, Hodgkin's disease, hepatitis, hemorrhage, protein loss in nephrosis, protein-losing enteropathy, burns, and protein synthesis reduction, as in liver diseases, malabsorption, and protein–calorie malnutrition, and by some drugs containing ammonium ion, dextran, oral contraceptives, salicylates, and pyrazinamide.

Conditions that increase globulins more than albumin include chronic infections, autoimmune diseases, sarcoidosis, hepatic cirrhosis, and paraproteinemia including myeloma.

Muscle mass provides most of the serum protein during food deprivation. Plasma proteins are catabolized by body tissues, serve a buffering function, and provide a transport system for many xenobiotics and drugs. Both albumin and globulins help maintain osmotic homeostasis. Globulins are much larger than albumins.

9.0.4 Bilirubin (Total and Direct)

The one-month-after-birth-to-adult reference range is: total, 0.18–1.2 mg/dL; indirect, 0.3–1.1; direct, 0.1–0.4. Total bilirubin in newborn is 2.0–6.0, at 48 h it is 6.0–7.0, and at 5 days it is 4.0–12 mg/dL.

Bilirubin is a degradation product of the pigmented heme part of hemoglobin (Section 2.11.5). Old, damaged, and atypical red blood cells are removed from circulation mostly by the spleen (and also to a degree by the liver and the bone marrow). The heme component is oxidized to bilirubin by the reticuloendothelial cells and released into the blood, where bilirubin adsorbs physically to albumin ("indirect" bilirubin) to be transported to the liver; there glucuronidation occurs, making it more water-soluble. The glucuronide is eliminated into the liver ducts and thence into the bile. Only small amounts of the glucuronide occur in blood ("direct" bilirubin), the bulk being excreted into the intestines, where it is converted into urobilinogens, oxidized to stercobilinogen, and excreted in the feces. A small amount in the intestines is reabsorbed because of microbial action, and it undergoes enterohepatic circulation, with some being excreted in the urine as urobilinogen and its oxidation product urobilin.

Bilirubin and its degradation products are pigments that provide the yellowish tinge of serum, the yellow-green color of bile, the brown hue of feces, and the yellowish aspect of urine. Very high serum bilirubin is correlated to jaundice, particularly in the newborn, when liver functions still may not be optimal, or in adults with hepatitis and cirrhosis. Obstruction of the bile duct produces pale stools and dark urine. Disorders in which the liver is unable to cope with bilirubin conjugation demands, through either excessive hemolysis, liver damage, or impaired uptake, manifest themselves in dramatic elevations in serum bilirubin.

Increases in indirect bilirubin are caused by: hemolysis (hemoglobinopathies, spherocytosis, glucose-6-phosphate dehydrogenase deficiency, autoimmunity, transfusion antibody/antigen reaction); red cell degradation (hemorrhage into soft tissue or body cavities, inefficient manufacture of red cells, pernicious anemia, sickle-cell anemia); defective liver cell uptake or conjugation (in viral hepatitis, in hereditary enzyme deficiencies such as Crigler-Najjar syndrome and Gilbert's disease, in liver immaturity, and in newborns); trauma in the presence of a large hematoma; severe exercise; severe congestive heart failure; high levels of 3-α-20-β-pregnandiol in mother's milk that inhibit uridine diphosphate glucuronyl transferase (Section 2.4); and many drugs (allopurinol, antibiotics, antibodies, antineoplastic drugs, barbiturates, caffeine, gallbladder dyes, indomethacin, propylthiouracil, steroids, sulfonamides, sulfonylureas, theophylline), and any hepatotoxic xenobiotics (such as chlorinated hydrocarbons) and drugs. Excessive indirect bilirubin may deposit in the brain to cause kernicterus, a complication of newborn hyperbilirubinemia and newborn jaundice (starts to manifest at 2–4 mg indirect bilirubin/dL). Fasting lowers indirect bilirubin concentrations except in people who suffer from Gilbert's syndrome.

Increases in direct bilirubin are caused by: intrahepatic disruption, often associated with increased alkaline phosphatase activity, viral hepatitis, alcoholic hepatitis, cytotoxic drugs such as antineoplastic drugs, hycanthone (schistosomiasis treatment), cirrhosis, toxins from poisonous fungi such as *Amanita phalloides*, paracetamol overdose, α_1-antitrypsin deficiency, and hypersensitivity (Section 13.3) to drugs such as chlorpromazine, halothane, isoniazid, methyldopa, and rifampicin, as well as agents that enhance elimination from the liver into plasma such as androgenic steroids and organic arsenicals; bile duct disease (biliary cirrhosis, cholangitis, biliary atresia); and extrahepatic bile duct obstruction (gallstones; carcinoma of the gallbladder, bile ducts, or pancreas head; bile duct stricture, from inflammation or from surgical incompetence). Impaired excretion of direct bilirubin will cause increased serum direct bilirubin.

The following clinical findings are associated with direct bilirubin content relative to the total: <20%, hemolysis or genetic factors; 20 to 40%, hepatic jaundice rather than posthepatic jaundice; 40 to 60%, either hepatic or posthepatic jaundice; and >50%, posthepatic jaundice rather than hepatic jaundice. Increased direct bilirubin has been associated with normal total bilirubin in up to one-third of patients with known liver disease. Nonpathological states also induce elevation in direct bilirubin: pregnancy in the third trimester, hormones such as contraceptives and methyl testosterone, Hodgkin's disease, total parenteral nutrition, and benign postoperative cholestasis.

Whenever impaired liver function is combined with bile duct obstruction as in cirrhosis, hepatitis, lymphoma, AIDS, liver metastasis, and hepatic cancer, both direct and indirect levels are elevated, usually with the direct bilirubin concentration more elevated relative to the personal baseline.

Total bilirubin >40 mg/dL indicates hepatocellular rather than extrahepatic obstruction. If the liver is healthy but excessive hemolysis occurs, fecal and urinary urobilinogen increase with only a moderate increase in serum bilirubin (indirect concentrations rarely higher than 5 mg/dL). Prolonged exposure to sunlight or ultraviolet light in a tanning salon reduces serum bilirubin, as does prolonged treatment with phenobarbitone, because of an increase in ligandin (Section 5. 1. 2) which binds bilirubin in the liver. A high-fat meal may decrease bilirubin. Ingestion of contrast media 24 h before measurement may interfere with the analysis. Foods containing yellow, absorbable pigments—yellow, orange, blue, and green items such as carrots, yams, oranges, lemons, blackberries, blueberries, and asparagus—will increase the yellow color of serum, thus confounding colorimetric analysis.

Samples in red-top Vacutainers should be stored immediately in a refrigerator in the dark out of fluorescent light or sunlight. The patient should fast for at least 4 h before sampling and not take any hepatotoxic drugs for 24 h. Routinely only total bilirubin is measured first.

"Early labeled" bilirubin is a test used to test the life span of red blood cells, which is typically 90 to 120 days. ^{15}N-Glycine administration produces ^{15}N-bilirubin at this time when the red cell is lysed. This may occur at 2 weeks for pernicious anemia and other megaloblastic anemias, erythroporphyria, thalassemia, sideroblastic anemia, lead poisoning, and shunt bilirubin.

The use of serum bilirubin and serum alkaline phosphatase activity to diagnose liver disease is common. Progressive increases in atypical readings indicate worsening; progressive return toward reference values implies recovery. Relatively constant but atypical bilirubin with increasing atypical alkaline phosphatase implies uncomplicated extrahepatic biliary obstruction, cholangitis, or cholangiolitis. Atypical bilirubin and moderately atypical or typical alkaline phosphatase imply diffuse hepatocellular damage or hemolytic conditions. Very high alkaline phosphatase with typical or moderately atypical bilirubin implies the likelihood of portal cirrhosis, liver abscess, secondary carcinomatosis of the liver, and sarcoidosis involving the liver. Typical bilirubin but very elevated alkaline phosphatase has been caused by obstruction of one major bile duct with an intact common bile duct. High relatively constant alkaline phosphatase with decreasing but atypical bilirubin may be caused by increasing liver damage superimposed on bile duct obstruction.

Hepatic scintigraphy with ^{99}Tc (technecium)–sulfur colloid allows detection of many hepatocellular diseases and cirrhosis by showing liver and spleen size and the degree of bone uptake of the nuclide. Little information is given on the nature of a lesion causing an obstruction. Ultrasonography can be used to detect liver disease by demonstrating hepatomegaly, atypical hepatic echoes, gallstones in the gallbladder, dilated intrahepatic radicles, bile duct obstruction (duct >6 mm), and sometimes ascites. Computed tomography imaging is very useful for detecting hypodensity in fatty infiltration or hyperdensity of the liver in hemochromatosis (iron overload) and primary lesions of the alimentary tract, spleen, and pancreas, but does not detect most diffuse hepatocellular, splenic, or pancreatic diseases. An abrupt cutoff to a duct implies malignancy, whereas a gradually tapering effect often represents a benign cause of obstruction. Direct cholangiography by instillation of contrast medium into the biliary tree while the patient is erect allows the clear-cut presence or absence of obstruction and the level of any obstruction (stone or tumor) to be determined.

Biliary elimination of xenobiotics in animals is regulated through molecular weight [31]; for example, above 325 for the rat, 400 in the guinea pig, and 475 in the rabbit. Rats probably have the lowest molecular weight threshold because of absence of a gallbladder and a high basal metabolic rate. Humans have a threshold nearer that of the rabbit. Organic cations above a molecular weight of 200 are excreted in the bile in all species. Most drugs excreted in the bile require a strongly polar group, as well as the molecular weight requirement.

Many xenobiotics therefore are eliminated as metabolites or Phase II conjugates, especially glucuronides and glutathione conjugates. Some compounds found in the bile of humans include phenol red indicator dye and drugs such as ampicillin, cephaloridine, clindamycin, diazepam, digitoxin, digoxin, erythromycin, meperidine, methotrexate, nortripyline, novobiocin, rifamide, rifamycin, sulfamethoxazole, tetracycline, and thiamphenicol.

There are species and gender differences in bile elimination in animals. The rabbit eliminates in its bile such xenobiotics as arsenic, lead, and indomethacin; the rat eliminates 2-acetylaminofluorene, 3,4-benzpyrene, butylated hydroxytoluene, *N*,*N*-dimethylaminoazobenzene, 7,12-dimethylbenzanthracene, 3-methylcholanthrene, PCBs, cadmium, mercury, and all the steroid hormones. Phenobarbital stimulates biliary elimination of xenobiotic metabolites in male (but not female) rats, in addition to enhanced bile flow, increased liver size, and liver content of ligandin, which binds bilirubin and many xenobiotic metabolites. Xenobiotics might be expected to perturb biliary and body functions. For example, 3,4-benzpyrene stimulated thyroxin glucuronide elimination in the rat bile, and pretreatment with this xenobiotic also enhanced biliary elimination in rats of the metabolites of 3,4-benzpyrene, 3-methylcholanthrene, 7,12-dimethylbenzanthracene, 2-acetylaminofluorene, or *N*,*N*-dimethylaminoazobenzene [31]. Inhibitors of mixed function oxidase enzymes such as piperonyl butoxide, SKF 525A, metyrapone, and emetine inhibit biliary excretion of the metabolites of these metabolites. The insecticide Mirex impairs biliary excretion of PCBs, imipramine, and sulfobromophthalein in the isolated perfused liver of the rat. The antibiotic novobiocin, which interferes with bilirubin glucuronidation, blocks rat biliary excretion of 3-trifluoromethyl-4-nitrophenol and warfarin. 2,3,7,8-Tetrachlorodibenzo-*p*-dioxin, although a potent inducer of rat mixed function oxidases, suppresses biliary excretion of indocyanine green, a dye that is not metabolized. Whether these events occur in humans has not been shown.

9.0.5 Alkaline Phosphatase and Gamma Glutamyl Transpeptidase

The adult alkaline phosphatase activity reference range is 20–90 U/L, Kind and King units; that of the newborn, 50–65; and that of the child, 20–150. There are differences between analytical procedures. For adults, the Bessey-Lowry method gives 0.8–2.3 U/mL; the Bodansky method, 1.5–4.5 U/dL; and the King-Armstrong method, 4–13 U/dL. For children the respective method ranges in the appropriate units are: 3.4–9.0, 5–14, and 15–30. Another range for adults is 80–280 IU/L, using international units of enzyme activity.

Phosphatases that cleave phosphate functional groups from compounds with a single phosphate group at a pH optimum of 9.0 are collectively called alkaline phosphatase. Liver, bone, proximal tubules of the kidney, lactating mammary glands, granulocytes of circulating blood, the placenta, and the intestine are the major sources. Cancers produce a distinctive form called the Regan enzyme. The bone enzyme (much from the synovial fluid) usually predominates; so serum levels increase during bone growth, increased bone destruction, or both. The liver component is thought to derive from the epithelium of the intrahepatic biliary ducts, and is maximal during obstruction and/or inflammation of the hepatobiliary tract. Intestinal contributions occur during digestion of high-fat meals.

Alkaline phosphatase isoenzymes from the bone, liver, and intestine have molecular weights of 92,400 to 95,800 atomic mass units, whereas those from the placenta have molecular weights of about 74,000. Hepatic and proliferating blood vessel isooenzymes (AP-1, α_2) are less (25%) heat-resistant at 56°C than are bone isoenzymes (AP-2, β_1), with the isoenzymes identified through electrophoresis or via total activity after heat treatment. The intestinal isoenzyme (AP-3, β_2), usually <20% of total alkaline phosphatase, is present in small quantities in blood group O and B individuals, and is increased in cirrhosis. Placental isoenzymes (five) are more stable to heat than to urea denaturation, and are increased in some cancer patients and during pregnancy. Smokers show heat-stable alkaline phosphatase activity levels ten times higher than the upper limit for nonsmokers.

A major isoenzyme of alkaline phosphatase is 5′-nucleotidase from hepatobiliary tissues with reference range 0–1.6 U/L or 0.3–3.2 Bodansky units (elevation indicates biliary cirrhosis, liver cancer, bile tract cancer, biliary obstruction, or choledocholithiasis). Normal levels in the presence of elevated total alkaline phosphatase indicate bone disease. 5′-Nucleotidase is not affected during pregnancy and during the postpartum period; so hepatobiliary disease may be diagnosed in these periods.

Another major isoenzyme of alkaline phosphatase is leucine aminopeptidase from many tissues, with the adult reference range 80–200 U/mL for males and 75–185 U/mL for females, with most from the hepatobiliary tissues, pancreas, and small intestine. Elevations occur during biliary obstruction, pancreatic disease, advanced pregnancy, and therapy with drugs such as estrogen and progesterone. Reference levels in the presence of elevated total alkaline phosphatase indicate bone disease.

Gamma glutamyl transpeptidase or GGTP (Section 2.11.4) is another major enzyme of alkaline phosphatase, and is from hepatobiliary tissues (predominant), renal tubules, and pancreatic epithelia, with minor amounts from the prostate gland, brain, and heart. Adult reference values are 6–37 U/L in men and in females over age 45, and 5.27 U/L for women under age 45. Marked increases occur during hepatobiliary disease, hepatitis, and cancers. Moderate increases are caused by liver cirrhosis, obesity, pancreatic or renal damage or neoplasms, congestive heart failure, acute myocardial infarction (after 4–10 days), type IV hyperlipoproteinemia, diabetes mellitus with hypertension, and epilepsy. Transient increases have been measured after ingestion of alcohol (in 60–80% of alcoholics detected with significant increases after >6 drinks, with reference range levels attained on abstinence after 2–6 weeks), barbiturates, and phenytoin, with lower levels caused by late pregnancy and oral contraceptives. Reference levels in the presence of elevated total alkaline phosphatase indicate bone disease.

The major clinical conditions marked by total alkaline phosphatase are: biliary obstruction, hepatobiliary disease, bone disease, and cancer; obstructive biliary disorders, with differentiation from hepatocellular disease; the assessment of the effect of renal diseases on bone metabolism; and signs of growth retardation in children.

Total serum alkaline phosphatase is elevated five times greater than the reference range by advanced pregnancy (reverting to reference range by the 20th day postpartum), biliary obstruction, biliary artresia, cirrhosis, hyperparathyroidism, infusion of albumin of placental origin, osteitis deformans, osteogenic sarcoma, and Paget's disease. Three- to fivefold elevations are caused by extrahepatic duct obstruction, granulomatous or infiltrative liver diseases, infectious mononucleosis, leukemia, metabolic bone diseases such as rickets and osteomalachia, and metastatic tumors in bone. Up to three times elevation can be produced in viral hepatitis, chronic active hepatitis, alcoholic cirrhosis, healing fractures, early pregnancy, and growing children, as well as by large doses of Vitamin D and congestive heart failure. Other agents causing increases include: ergosterol, chlorpropamide, and anticonvulsant drug administration; and from liver nodules caused by tumors, abscesses, cysts, parasites, amylosis, tuberculosis, sarcoidosis, or leukemia. Normal total alkaline phosphatase is seen in alcoholism with elevated SGPT.

Reduced levels of total alkaline phosphatase occur in achondroplasia, celiac disease, cretinism, excess Vitamin D ingestion, hypophosphatasia, hypothyroidism, kwashiorkor, malnutrition, milk-alkali (Burnett's) syndrome, pernicious anemia (one-third of patients), scurvy, placental insufficiency, and osteoblast damage caused, for example, by bone destruction and deposition of radioactive materials, clofibrate, or propanolol therapy. Because collection of blood using anticoagulants such as EDTA, fluoride, and oxalate decreases serum alkaline phosphatase, heparin is the recommended anticoagulant.

9.0.6 Glutamic-Oxaloacetic Transaminase (SGOT) or Aspartate Aminotransferase (AST)

Adult and >7 years reference range is 8–46 U/L in men and 7–34 in women. Newborn reference range is 16–72; 6 months, 20–43; one year, 16–35; and 5 years, 19–28.

SGOT now has been officially renamed aspartate aminotransferase (AST).

The enzyme catalyzes the reversible transfer of an amino group between aspartic acid and α-ketoglutaric acid to form glutamic acid, a process occurring in the matrix of mitochondria (Section 2.11.4); thus AST is mostly in the white blood cells. Therefore, hemolysis must be prevented in blood samples. AST is found mostly in tissues of high metabolic activity such as the liver and the heart, but skeletal muscle, kidneys, pancreas, lungs, spleen, and brain also contribute. The circulating half-time is 17 ± 5 h. The personal baseline level varies <10 U/day in the same person if healthy.

The serum enzyme activity rises whenever there is cellular damage to the tissues where AST is found. Damaged heart muscle produces a serum increase 6 to 8 h after the damage, with peak values (4–10 times baseline) at 24 to 48 h and with reversion to baseline values at 72 to 96 h. This peak occurs after that in the serum for creatine phosphokinase (rise and fall within 48 h), and before that of lactate dehydrogenase, the latter rising 12 h or more after the damage to remain elevated for a week or more. This behavior of the three enzymes together is a good proof for the occurrence of myocardial infarction.

Many conditions elevate AST activity. For activities greater than five times baseline, the following might be suspected: acute hepatocellular damage, acute pancreatitis, cardiac massage, cardiac surgery, crushing injuries, infectious mononucleosis, irradiation treatments, myocardial infarction, severe burns, and shock. Activities three to five times baseline suggest: biliary tract obstruction, cardiac arrhythmias, chronic hepatitis, congestive heart failure, dermatomyositis, heart angina, liver tumors, and muscular dystrophy. Activities up to three times baseline are caused by: asthma, cirrhosis, fatty liver, cerebrovascular accident, delirium tremens, gout, hemolytic anemia, hornet stings hypothermia, pericarditis, pregnancy concurrent with abnormal metabolism of pyridoxine, pulmonary infarction, and salicylates. Strenuous activity causes a peak enzyme activity 24 h later.

In infective hepatitis, the serum AST activity peaks at greatest patient malaise and liver tenderness. The rise parallels that in serum iron (compare with biliary obstruction). Liver damage stimulates enzyme activity when caused by many industrial factors (chlorinated and brominated chemicals, carbon monoxide poisoning, heat stroke, and inhaled calcium dust) and drugs [clofibrate, desferrioxamine, erythromycin, heparin, opiates, polycillin, prostaphlin, rifampicin and isoniazid therapy especially for slow acetylators (Section 5.1.4), and salicylate].

Decreased levels occur in beriberi, severe liver disease, chronic hemodialysis, and uremia (parallel to blood urea nitrogen level), and in uncontrolled diabetes mellitus with acidosis.

9.0.7 Glutamic-Pyruvic Transaminase (SGPT) or Alanine Aminotransferase (ALT)

The adult reference range varies among methods and laboratories: 10–30 IU/mL; 1–36 U/mL; 5–35 Sigma Frankel U/mL; 5–25 mU/mL—Wroblewski; 8-50 mU/mL at 30°C—Karmen; and 4–36 U/L at 37°C—SI units.

SGPT now has been officially named alanine aminotransferase (ALT). ALT catalyzes the reversible transfer of an amino group between alanine and α-ketoglutarate to form glutamate (Section 2.11.1). Hepatocytes are the predominant cell type containing ALT, although heart, kidneys, pancreas, and skeletal muscle have moderate amounts also. The circulating half-time is 47 ± 10 h. Because the use of heparin anticoagulant gives 70% of the true value, EDTA or other anticoagulants must be used in taking blood samples.

Elevated levels (5–20 times baseline) are considered a sensitive marker of liver damage, including that of alcohol. The marker is used to differentiate between hemolytic jaundice and jaundice due to liver disease. Muscular dystrophy, severe muscle trauma, myocardial infarction, congestive heart failure, pancreatitis, infectious mononucleosis, and renal failure also cause moderate elevations. A sudden drop after extreme elevation (as observed for severe viral or toxic hepatitis) is an ominous sign, caused by so much damage that no additional source of ALT remains. Gradually declining levels after elevation imply recovery. Salicylates can cause increased (plasma salicylate >25 mg/dL) or decreased levels. High dietary sucrose, clofibrate therapy, and carnitine deficiency increase activities.

Very low levels are found in the newborn, with a peak in the infant about 5 days after birth. Much of the decrease is caused by pyridoxal-5′-phosphate depletion. In adults, ALT generally parallels AST. The AST/ALT ratio is <2 in alcoholic liver damage and >2 in nonalcoholic liver damage. The increase in AST/ALT is less marked for myocardial necrosis, chronic hepatitis, cirrhosis, hepatic metastases, and liver congestion, but is more marked in liver necrosis and acute hepatitis.

9.0.8 Lactate Dehydrogenase (LDH)

The adult reference range is: 80–120 U—Wacker; 71–207 IU/L; and 150–450 U—Wroblewski. The reference range percentages for the isoenzymes are: LDH-1, 29–37; LDH-2, 42–48; LDH-3, 16–20; LDH-4, 2–4; and LDH-5, 0.5–1.5.

LDH catalyzes the reversible intracellular conversion of lactic acid to pyruvate in gluconeogenesis (Section 2.4). Many tissues contain LDH, a tetramer. High elevations (10–40 times baseline) are observed for megablastic anemias, metastatic cancers, shock, anoxia, hypoxia, and renal infarction. Moderate increases (4–10 times baseline) are caused by myocardial (4–10 times baseline) and pulmonary infarctions, hemolytic conditions, leukemias, sprue, infectious mononucleosis, and muscular dystrophy. Mild elevations (2–4 times baseline) result for liver diseases, nephrotic syndrome, hypothyroidism, and cholangitis. Slight increases (less than twice baseline) occur in delirium tremens, hepatitis, obstructive jaundice, and cirrhosis.

Numerous drugs elevate LDH (e.g., anabolic steroids, anesthetics, aspirin, alcohol, fluorides, narcotics, clofibrate, mithramicin, and procainamide). Childbirth, skin diseases, burns, trauma, muscle atrophy, pneumonia, hornet stings, and laboratory hemolysis of red blood cells also increase the activity. The total LDH activity is unchanged by some cases of pulmonary infarction, pericarditis, chronic lymphatic leukemia, and aleukemic leukemia. Activities decrease upon X-ray irradiation.

Analysis for the five LDH isoenzymes has proved very useful for diagnosis of specific organ damage. Prevalent forms are: in the heart and red blood cells, mostly LDH-1,2; in the brain, LDH-1,2,3; in the kidneys, LDH-3,4; and in the liver and skeletal muscle, LDH-4,5. LDH-3 is also contained in the thyroid, adrenal, thymus, pancreas, spleen, lungs, lymph nodes, and white blood cells. The ileum secretes LDH-5. The lung contains LDH-3,4,5. These leak into the plasma on damage. The technique has been used to distinguish myocardial infarction (high LDH-1 with LDH-1/LDH-2 $>$ 1.0 in over 80% of myocardial infarcts within 48 h, although acute renal infarction, pernicious anemia, and hemolysis also produce the same change) from lung or liver problems, to diagnose myocardial infarction during the postoperative period or during severe shock, and to show hemolysis during bone marrow hypoplasia. Typically, LDH-2 $>$ LDH-1. After organ damage, the ratios are elevated only for about a week, even though total LDH may still be elevated after this. LDH-3 is a classical marker for cancer presence in over 50% of cancer patients.

9.0.9 Blood Urea Nitrogen (BUN)

Reference values are: adult, 6–20 mg/dL; newborn, 4–18; 1 week, 8–25; child, 5–18.

Urea is a small polar molecule formed in the liver from ammonium ion (Section 2.11.1), and is the major nonprotein nitrogenous end product of protein catabolism. Ultimately urea is excreted by the kidneys.

BUN concentrations reflect the balance between the production and the excretion of urea. Changes in protein intake, fluid balance, liver function, and renal excretion will affect concentrations; but BUN is less sensitive than creatinine to kidney clearance changes. The most common cause of increased BUN is inadequate excretion due to kidney disease or urinary tract obstruction, the latter often caused by prostate enlargement. The BUN level rises when the equivalent of one kidney is lost, or when glomerular clearance is $<$10 mL/min. A BUN level of 50 to 150 mg/dL indicates serious impairment; 150 to 250 mg/dL implies seriously impaired function. The latter concentration range may be accompanied by confusion, disorientation, and convulsions.

Some human factors that elevate BUN are advanced age, advanced pregnancy, burns, dehydration, excessive protein ingestion, fasting, fever, hypovolemia, infections, sepsis, severe crushing injuries, shock, and starvation. Some pathological states that increase BUN include: Addison's disease, bleeding in the gastrointestinal tract, congestive heart failure, diabetes mellitus, gout, kidney diseases, malignancies, myocardial infarction, nephrotoxic agents, pancreatitis, tissue necrosis, and urinary tract obstruction.

Some drugs that elevate BUN are: acetominophen; antibiotics such as amphotericin B, cephalosporins, and aminoglycosides; aspirin; cancer chemotherapeutic agents; codeine; dextran; guanethidine (ismelin); indomethacin (indocin); lithium carbonate; methyldopa (aldomet); morphine; pargyline (eutonyl); propranolol (inderal); sulfonamides; sulfonylureas; and thiazide diuretics.

Decreased BUN is caused by: amyloidosis; fasting; hypertension; inadequate dietary protein, as, for example, in starvation, malnutrition, low protein/high carbohydrate diet, and malabsorption syndromes; nephrotic syndrome; pregnancy; severe liver disease; and water overload (often it is as low as 6–10 mg/dL). Drugs that decrease BUN include intravenous dextrose, phenothiazines, and thymol.

On a typical diet, about 50 to 60 g of urea is cleared by the kidney, and 24 to 35 g of urea appears in the urine every day; that is, 40 to 50% is reabsorbed. The standard clearance is 41 to 65 mL/min.

9.0.10 Creatinine

Reference ranges are: adult males, 0.6–1.7 mg/dL; adult females, 0.5–1.0 mg/dL; children to age 6, 0.3–0.6; children 6 to 18, 0.4–1.2.

Creatinine is the end product of creatine metabolism predominantly in skeletal muscle, even though creatine is synthesized mostly in the liver (Section 2.11.6). The creatinine present in blood reflects skeletal muscle mass. Serum creatinine is a more sensitive marker of kidney function than is BUN. Daily creatinine generation is relatively constant unless crushing injuries or degenerative diseases cause massive muscle damage, or unless massive muscle wasting occurs, as is common for the elderly.

Creatinine is elevated by: kidney damage; chronic nephritis; dialysis (10 mg/dL is the warning level); diets high in cooked meat; high levels of vitamin C; muscle diseases such as gigantism and acromegaly; nephrotoxic antineoplastic agents such as methotrexate, cisplatin, cytoxan, mithramycin, and semustine; salicylate therapy; severe congestive heart failure; trauma; uremia; and urinary tract obstruction. Decreases are associated with muscular dystrophy and with the last trimester of pregnancy before the final 6 weeks.

Diagnostically, creatinine generally is considered along with plasma BUN. An elevated BUN and a typical creatinine imply a nonkidney cause for the high BUN. BUN increases more steeply than creatinine as kidney function declines, and falls more rapidly with dialysis. With severe kidney impairment, BUN still increases, but creatinine tends to plateau with excretion of the latter in the bile and feces. A high plasma urea/creatinine ratio signals sodium and water depletion, protein catabolism, and oligonuria (prerenal, failure congestive heart failure, and severe water depletion). Low ratios with typical urea and creatinine imply excess fluid intake and a low-protein diet; low ratios with raised plasma urea and creatinine signal liver failure and recent hemodialysis or peritoneal dialysis.

The amylase/creatinine clearance ratio also is used diagnostically to indicate macroamylasemia at <1% and acute pancreatitis at >5%. Normal ratios are 1 to 5%.

Urinary creatinine and clearance are discussed in Section 6.2.2.

9.0.11 Uric Acid

Reference ranges are: adult males, 3.5–8.5 mg/dL; adult females, 2.6–7.3 mg/dL; children, 2.0–5.5. The serum uric acid ratio for women/men is about 0.85 until after menopause.

Uric acid is the end product of purine metabolism (Section 2.11.7). Purines are constituents of the nucleotides in nucleic acids. Most uric acid is synthesized in the liver, and about two-thirds is excreted by the kidneys (reflecting only 10% not reabsorbed). About one-third of uric acid excreted is in the feces. The serum level reflects this balance.

The major clinical diagnoses for elevated uric acid are gout and kidney stones. Lack of uricase also causes accumulation. Elevated levels also are seen after ingestion of foods containing purines such as legumes, meats, yeasts, and yogurt and foods containing xylitol; and during fasting, hypertension, malnutrition, severe exercise, shock, starvation, and stress. Decreased kidney function usually is implied by simultaneous elevations in serum urea, creatinine, and uric acid. Urate varies day to day and with the seasons for the same person.

Increased uric acid levels (hyperuricemia) also are observed for: acute tissue destruction (as in infection, starvation, and strenuous exercise); chemotherapy and radiation therapy; diabetic ketoacidosis; Down's syndrome; eclampsia; factors decreasing excretion (lactic acidosis, ketoacidosis, renal failure, and congestive heart failure); hyperparathyroidism; hypertension; Launois-Bensaude adenolipomatosis; leukemia; lymphomas; polycythemia; psoriasis (one-third); sickle cell and pernicious anemia; Tangier disease; Type III hyperlipidemia; von Gierke's disease; and many drugs [alcohol, aminophylline, antibiotics such as gentamicin, ascorbic acid, aspirin (<2 g/day), dextran, diazoxide (hyperstar), diuretics except for spironolactone, mercurials and dyrenium, edecrin, epinephrine, ethacrynic acid, furosemide, griseofulvin, methyldopa, phenothiazines, pyrazinamide, rifampin, ticrynafen, and thiazide diuretics]. Lead, chronic beryllosis, and strychnine poisonings also elevate uric acid, as do alcoholism and metabolic acidosis.

Decreased uric acid levels are seen with: Fanconi's syndrome, Wilson's disease, yellow atrophy of the liver, some cases of acromegaly, pregnancy, and some drugs (acetohexamide, ACTH, allopurinol, atophan, cinchophen, clofibrate, cortisone, coumarins, dicoumarol, dymelor, estrogens, ethyl biscoumarate, imuran, mannitol, marijuana, phenylbutazone, probenecid, salicylates, sulfinpyrazone, sulfoxyphenylpyrazolidine, taractan, and thiophenylpyrazolidine).

About 0.97% of patients with neoplasms show low urate. Serum urate declines in parallel to an increase in LDH after acute myocardial infarction, with return to the baseline by 6 to 8 days. Serum uric acid tends to be higher in blood group B humans and lower in those in group AB. Uric acid levels are higher in Blackfoot and Pima Indians, Filipinos, and Maori. Very high levels, above 11 to 13 mg/dL, are associated with mental deficiency and self-

TABLE 9.1. Reference values for complete blood count [32].

CBC Component	Newborn	1 Month	6 Months	1–10 Years	Adult Male	Adult Female
Red blood cells (RBC)	4.8–7.1 million/mm^3	4.1–6.4 million/mm^3	3.8–5.5 million/mm^3	4.5–4.8 million/mm^3	4.6–6.2 million/mm^3	4.2–5.4 million/mm^3
Hematocrit	44–64%	35–49%	30–40%	35–41%	40–54%	38–47%
Hemoglobin	14–24 g/dl	11–20 g/dl	10–15 g/dl	11–16 g/dl	13.5–18 g/dl	12–16 g/dl
Red cell indices						
MCV*	96–108 μm^3	82–91 μm^3	—	—	80–94 μm^3	81–99 μm^3
MCH†	32–34 pg	27–31 pg	—	—		27–31 pg
MCHC‡	32–33%	32–36%	—	—		32–36%
Stained red cell examination	Normochromic and normocytic for all age groups and both sexes					
White blood cells (WBC)	9000–30,000/mm^3	6000–18,000/mm^3	6000–16,000/mm^3	5000–13,000/mm^3	5000–10,000/mm^3	
Differential WBC						
Neutrophils	45% or less by 1 wk	40% or less by 4 wk	32%	60% after age 2 yr		54–75% (3000–7500/mm^3)
Bands	—	—	—	—		3–8% (150–700/mm^3)
Eosinophils	—	—	—	0–3%		1–4% (50–400/mm^3)
Basophils	—	—	—	1–3%		0–1% (25–100/mm^3)
Monocytes	—	—	—	4–9%		2–8% (100–500/mm^3)
Lymphocytes	41% or more by 1 wk	56% by 4 wk	61%	59% after age 2 yr		25–40% (1500–4500/mm^3)
T-lymphocytes	—	—	—	—		60–80% of lymphocytes
B-lymphocytes	—	—	—	—		10–20% of lymphocytes
Platelets	140,000–300,000/mm^3	150,000–390,000/mm^3	200,000–473,000/mm^3	150,000–450,000/mm^3	150,000–450,000/mm^3	

* Mean corpuscular volume.
† Mean corpuscular hemoglobin.
‡ Mean corpuscular hemoglobin concentration.

mutilation in males. Serum urate is increased in 80% of patients with elevated triglycerides.

9.1 COMPLETE BLOOD CELL COUNTS MARKERS

The reference ranges for a complete blood count (CBC) are provided in Table 9.1 [32].

A CBC includes quantification of the cellular elements of blood, evaluation of red cell indices, and determination of the state of the cells by microscopic examination after differential staining. The CBC consists of a white blood cell count (WBC); a differential white cell count (Diff); a red blood cell count (RBC); hematocrit (HcT); hemoglobin (Hb); red cell indices such as mean corpuscular volume (MCV), mean corpuscular hemoglobin (MCH), and mean corpuscular hemoglobin concentration (MCHC); a stained red cell examination (film or peripheral blood smear); and a platelet count.

Reference values vary across the life cycle and with gender (Table 9.1). In the newborn, the number of red blood cells is high, and it decreases after birth along with hematocrit and hemoglobin. During childhood, red cells increase although hemoglobin may decrease slightly. Before puberty, males and females have the same red cell numbers and hemoglobin. After puberty, values increase in males to age 40 to 50, decline slowly to age 70, and decrease rapidly thereafter. In females, the drop in hemoglobin and hematocrit initiated at puberty reverses at about age 50, but the values never rise to prepubertal levels

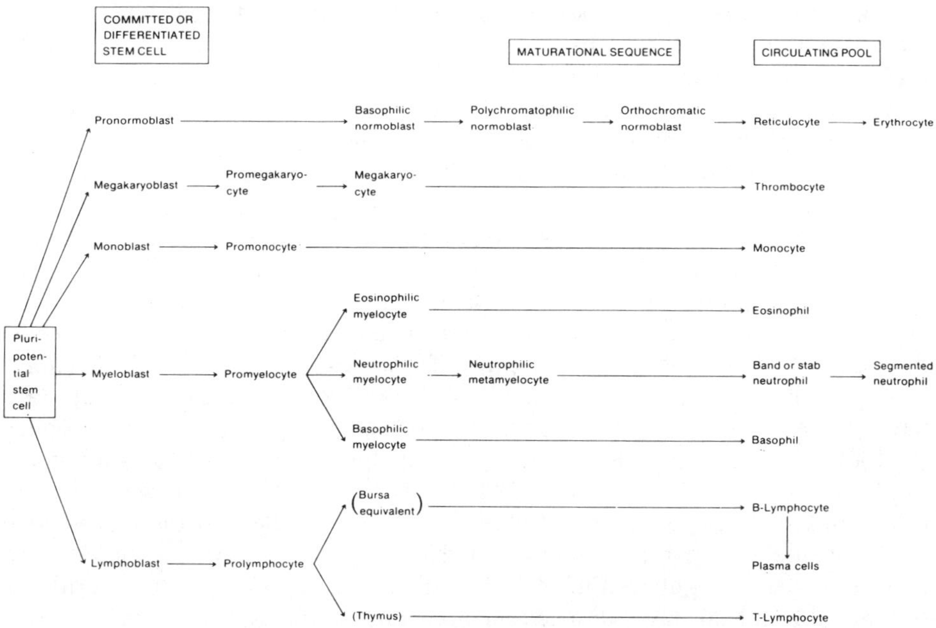

FIGURE 9.1 Theory of formation and maturation of blood cells (hematopoiesis). (From Price and Wilson, *Pathophysiology*, 3rd ed., McGraw-Hill, New York, 1986, p. 181.)

or to those of males of the same age. Menstruation and the excess androgens in males are the major factors, as male castration causes hemoglobin and hematocrit to decrease to the values found in women of the same age.

The origin and the maturation of blood cells are depicted in Figure 9.1. The number of red cells declines in both genders with old age. The number of white cells varies with the health of the individual, and reflects also the impact of the local environment or workplace. White cell numbers are high (10,000–20,000/mm^3) in newborns and infants, and gradually decrease to adult values at about age 21. In adults, there is a circadian rhythm with an early morning minimum and a late afternoon maximum.

The CBC is an essential component of a complete physical examination, but especially on admission to the hospital or before surgery. The CBC also helps to indicate the following: suspected hematologic disorders, neoplasms, or immunologic (e.g., T-lymphocyte count in AIDS) problems; history of hereditary hematologic disorders; suspected infections; suspected effects of physical and emotional stress; responses to drug therapy and blood dyscrasias as side effects. Also it is used in monitoring the progression of nonhematologic disorders such as chronic obstructive pulmonary disease, malabsorption syndromes, malignancies, and kidney diseases.

The venipuncture sample should be contained in a lavender-topped Vacutainer. A capillary sample suffices for children and infants, or for adults when venipuncture is not feasible.

9.1.1 WBC

The adult reference range is 5,000–10,000. The WBC, relative to the reference range, is defined for elevation as slight at 11,000–20,000, moderate at 20,000–30,000, and severe at >50,000. Similarly, for decreases, slight is 3,000–4,500, moderate is 1,500–3,000, and severe is <1,500. See Table 9.1 for WBC reference ranges across the life cycle.

The white blood cell count measures the number of white cells or leukocytes per cubic millimeter of whole blood. White cells constitute the body's major defense against "foreignness" relative to its usual transport, anabolic, and catabolic processes. White cells protect against foreign organisms, xenobiotics, pollens, mutated proteins of the host, and tissues. Leukocytosis in general is found in infection, inflammation, leukemia, and parasitic infections. Leukopenia occurs in bone marrow depression, severe infection, viral infections, autoimmune diseases, malignancies, and malnutrition. WBC is a nonspecific marker. All white cells are hardly ever affected except in hemoconcentration.

The major cell types quantitated in the differential WBC in adults are neutrophils (54–75%), monocytes (2–8%), eosinophils (1–4%), basophils (0–1%), band neutrophils (0–8%), and lymphocytes (20–40%), all being produced in the bone marrow, with the lymphocytes also being generated at other sites such as the thymus, spleen, and tonsils. They do their protective work outside of the bloodstream and thus are in transit in the blood. The endocrine system regulates the white blood cell system. The cell life span varies between 13 and 20 days, destruction occurring in the lymphatic system with many ghosts excreted in the feces. Lymphocytes and monocytes are called agranulocytes; the rest of the white cells are called granulocytes because they contain granules in their cytoplasm. Neutral stains reveal neutrophils; acid stains, eosinophils; and basic stains, basophils.

Elevated neutrophils are indicative of infectious, inflammatory, and necrotic processes. An increase in immature neutrophils, that is, "bands" and "stabs," is the result of a body response to a pathogenic process. Increases in eosinophils occur in allergic responses and parasitic infections; basophils increase in leukemias, Hodgkin's disease, and polycythemia vera. Monocyte numbers are stimulated in chronic inflammatory and infectious states, and during recovery from acute infections. Increased lymphocytes also appear in chronic inflammatory and infectious processes, as well as in lymphomas and lymphocytic leukemias. Chapter 13 examines molecular immunology further.

9.1.2 WBC: Neutrophils and Monocytes

Neutrophils and monocytes are the most mobile and active cells. They ingest foreign material by phagocytosis and they can degrade various proteins and lipids such as those found in bacterial cell membranes. Neutrophils are increased by: stresses (such as allergies, childbirth, exercise, surgery, and temperature extremes), hemorrhage, hemolysis, infectious diseases, inflammatory disorders (such as drug reactions, gout, myositis, rheumatoid arthritis, rheumatic fever, and vasculitis), tissue necrosis (abscesses, burns, crushing injuries, and malignancies), metabolic disorders (Cushing's syndrome, diabetic ketoacidosis, eclampsia, thyroid crisis, and uremia), venoms, xenobiotic exposure (arsenicals, benzene, heavy metals, mercury, potassium chlorate, and turpentine), myelocytic leukemia, and drugs (ACTH, digitalis, epinephrine, heparin, histamine, and lithium). Decreases in neutrophils ($<500/mm^3$ will increase susceptibility to bacterial infections) are caused by: acromegaly, Addison's disease, anaphylaxis, anorexia nervosa, bone marrow activity depression (caused by Felty's syndrome, Gaucher's disease, hypersplenism, ionizing radiation exposure, myelofibrosis, old age, overwhelming infection, pernicious anemia, toxic chemicals, and viruses), disseminated lupus erythematosus, folic acid deficiency, malnutrition, malignancies, starvation, thyrotoxicosis, vitamin B_{12} deficiency, and certain drugs (alcohol, aminophylline, antineoplastic agents, barbiturates, butazolidin, chloramphenicol, chlorpromazine, dilantin, dinitrophenols, mesantoin, PBZ, penicillin, phenacetin, phenurone, pyramidon, quinine, streptomycin, and sulfonamides). Immature neutrophils ("bands") increase in antineoplastic drug administration, infections, and any conditions causing neutrophilia.

Monocytes, the largest cells in normal blood, are increased in: carcinomas, cirrhosis, collagen diseases, Gaucher's disease, hemolytic anemias, Hodgkin's disease, infections, ionizing radiation therapy exposure, leprosy, lipid storage disease, lymphomas, monocytic leukemia, polythemia vera, regional enteritis, sarcoidosis, systemic lupus erythematosus, thrombocytopenic purpura, tuberculosis, and ulcerative colitis. They produce interferon, an antiviral agent. Monocytes are decreased in hairy cell leukemia and after prednisone treatment. Monocytes also produce a number of soluble mediators, called monokines, such as tumor necrosis factor-α (TNF-α) and interleukin-1-β (IL-1-β), which are important to the initiation and regulation of the immune response. For example, IL-1-β facilitates T-lymphocyte proliferation, and interleukin-8 is a chemoattractant for T-lymphocytes and neutrophils. Agents such as gram-negative bacterial endotoxin, phorbol myristate acetate, and gram-positive bacterial components induce the release of these two monokines, as do such other events as cell-to-cell adhesion and contact of tumor cells by monocytes.

9.1.3 WBC: Eosinophils

The function of eosinophils is still unknown, but it is thought that they detoxify foreign proteins that emanate from the lungs and the intestinal tract, especially in the later stages of inflammation. They obey a circadian rhythm that reaches a minimum in the morning and a maximum after midnight. Eosinophils increase in: Addison's disease, allergic responses, asthma, autoallergies, autoimmune diseases, chorea, chronic inflammatory diseases, dermatoses, Hodgkin's disease, hypersensitivity, leprosy, malignancies, parasitic infestations, pernicious anemia, polycythemias, sarcoidosis, sickle cell anemia, splenectomy, and ulcerative colitis. Eosinophils decrease in: acromegaly, congestive heart failure, Cushing's syndrome, disseminated lupus erythematosus, electric shock treatment, cases of elevated hormones [such as ACTH (basis of the Thorn ACTH test), adrenaline, and thyroxine], cases of elevated steroids, hyperplastic anemia, hypersplenism, infectious mononucleosis, and stress.

9.1.4 WBC: Basophils

Basophils, also called mast cells, are only a little better understood than eosinophils. Basophils contain heparin, histamine, and serotonin, and are thought to stimulate blood flow to injured tissues, simultaneously preventing excessive clotting. They are used to study allergic processes. Basophils are increased in: chronic hypersensitivity, Hodgkin's disease, ionizing radiation treatment, leukemia, nephrosis, polycythemia vera, and ulcerative colitis. Basophils decrease in: acute allergic processes, chronic steroid therapy, hypersensitivity, hyperthyroidism, and stress after myocardial infarction and during bleeding peptic ulcer.

9.1.5 WBC: Lymphocytes

Lymphocytes are important in immunity. The T-lymphocytes (60–80% in adults) oversee cellular immunity and interact directly with the antigen; the B-lymphocytes (10–20%) produce antibodies and are responsible for humoral immunity by distributing these antibodies to all body fluids; and the null cells (5–20%) are of unknown function. Diseases that implicate lymphocyte failure to protect manifest as a hypersensitivity and a susceptibility to xenobiotics, and as autoimmunity (development of immune reactions to the individual's own cells). The majority of lymphocytes are located in the spleen, lymph nodes, and other lymphatic tissues. Lymphocytes increase in: Addison's disease, Bantis' disease, Felty's syndrome, infections (bacterial and viral), infectious mononucleosis, ionizing radiation treatment, lead exposure, lymphocytic leukemia, lymphomas, lymphosarcomas, malnutrition, myeloma, rickets, thyrotoxicosis, toxiplasmosis, ulcerative colitis, and Waldenstrom's macroglobulinemia.

Lymphocytes decrease (<500/mm^3 means a great susceptibility to viral infections) after administration of high doses of adrenal corticosteroids and antineoplastics, ionizing radiation treatment, and massive transfusions; and in patients afflicted with AIDS and HIV, aplastic anemia, burns, bone marrow failure, Gaucher's disease, hemolytic disease of the newborn, Hodgkin's disease, hypersplenism, immune deficiency diseases, pernicious anemia, pneumonia, rheumatic fever, septicemia, thrombocytopenia purpura, toxic chemical exposures (benzene, bismuth, DDT), and transfusion reactions.

T-lymphocytes develop from the stem cells of bone and migrate to the thymus, where they proliferate and mature (Figure 9.1). Most die on maturation, but a small proportion reach the peripheral tissues as mature T-cells. The thymus functions primarily during fetal life, and the newborn has a fully functional cellular immunity system. There are two subsets of T-cells: helper (50–65% in adults) and suppressor (20–35%) cells, usually in a ratio of 2:1, respectively, for each adult individual. Helper cells promote the proliferation of T-lymphocytes, stimulate B-lymphocyte reactivity, and activate macrophages, thus increasing their bactericidal and cytotoxic functions. Suppressor T-cells control the magnitude of the immune response. The balance between the two subsets determines the ability of an individual to survive physical, chemical, biochemical, and foreign matter–induced stress. Therefore, they are the chief CBC markers of exposure to xenobiotics.

Increased T-lymphocyte cell densities are observed in: acute lymphocytic leukemia, multiple myeloma, chronic beryllium disease, infectious mononucleosis, and Graves' disease. Decreases are caused by: AIDS and HIV infection, chronic fatigue syndrome, chronic lymphocytic leukemia, DiGeorge's disease, Hodgkin's disease, long-term therapy with immunodepressant drugs, Nezelof's syndrome, severe combined immunodeficiency (SCID), Waldenstrom's macroglobulinemia, and Wiskott-Aldrich syndrome. T-cell activity often is assessed through hypersensitivity skin tests, the sheep erythrocyte rosette test, and reactivity with monoclonal antibodies.

B-lymphocyte precursors are found in the fetal liver and bone marrow; the locus of maturation of B-lymphocytes is still unknown in humans. The most differentiated forms of B-lymphocytes are the plasma cells. The latter carry immunoglobulins (Ig) on their surfaces that serve as receptors for specific antigens (IgG, IgM, IgA, IgD, and IgE). Not only do these antigens have to react with surface Ig on B-lymphocytes, but also B-lymphocytes must interact with T-helper lymphocytes. The activated B-lymphocytes transform then into immunoblasts which divide into plasma cells that produce antibodies, and/or into memory cells, often called small lymphocytes, that can recognize the antigen directly, thus reducing the time to elicit an immune response ("sensitization").

Increased B-lymphocytes are measured in: acute lupus erythematosus, chronic lymphocytic leukemia, DiGeorge's syndrome, multiple myeloma, and Waldenstrom's macroglobulinemia. Decreases are found in acute lyphocytic leukemia, X-gene–linked agammaglobulinemia, and SCID. B-lymphocytes are visualized by fluorescent labeling using fluorescein dye after reaction with heterologous antisera. Both types of lymphocytes can be differentiated by electron microscopy because T-cells are smooth, and B-cells have irregular surfaces and projections.

The ability of a lymphocyte to transform into an immunoblast also may be impaired. This possibility is assessed by exposing lymphocytes to mitogens used for that purpose, as, for example, phytohemagglutinin and concanavalin A for T-lymphocytes and pokeweed mitogen for both B- (more) and T-cells. These agents also are extensively used in the research area of cytogenetics (Section 9.3.2). About 72 h after stimulation, radiolabeled thymidine is added, and the rate of uptake into cellular DNA indicates the ability of the lymphocytes to establish immune capability. Pregnancy, oral contraceptives, transfusions, and steroid ingestion may cause decreased responses, as can prior radioisotope administration. A stimulation index of greater than 10 implies immunocompetence.

After this, antigen-specific tests can be performed if a viral, a microbiological (for example, gram-negative or -positive bacteria), or a human-tissue rejection mechanism is suspected. A stimulation index of greater than 3 indicates prior exposure to the antigen. Mixed lymphocyte culture techniques also are used to allow foreign antigens to be recognized before an organ transplant. Nonresponsiveness (stimulation less than 3) indicates good histocompatibility.

9.1.6 WBC: White Cell Enzymes

White cell enzymes mostly are analyzed to confirm leukemias through the activity of leukocyte alkaline phosphatase (reference range 13–130 U) originating from mature neutrophils (increases in leukemoid reactions to infections, myelofibrosis, and polycythemia vera; and decreases in chronic granulocytic leukemia), and enzymes found in mature granulocytes stained by the periodic acid–Schiff (PAS) stain to visualize compounds oxidized to aldehydes (mostly cytoplasmic glycogen).

9.1.7 RBC

The mature red blood cell or erythrocyte has an average life span of about 120 days. The RBC is a biconcave disk in shape that can survive passage through the strictures of the capillaries. RBCs lack a nucleus and mitochondria, and thus cannot synthesize protein. Their primary function is to transport oxygen as a hemoglobin complex from the lungs to the tissues and to transfer carbon dioxide out of these tissues back to the lungs.

Old, damaged, and atypical red blood cells are removed mainly by the spleen but also by the liver and red bone marrow. The iron from hemoglobin is transported by plasma transferrin (made in the liver) back to the bone marrow, or is stored in the liver and the spleen as ferritin and hemosiderin. The transferrin is only about 20 to 55% saturated. If protein homeostasis is disordered but iron stores are normal, the percentage saturation will be high. In processes where total body iron is low and transferrin increases, the % saturation will be high. In iron overload as in hemachromatosis, lead poisoning, multiple blood transfusions, and severe hemolysis, both serum iron and %

saturation of transferrin will be high. If serum is exposed to enough iron, so that all iron is chelated by transferrin, the amount of iron taken up to saturation is the total iron binding capacity.

Serum ferritin begins very high in the newborn (>100 μg/L), decreases sharply to 10–15 μg/L soon after birth, and plateaus for both genders at about 25μg/L between the ages of 5 and the end of puberty. After adolescence males always have higher values than females of the same weight, although after menopause concentrations in females increase sharply.

The bilirubin component (Section 9.0.4) of hemoglobin is transported by plasma albumin to the liver, conjugated, eliminated in the bile, and excreted in the feces, or some is returned through enterohepatic circulation. The number, structure, color, size, and shape of red cells, as well as the types and amount of hemoglobin contained, their fragility (leakability), and atypical components, usually are noted.

The red cell count is expressed in RBCs/mm^3. Erythropoiesis in the bone marrow maintains a population of about 25×10^{12} circulating RBCs or 5 million/mm^3 in adults. The production rate is about 2 million cells/sec, with eightfold stimulation possible. The production is regulated by the level of tissue oxygenation through the action of erythropoietin, whose precursors are found mostly in the kidney and, to a much lesser extent, in the liver.

Erythropoiesis from tissue hypoxia is caused by acute blood loss, anemias, compromised blood flow to the kidneys, hemolysis, impaired oxygen binding to or release from Hb, impaired oxygen–carbon dioxide exchange in the lungs and tissues, low hemoglobin, severe diarrhea, and conditions causing pulmonary edema.

Decreased RBCs occur when insufficient erythropoietin is produced, and in cases of bone marrow disorders, people lacking kidneys or requiring dialysis, drug and toxic chemical effects, ionizing radiation treatment, malignancies, hypothyroidism, insufficient iron, deficiency in vitamin B_6 and B_{12}, and low intake of folic acid.

The red cell count is affected by many factors. Decreases are caused in: blood loss, chronic inflammatory diseases, excessive blood cell destruction as in hemolytic anemia, hemodilution as occurs during pregnancy, impaired erythropoiesis, and the administration of many drugs (e.g., acetaminophen and its compounds, antineoplastics, arsenicals, hydantoin derivatives, mercurial diuretics, monoamine oxidase inhibitors, nitrites, penicillins, pyrazolone derivatives, radioisotopes, sulfonamides, sulfones, sulfonylureas, tetracyclines, thiazide diuretics, and thiocyanates and their precursors). Sampling in the supine position causes a low count.

Increases occur in anxiety, at high altitudes, in chronic pulmonary disease with hypoxia and secondary polycythemia, with dehydration from excessive exercise, in hemoconcentration, with pain, in polycythemia vera, and after drug administration such as methyl dopa and gentamicin.

Red cell precursors in the bone, which are nucleated, are called normoblasts (basophilic, polychromatophilic, and orthochromatic in order of increasing age). The precursor cell is the pronormoblast. The nucleus gradually decreases while the hemoglobin concentration increases. At the point of nuclei loss but with fragments of mitochondria and other organelles present, orthochromatic normoblasts enter the bloodstream as reticulocytes (adults have between 0.5 and 2% of total blood cells with higher levels for pregnant women and for infants younger than 2 months—up to 3.2% at birth).

Within 4 days of entering the bloodstream, the reticulocyte becomes a mature blood cell. Under anemic, hemolytic (for example, caused by exposure to the gas phosgene), and hypoxic stress, increased reticulocytes may be produced in the peripheral circulation. Pernicious anemia, severe iron deficiency anemia, and thalassemia cause ineffective erythropoiesis leading to lower reticulocytes because the cells never mature enough to be released into the circulation. Increased reticulocytes are observed to compensate for blood loss and in response to vitamin B_{12} therapy, as well as in hypoxia and anemia. A small blood sample is mixed with a supravital stain such as brilliant cresyl blue, and the smear is observed under the microscope for reticular material, which stains gray-blue.

However, a major problem in using reference ranges is illustrated by the following example. A "normal" reticulocyte count in the presence of a "normal" hemoglobin signifies typical bone marrow activity, whereas a "normal" reticulocyte count in the presence of low hemoglobin implies an inadequate bone marrow response to anemia. The latter could be caused by defective erythropoietin production, bone marrow function, or hemoglobin formation. After blood loss or effective therapy for anemia, increased reticulocytes peaking at 4 to 7 days after the loss indicate that the bone marrow is normally responsive and is attempting to replace cells lost or destroyed; the levels will fall again once hemostasis is achieved. A permanent increase must be looked into further. Again personal baseline levels are necessary for one to be able to interpret these data, as well as an understanding of which parameters to regard as primary and which as secondary, necessitating mechanistic knowledge.

9.1.8 RBC: Hematocrit

The hematocrit is the percentage of red blood cell volume of whole blood volume. In the newborn, hematocrit is 44–64%; at 1 month, 35–49%; at 6 months, 30–40%; at 1–10 years 35–41%; in adult males, 40–54%, and in adult females, 37–47%. Factors influencing RBCs will affect the hematocrit because RBCs comprise 99% of the total cells of the blood. Abnormally oversized RBCs, very elevated WBCs, and hyperosmotic conditions, as found in elevated blood glucose and sodium, can cause increased hematocrits. The hematocrit's chief clinical use is to signal known or suspected anemia, fluid imbalances, and hematologic status during pregnancy together with hemoglobin. The hematocrit increases at high altitudes and consistent exercise, and decreases after age 50.

9.1.9 RBC: Hemoglobin

Hemoglobin content reflects the number of RBCs. Reference ranges are: adult male, 13.5–18 g/dL; adult female, 12–16 g/dL; the newborn, 14–24; at 1 month, 11–20; at 6 months, 10–15; and at 1–10 years, 11–16. Hemoglobin is the primary intracellular protein of RBCs; it binds oxygen in the pulmonary artery for transport to tissues (1.34 mL of oxygen/g hemoglobin is the capacity at 37°C), and binds tissue carbon dioxide for transport back to the lung for exhalation of carbon dioxide.

Hemoglobin consists of two proteins, heme and globin. Heme has a red porphyrin pigment (Section 2.11.5), which contains iron. The globin portion comprises four polypeptides, each with a heme. Oxygen and carbon dioxide binding depend not only on the heme group and iron, but also on the ability of the globin chains to shift in the proper manner. Hemoglobin also functions as an acid/base buffer that combines with hydrogen ions and with bicarbonate ions from the breakdown of carbonic acid (fueling the bicarbonate/carbonate buffer system of the blood and tissue). Chloride ions are retained in RBCs when bicarbonate is eliminated into the plasma by RBCs. The major clinical use of hemoglobin is to evaluate anemia in conjunction with hematocrit. Increased hemoglobin is shown by people living at high altitudes, and it is enhanced by any factor that increases RBCs.

9.1.10 RBC: Aberrant Hemoglobin

Hemoglobin types are evaluated electrophoretically. At birth, fetal hemoglobin, HbF, has two alpha and two gamma globin chains. Within a few months, HbF largely disappears and is replaced with adult Hb (HbA), which has two alpha and two beta globin chains. HbA is 95 to 97% of total adult hemoglobin. HbA_2, about 2 to 3%, has two alpha and two delta chains. Traces of HbF (1–2%) occur throughout a person's life. Genetic abnormalities of Hb resulting in decreased production rates of alpha or beta globin chains are called thalassemias. Hemoglobinopathies are characterized by atypical amino acid sequences in the globin chains. Lack of the alpha globin chain causes death through nonrelease of oxygen to tissues from the gamma chains. Sickle cell disorders occur because of double beta gene defects that produce hemoglobin S (HbS), resulting in the characteristic sickle RBCs. Affected individuals have shorter than normal life spans, and their tissue oxygenation is impaired. The gene for HbS is most prevalent in Black populations.

The heme part of hemoglobin also may be defective. Methemoglobin (HbM) is formed when the iron in heme is oxidized to the ferric state instead of a ferrous form, thus impairing its oxygen-combining ability. Methemoglobinemia can be genetic or environmental. The latter type is caused by: excessive ionizing radiation; drugs such as nitrates, lidocaine, and phenacetin; and exposure to chemicals such as anilines, nitrobenzenes, nitric oxide, nitrogen trifluoride, propylene glycol dinitrate, *n*-propyl nitrate, and xylidines (Section 21.4.13). HbF is more prone to methemoglobinemia than HbA. Placental transfer is therefore important for expectant mothers exposed to chemicals causing methemoglobinemia.

9.1.11 RBC: Red Cell Indices

Red cell indices are also calculated: mean corpuscular volume (MCV)—the volume of Hb in each RBC (80–94 μm^3 in males; 81–99 in females); mean corpuscular hemoglobin (MCH)—the weight of Hb in each RBC (27–31 pg in males and females); and mean corpuscular hemoglobin concentration (MCHC)—Hb concentration in the red blood cells [32–36% (weight/weight) in males and females].

RBC, hematocrit, and Hb concentration are required to calculate the above parameters. A stained blood smear is used to assess RBC size. These indices identify and classify types of anemias, depending on RBC size and Hb content. Cell size is said to be normocytic (6–8 μm in diameter), microcytic (<6 μm in diameter), or macrocytic (>8 μm in diameter). Hemoglobin content is described as normochromic, hypochromic, or hyperchromic.

MCV of 82 to 92 cubic μm, MCH of 25 to 30 pg, and MCHC of 32 to 36% define normocytic, normochromic anemia, some causes of which are aplastic anemia, hemolysis, hemorrhage, hereditary spherocytosis, ionizing radiation, and sepsis. MCV of $<80\,\mu m^3$, MCH of 20 to 25 pg, and MCHC of 27% characterize microcytic, normochromic anemia; some of its causes are infections, liver disease, malignancies, and renal disease. MCV of 50 to $80\,\mu m^3$, MCH of 12 to 25 pg, and MCHC of 25 to 30% define microcytic, hypochromic anemia; some causes are iron deficiency, lead poisoning, rheumatoid arthritis, and thalassemia. MCV of 95 to $150\,\mu m^3$, MCH of 30 to 50 pg, and MCHC of 32 to 36% characterize macrocytic, normochromic anemia; some causes are deficiencies of folic acid and vitamin B_{12}, some drugs, and pernicious anemia.

The stained red cell smear also is used to assess RBC shape, inclusions, and atypical cell contents such as Heinz bodies (denatured Hb), Howell-Jolly bodies (fragments of residual DNA), Cabot's rings, basophilic stippling (residual cytoplasmic RNA), and siderotic granules (iron/hemosiderin granules). Both Heinz bodies and Cabot's rings are caused by: α-thalassemia, glucose-6-phosphate dehydrogenase deficiency, hemolytic anemias, splenectomy, and administration of drugs such as analgesics, antimalarials, antipyretics, furacin, furadantin, phenylhydrazine, sulfonamides, tolbutamide, and excess vitamin K. Basophilic stippling (usually identifying reticulocytes) occurs in anemia due to liver disease, lead poisoning, and thalassemia. Howell-Jolly bodies appear in intense hemolysis or inefficient erythropoiesis. Siderotic granules characterize abnormal iron metabolism and abnormal Hb manufacture.

9.1.12 RBC: Erythrocyte Sedimentation Rate

The erythrocyte sedimentation rate measures the rate at which RBCs settle. Reference rates are: males < 50 years, 0–7 mm/h Wintrobe units; males > 50, 5–7; females < 50 years, 0–15; females > 50, 25–30.

Increased rates occur in the following cases: in inflammatory, infective, and necrotic processes; when the globin/albumin ratio increases; during acute heavy metal poisoning; when high fibrinogen is present; for people having severe anemias, nephritis, thyroid disorders, pregnancy, collagen disorders, and malignancies; and after administration of drugs such as dextran, methyldopa, oral contraceptives, penicillamine, procainamide, theophylline, and vitamin A.

Decreased rates occur when the plasma is very viscous, or if cholesterol or lipid levels are very high. Such decreases may result from congestive heart failure, cryoglobulinemia, degenerative joint disease, polycythemia vera, and sickle cell disease, and after drug administration of adrenal corticosteroids, quinines, and salicylates.

9.1.13 RBC: Osmotic Fragility Test

The osmotic fragility test for RBCs is performed by exposing RBCs to increasingly dilute saline solutions. The composition of the solution causing swelling and rupture is noted. Spherocytes (RBCs that are not biconcave) and RBCs with damaged membranes burst quickly in slightly hyperosmotic conditions (<0.3% saline). Some causes are: autoimmune anemias, burns, disseminated intravascular clotting, heme pathway enzyme deficiencies, hemolytic anemias, hereditary spherocytosis, hypotonic transfusions, infections by parasites, prosthetic heart valves, transfusions with incompatible blood, and toxins (microbial and chemical).

Decreased fragility at >0.5% saline is produced by: hereditary anemias such as sickle cell, hemoglobin C, and thalassemias; iron-deficiency anemias; liver diseases; obstructive jaundice; polycythemia vera; and splenectomy.

9.1.14 RBC: Red Cell Enzymes

Red cell enzymes sometimes are monitored to assess whether the RBC energy source of the glycolysis/pentose pathway is working. Deficiencies have been found for glucose-6-phosphate dehydrogenase (reference range is 4.3–11.8 IU/g Hb and 125–281 U/dL RBCs; 15% of African Americans have a type A variant that cannot resist oxidative stressors; ingestion of fava beans causes hemolysis for individuals with the Mediterranean type variant) and for pyruvate kinase (reference range is 2.0–8.8 U/g Hb and 0.3–0.91 mg/dL RBCs; RBCs lacking this have a low affinity for oxygen, and RBCs hemolyse). Both conditions are hereditary.

9.1.15 Platelet Indices

Failure of hemostasis leads to hemorrhage. There are three major hemostatic processes: vascular activity, platelet function, and coagulation. Vascular activity concerns the constriction and the expansion of muscles within the walls of blood vessels in response to vascular damage. This only can be effectively done in the arterioles because large vessels and very small vessels cannot constrict or expand readily. This process provides only temporary relief.

Circulating platelets (thrombocytes) do not have nuclei. They are formed in the bone marrow under the influence of "thrombopoietin" from megakaryocytes, which are large multinucleated cells. Up to tenfold production is possible under hemostatic stress or bone marrow stimulation. Their lifetime in the blood is about 10 days. About two-thirds circulate, and most of the rest stay in the spleen, which destroys old or damaged platelets. For conditions with an enlarged spleen (for example, in chronic liver diseases such as cirrhosis; connective tissue diseases such as rheumatoid arthritis and lupus erythematosus; acute infections such as infectious mononucleosis and miliary tuberculosis; and myeloproliferative diseases such as leukemias, hemolytic anemias, and lymphomas), excessive bleeding occurs because most of the platelets are trapped in the enlarged spleen.

People with too few platelets or platelets that are poorly functional experience numerous, pinpoint hemorrhages (petechiae), multiple small bruises (ecchymoses), and slow bleeding or serum oozing from venipuncture sites, shaving cuts, and mucosal surfaces. Platelet count, bleeding time, platelet aggregation, platelet survival time, clot retraction, and capillary fragility usually are monitored.

Platelets protect blood vessels from endothelial damage by microtraumas, and they initiate repair in damaged blood vessel walls through the formation of platelet plugs. Blood vessel damage causes platelets to adhere to the altered surface; and this requires calcium ion (Coagulation Factor IV), fibrinogen (Coagulation Factor I), and von Willebrand's factor (associated with Coagulation Factor VIII). Platelet adherence causes release of ATP, ADP, calcium ion, and serotonin.

If enough of the surface is damaged, platelet aggregation occurs to form a plug that controls bleeding until a clot can form. Prostaglandins are generated that promote adherence (this being inhibited by aspirin). Different prostaglandins are produced by the endothelial cells lining the blood vessels to inhibit platelet aggregation. Thrombin generated by the coagulation sequence causes release of platelet factor 3 from platelets to enhance coagulation, and hence to generate more thrombin. Released platelet Factor 4 enhances these platelet/coagulation processes by neutralizing the anticoagulant heparin.

There are 12 clotting factors. There is no Factor VI because it has been shown to be activated Clotting Factor V (Clotting Factor Va; accelerator globulin or proaccelerin). Coagulation involves interaction of plasma proteins to form a stable fibrin gel, ultimately leading to clot formation. At least 30 compounds are involved in the process, with each of the 12 clotting factors essential for its specific step, the whole process proceeding sequentially.

There are three major clotting sequences, namely, the intrinsic (blood contacts injured vessel walls), extrinsic (blood contacts damaged tissues), and common final pathways [involving conversion of Factor X (autoprothrombin III or Stuart factor) to Factor Xa—activated Factor X—in the presence of calcium ion (Factor IV) and platelet phospholipid, followed by prothrombin-to-thrombin conversion, fibrinogen-to-fibrin metamorphosis, and then, under influence of the fibrin stabilizing factor (Clotting Factor XIII), formation of an insoluble fibrin clot].

The intrinsic clotting process involves, in order: Factor XII (Hageman factor) to XIIa, Factor XI (plasma thromboplastin antecedent) to XIa, Factor IX (Christmas factor, autoprothrombin II) to IXa, and Factor VIII (antihemophilic factor, autoprothrombin II) to VIIIa.

The extrinsic clotting process involves in order: Factor III (tissue thromboplastin) converted to IIIa, and Factor VII (proconvertin, antiprothrombin I) to VIIa.

Calcium ion is necessary for activation of Factors VII, IX, X, and XI; for the conversion of Factor II (prothrombin) to thrombin; and for fibrin formation. Citrate, oxalate, and EDTA are anticoagulants because they bind calcium ion and prevent it from participating in the clotting process.

Both platelet activation and coagulation are controlled through inhibitors. The maintenance of adequate blood flow aids in diluting and removing clotting factors and in dispersing aggregated platelets. The two control processes are linked. Fibrin strands are broken down by the proteolytic enzyme plasmin, which is generated from its circulating precursor plasminogen through the actions of such compounds as Factor XII, urokinase, and streptokinase. Plasmin also attacks fibrinogen and degrades Factors V, VIII, and XIII. The degradation products interfere with platelet aggregation, reduce prothrombin, and inhibit the conversion of soluble to insoluble fibrin. Plasmin is directly antagonized in the circulation by antiplasmin and α_1-antitrypsin.

Another anticlotting/platelet mechanism acts through neutralizing the clotting ability of thrombin. The most important inhibitor is antithrombin III (heparin cofactor), which inhibits thrombin (Factor IIa) and activated factors X, XI, and XII and plasmin. Heparin greatly augments the activity of heparin cofactor. Platelet Factor 4, which is released when platelets are broken down by the reticuloendothelial system, inhibits heparin cofactor.

Deficiency of von Willebrand's factor, which is associated with clotting Factor VIII, leads to improper adherence of platelets with the result of a prolonged bleeding time.

9.1.16 Platelet Indices: Platelet Count

Platelet count (adult reference range 150,000–450,000/mm^3) may be interfered with by severe red cell fragmentation, by excessive WBCs above 100,000/mm^3, if the diluting fluid contains extraneous particles, if the plasma sample is allowed to sit too long before counting, by repetitive venipunctures which may activate coagulation, by severe sample agitation, or if the platelets adhere to one another. Individuals with platelet counts $<$15,000 to 20,000 may bleed spontaneously. Those with counts between 50,000 and 100,000/mm^3 may bleed in a prolonged manner on surgical, dental, obstetrical, or invasive diagnostic procedures.

Platelet dysfunction is defined as a long bleeding time ($>$6 min using the Ivy or Template methods) for a platelet count $>$100,000/mm^3. Counting can be done microscopically or electronically. Increased platelets are caused by: anemias (posthemorrhagic and iron deficiency), carcinomatosis, childbirth, chronic heart disease, chronic pancreatitis, cirrhosis, drugs such as adrenaline, hemorrhage, leukemias (chronic), polycythemia vera, splenectomy, surgery, trauma, and tuberculosis.

Decreased production of platelets is caused by: bone marrow malignancies, Fanconi's syndrome, histiocytosis, ionizing radiation, leukemias (acute), uremia, viral infections, vitamin B/folic acid deficiencies, and drugs such as alcohol, anticonvulsants, antineoplastics, carbamates, chloramphenicol, chlorothiazides, isoniazid, pyrazolones, streptomycin, sulfonamides, and sulfonylureas. Increased destruction of platelets is caused by: antibody/HLA antigen reactions; burns; chronic cor pulmonale; congenital infections such as adventitious infections of AIDS, cytomegalovirus, herpes, syphilis, and toxoplasmosis; disseminated intravascular coagulation; hemolytic anemias; hemolytic disease of the newborn; idiopathic thrombocytopenia purpura; immune complex formation; lymphomas; meningococcemia; miliary tuberculosis; Rocky Mountain spotted fever; sarcoidosis; splenomegaly due to liver disease; and drugs such as aspirin, aromatics, DDT, digoxin, gold salts used for arthritis, heparin, quinidine, quinine, and thiazides.

9.1.17 Platelet Indices: Bleeding Time

Prolonged bleeding (>6 min using the Ivy and Template methods) after a superficial injury implies low platelet number, inadequate function, or both. Prolonged bleeding occurs for <10,000 platelets/mm^3. Aspirin can prolong bleeding time as long as 5 days after a single 300 mg dose. Diseases causing prolonged bleeding are: aplastic anemia, Bernard-Soulier syndrome or giant platelet syndrome, connective tissue diseases, disseminated intravascular coagulation, Glanzmann's disease, hepatic cirrhosis, hypersplenism, hypothyroidism, leukemias, malignancies such as Hodgkin's disease and multiple myeloma, measles, mumps, scurvy, and von Willebrand's syndrome. Some drugs that increase bleeding time are: alcohol, analgesics, anticoagulants, aspirin and derivatives, chlorothiazides, high molecular weight dextran, mithramycin, streptokinase, sulfonamides, and thiazide diuretics. Abstinence from all these drugs must be observed by patients for 5 days before the test. Bleeding times greater than 10 min require a pressure dressing to stop the bleeding.

9.1.18 Platelet Indices: Platelet Aggregation Test

Platelet aggregation and precipitation (usually clearing occurs within 5 min) are measured by treating platelet-rich plasma with known inducers of platelet aggregation such as adrenaline, collagen, ristocetin, and thrombin. The test is dependent on the existence of platelet ADP. Individuals with advanced alcohol-related conditions, dysproteinemias, myeloproliferative disorders, severe liver disease, or uremia often depress the effects of collagen, adrenaline, and directly added ADP. Absence of von Willebrand's factor cannot be detected through addition of adrenaline, collagen, or directly added ADP, which all react, but is detected by no reaction with ristocetin.

Other factors that may impair platelet aggregation include: giant platelet syndrome, Glanzmann's disease, idiopathic thrombocytopenia purpura, infectious mononucleosis, and drugs such as aminophylline, antihistamines, anti-inflammatory drugs, caffeine, dipyridamole, phenothiazines, phenylbutazone, salicylates, sulfinpyrazone, and tricyclic depressants.

9.1.19 Platelet Indices: Platelet Survival Test

This test measures the survival time of circulating platelets, which is usually 10 days. The individual's platelets are labeled with radioactive chromium, and then the label is remeasured daily for 10 days. Any condition causing disseminated intravascular coagulation such as abruptio placenta, burns, crushing injuries, overwhelming sepsis, severe shock, surgical trauma, and tissue infarction, or any condition causing vascular injury such as hemolytic uremia syndrome, intravacular prosthetic devices, thrombotic thrombocytopenia purpura, and vasculitis, will cause increased platelet destruction. Any other factors decreasing platelet count will reduce the survival time.

9.1.20 Platelet Indices: Clot Retraction Test

A normal fresh clot incubated at 37°C usually shrinks to half its original size within 1 h to produce a firm cylindrical fibrin clot that contains all the RBCs, and is sharply demarcated from the clear serum. If hematocrit is low, the clot is small and the serum volume high. If platelet dysfunction occurs or there are excess platelet numbers, there is little serum, and a soft, plump, and a poorly demarcated clot is observed. Hemoconcentration and polycythemia produce poor clot retraction.

If fibrinogen is low, often for conditions causing disseminated intravascular coagulation, there may be no clot, or RBCs may spill into the serum when retraction begins. Clot retraction does not occur if more than 90% of platelet activity is neutralized, a common condition for drugs that have produced platelet antibodies or in immune disorders.

9.1.21 Platelet Indices: Rumple-Leeds Capillary Fragility Test (Tourniquet Test)

This test indicates the ability of capillaries to resist rupturing under pressure due to abnormalities in the blood vessel walls or excess platelets. A blood pressure cuff is set at 100 mm Hg pressure on the patient's arm for 5 min. The number of petechiae resulting in a 2-inch circle are measured (fewer than 10 is normal). Results can also be reported as Grade 1, 0–10 petechiae; Grade 2, 10–20; Grade 3, 20–50; and Grade 4, >50. The test identifies "easy bruisers" and assesses capillary integrity. It should not be performed on people with spontaneous petechiae or large ecchymoses, or those known to have disseminated intravascular coagulation.

9.2 URINE MARKERS

Urine contains 95% water and 5% solids. Urine formation begins in the glomerular capillaries of the kidneys with dissolved substances passing into the proximal tubule because of blood pressure and the pressure in Bowman's capsule (Section 6.2.1). As the filtrate passes along the tubule, more solutes are eliminated from the capillary blood, and secretions are received from the tubular epithelial cells, the latter also reabsorbing some solutes and water. Urine concentration and dilution occur in the renal medulla. Sodium excretion also is a major function of the kidney. The major urine solids are urea and sodium chloride.

Urinalysis is an essential procedure for hospital admissions and physical examinations. Physicians since ancient times have reported on urine color, odor, turbidity, volume, and sweetness. The sweetness of urine once was gauged by its ability to attract ants.

Today, dipsticks, tapes, and tablets are used for many direct-reading tests based on colorimetry. Dipsticks are excellent screening tools for bilirubin, glucose, hemoglobin, ketones, white cell esterase, nitrite, pH, protein, and urobilogen, among others. These dipsticks work by producing a color at a critical concentration of the target chemical, or by the depth of color (necessitating color comparison standards). Multiscreening tests on one dipstick also are popular, for example, for pH, protein, and glucose. Other tablets and treated slides are available to detect bacteria, cystinuria, mucopolysaccharide, phenylketonuria, and salicylate. Precise timing and adherence to directions are essential. All such direct-reading devices should be stored in the dark in a closed container in a refrigerator together with a desiccant. One must know any positive and negative interferences to be able to interpret the readings. The effects of diet, human factors, and life-style on urine production, as well as clearance tests of urine, and the physiology of urine production were considered in Section 6.2.4.

Routine urinalysis provides the following typical results on healthy subjects:

General characteristics:

- Color: Yellow-amber indicates high specific gravity, concentrated urine. Colorless indicates a dilute urine of low specific gravity.
- Turbidity: clear to slightly hazy.
- Odor: faintly aromatic
- Specific gravity: 1.0015–1.035 for normal fluid intake.
- pH: 4.5–8.4 with an average of 6.0. Females have a more alkaline urine than males.

Chemical determinations:

- Negative for bilirubin, blood or hemoglobin, glucose, ketones, leukocyte esterase, nitrite, and protein using dipsticks.
- Urobilinogen: 0.1–1 Ehrlich U/2 h; 1–4 mg/day; 0.1–1 Ehrlich U/mL.

Microscopic examination of urine sediment (RBCs, WBCs, epithelial cells, crystals, casts, mucus, bacteria):

- Casts: negative; occasional hyaline or granular casts.
- RBCs: negative or rare (0–3 using a high-powered field).
- Crystals: negative or occasional.
- WBCs: negative or rare.
- Epithelial cells: few
- Bacteria: occasional
- Mucus: occasional

Routine urinalysis involves macroscopic analysis for overall physical and chemical characteristics and microscopic analysis of insoluble solids (urine sediment). Urine samples for these parameters usually are performed on the first morning void, which must be examined within 1 h of collection. Urinary sediment begins to deteriorate 2 h after collection. Samples should be shielded from light because bilirubin and urobilinigen are photooxidized. Refrigeration is necessary for samples when they cannot be examined promptly, with the proviso that the results may not be valid on such refrigerated samples.

9.2.1 Color

The yellowish color of urine is caused by the pigment urochrome produced by metabolism. Highly yellow urines are concentrated and of high specific gravity, whereas colorless urines are dilute and of low specific gravity. High fluid intake in healthy people causes dilute urines. In an untreated diabetic, the urine may be colorless because of diuresis from excessive glucose. The specific gravity may be high if excess glucose is in the urine. Similarly, deeper-colored urine may not always indicate concentrated urine, especially if excess bilirubin is present. The color should be assessed in a good light against a white background.

If excess biliverdin (oxidation product of bilirubin) is present in fresh urine, a yellow or green foam appears on shaking. Blood in the urine is signaled by black/brown/red/pink colors with cloudiness. Hemoglobin and myoglobin (produced from severe muscle damage) in the urine can produce the same colors without the cloudiness. Foods such as beets, rhubarb, asparagus, and carrots can produce colored urine; so dietary and medical histories must be known in order to interpret findings. Urine allowed to stand longer than 30 min darkens because of oxidation of urobilogen to urobilin.

Drugs such as cascara and senna in acid urine turn urine reddish-brown, and red in alkaline urine. Other drugs turn urine orange (pyridium and amidopyrine), orange to orange-red (pyridium and ethoxazene), orange to purple-red (chloroxazone), orange-yellow (salicylazosulfapyridine, anisindione, and phenindione in alkaline urine), rust-yellow (sulfonamides and nitrofurantoins), pink/red/red brown (dilantin, doxidan, Ex-Lax, and phenothiazine), magenta (Ex-Lax), red (amidopyrine, aniline dyes, desferol, neotropin, phenolphthalein, and pyridium in acid urine; prontosil, and PSP and BSP dyes in alkaline urine), purple-red (Ex-Lax in alkaline urine), dark brown (phenolic dyes and phenylhydrazine), brown black (cascara and Jectofer), bright yellow (riboflavin or pyridium in alkaline urine), blue or green (methylene blue dye and amitripyline), dark color (iron salts), pink to brown (phenothiazine tranquilizer), and pale blue (triamterene).

If the urine is red, it must be tested for hemoglobin. An orange color also can arise from concentrated urine, restricted fluid intake, excess sweating, fever, and the presence of bile pigments. Brownish yellow or greenish yellow may indicate bilirubin and stale urines. Red or a reddish color indicates blood, hemoglobin, or myoglobin. A port wine color could be due to methemoglobin/oxyhemoglobin and porphyrins. Dark brown may indicate hemoglobin, Lysol poisoning, or melanin. Black urine occurs in alkaptonuria.

9.2.2 Turbidity (Appearance, Clarity)

Urine is usually clear or slightly cloudy. In alkaline urine, the cloudiness usually is caused by the precipitation of phosphates and carbonates. In acidic urine, cloudiness may be due to the precipitation of urates, uric acid, or calcium oxalate. Accumulation of uroerythrin may produce a pink or reddish haze in acid urine. More commonly, cloudiness can be caused by WBCs, RBCs, bacteria (often fishlike odor), casts, pus, and epithelial cells, ascertainable through microscopic examination. Mucus, yeasts, sperm, lymph, fat globules, prostatic fluid, menstrual and vaginal discharges, fecal material, and external contamination from talcum powder, dust, or antiseptics may be sources of cloudiness.

9.2.3 Odor

A fresh urine specimen from a healthy person smells faintly aromatic. The odor of ammonia predominates on standing. Urine with a fruity odor may indicate ketonuria due to uncontrolled diabetes or starvation. Mousy smells signal phenylketonuria (PKU). A maple syrup odor is associated with maple syrup disease. A fishy smell is associated with bacterial infection in fresh urine or bacterial growth in old samples. A sweet acetone smell occurs in diabetic ketosis. An asparagus smell means ingestion of asparagus. Lack of an odor in fresh urine is found in acute renal failure due to acute renal necrosis and ammonium ion secretion inhibition.

9.2.4 Specific Gravity

Specific gravity is the density of a substance divided by the density of pure distilled water at the same temperature. Thus because it contains dissolved solids, the specific gravity of urine is greater than 1.000. The presence of large molecules such as proteins, glucose, or urea will affect specific gravity more than small ions such as sodium and chloride. The specific gravity of the glomerular filtrate is usually 1.010 as it enters Bowman's capsule. A consistent urine specific gravity of this value indicates loss of concentrating ability in the proximal tubules (isothenuria). Overhydration, hypertension, renal disease, and diabetes insipidus cause low specific gravities. High specific gravities can be caused by dehydration, fever, proteinuria, uncontrolled diabetes mellitus, nephrosis, vomiting, diarrhea, intravenous dextran or other high molecular weight fluids, and patients who have received radiological contrast media. The early morning void generally has the highest specific gravity.

9.2.5 pH

The pH is defined as the negative logarithm of the hydrogen ion activity (see Sections 1.5 and 1.6). The pH of urine reflects the kidney's ability to regulate the acid–base balance of the body. When too much acid is present (as in respiratory and metabolic acidosis), the urine becomes more acidic (lower pH or higher hydrogen ion concentration). Alkaline urine ($pH > 7$) is excreted during metabolic and respiratory alkalosis. The pH also is affected by diet.

Bicarbonate ions are reabsorbed and hydrogen ions secreted in exchange for sodium ions in the renal tubules. Excess hydrogen ions are excreted as ammonium ions. Disorders of these processes will lead to changes in urine pH and the dominant ions excreted. In instances of prolonged vomiting or excessive use of diuretics, acidic urines are produced to conserve potassium ions.

Diets high in berries, tomatoes, protein, and meat will be acidic, whereas vegetarians (especially legume eaters), milk drinkers, and citrus fruit eaters produce an alkaline urine. Drugs in the ammonium salt form will produce acid urines, whereas sodium, potassium, and lithium salts of drugs will yield alkaline urine. Dietary control is used to control urinary tract infections through pH control. Acid urine inhibits the growth of organisms that utilize urea as a nitrogen and a carbon source. Also acid urine helps to prevent formation of calcium phosphate, calcium carbonate, and magnesium phosphate kidney stones. Other types of kidney stones are less likely for alkaline urine (uric acid, cystine, and calcium oxalate). Acidic drugs for treating urinary tract infections may be more effective for alkaline urine than for acidic urine because these drugs are more soluble in the salt form (for example, kanamycin, streptomycin, neomycin, and sulfonamides).

Urine following a meal is usually less acidic than normal because of gastric secretions; early morning urine tends to be more acidic because of mild respiratory acidosis. Thus, urine samples should be collected at the same time each day after a 12-h fast for pH evaluation.

9.2.6 Protein

Natural proteins in urine include Tamm-Horsfall glycoprotein excreted by the distal renal tubules, small amounts of albumin (mostly reabsorbed in proximal tubules), microglobulin, immunoglobulin light chains (Bence Jones protein), and enzymes and proteins from tubular epithelial cells, leukocytes, and other cells shed by the urinary tract. Over 200 urinary proteins have been identified, one-third of the amount being albumin.

People with healthy kidneys exhibit proteinuria in certain situations: after cold exposure, fever, congestive heart failure, ingestion of a large amount of protein, severe emotional stress, and strenuous exercise; during pregnancy and the premenstrual state; in mothers after infant delivery and in their newborn children; and upon assuming the erect position after being supine for certain individuals (3–5%).

Persistent proteinuria indicates renal disease or systemic disorders that increase serum low molecular weight proteins. For kidney damage, glomerular damage can be distinguished through change in creatinine clearance (Section 6.2.2) from tubular damage (specific gravity consistently near 1.010). If the glomerular damage is severe, globulins which are larger than albumins will also be detected. Tubular damage is reflected by the greater presence of urinary proteins that usually are absorbed by the tubules, for example, albumin.

Excess myoglobin in serum, which occurs when there is extensive destruction of muscle fibers, not only causes proteinuria but also can lead to acute renal tubular necrosis. Bence Jones proteins in the urine occur in 40% of people with multiple myeloma, a neoplastic disorder of plasma cells. This may also lead to kidney damage. Bence Jones proteins also appear in tumor metastasis in amyloidosis, bone, chronic lymphocytic leukemia, and macroglobulinemia.

Proteinuria during the later months of pregnancy may indicate complications in utero. All proteinuria must be followed up with confirmatory tests to assess the cause.

Proteinuria occurs in the following diseases: cancer of the kidney, kidney stones, nephritis, nephrosis, polycystic kidney, and tuberculosis. Proteinuria does not occur with all kidney diseases. Sometimes nonrenal proteinuria is observed in the following: abdominal tumors, acute infections, ascites, cardiac disease, convulsive disorders, fever, hyperthyroidism, intestinal obstruction, liver disease, severe anemias and leukemias, toxemia, trauma, and toxic effects of drug therapy, lead, mercury, opiates, phenol, phosphates, sulfosalicylic acid, and turpentine.

Proteinuria and the detection of large numbers of WBCs usually indicate infection somewhere in the urinary tract. If RBCs also are present, this usually means a noninfectious inflammatory disease of the glomeruli. Casts in urine are associated with proteinuria.

9.2.7 Glucose

Glucose is almost absent from urine in healthy people in spite of being present in the glomerular filtrate. Most of the glucose in the latter is reabsorbed in the proximal tubules of the kidney by an active carrier process. This process can be overwhelmed by high plasma glucose concentrations above 160 to 200 mg/dL, as found in diabetes mellitus. A high glucose intake in healthy people can cause glucose excretion. Thus, urine samples for glucose status are best taken before meals or snacks. The first morning void usually has a high level of glucose.

High blood sugar can cause glucose to appear in the urine. Some diseases known to promote this are: acromegaly, advanced cystic fibrosis, brain tumor, carcinoma of the pancreas, Cushing's syndrome, diabetes mellitus, gestational diabetes, glycogen storage disease, hemachromatosis, hyperthyroidism, massive metabolic derangement (as produced by advanced liver disease, cardiogenic shock, sepsis, severe burns, and uremia), obesity, pheochromocytoma, severe chronic pancreatitis, and drugs that cause hyperglycemia (such as ACTH, adrenal corticosteroids, dextrothyroxine, excessive intravenous glucose, and thiazides). When renal tubular reabsorption is impaired, glucose can appear in the urine without blood hyperglycemia; and excess bicarbonate, phosphate, sodium, and water also appear in the urine. The major causes for this glucose excretion are: renal tubular dysfunction as found in cystinosis, Fanconi's syndrome, galactosemia, lead poisoning, and multiple myeloma; and pregnancy, as distinct from gestational diabetes.

Certain drugs produce false positives on the Clinitest tablets or Benedict's solution used for glucose tests. Some drugs that interfere are: ascorbic acid, cephalosporins, chloral hydrate, levodopa, morphine, Neggram, para-aminobenzoic acid, paraldehyde, penicillins, radiological contrast media, salicylates, skelaxin, streptomycin, and terramycin. Allowing urine samples to sit at room temperature also may produce glucose that is not present in fresh urine. The presence of fructose, galactose, lactose, pentose, and sucrose in urine produces false positive results. Fructose may appear after parenteral feedings or in some genetic diseases (also galactose for the latter). Lactose appears in normal pregnancies and lactation, in lactase deficiency states, and in intestinal diseases such as celiac disease, kwashiorkor, and tropical sprue. Pentose excretion occurs after ingestion of large amounts of fruits. Sucrose appears after candy ingestion and in sucrase intestinal deficiency in sprue.

A diagnosis of glycosuria demands knowledge of drug and food ingestion before a pathological state can be identified.

9.2.8 Blood, Hemoglobin, or Heme

RBCs (hematuria) or hemoglobin (hemoglobinuria) may be present in urine because of "occult blood" from bleeding in the urinary tract (for example, cystitis), massive hemorrhages, extensive hemolysis, or overload of the reticuloendothelial system. Proteinuria also is observed after bleeding elsewhere in the body, and RBCs and hemoglobin both are found. Significant proteinuria may indicate serious kidney disease. If RBCs are not detected, myoglobinuria may be occurring. The latter may often be seen after traumatic muscle injuries, muscle disorders such as arterial occlusion in muscle and muscular dystrophy, and toxicities due to carbon monoxide or fish poisoning. Both RBCs and hemoglobin can be detected by dipsticks.

Hematuria is relatively common in healthy people after strenuous exercise, in heavy smokers, and through menstrual blood contamination. It is also caused by: acute appendicitis; acute systemic febrile and infectious diseases; acute tubular necrosis (occasionally); anticoagulant therapy; bleeding disorders; blood dyscrasias; cystitis; diverticulitis; glomerulonephritis; hydronephrosis; kidney stones; lower urinary tract infection, inflammation, bleeding, trauma, and damage; lupus erythematosus; malignant hypertension; malignant nephrosclerosis (occasionally); polyarteritis; polycystic kidney disease; pyelonephritis; renal vein thrombosis; salpingitis; subacute bacterial endocarditis; tumors involving the colon, kidney, pelvis, rectum, and urinary tract; and drugs that cause bleeding such as anticoagulants, coumarin, cyclophosphamide, salicylates, and sulfonamides.

Hemoglobin is not normally found in urine except in certain individuals with weak small blood vessel walls. Hemoglobinuria can be caused by: crushing injuries, extensive burns, hemolysis of RBCs (hemosiderin is excreted also a few days after the hemolysis), hemolytic anemias, malaria, poisonous mushrooms, post-surgery prostate exudates, severe infections, snake venoms, transfusion reactions, trauma to RBCs by prosthetic devices, trauma to muscles and blood vessels, and drugs that are kidney-toxic (bacitracin and amphotericin) or that cause hemolysis (e.g., aspirin) and alkaline urine when RBCs are hemolysed. People taking high doses of vitamin C may give a false negative effect, whereas drugs giving false positive results include bromides, copper salts, iodides, and oxidizing agents.

9.2.9 Bilirubin and Urobilogen

The breakdown of RBCs was discussed in Sections 6.1.1 and 9.0.4. RBCs are broken down in the spleen, and less so in the liver, to iron, protein and protoporphyrin. The latter is converted to bilirubin, most of which is adsorbed to albumin with the rest unconjugated (Section 9.0.4). The latter is conjugated in the liver with glucuronic acid, eliminated into the bile ducts, stored in the gallbladder, and eliminated into the intestine. In the intestine, bilirubin is converted to urobilinogen by the microflora and fauna. About half of the urobilinogen is excreted in the feces, where it is converted to urobilin; the rest undergoes enterohepatic circulation, with a small amount (>4 mg/day) excreted in the urine.

Bilirubin in the urine is found in alkalotic states, diseases with biliary tract obstruction, ingestion of bananas, and liver diseases (for example, cirrhosis, hepatitis, prejaundice, and jaundice) (see Section 9.0.4), but not when the liver is so impaired that it cannot conjugate bilirubin, and not in hemolytic disorders. Excessive urobilinogen also may be detected for persons in alkalotic states and in cases of liver disease, hemolytic disorders, malaria, and congestive heart failure with liver congestion, though not for complete obstruction of the common bile duct.

If urobilinogen is absent but there is blood in the stool, carcinoma involving the head of the pancreas may be indicated. Decreased urobilinogen occurs in acid urines, severe diarrhea, and severe inflammatory diseases, and with drugs that kill or inhibit the actions of microflora and fauna in the intestines.

Urobilinogen levels are subject to circadian control, peak excretion being from 1200 to 1600 h. Comparison should be made on samples collected at the same time of day.

Because bilirubin is easily oxidized by air and light, fresh urine samples only must be used for this test. Large amounts of ascorbic acid and nitrates in the urine cause false negative results.

9.2.10 Ketone Bodies Including Acetone

Ketone bodies result from the metabolism of fatty acids and fats (Section 2.6), and consist of three main compounds, acetone, β-hydroxybutyric acid, and acetoacetic acid. The last two compounds are readily converted to acetone. Negligible amounts of these compounds appear in the urine of healthy individuals. When fat becomes the predominant body fuel instead of carbohydrates because of inhibition of carbohydrate absorption or metabolism, the result is acidosis with ketone bodies in the urine. Ketonuria is mostly associated with diabetes, ketoacidosis, and poor response to oral hypoglycemic agents after insulin treatment withdrawal, especially if infections are present.

Ketonuria appears in connection with: acute illnesses (15% of nondiabetics), anesthesia administration (appearing afterward), anorexia, carbohydrate-free diets, diarrhea, fasting, fever, high-protein diets, high-fat diets, prolonged vomiting, starvation, stress, and administration of drugs such as ether, insulin, isopropyl alcohol, levodopa, metformin, paraldehyde, phenformin, phthaleins, and pyridium.

9.2.11 Nitrite

Bacteria convert urinary nitrate to nitrite. A positive nitrite test must be confirmed by a regular urine culture to identify the bacteria. However, not all bacteria reduce nitrate to nitrite. Gram-negative bacteria do, but yeasts and gram-positive bacteria may not. There may not be enough nitrate either (especially for persons who do not eat enough green vegetables). If excess urinary ascorbic acid, antibiotics, or bacteria are present, the nitrite may be further reduced to nitrogen (bubbles may be seen). The best urine samples for testing are those that have been in the bladder overnight, using the midstream portion to avoid bacterial contamination. False positive results may be found with unsterilized containers and with the metabolites of azo dyes. False negative results may occur on freshly voided random samples or samples withdrawn by catheter, or for high specific gravity urines.

9.2.12 Leukocyte Esterase

This test detects the presence of neutrophils. If the dipstick is positive, confirmation by regular urine culture is required. Vaginal secretions (use the midstream urine sample to minimize this interference), trichomonas, parasites, heavy mucus, and concentrated urinary yellow pigments cause false positive results. False negative results occur in the presence of high urinary protein and ascorbic acid. A urine sample that is positive for both nitrite and leukocyte esterase should be cultured for pathogenic bacteria.

9.2.13 Microscope Analysis of Urinary Sediment

This analysis involves microscopic examination of RBCs, WBCs, epithelial cells, casts, crystals, bacteria, and mucus. About 10 mL of well-mixed urine is centrifuged at 2000 rpm for 5 min, and the residue is examined. In an Addis count, all urine for 12 h is collected and centrifuged, with the residue examined.

The reference range for RBCs is 0 to 3 using the high-powered field. Disorders associated with RBCs in urine for hematuria are discussed in Section 9.2.8.

The reference range for WBCs is 0–4 using the high-powered field. WBCs are hardly found in urine. Pyuria generally indicates renal or genitourinary tract diseases, especially bacterial infections in the renal/genitourinary tract as in cystitis and pyelonephritis, and such noninfectious disorders as glomerulonephritis, lupus nephritis, renal calculi, and tumors. Contamination with genital secretions also may cause pyuria, especially in females. Alkaline urine lyses WBCs in 1 to 2 h. Leukocyte esterase will be positive in the presence of neutrophils (Section 9.2.12).

A few epithelial cells are normal in the urine. Urinary epithelial cells derive from the squamous epithelial linings of the male and female urethras and the vagina, transitional epithelial cells of the linings of the renal pelvis, bladder, and upper urethra, and the cell linings of the renal tubules. Large consistent numbers of epithelial cells, especially those of renal tubular origin, are pathological. Renal transplant rejection, any ischemic injury to the kidney, glomerulonephritis, pyelonephritits, and any kidney damage done by toxins and drugs may be indicated by pyuria.

Oval fat bodies (cells that contain lipoproteins, triglycerides, and cholesterol) may be seen in renal tubular epithelial cells. Histiocytes are fat-containing cells that are larger than oval fat bodies and are characteristic of lipid storage diseases and nephrotic syndrome. Melanin (black) in tubular epithelial cells indicates malignant melanoma that has spread to the genitourinary tract. Hemosiderin and hemoglobin also may occur. Large clumps or sheets of transitional epithelial cells indicate carcinoma in the area from the renal pelvis to the bladder.

Occasional casts (hyaline or granular) are normal in the urine also. Casts are cylindrical gels that form in the renal tubules and collecting ducts. Tamm-Horshall protein, a glycoprotein secreted by distal renal tubular cells, is the major constituent and forms a clathrate, which traps other formed elements such as RBCs, WBCs, bacteria, fats, and urates. Usually healthy individuals excrete only a few casts. Low urine pH, high urine protein, increased solute excretion, and decreased urine flow are favorable conditions for casts to appear in the urine of healthy people. Any factors producing these conditions may also produce casts. Otherwise, excessive casts are signs of widespread kidney disease involving the renal tubules. Casts are classified into various types: broad—greater than five RBCs in width; medium broad—three to four RBCs;

and narrow—one to two RBCs, with the broad category indicative of severe renal damage. They may be further characterized as crystal, epithelial cell, fatty, granular, hyaline, red blood cell, waxy, and white blood cell (the latter only from kidney tubules). All casts present in excessive numbers indicate that further investigation of their cause is necessary.

Occasional crystals in the urines of healthy people are expected (uric acid, urate, phosphates, or calcium oxalate). There are many types of crystals, many not being of major clinical significance. The major crystals found at a given pH are: ammonium biurate (thorny yellow-brown apples; alkaline pH), amorphous phosphates (white; alkaline–neutral), amorphous urates (brick or yellow-brown; acid), ampicillin (colorless; acid–neutral), calcium carbonate (colorless dumbbells; alkaline), calcium oxalate (colorless envelopes; all pHs), calcium phosphate (colorless; acid-neutral), cholesterol (colorless notched plates; acid), cystine (colorless; acid), leucine (yellow; acid–neutral), radiological dye (colorless; acid), struvite or triple phosphate ($MgNH_4PO_4$—colorless/white), sulfonamides (green; acid–neutral), tyrosine (colorless/yellow; acid-neutral), and uric acid (yellow/brown; acid).

The only crystals of any known clinical significance are: uric acid (gout, leukemias, and lymphomas during drug therapy), calcium oxalate (Crohn's disease, ethylene glycol toxicity, high doses of vitamin C, hypercalcemia, severe chronic renal disease), cystine (cystinuria, an inherited metabolic defect preventing reabsorption of cystine by the proximal tubules), struvite (urinary tract infection), and leucine and tyrosine (severe liver disease).

The pH of urine, its temperature, the concentrations of precursor substances, the age of the samples, and whether they have been stored in a refrigerator are important variables in the interpretation of a microscope crystal analysis.

Bacteria, yeast, mucus, meat fibers, pus, vegetable fibers, spermatozoa, and parasites have all been detected in the urinary sediment. Bacteria are not important unless accompanied by excessive white blood cells and excessive nitrite. Parasites are often of vaginal origin (*Trichomonas vaginalis*), but a true urinary parasite is *Schistosoma hematobium*. Yeast, mucus, and spermatozoa usually are benign. The pathogen *Candida albicans* is sometimes observed in samples contaminated with vaginal secretions or in urines of diabetics.

9.3 SIGNIFICANCE OF SELECTED HEALTH SURVEILLANCE MARKERS

9.3.1 Introduction

The factors affecting medical monitoring and medical surveillance also influence health surveillance monitoring. Whereas medical monitoring involves detections of markers known to be related to adverse effects in impaired tissues, health surveillance utilizes markers predictive, or thought to be predictive, of adverse effects [33]. The World Health Organization [33] defines adverse effects as "changes that occur with intermittent or continued exposure and that result in impairment of functional capacity (as determined by anatomical, physical, biochemical or behavioral parameters), or in a decrement of the ability to compensate additional stress; changes that are irreversible during exposure or following cessation of exposure if these changes cause detectable decrements in the ability of the organism to maintain homeostasis; and changes that enhance the susceptibility of the organism to the deleterious effects of other environmental influences."

Research is continuous on health surveillance markers until some of them become medical monitoring or medical surveillance markers when more is known about their etiology. Thus the distinction between medical monitoring/ medical surveillance and health surveillance markers can be academic rather than real. Health surveillance markers may then be related to both dose-effects (effects that are not adverse) and dose-responses (adverse effects) through dose. Equally, they may be purely qualitative.

Health surveillance has had a long history in occupational medicine, and the designation has been increasingly applied to predictive markers of health effects associated with exposure to hazardous wastes. Frequently health surveillance and medical monitoring together are termed "medical surveillance." Some investigators also term this "health surveillance." The health surveillance indicators of absorption of xenobiotics may be the same as biological monitoring markers, but health surveillance markers also may be predictive of health effects, adverse or otherwise. In fact, some investigators like to term research on the predictive markers of adverse effects "biological effect monitoring."

Health surveillance thus is part of preventive medicine as well as environmental hygiene. The definition of health surveillance agreed to by many [33] is: "The periodic medico-physiological examination of exposed workers with the objective of protecting and preventing occupationally related disease. The detection of established disease is outside the scope of this definition." The implication is that health surveillance is distinct from medical monitoring and medical surveillance of disease states. This definition is related only to the occupational environment, which to the present author, is too restrictive a sphere because the potentially adverse effects of the workplace are a specialized case of the effects of environmental pollution, and nonworkplace exposeres may exacerbate the effects of workplace exposures.

Like medical monitoring markers, markers used in health surveillance can be nonspecific or specific. Specific markers are useful if specific chemical exposure information is available by environmental analysis or through accurate hazardous material data sheets. Nonspecific markers are important when there is exposure to many chemicals, for intermittent exposures, when there are physical factors, and in signaling whether further investigation is necessary in the absence of specific chemical exposure information. The emphasis in health surveillance as in medical monitoring is on the individual rather than the group (biochemical epidemiology). Under such conditions, acute effects are easier to deal with than chronic effects, where group analysis lends validity for responses to a common source. The causes of chronic effects in individuals are often difficult to assign because of subjective recall, interactions, and nonspecificity problems.

9.3.2 Chromosomal Markers

Gross alterations in chromosomes (bundles of intertwined DNA) include overt breakage and chromosomal rearrangement within the cell (structural chromosomal aberrations), as well as switching of parts of a single chromosome (sister chromatid exchange or SCE) or loss of nuclear material during division to form at least one other small nucleus (micronucleus). Such changes can be visualized by looking at chromosomes through a light microscope [34]. These alterations are called cytogenetic changes, and the general process is clastogenesis.

The usual human chromosome complement (karyotype) contains 46 chromosomes: 22 pairs of autosomes and two sex chromosomes (XX in females; XY in males). Each chromosome at mitosis assumes an X-shape joined at the centromere and characterized by two long (q) and two short (p) arms (telomeres). There are seven major types of chromosomes based on size. Newborns show frequencies on the order of 0.6% for chromosomal aberrations (numerical and structural). In human spontaneous abortuses, this frequency is about 50%. Because red blood cells do not have nuclei but circulating leukocytes do, white blood cells (Sections 9.1.1–9.1.6) are the preferred blood cells for cytogenetic studies. In urine, epithelial cells are the major ones used to evaluate effects on the kidney (Section 9.2.13). A dose–response must be induced by a genotoxic agent (often an activated form of the exposing agent); the effect is then linked to a disease by correlation, a process that does not uniquely identify cause and effect.

Lymphocytes (T- and B-cells) are culturable, carry nutrients and metabolites throughout the body, and are sensitive to exposures throughout the body (Section 9.1.5). This last property allows these cells to be utilized as indicators of exposure, and as surrogate cells that may predict effects in other cells of the body. The majority of lymphocytes are in the G_0 stage of the cell cycle (unreplicated chromosomes). The division stimulant *in vitro* usually is phytohemagglutinin, which means that mostly T-cell types are stimulated to divide through the other steps of the cell cycle [G_1 (chromosomes behave like an unreplicated single DNA double helix or one chromatid); S (DNA replication); G_2 (chromosomes are analogous to two DNA double helices, that is, two sister chromatids); and mitosis (chromosomes separate under the control of a critical level of a serine-threonine protein kinase produced by a control gene analagous to cell division cycle gene *cdc*-2 of *Schizosaccharomyces pombe* and human T-lymphocytes, and two other protein types, the cyclins and the phosphatases to deactivate *cdc*-2)].

The circulating lymphocyte is not a proliferating cell, and this explains why chromosome-type aberrations can be detected years after chromosomal damage. The short-lived lymphocyte has a half-life of about 12 months, whereas long-lived ones may last over 20 years. Any aberrations observed in humans depend on at least three competing processes: prolonged induction time of lesions, continual repair processes, and rate of removal and redistribution of lymphocytes from the circulating pool. The last is much influenced by viruses and immunosuppressive diseases and infections.

Ionizing and ultraviolet radiations and the four radiomimetic chemicals can directly fragment DNA and induce structural chromosomal aberrations independent of division or division cycle. Most chemicals, however, form covalent adducts to the DNA, distort the DNA helix (intercalating agents), or interfere with DNA precursor metabolism or repair. Such chemicals induce SCEs and micronuclei, and can be expressed only after at least one cell division after the molecular lesion occurs. The dose rate and potency are important, but the agents that break DNA directly may not show dose-effects. The persistence of any lesions depends on repair and metabolic processes, the organ affected, and the lifetime of the cells.

Structural chromosomal aberrations are stable or unstable relative to their ability to persist in dividing cell populations. Unstable aberrations (dicentrics, triradials, rings, deletions, and other asymmetrical aberrations) cause cell death through prevention of cell division or loss of vital genetic information during cell division. Stable aberrations consist of balanced translocations, inversions, and other symmetrical rearrangements and are propagated through many divisions. There are as many asymmetrical rearrangements as symmetrical ones, as demonstrated through staining studies to produce banded chromosomes.

About half of the people carrying a constitutional translocation in the gametes of germ cells eventually produce viable progeny. The role of stable rearrangements in cancer is still unclear, though many postulate a role in the etiology or progression of cancers. For example, Burkitt's lymphoma is associated with a specific translocation involving the long arm of chromosome 8 with the long arm of chromosome 14. An oncogene, *c-myc*, has been mapped distal to the breakpoint on chromosome 8 in lymphoma patients and is translocated to chromosome 14 at a site very close to the genes coding for one of the heavy-chain immunoglobulins. Chromosomal rearrangements involving other oncogenes also have been observed in some other cancers [35].

SCEs result from the breakage and rejoining of DNA without any observable distortion of the chromosome. The SCE-forming lesion, to be detectable, must persist *in vivo* until the blood is withdrawn and then *in vitro* until the cultured lymphocyte begins DNA synthesis.

To visualize chromatid exchange, cells are grown in bromodeoxyuridine, which quenches the fluorescence of the fluorochrome Hoechst 33258 or diminishes the uptake of Giemsa stain into chromatin. At least four strands of DNA (two double helices) must be broken, with a switch of those strands from one to the other arm of the same chromosome and rejoining of those strands in their new location. This exchange process may cause errors in the genetic code (molecular mutations), but also may cause no errors.

Although the incidence of SCEs and mutations are often correlated, this ratio varies with the type of chemical and the type of cell. The relationships of the induction of SCEs to the induction of transformation *in vitro* and to the induction of tumors *in vivo* appear to be similar. Diseases such as Bloom's syndrome and multiple sclerosis increase SCEs. Xeroderma pigmentosum sensitizes SCE formation in the presence of ultraviolet light or alkylating agents. Other sensitizations have been noted for Fanconi's anemia, Bloom's syndrome, and ataxia telangiectasia. Increased SCEs are caused by exposure to cigarette smoke, viruses, alcohol consumption, oral contraceptives, and antineoplastic agents. Interlaboratory variations are large. Pregnancy, protein malnutrition, the beginning and end of menstruation, and advancing age increase SCEs. There are no significant differences in SCE frequencies in adults of both genders for Caucasians, African Americans, Chinese, and American Indians.

Micronuclei are formed by condensation of acentric chromosomal fragments or by whole chromosomes left behind (lagging chromosomes) during anaphase [36], as a result of spindle defects or lack of a centromere. Micronuclei thus indicate the previous existence of chromosomal aberrations. 5-Bromodeoxyuridine is used to mark divided and nondivided nuclei after stimulation. However, 5-bromodeoxyuridine can induce micronuclei by itself. Another method for denoting divided nuclei uses cytochalasin B to block cytokinesis in the presence of phytohemagglutinin. Thus, lymphocytes undergo one cell division only, not the 2–4 that phytohemagglutinin alone induces. Reference information on micronuclei incidence still is not available. Micronuclei have been produced by exposure to antineoplastic agents.

Other types of cytogenetic assays include aneuploidy and nuclear aberrations. Aneuploidy occurs when the karyotype is increased or decreased by one or more chromosomes compared with the usual human diploid karyotype. Polyploidy occurs when the entire complement of chromosomes in a cell is increased. Some diseases caused by aneuploidy include Down's and Klinefelter's syndromes. Some tumors may be caused by aneuploidy, and vice versa.

9.3.3 Mutagenesis and Cancer: Overview

It is postulated that cancer is a multistep process initiated by mutations in somatic cells. Mutations in germ cells also are associated with the potential for induction of transmissible genetic diseases, such as those producing developmental backwardness, physical and mental retardations, and reproductive loss. Detection of mutations thus may constitute a predictive biological monitoring marker for the potential development of cancer.

"Point" mutations or "gene-locus" mutations are small changes in a DNA sequence through addition and deletion of a small number of DNA base pairs (Section 10.1.1) or through substitution of incorrect base pairs. (Six are possible: AT → GC, GC → AT, AT → TA or CG, and GC → CG or TA, where A is adenine, T is thymine, G is guanine, and C is cytosine.) These mutations may arise from a new triplet codon; or if the codon for protein synthesis termination is generated in the messenger RNA (DNA coding sequences ATC, ACT, and ACC); or if there is prevention of DNA transcription; or if RNA maturation is prevented.

Addition or deletion of base pairs when the base-pair change is not a multiple of three is termed "frameshift" mutation. Addition or deletion of three base pairs (or multiples of three) could add or delete amino acids from a coded protein. The term "small" is used when fewer than ten DNA base pairs are changed; ten or more DNA base changes are termed "large additions" or "large deletions"; changes $>10^4$ cause visual chromosomal abnormalities (Section 9.3.2).

The link between macroscopic aberrations and DNA mutations is frequently assumed rather than proven. Often several factors need to be present before definite chromosomal abnormalities can be observed under the light microscope, and it is often not clear which factors are the most important, especially in genetic diseases that display multifactorial causality. Conversely, there may only be a sensitivity problem (for example, enough contrast to detect visible changes may require much cell division) or a duration of propagation problem (for example, damage done may need expression before visible changes can occur as for lymphocytes in the G_0 state).

The observation of cell mutants that differ in appearance from typical, characteristic cells has been complemented at the molecular level by the finding that mutant cells contain DNA with atypical nucleotide bases. Agents known to cause higher frequencies of cellular mutants are: physical agents such as ionizing radiation, ultraviolet radiation, and hyperthermia; many chemicals in the diet and the environment; and some viruses. The relationship of initial mutation events in DNA to the altered DNA bases of cancers is still unclear. The repair and protective defenses of the human body are such that one single mutation in a nucleotide base will not generally lead to a mutant DNA, let alone a mutant cell. Even a stable mutation may not cause a cancer.

Yet in health surveillance for exposure to xenobiotics, DNA adducts (DNA with atypical nucleotide bases produced through reaction with the xenobiotic, its metabolites, or activated intermediates) have been postulated to be the earliest predictive markers for a genotoxin (Chapters 10 and 11). The mutant DNA must survive any repair processes, be stable enough to be propagated through cell division cycles, and yet not be so toxic that the cell is killed or impaired. Even if DNA mutants are detected, the advent of cancer is not automatic; not all chemical mutagens are carcinogens. Also, not all carcinogens are mutagenic. Clearly the links between the molecular and the cellular levels are the keys to an understanding of how cancers form.

In contrast to chromosomal aberrations, mutational changes usually are observed indirectly by observing some phenotypic property of the cell or colony of cells altered by the mutation under defined conditions. This may include "forward mutations," involving loss of a normal function, or "back mutations" or "reversions," involving the regaining of a normal function. The three conditions required to observe DNA mutations are: the frequency of atypical phenomena is affected by mutagenic stimuli; the occurrence is a spontaneous event independent of selective conditions; and the phenotype is heritable. Some changes monitored include: morphologic changes such as colony size, shape, and light emission or color in microbiologic systems; wing veination or absence of bristles in *Drosophila melanogaster*; coat color or marking in mice. The genetic basis of these changes has to be demonstrated by mating and back crossing, techniques of classical genetics. Electrophoretic and HPLC changes in proteins and amino acids are increasingly popular techniques for monitoring atypical nucleic acid species [37]. In all these studies, the "unexposed" reference group determines the sensitivity of any changes. Dose–response studies are essential to ensure conditions favorable to expression of mutagenic changes rather than nonexpression caused by toxicity.

Since 1975, the major system for mutagenesis testing has been bacterial, utilizing *Salmonella typhimurium* because of its simplicity, low cost, and speed. The *his* operon in several mutant strains [TA97, TA98 (its predecessor without the ampicillin resistance pKM101 plasmid was TA1538), TA100 (its predecessor without pKM101 plasmid was TA1535), and TA102] is reverted by base-pair substitution, addition, or deletion mutations [38]. The most often used form of the test involves a mutant strain that lacks the phosphoribosyl ATP synthetase required for histidine synthesis, and that cannot grow in a histidine-deficient medium unless a reverse or back mutation occurs. TA100 and TA1535 strains indicate base-pair substitution back mutations, whereas the TA97 and TA98 strains detect frameshift mutations. TA102 strains are sensitive to compounds such as cross-linking and oxidizing agents (such as glyoxal, ultraviolet radiation, and formaldehyde), which are not detected well by the other strains.

Many xenobiotics require biotransformation to be mutagenic, for example, by the endoplasmic reticulum or, much less frequently, by glutathione conjugation. Rat liver microsomes (S_9 fraction—isolated by centrifugation at 9000*g*) thus are usually added to the growth medium containing the mutant strain and the test chemical, and the number of bacterial colonies that are produced is compared with that produced for no microsomal additive and with that of control cultures. A mutagenic response usually is defined as one above a signal-to-noise ratio greater than two relative to control cultures. Positive controls have to be included to assure quality assurance and control. Dimethylsulfoxide is the general solvent for the test chemical or medium to be evaluated because of its membrane-penetrating and broad-range solvent properties. The enzymes and potencies of S_9 fractions vary markedly with inducing agent and from animal to animal with the same inducing agent.

Many chemicals in the absence or the presence of the S_9 fraction have been shown to be mutagenic, and they have been the subject of many books and reviews. Of the 2622 chemicals in the U.S. EPA's Gene-Tox data base in 1986 [39], 1078 had been evaluated in *Salmonella*; and, of these, 603 (56%) were positive, 148 were negative (13.7%), and 327 (30.3%) were unassignable.

An assay for forward mutation to 8-azaguanine drug resistance also has been developed [40]. Most of the data obtained with this technique involve the TM677 strain of *Salmonella typhimurium*. Mutagenicity is scored as the number of 8-azaguanine–resistant colonies formed relative to control colonies. All types of base-pair exchanges, frameshift alterations, large deletions, and insertions are theoretically detected [41], making the forward mutation assay more flexible than the reverse mutation bioassays.

The major mammalian test for mutations is a staple of reproductive investigations with rodents—the dominant lethal test. The male is exposed to a single dose of the test compound and then mated with two untreated females weekly for 8 weeks. The females are exsanguinated before term, and the number and morphology of live embryos and the number of corpora lutea are determined. The mouse specific locus bioassay correlated 64.3% (random concordance was 54.1%) to the *Salmonella* assay, whereas the heritable translocation assay correlated 71.4% (compared with 65.3% for random concordance), both being statistically insignificant differences. *In vitro* diploid human lymphoblast and animal and human fibroblast cell lines also are being increasingly used as screening techniques.

Cancer is defined as existing when: (a) tumors (localized masses of cells growing and dividing uncontrollably) are observed that are not in controls; (b) the tumor incidence is significantly greater than in controls; (c) the tumors develop earlier than in controls; and (d) an increased multiplicity of tumors is seen that is not found in controls. On the molecular level, two mechanisms for carcinogenicity have been proposed: genetic (DNA-reactive) and epigenetic (no direct interaction with DNA). Both are postulated to have oncogenic control; that is, control of mitosis and growth is lost. Mutation is not always bad, however; the selection of cells that are better able to survive their environment through mutations has been postulated to be the basis of evolution, and thus an advantageous trait. Development of hardier crop species is a familiar example.

Conversion of a cell to a neoplastic cell can occur through activation of the xenobiotic or a metabolite to an electrophilic species within cells; through covalent bonding to alter critical macromolecules to form adducts (Chapter 10); through DNA miscoding, errors in replication of DNA, codon transposition, and combinations of these events; through interactions with proteins that regulate gene expression, including enzymes that methylate DNA; and by multiplication of altered cells that are not so changed that they die or cannot undergo division.

Cells that are neoplastic may be dormant until activation (promotion) by promoters, the latter being xenobiotics, their metabolites, or dietary constituents or their intracellular transport forms. At the macroscopic level, benign or preneoplastic lesions (a mass of cells that are clearly different from the surrounding ones, but which are growing and dividing in a controlled way) may become malignant. Genotoxic carcinogens are thought not to exhibit safe threshold doses. Epigenetic carcinogens sometimes do, and also those carcinogens that depend on other promoters for expression of neoplastic behavior. Certain cancers also have a viral cofactor, especially for those chemicals that cause immunosuppression (causing leukemias, lymphomas, or sarcomas).

The sensitivity of the *Salmonella* test relative to carcinogenicity in any animal strain for the chemicals in the U.S. EPA's Gene-Tox data base in 1986 was about 79.9%, the specificity 66.6%, and the accuracy 79.4% [39]. The carcinogens that were not mutagenic included: acetamide, aldrin, 3-amino-1 H-1,2,4-triazole, aniline, auramine O, benzyl violet 4B, butylated hydroxyanisole, carbon tetrachloride, cycasin, *p,p'*-DDE, DDT, diethylstilbestrol, 1,2-dimethylhydrazine, diphenylnitrosamine, ethyl carbamate, FD and C Citrus Red No. 2, hexachloroethane, 1'-hydroxysafrole, natulan, pararosaniline, Ponceau 3R, safrole, sodium saccharin, succinic anhydride, thioacetamide, thiourea, trifluralin, 1,8,9-trihydroxyanthracene, and Trypan blue. The noncarcinogens that were mutagenic were Dexon and α-naphthylamine. The chemical carcinogens that were not mutagenic included the following chemical classes: antimetabolites, aromatic azo compounds, carbamyls and thiocarbamates, halogenated compounds, steroids, cross-linking agents, inorganics, and promoters. Some mutagens that were not carcinogens included quercetin, glutathione, and cystine.

When the known carcinogens of the National Toxicology Program were evaluated for correlation to *Salmonella* mutagenicity, the *Salmonella* test detected 24 out of 44. Mutagenesis in mouse lymphoma cells and chromosomal aberrations and sister chromatid exchanges in Chinese hamster ovary cells were no better bioassays, either alone or in combination with *Salmonella* results [42, 43]. The mouse bone marrow test for chromosomal aberrations or micronuclei detected some known carcinogens that the *Salmonella* assay did not detect [44].

The third major data base for chemical carcinogens [44], the International Agency for Research on Cancer (IARC), now utilizes the results of short-term genetic toxicity in its ranking decisions. Group 1 denotes human carcinogens; group 2 indicates probable human carcinogens with subgroup A being high probability (37 chemicals) and subgroup B low probability (158 compounds);

group 3 constitutes unassignable human carcinogens; and group 4 denotes probable human noncarcinogens (only one chemical, caprolactam).

Other *in vitro* short-term tests that complement bacterial mutagenesis, mammalian mutagenesis, micronucleus, and sister chromatid exchange bioassays include the hepatocyte primary culture DNA repair assay and the cell transformation assay [45]. If only one short-term bioassay is positive, the connection to carcinogenicity is regarded as tenuous. However, if the chemical structure is suggestive of similarity to a known carcinogen [46], or if at least two of the *in vitro* short-term tests are positive, limited *in vivo* assays should be performed. These include the skin neoplasm induction bioassay in mice, pulmonary neoplasm induction in mice, breast cancer induction in female Sprague-Dawley rats, and altered foci induction in rodent liver [45]. Proven activity in more than one of these limited *in vivo* bioassays is unequivocal evidence of carcinogenicity, whereas two positive tests in the *in vitro* short-term bioassays and one positive limited *in vivo* bioassay indicate potential carcinogenicity. Positive tests in one each of the *in vivo* and *in vitro* bioassays indicate that the agent is highly suspect but more testing is required. A negative test in any bioassay is not proof of noncarcinogenicity.

Chronic *in vivo* dose–response bioassays at the maximally tolerated dose using at least two different animal species are finally utilized as a last resort to confirm uncertain results in the other bioassays above; to confirm the results for chemicals that are negative in the initial stages of testing, but where extensive human exposure is likely; and to confirm that an epigenetic mechanism is not present [45].

Most compounds affect human health in three ways: deficiency may cause adverse effects; sufficiency will allow normal functioning; and excess may result in toxicity—either acute, chronic, or both. The thresholds for these effects vary widely among compounds. Also, although selenium as selenite or selenate is an essential element, excess selenium sulfide ingested by female and male Fischer 344 rats and by female B6C3F1 mice causes liver cancer, but does not do so on skin administration, according to studies by the National Toxicology Program. Chemical speciation, oxidation state, and bioavailability considerations obviously are important; yet most toxicologists persist in defining metal carcinogenicity in terms of the elements rather than particular compounds. Thus elements such as arsenic, beryllium, cadmium, chromium, cobalt, lead, nickel, zinc, and iron-carbohydrate are declared carcinogenic in animals, with arsenic, cadmium, chromium, and nickel being the human carcinogens [47, 48]. Interactions of organics and inorganics often cause the results of studies to be uninterpretable, especially where multicomponent exposures occur.

Carcinogenicity may also be dependent on the diet (or lack of it). For example, hepatic lesions developed in male Fischer-344 rats fed AIN-76a diet [49], but not in Sprague-Dawley rats for which the diet was optimal. Human diets are so diverse that it is difficult to prove whether a toxicant is wholly responsible for any observed cancers in epidemiological studies of people exposed to ambient chemicals, especially if the "unexposed" population is not truly unexposed or is not truly matched for interfering cofactors (Chapter 23). The cause-and-effect situation is easier to deal with in the workplace than in broader populations because the exposures are higher in the more confined, windless, conditions, and because other workers doing the same work routine may show the same effects. The frequency of common affliction in environmental exposure and disease is also the basis of epidemiology.

Nevertheless, Ames [50] has postulated that the diet is an important determinant of human cancer because it can contain known procarcinogens, carcinogens, and anticarcinogens, either present naturally or produced by cooking. Any factors that influence the control of the division and growth cycles may promote, initiate, inhibit, or antagonize cancer. The roles of mitogenesis (induced cell division) as related to promoters and/or selective growth of preneoplastic cells also can be important [51], but their influence is hard to detect because of long latency periods in conjunction with multicomponent exposures.

9.3.4 Mutagenesis as a Biological Marker

Yamasaki and Ames published the first paper on the XAD-2 concentration technique for urine mutagens using *Salmonella* in 1977 [52]. Sulfatase and β-glucuronidase enzymes are generally used to hydrolyze conjugates in these studies. Many investigators have detected mutagenic urines after human exposure: to chemicals during antineoplastic drug therapy [53–60] or after occupational exposure of nurses and pharmacists [61–68]; to tobacco smoke [52, 69–76]; to halothane-exposed anesthesiologists [77]; by skin exposure in children wearing sleepwear containing Tris-BP flame retardant [78]; to the chemicals used or produced during rubber manufacture [79]; to the chemicals of an ink factory and a pharmaceutical factory [80]; to the pitch used in carbon electrode production [81]; to the chemicals exposing workers in the sewers of New York State [82]; to coal dust [83]; to the chemicals produced during coal liquefaction [84]; and to individual chemicals such as epichlorhydrin [85], metronidazole [53], niridazole [53], and nitrofurantoin [86]. Eating fried pork and bacon may result in mutagenic urine [87, 88]. People with hepatic cirrhosis [89] and bladder cancer [90, 91] also show mutagenic urine.

Reproducible interlaboratory quantitative mutagenicity has been difficult to achieve because investigators prepare the XAD-2 column differently, poor quality assurance and quality control are utilized, and urine matrices, isolation methods, and inducers of S_9 fractions and S_9 fractions themselves also vary. The concentration technique for the column chromatography step must be optimized for the task at hand, with due concern for using a column washing technique that minimizes toxicity or histidine interference, and for whether passing through more than one column is necessary [60].

Biological fluids other than urine also have been utilized to demonstrate *Salmonella* mutagenicity, for example, bile, serum, gastric fluid, human breast fluid, and peritoneal fluid [92]. Most of these fluids are obtained invasively; so their use is limited. Feces contain mutagens in the ether-extractable fraction, the major mutagen being a pentaene diol of mass spectrometric molecular ion m/z 251 [93]. The compound is the (*S*)-3-(1,3,5,7,9-dodecapentaenyloxy)-1,2-propanediol, produced by colonic bacteria. The polyene concentration has been correlated with the risk of colon cancer. About 3% of the people of North America excrete feces that on extraction with ether have high mutagenic activity [94, 95]. The polyene is unstable in air and in acid conditions.

Organisms other than *Salmonella* have been used for mutagenicity determinations. *Escherichia coli* WP2 *uvr*A strain was used as a base-pair indicator strain for urine from rubber industry workers [79], and from the workers in a factory where pharmaceuticals and veterinary products were synthesized [96]. The fly, *Drosophila melanogaster*, also has been extensively used for mutagenesis assays.

9.3.5 Interrelationships Among the Genotoxicity Bioassays

This topic has been reviewed elsewhere [97, 98].

Ethylene oxide is mutagenic in bacteria, plants, fungi, and insects, causes mononuclear-cell leukemia in rats and probably in humans, and increases the frequencies of sister chromatid exchanges and structural chromosomal aberrations in human peripheral blood lymphocytes [98, 99].

When patients are treated with alkylated cytostatic drugs, their urines are mutagenic to bacteria; and the frequencies of sister chromatid exchanges, chromosomal aberrations, and the occurrence of micronuclei in their peripheral blood lymphocytes increase [98]. *In vitro* testing of the mutagenic urine excreted by patients receiving cyclophosphamide relative to human peripheral blood enclosed in dialysis bags resulted in elevation of sister chromatid frequencies of peripheral lymphocytes in the blood [101]. The present author has utilized an *in vitro* micronucleus bioassay involving peripheral lymphocytes for urines of patients administered antineoplastic drugs (198).

Nurses, who are exposed to far lower doses of neoplastic drugs than patients who are administered drugs, often do not show chromosomal aberrations or sister chromatid exchanges in spite of mutagenic urine [68, 99, 100], although the findings vary with hygienic practices, frequency of handling, protective equipment and clothing, exposure duration, and drug type. The cofactors involved in the correct interpretation of such studies often may be unknown to the designers of the studies.

The urines of tobacco smokers and chewers are mutagenic, but they induced no bone marrow micronuclei on injection into mice, nor did they show significant induction of 8-azaguanine resistance in Syrian hamster V79 cells [74].

9.3.6 Medical Markers of Cancer

The major medical markers for cancer have the disadvantage that they depend on the presence of the cancer itself. However, such markers are invaluable in assessing how effective treatment has been and whether remission has occurred, and in diagnosis. The major markers used have been serum carbohydrate antigens (CA), notably CA-50 [102, 103] and carcino-embryonic antigen or CEA [104], most being detected by monoclonal antibodies (Chapter 11 and Section 13.2). High specificity for cancer type has been claimed—for example, CA-15.3 for breast cancer [105]; CA-125 for ovarian cancer [106]; and CA-50 for colorectal cancer, pancreatic cancer, and cancer of the bile duct [102, 107].

CA-50 exceeding the mean plus three standard deviations for noncancer patients has been found [102] in 50% of patients with early, localized tumors for colorectal adenocarcinomas (75% of advanced cases), in 69% of those with other gastrointestinal carcinomas, in 75% of those with corporeal uterine cancer (88% with cervical cancer), in 90% of those with prostatic cancer, in 52% of those with lung cancer, and in 26 to 67% of those with breast, ovarian, kidney, and urinary bladder carcinoma. CA-50 was unrelated to CEA, the latter also being increased in noncarcinogenic inflammatory diseases such as ulcerative colitis [108].

About 50% of cancer patients show no reaction with CEA [108], a marker first reported in 1965. Because CEA is a component of the glycocalyx of normal epithelial cells, its presence signals a rapid cellular proliferation with disruption of the basement membrane, which increases the blood CEA, a condition often shared by inflammatory diseases such as pneumonia (46%), hepatitis (40%), and chronic obstructive lung disease (57%) that are nonmalignant [109]. Some CEA sensitivities for tumor sites are: gastrointestinal tract, 30%; stomach, 72%; pancreas, 88%; breast, 24%; and respiratory tract, 30% [109].

Although the CA-125 marker appears most diagnostic of ovarian cancer, it has been detected [110] in patients with cancers of the breast (18%), lung adenocarcinoma (43%), lung squamous cell carcinoma (19%), lung small cell carcinoma (25%), all types of lung cancer (33%), colorectal cancer (7%), ovarian cancer (43%), and other types of cancer (19%). Reliance on so-called specific markers for diagnosis of a particular cancer type may be misplaced, not only because they are related to other cancers (false positives) but also because not all people with a cancer type contain the marker (false negatives).

Thus batteries of CA-markers have been utilized to define which people may have cancer, and then specific CA types have been used to indicate the probable tumor site. Even this approach has drawbacks. For instance, Marechal et al. [104] reported CEA, neuro-specific enolase (a "specific" blood enzyme marker for small cell lung cancer), CA-125, CA-19.9, and CA-50 in 38, 23, 54, 41, and 44%, respectively, of the sera from 96 patients with advanced lung cancer. The incidences of false positives in a cohort of 60 patients with nonneoplastic diseases of the lung were: CEA, 3.3%; enolase, 6.7%; CA-15.3, 5%; CA-19.9, 13.3%; CA-50, 33.3%; and CA-125, 53.3%. CEA $>$ 2.5 ng/mL serum was detected in 7.8% of smokers (118/1512) in one study, whereas another investigator detected CEA above 2.5 ng/mL in 11% (19/176) of random samples, most of whom smoked. The cancer status of the smokers in both studies was unknown.

Serum and urinary α-transforming growth factor [111] and plasma sialyltransferase [112] also have been suggested as generalized markers for tumors, as have serum B-protein [113], serum α-fetoprotein [114], and serum cancer procoagulant [115]. Specificity for the α-transforming growth factor marker varied [111] between 14% (pancreatic cancer) and 50% (lung and colon cancers). Similarly, mean plasma sialyltransferase $>$ 1200 U occurred [112] for patients with cancers of the lung, colon, ovaries, cervix, pancreas, prostate, and gastrointestinal tract, but not for breast cancer (mean was 757 vs. control average of 837).

B-protein specificity was better [113] than this, with specificities of 88, 89, 90, 91, 88, 78, 83, 90, and 87% for cancers of the head, neck, gastrointestinal tract, genitourinary tract, respiratory tract, reticulo-endothelial tissues, the skin, breast, and other sites, respectively. The average specificity in over 6000 cancer patients was about 90%. The positives in controls with a variety of noncarcinogenic conditions varied between 5.8 and 12%. Women in the middle to late second trimester through to the end of the third trimester of pregnancy (93% of women) and people severely burned also show elevated B-protein levels.

α-fetoprotein >10 ng/mL serum appears to be indicative of cancer in the liver (80%), but especially teratocarcinomas (>500 ng/mL usually indicates hepatoma) and cancer in testicular germ cells; but elevation occurs also after fetal distress, during pregnancy, and in the presence of neural tube defects, hepatitis, and primary biliary cirrhosis [114]. α-fetoprotein was first reported in 1972. CEA and α-fetoprotein are considered the classic markers for cancer.

A newer marker, a cancer procoagulant as detected with an enzyme-linked immunosorbent assay (ELISA), has been tested on 54 cancer patients—29 with gastrointestinal, 22 with lung (including one with asbestosis), and 3 with urogenital cancer, relative to 20 people with benign cancer and 54 people with no cancer [115]. All of the 13 early-stage cancers were positive (>0.57 microgram/mL) and 31/41 (76%) of the late stage cancers were positive, with an overall 81% sensitivity and 88% specificity. For the sera from the people with no cancers and those with benign lesions, the positives were 90% and 20%, respectively. The early-warning nature of this new marker is promising, but more investigations are required to define its drawbacks. The cancer procoagulant is thought to be an oncofetal protein. Hepatin, citrate, and sodium fluoride anticoagulants provided nonsignificantly different answers, but EDTA anticoagulant caused results to be generally 50% lower and with high variability. Extensive hemolysis and lipemic serum (countered by Liposolve usage) produced false positives.

The only proven reliable early-warning marker is the screening Papanicolou smear for squamous cell carcinoma of the cervix [116]. Other even less specific markers include [114]: chorionic gonadotropin (for germ cell cancer but also elevated during pregnancy), calcitonin [cancers of the thyroid (confirm with pentagastrin provocation test), lung, breast, and pancreas], prostatic acid phosphatase (prostate leukemia), acute lymphocytic leukemia antigen (leukemia), creatine kinase BB (lung, colon, ACTH-producing tumors), lactate dehydrogenase (seminoma and non-Hodgkin's lymphoma), gross cystic disease protein (breast cancer), and lipid-bound sialic acid (lung, breast, prostate, melanoma, carcinoma, and lymphoma cancers).

The relationships of these medical markers to markers discussed in Sections 9.3.1 through 9.3.5 are unknown. The relationships with DNA and protein adducts (Chapters 10–12) are still unresearched.

A whole journal issue recently was devoted to bladder cancer screening in high-risk groups [117]. Exposure to most aromatic amine dyes and nitrogen-containing aromatics is suspected to cause this type of cancer, as well as such industrial processes as the Soderberg process for aluminum. Urine cytology [118], monoclonal antibody markers utilizing flow cytometry [119], urinary autocrine motility factor and tumor cell collagenase stimulating factors [120], and hematuria by dipstick and cytoscopy [121] are the major medical monitoring screening markers. The immunoassay detection of cytokeratin via flow cytometry of bladder epithelia, of ABH antigens in the urothelium, and of tumor-associated antigens has been reported [119]. The tumor-associated antigens are produced by cancerous cells but not by noncancerous ones, and have been extensively studied because of the sensitivity and specificity of the method [117].

The influence of slow acetylation (Section 5.1.4) on increase of bladder cancer incidence is also important [122]. Over 50% of new cases occurred in the elderly >70 years of age, the rate among men being 2.5 times greater than in women, and with a 37% greater incidence in Whites than Blacks [123].

9.3.7 Urinary Thioethers

These are the ultimate urinary end products of the glutathione conjugation pathway, which was discussed in Sections 2.11.4 and 5.1.2. Deactivation of electrophilic deactivating centers in xenobiotics, their activated forms, or their activated metabolites is one of the prime functions of glutathione (Glu–Cys–Gly).

The test considered here is utilized in the total thioethers form rather than individual thioethers for specific chemicals. The total urinary thioether content is related to the glutathione available for conjugation rather than to total body glutathione. Thus, excessive total thioethers may indicate a stress on the glutathione conjugation system, whose chief function is thought to be protection against oxygen toxicity associated with mitochondria [124]. The role of glutathione in human cellular detoxification and repair of cellular injury by chemical agents, ionizing radiation, hyperthermia, and oxygen toxicity has been reviewed [125, 126]. Stress on available glutathione occurs at high exposures of chemicals or physical agents or after multicomponent chemical exposures.

A definite case of saturation of urinary thioethers occurs as a response to antineoplastic drug therapy [59] involving cyclophosphamide, which produces in situ acrolein which is excreted as a urinary thioether [125].

A review on the utility of the total urinary thioethers assay is available [127]. Urinary thioethers result after human exposure to acrylamide, acrylonitrile, allyl alcohol, aniline, benzene, benzyl chloride, biphenyl, carbon disulfide, epichlorhydrin, ethylene dichloride, glycidol, mesityl oxide, methyl acrylate, naphthalene, phenyl glycidyl ether, styrene, vinyl chloride, vinylidene chloride, and *o*-xylene, as well as such complex mixtures as tobacco smoke, antineoplastic drugs during their handling, gasoline, chemical waste incinerators [127], and rubber-plant chemicals [128, 129].

The total thioethers assay was bedeviled by analytical problems until 1980 [127]. The accepted method involves [59] ethyl acetate extractions of acidified urine in the presence of excess salt and evaporation of the ethyl acetate to produce the thioethers, which then are redissolved in water. The sample is split into halves, one half undergoing Ellman reaction with 5,5′-dithiobis-(2-nitrobenzoic acid) and the other half being subjected to alkaline hydrolysis before Ellman reaction. The difference between the two Ellman steps is the total urinary thioether content free of interference from cystine and cysteine conjugates. The normal upper limit [95th percentile) has been found to be 5.9 mmol SH/mole creatinine in Europeans [127] and white Americans [59].

The generation of an electrophile is postulated to be an important initial step toward generation of a moiety that can attack cellular macromolecules including DNA. Most electrophiles with reactive functional groups will form glutathione conjugates, but not compounds such as biphenyl, though PCBs are conjugated [127]. The glutathione conjugates can be excreted in the urine or eliminated in the bile, depending on their molecular weight and water solubility. For example, aflatoxins and bromosulphthalein and such toxic metals as cadmium, mercury, zinc, silver, and copper are found in the bile as glutathione conjugates [130]. The biliary glutathione conjugates generally are hydrolyzed by the enteric flora and fauna in animals including humans [131] with enterohepatic circulation then possible, as well as excretion in the feces for those not hydrolyzed. High glutathione and glutathione transferase and glutathione peroxidase activities are also found in human intestinal mucosa, which are available to react with hydrolyzed species [132].

A thiomethyl shunt pathway is available as an overflow pathway to thioether formation, should the final cysteine thioether *N*-acetyltransferase reaction in the microsomes be inhibited [133]. The shunt pathway involves a cysteine conjugate β-lyase and then a thiol *S*-methyltransferase to produce thiols and methyl thiols, respectively [133]. Methyl chloride in humans mostly is excreted as a thiol rather than as a thioether [127].

It might be noted that the human placental form of glutathione-*S*-transferase (GST-Π), analagous to GST-P or GST 7-7 in rats, has been noted [134] as a new immunohistochemical marker for human colonic carcinoma (53%) and adenocarcinoma (38%), but not for adenomas (11%) and normal mucosa (10%). The enzyme is also found [135] in squamous non–small cell carcinoma (70%) and differentiated adenocarcinomas of the lung (100%).

People with deficiencies of glutathione synthetase show decreased tissue glutathione, accumulate 5-oxoproline in blood plasma and cerebrospinal fluid, and excrete massive amounts of 5-oxoproline in their urine [136]. Such people evidence defective brain function, marked acidosis, and a tendency to hemolysis (also shown by patients with glucose-6-phosphate dehydrogenase and oxidized glutathione reductase deficiencies). GSH deficiency also results in the same symptoms. People with γ-glutamylcysteine synthetase deficiency exhibit increased hemolysis and brain dysfunction, as well as peripheral neuropathy, myopathy, and aminoaciduria. Patients with γ-glutamyl transpeptidase deficiency also show brain dysfunction, as well as urinary excretion of glutathione, γ-glutamylcysteine, and cysteine conjugates.

Urinary mutagenesis and thioether excretion appear correlated in tobacco smokers [137]. Saturation of urinary thioether levels appeared in heavy smokers, who also had the most mutagenic urine. In nonsmokers, the enzymes in the liver need to be induced, as also demonstrated for new workers in rubber plants [129].

9.3.8 Urinary Glucuronides and D-Glucaric Acid

The glucuronic acid metabolic pathway, where individual xenobiotics are excreted as specific glucuronides, was discussed in Section 5.1.1. The two medical monitoring assays considered here are urinary β-glucuronidase, as related to the analysis of total glucuronides, and urinary D-glucaric acid, the nonspecific end product of the glucuronic acid metabolic pathway.

Activities of urinary β-glucuronidase reflect not only liver contributions but those also of the kidney and bladder, thus also affecting urinary concentrations of D-glucaric acid produced from D-glucuronic acid. The intestinal flora also possess high activities of the enzyme, thus facilitating enterohepatic circulation.

To estimate total glucuronides, the β-glucuronidase activity first must be measured in the urine at pH 5 in acetate buffer, and then an excess amount of β-glucuronidase added if the initial enzyme determination is close to zero. The amount of added enzyme reacted is related to the mass of glucuronides present in the urine. The glucuronides of 17-hydroxycorticosteroid have been quantitated [138]. Hydrolysis of glucuronides occurs at pH values below 2 or above 12. Glucuronidation to form *O*-, *N*-, *S*-, and *C*-β-glucuronides [139] from compounds with hydroxy-, amino-, sulfhydryl, and nucleophilic carbon centers, respectively, is the major backup metabolic pathway of the body. This pathway is suitable because tissue glycogen is the ultimate source of the glucose utilized for the synthesis of uridine-5′-diphospho-α-D-glucuronic acid, which is the key activated high energy nucleotide required for glucuronidation. Some compounds known to produce glucuronides during metabolism are: *N*-acetyl-*N*-phenylhydroxylamine, *o*-aminobenzoic acid, bilirubin, disulfiram, estrone, α-ethylhexanoic acid, hexobarbital, meprobromate, methylphenylcarbinol, 2-naphthylamine, phenylbutazone, progesterone, sulfadimethoxine, thiophenol, trichloroethanol, and tripelennamine [138].

Glucuronides below a molecular weight of 250 are cleared through the urine, and those above 350 through the bile. Mixed routes occur for molecular weights between 250 and 350. Deficiency of β-glucuronidase causes mild mental retardation with gingivitis, organomegaly, and, sometimes, corneal clouding.

Although urinary D-glucaric acid concentration does depend on the activity of the hepatic cytochrome P-450 enzymes, the kidney and bladder cytochrome P-450 enzymes also contribute. The presence of urinary β-glucuronidase also suggests that the glucuronides have been hydrolyzed, and that D-glucaric acid content truly reflects the total D-glucuronic acid precursor. The amount of D-glucaric acid also correlates with the total amount of cytochrome P-450 enzyme-inducing drugs administered.

Although an extensive literature exists since D-glucaric acid's discovery as a marker in 1963 [140], it was only in 1983 that the analytical chemistry difficulties in using it were solved [141]. The method of analysis is based on converting D-glucaric acid to its lactone by boiling at pH 1 to 3. The lactone inhibits limpet β-glucuronidase, and the degree of inhibition using phenolphthalein glucuronide as substrate pH 3.8 is proportional to the D-glucaric acid converted to the lactone. The interrun and intrarun coefficients of variation were 7 to 9% and 4 to 6%, respectively. The reference European values for 402 males were 26.9 ± 8.7 μmol/day compared with 29.7 ± 8.4 for females [142]. For the same analytical technique, the values for white American males and females varied [59] between 14 and 54 μmol/day with an arithmetic mean and associated standard deviation of 30.9 ± 11.0 μmol/day, indistinguishable from the European data. The corresponding creatinine-normalized quantity, 20 to 50 μg/g creatinine, showed less interpersonal variation than the daily excretion rate [59].

Compounds found to increase urinary D-glucaric acid in humans include:

acetanilide [143], cyclophosphamide [59], diphenylhydantoin [143], anticonvulsant drugs [144], organochlorine pesticides [145], phenobarbitone [146], 2,3,7,8-TCDD [147], endrin [148–150], and PCBs [151]. A review is available [152].

Times Beach, Missouri residents potentially exposed to 2,3,7,8-TCDD and estrogen therapy exhibited a nonsignificant increase in D-glucaric acid excretion [152] although the effect of smoking was unclear [153]. Alcoholism, early-stage renal disease of children, and liver diseases increase urinary D-glucaric acid, whereas congestive heart failure, starvation, fasting, severe burns, favism, and dystonic reactions to antiemetics decreased the concentration in urine [152].

Dietary calcium D-glucarate in rodents is postulated to serve as an efficient slow-release source of D-glucaro-1,4-lactone, which inhibits serum β-glucuronidase that is essential for hydrolysis of glucuronides of estradiol and 17-ketosteroids, the latter reflecting the endogenous levels of androgens [154, 155]. Dietary calcium D-glucarate inhibited by 70% the mammary tumor development in Sprague-Dawley rats elicited by 7,12-dimethylbenz(a)-anthracene. The applicability to humans who cannot use glucuronic acid to synthesize ascorbic acid (vitamin C in humans) as rodents can is unknown.

9.3.9 Urinary Porphyrins

Many books and reviews exist on the use of urinary porphyrins (Section 2.11.5) as a screening tool [152, 156, 157].

During heme biosynthesis in the liver, uroporphyrinogen, a tetrapyrrole with eight carboxyl groups, is stepwise decarboxylated to hepta-, hexa-, pentaporphyrinogens, and then to coproporphyrinogen [152]. Each of these porphyrinogens may auto-oxidize to the corresponding porphyrin. All of these moieties are found in the plasma and are excreted in small amounts in the urine and feces, depending on their molecular weight. Liver damage induces coproporphyrinuria, which leads to chronic porphyria (Types A, B, and C), latent porphyria, and then overt porphyria cutanea tarda [152].

The last is defined when both uro- and heptacarboxylicporphyrin are raised significantly, and when 45 to 80% is uroporphyrin and 15 to 35% is heptacarboxylicporphyrin. Porphyrinuric levels of total porphyrins are considered [156] to be 200 to 1400 μg/L. Type A porphyria (mildest form, which has two subtypes) is defined when the ratio of copro- to uroporphyrin is greater than 1 (200–600 μg/L of total porphyrins); Type B porphyria occurs when the uro- to coproporphyrin ratio is between 2 and 6 (200–600 μg/L of total porphyrins); and when the latter ratio is 6 to 7, it defines Type C (400–1400 μg/L of total porphyrins), whereas porphyria cutanea tarda or Type D porphyria (>600 μg/L and with skin problems) occurs when the ratio is >7.

Porphyria can be caused by: alcoholism; liver disease; exposure to halogenated aromatic hydrocarbons such as 1,4-dichlorobenzene, hexachlorobenzene, hexabromobenzene, octachlorostyrene, PBBs, PCBs, and 2,3,7,8-tetrachlorodibenzo-*p*-dioxin (2,3,7,8-TCDD), and exposure to halogenated aliphatics such as allyl chloride (possibly), lindane, methyl chloride, and vinyl chloride (Type A porphyria); estrogen; heavy metals; hepatotoxic drugs; hormones; and lead [156]. The lack of uroporphyrinogen decarboxylase can be genetic. A genetic defect is required for liver disease, alcohol ingestion, and estrogen exposure to produce hepatic porphyrias. The nonaromatic compounds require much higher molar doses to produce porphyria than do halogenated aromatic substances [156].

Total porphyrin content integrates over all of these factors to constitute a nonspecific medical monitoring marker in the same fashion as for total thioethers or glucuronides. The difference is that porphyria involves elevated concentrations of naturally occurring compounds, whereas total thioethers and glucuronides are xenobiotic-derived and endogenously derived. In both cases preexposure and postexposure sampling are essential for one to be able to interpret the results.

The pattern of porphyrins present is related to the specific biochemical steps inhibited. Greater uro- and heptaporphyrins and lesser coproporphyrins usually are observed as liver damage progresses from exposure to halogenated aromatic hydrocarbons [152], and these porphyrins can be detected in both plasma and urine. The change of porphyrin pattern qualifies as a biological marker of adverse effect, whereas an irreversible change in total porphyrins occurs when the damage to the liver becomes adverse. Early chronic porphyria thus is reversible, but overt porphyria cutanea tarda is not. Irreversible porphyria occurs mostly after chronic exposures but infrequently after acute exposures unless the dose is high enough to produce overt damage, a condition sometimes occurring in suicide and poisoning cases.

A 1978 study of 115 urine samples form people exposed at Seveso, Italy in the 1976 release of chlorinated phenols containing 2,3,7,8-TCDD showed 84% with an atypical pattern but only 23% with increased porphyrins [158, 159]. PBBs from Firemaster BP-6 in the families affected by a 1973 cattle-feed contamination incident in Michigan caused 47% atypical patterns of 142 samples but no raised levels [160]. The effects were dose-related as well as dependent on time after exposure. The Seveso and Michigan subjects were sampled two years after the original exposure incidents. Victims of the 1968 Yusho incident in Japan involving PCB contamination of rice oil, however, showed no atypical porphyrin patterns ten years after that incident [161]. The same result has been observed for PCBs in some occupational studies [162]. Of 22 people exposed to 2,3,7,8-TCDD–contaminated 2,4,5-trichlorophenoxyacetic acid herbicide, 64% exhibited atypical patterns, and 50% elevated porphyrins [163]. Times Beach, Missouri residents exposed to 2,3,7,8-TCDD–containing soils showed high urinary uroporphyrins and total porphyrins [164]. Of 40 persons with vinyl chloride disease, 75% revealed atypical patterns [165].

The classic case of porphyria cutanea tarda is a mass poisoning in Turkey between 1955 to 1959 due to the consumption of wheat treated with 0.1% hexachlorobenzene used as a fungicide [163]. Over 3000 children were affected. Their symptoms included red or brown urine, undernourishment, enlarged livers, positive liver function tests, sores and blisters, dark pigmentation, hirsutism, and a 10% mortality rate. Even after ten years, many exhibited atypical liver function and skin problems in the summer.

The chronic effect of lead exposure on children and adults is reflected by blood zinc protoporphyrin accumulation as a result of displacement of zinc in such zinc-containing enzymes as red cell, spleen, and liver porphobilinogen synthase, bone mitochondrial ferrochelatase, and liver, renal, bone, and spleen cytosolic δ-aminolevulinic acid dehydratase (ALAD) and mitochondrial synthase (ALAS) [166]. The activities or concentrations of these biological monitoring markers are also dependent on the concentration of dietary and occupational exposures to zinc, especially for young children where zinc deficiency is common. Peaks in zinc protoporphyrin usually lag peaks in blood lead by about 3 months, as this is the average lifetime of red blood cells. A divalent iron/zinc/lead interaction also may be important at low exposure concentrations of lead, suggesting that adequate iron and zinc in the diet must be maintained to prevent toxicity. The effect of lead on the accumulation of blood protoporphyrin was first reported in 1936, and the effect of lead on the utilization of iron in 1948 [166]. Use of the term "free erythrocyte protoporphyrin" or FEP to describe the zinc protoporphyrin concentration arose through the analytical chemistry artifact produced when bloods were acidified to produce protoporphyrin in the older analytical methods. This is similar to the analytical artifacts produced when acidification of urines hydrolyzes conjugates. Normalization with hermoglobin concentration is performed to correct for blood volume changes.

The inhibition of blood and renal ALAD isoenzymes and the resultant accumulation of urinary ALA also have been utilized as biological monitoring markers for low level lead exposure [167] to complement the accumulation of urinary and blood protoporphyrins. A predisposition to lead poisoning has been suggested in individuals with ALAD 1-2 and 2-2 phenotypes, with the $ALAD_2$ allele being more prevalent in Latin Americans, Chinese, and Ashkenazi Jews than in Caucasians and Blacks [167]. Other cations that affect ALAD activity *in vitro* include Al^{3+}, Ag^{+}, Hg^{2+}, Ga^{3+}, and Cu^{2+}, but apart from aluminum overload in dialysis patients there is little evidence for effects of these metal cations in humans. Uroporphyrinogen decarboxylase and coproporphyrinogen oxidase, which both contain thiol groups, have been implicated in the accumulation of specific porphyrins in the urine [168]. Hg^{2+} inhibits uroporphyrinogen decarboxylase more than Fe^{2+} or Pb^{2+}, the lead readily inhibiting only those enzymes with vicinal thiols at the catalytic site such as ALAD [168]. The activity of coproporphyrinogen oxidase is affected more by administration of lead *in vivo* than *in vitro*, implying that changed cellular/organelle permeabilities or indirect effects are responsible for the accumulation of protoporphyrinogen IX.

Prolonged exposure to organic and inorganic mercurials produces porphyria, caused by effects on renal mitochondria [169]. Arsenate exposure in rats causes porphyria by acting on the liver and the kidney [169]. Japanese quails are the preferred animal models for porphyria [163].

Reference ranges for uroporphyrin, coproporphyrin, and protoporphyrin are, respectively [170]: in 24-h urines—3–24, 14–78, and below detection in μg/day; in feces—1–6, 3–24, and 12–85 μg/g dry weight; in blood plasma—0–0.1, 0–0.2, and 0–0.8 μg/dL; in red blood cells—0–0.1, 0–2, and 5–36 μg/dL; and in the liver—0–0.1, 0–0.3 and 0.2–1.3 μg/g dry weight.

9.3.10 Screening with Multiple Nonspecific Medical Monitoring Markers

Sections 9.3.1 through 9.3.9 illustrate the many difficulties of individual nonspecific health surveillance tests. Multiple marker screening on the same biological sample (such as the blood tests used by physicians) has not been much attempted because of costs and sample deterioration. Screening with different markers at different times cannot be compared because the biological status of the human may have changed.

Nevertheless, no correlation between D-glucaric acid (stimulated) and total porphyrins (no effect) for the same urines was seen in workers in the Netherlands exposed to endrin [171], though there was a correlation [172] with D-glucaric acid and urinary concentrations of anti-12-hydroxyendrin (0.13 μg/g creatinine was the threshold below which hepatic enzyme induction was not stimulated). Higher D-glucaric acid (not elevated above the upper reference range, however) and total thioether levels (many above the upper reference range) in urine were noted for workers in a pesticide plant in the Netherlands [173]. Elevated thioethers were found in the smokers in the cohort, whereas levels of D-glucaric acid were not increased [173].

No differences in urinary D-glucaric acid were observed for chemical and coke plant workers in spite of production of mutagenic urine [174]. This study utilized an unoptimized method for D-glucaric acid. The relationship between urinary thioethers and mutagenic urine for smokers was discussed in Section 9.3.7 [137].

Workers exposed to mineral oils in a steel plant showed no elevation in urinary D-glucaric acid but produced mutagenic urine [175]. Workers exposed to chemicals involved with the manufacture of 2,4,6-trinitrotoluene had mutagenic urine but no increased thioether excretion [176].

A study comparing D-glucaric acid, thioethers, and urine mutagenicity for the urines of patients given antineoplastic drugs, notably cyclophosphamide, found no correlation between thioethers and D-glucaric acid, irrespective of preexposure baseline correction [59]. However, the ratio of post- to pre-exposure D-glucaric acid was significantly correlated to the ratio of post- to preexposure thioethers, but mostly because both parameters were saturated at the high doses utilized for chemotherapy, an observation also found for urinary thioethers of heavy smokers [137]. It was suggested [59] that a dose-effect might be detected at lower doses of antineoplastic drugs, and that drug side effects might be minimized by studying this relationship. The urines of patients administered cyclophosphamide and adriamycin could be distinguished by use of the forward and reverse mutation assays of different *Salmonella* strains. There appeared to be no correlation between the concentrations of urinary thioethers, D-glucaric acid, and urinary mutagenicity.

Lead exposure has occasioned the most extensive comparison of nonspecific parameters, usually with blood lead. Such parameters as blood zinc protoporphyrin, blood and urinary ALAD and ALAS, and urinary ALA were discussed in Section 9.3.9 [166–168]. Children one year of age showed [177] a nonlinear dose-related depression of hematocrit reflecting anemia (<35% hematocrit) above blood lead values of 20 μg/dL (defined as background) in an Idaho study. Heme synthesis begins to be inhibited between 10 and 20 μg/dL blood lead (178, 179); vitamin D metabolism at <25 μg/dL of blood lead [180]; peripheral nerve conduction velocity at 20 to 30 μg/dL [181]; and cognitive function at 15 to 20 μg/dL [182]. Some other relationships for adult U.S. workers relative to blood lead in mg/dL include [183]: anemia, >14; blood urea nitrogen [BUN], >20. However, anemia was found in 5% of lead smelter and chemicals workers with blood leads between 40 and 59 μg/dL, in 14%

between 60 and 79, and in 36% above 80; 13% between 40 and 79 μg/dL showed extensor muscle weakness or gastrointestinal symptoms; and BUN was elevated in all but three workers of greater than 4 years work experience. The "safe" blood lead level (no atypical symptoms) for these markers in these workers was about 40 μg/dL. Most of the occupational and environmental exposures are to lead/lead oxide. These data reflect much interindividual variation.

9.3.11 Modified Urinary Purines and Pyrimidines

Dimethyl sulfate, an animal alkylating carcinogen, causes urinary excretion of 7-methylguanine and 1- and 3-methyladenine in rats [184], these constituting 0.16% of the urinary excretion of labeled compounds originating from labeled inhaled dimethylsulfate over 2 days. 7-Methylguanine is a normal constituent of mammalian urine, but 3-methyladenine is not [185]. Similarly, enhanced 7-methylguanine and 1-methylnicotinamide in 24-h urines have been found in rats treated with the animal carcinogens dimethylnitrosamine, 1,2-dimethylhydrazine, methyl methanesulfonate, and *N*-methyl-*N*′-nitrosoguanidine, but not O^6-methylguanine [185].

The elevation of four modified nucleosides and bases in mouse urine after tumor induction by 3-methylcholanthrene was regarded as an early marker of tumor development [186]. These bases were N^4-acetylcytidine, 1-methyladenosine, 5-(β-D-ribofuranosyl)-uracil or pseudouridine, and N^2-methylguanine. Mice with fully developed tumors excreted elevated levels of another nine modified bases and nucleosides.

Human cancer patients also excrete higher levels of modified nucleosides and bases [187–189]; their excretion is related to the activity of human leukemias [188, 190]. Urinary pseudouridine, which is mostly a degradation product of transfer RNA, was increased in patients (16/23) with hepatocellular carcinoma but not for those who were healthy or who had liver cirrhosis [191]. Nine of the 13 patients in Japan who had serum α-fetoprotein below 400 ng/mL showed elevated pseudouridine levels [191]. Clearly more research needs to be done in this area, especially with alkylating anticancer drugs.

Twenty aflatoxin B1 (AFB1)–exposed subjects via the diet in Guangxi Province of China excreted AFB1-N^7-guanine in the urine as well as AFB1 itself [192]. The AFB1 was excreted at 0.1 to 10 μg of AFB1 equivalents/day. AFB1-N^7-guanine was also detected (118/983) in the urine of agrarian people in Kenya [193]. A GC/MS quantitation of urinary 3-methyladenine as a marker of exposure to methylating agents in nine people resulted in levels of 4.5 to 16 μg/day [194].

HPLC analysis of urinary free thymine glycol (0.39 nmol/kg/day) and thymidine glycol (0.10 nmol/kg/day) has also been used as a marker of oxidative DNA damage caused by ionizing radiation and other oxidative agents [195]. Carcinogens may cause indirect DNA damage by being responsible for the formation of free radicals and superoxides that react with DNA and cause molecular lesions, such as thymine glycol [196]. Agents that cause proliferation of peroxisomes or stimulate the arachidonic acid cascade will generate superoxides and hence stimulate excretion of thymine glycol [197].

Further Reading

Blood and Urine Markers

Cella, J. H., and Watson, J. 1989. *Nurse's Manual of Laboratory Tests*, F. A. Davis, Philadelphia, PA, pp. 1–87, 130–207, and 289–311.

Fischbach, E. T. 1988. *A Manual of Laboratory Diagnostic Tests*, 3rd ed., J. B. Lippincott, Philadelphia, PA, pp. 13–69 and 79–160.

Tietz, N. W. 1986. *Textbook of Clinical Chemistry*, W. B. Saunders, Philadelphia, PA, pp. 356–386, 387–409, and 478–518.

Health Surveillance Markers

Brewster, M. A. 1988. Biomarkers of xenobiotic exposures. *Ann. Clin. Lab. Sci.* **18**: 306–317.

Thilly, W. G., and Call, K. M. 1986. Genetic toxicology. In *Casarett and Doull's Toxicology: The Basic Science of Poisons*, 3rd ed., C. D. Klaassen, M. O. Amdur, and J. Doull (eds.), Macmillan, New York, pp. 174–194.

References for Part 3 (Chapters 7–9)

1. Snedecor, G. W.; and Cochran, W. G. 1989. *Statistical Methods*, 8th ed.; Iowa State University Press, Ames, IA.
2. Hansen, H. J.; Snyder, J. J.; Miller, J. J.; Miller, E.; van de Voorde, J. P.; Miller, O. N.; Hines, L. R.; and Burns, J. J. 1974. Carcinoembryonic antigen (CEA) assay: a laboratory adjunct in the diagnosis and management of cancer. *Human Pathol.* **5**: 139–147.
3. Stevens, D. P.; and MacKay, I. R. 1973. Increased carcinoembryonic antigen in heavy cigarette smokers. *Lancet* **II** (7840): 1238–1239.
4. Alexander, J. C.; Jr.; Siverman, H. A.; and Chretien, P. B. 1976. Effect of age and cigarette smoking on carcinoembryonic antigen levels. *J. Am. Med. Assoc.* **235**: 1975–1979.
5. Meeker, W. R.; Jr.; Kashmiri, R.; Hunter, L.; Clapp, W.; and Griffen, W.O.; Jr. 1973. Clinical evaluation of carcinoembryonic antigen test. *Arch. Surg.* **107**: 266–274.
6. U.S. Surgeon General. 1979. *Smoking and Health*, U.S. Dept. Health, Education and Welfare.
7. National Research Council. *Environmental Tobacco Smoke: Measuring Exposures and Assessing Health Effects*, National Academy Press, Washington, DC, pp. 133–159.
8. Young, D. S. 1984. The effects of frequently prescribed drugs on common laboratory procedures. In *Practice of Medicine,* Vol. 1, J. A. Spittell, Jr. (ed.), J. B. Lippincott, Philadelphia, PA, Chap. 26, pp. 1–21.
9. Freed, C. R.; and Yamamoto, B. K. 1985. Regional brain dopamine metabolism: a marker for the speed, direction, and posture of moving animals. *Science* (U.S.A.) **229**: 62–65.
10. Wightman, R. M.; May, L. J.; and Michael, A. C. 1988. Detection of dopamine dynamics in the brain. *Anal. Chem.* **60**: 769A–779A.
11. Maugh, T. H.; II. 1981. Biochemical markers identify mental states. *Science* **214**: 39–41.
12. Rinkel, M.; and Denber, H. (eds.). 1958. *Chemical Concepts of Psychosis*, McDowell and Obolensky, New York.
13. Anon. 1982. Excretion of β-phenethylamine is elevated in humans after profound stress. *Science* (U.S.A.) **215**: 1127–1129.

14. Sabelli, H. C.; Fawcett, J.; Gusovsky, F.; Javaid, J.; and Jeffriess, H. 1983. Urinary phenyl acetate: a diagnostic test for depression. *Science* (U.S.A.) **220**: 1187–1188.
15. Hryhorczuk, L. M.; Novak, E. A.; and Gershon, S. 1984. Gut flora and urinary phenylacetic acid. *Science* **226**: 996 (letter). Also reply by H. C. Sabelli and J. Fawcett.
16. Davis, K. L.; Davidson, M.; Mohs, R. C.; Kendler, K. S.; Dacis, B. M.; Johns, C. A.; DeNigris, Y.; and Horvath, T. B. 1985. Plasma homovanillic acid concentration and the severity of schizophrenic illness. *Science* (U.S.A.) **227**: 1601–1602.
17. Anon. 1982. Schizophrenia: dopamine β-hydroxylase activity and treatment response. *Science* (U.S.A.) **216**: 1423–1425.
18. Kolmodin-Hedman, B.; and Swensson, A. 1975. Problems related to shift work. A field study of Swedish railroad workers with irregular work hours. *Scand. J. Work Environ. Health* **1**: 254–262.
19. Kalimo, R.; Lehtonen, A.; Daleva, M.; and Kuorinka, I. 1980. Psychological and biochemical strain in firemen's work. *Scand. J. Work Environ. Health* **6**: 179–187.
20. Daleva, M.; Piperova-Dalbokova, D.; Hadjiolova, I.; and Mincheva, L. 1982. Changes in the excretion of corticosteroids and catecholamines in tractor-drivers. *Int. Arch. Occup. Environ. Health* **49**: 345–352.
21. Hochachka, P. W. 1986. Defense strategies against hypoxia and hypothermia. *Science* (U.S.A.) **231**: 234–241.
22. Leonard, P. J. 1973. The effects of age and sex on biochemical parameters in blood of healthy human subjects. In *Reference Values in Human Chemistry*, G. Siest (ed.), Karger, Basel, Switzerland.
23. Mourant, A. E.; Kopec, A. C.; and Domaniewska-Sobczak, K. 1978. *Blood Groups and Diseases*, Oxford University Press, Oxford, UK.
24. Wallach, J. 1986. *Interpretation of Diagnostic Tests: A Synopsis of Laboratory Medicine*, 4th ed., Little, Brown, Boston, MA.
25. Liu, P. I. 1986. *Blue Book of Diagnostic Tests*, W. B. Saunders, Philadelphia, PA.
26. Fischbach, F. T. 1988. *A Manual of Laboratory Diagnostic Tests*, 3rd ed.; J. B. Lippincott, Philadelphia, PA.
27. Eastham, R. D. 1985. *Biochemical Values in Clinical Medicine*, 7th ed.; John Wright and Sons, Bristol, UK.
28. Bone, R. C.; and Griffin, K. A. 1990. *The Rush Internal Medicine Handbook*, Year Book Medical Pub.; Chicago, IL.
29. Cella, J. H., and Watson, J. 1989. *Nurse's Manual of Laboratory Tests*, F. A. Davis, Philadelphia, PA.
30. Holroyd, S. V.; Wynn, R. L.; and Requa-Clark, B. 1988. *Clinical Pharmacology in Dental Practice*, 4th ed.; C. V. Mosby, St. Louis, MO.
31. Levine, W. G. 1978. Biliary excretion of drugs and other xenobiotics. *Ann. Rev. Pharmacol. Toxicol.* **18**: 81–96.
32. Cella, J. H.; and Watson, J. 1989. *Nurse's Manual of Laboratory Tests*, F. A. Davis, Philadelphia, PA.
33. Notten, W. R. F.; Herber, R. F. M.; Hunter, W. J.; Monster, A. C.; and Zielhuis, R. L. eds.; 1988. *Health Surveillance of Individual Workers Exposed to Chemical Agents*, Springer-Verlag, Berlin.
34. Carrano, A. V. 1986. Chromosomal alterations as markers of exposure and effect. *J. Occup. Med.* **28**: 1112–1116.
35. Slamon, D. J.; de Kernion, J. B.; and Verma, I. M. 1984. Expression of cellular oncogenes in human malignancies. *Science* (U.S.A.) **224**: 256–262.
36. Carrano, A. V.; and Natarajan, A. T. 1988. Considerations for population monitoring using cytogenetic techniques. *Mutat. Res.* **204**: 379–406.

37. Fini, C.; Floridi, A.; Finelli, V. N.; and Wittman-Liebold, B. eds. 1990. *Laboratory Methodology in Biochemistry: Amino Acid Analysis and Protein Sequencing*, CRC Press, Boca Raton, FL.
38. Ames, B. N.; McCann, J.; and Yamasaki, E. 1975. Methods for detecting carcinogens and mutagens with the *Salmonella*/mammalian microsome mutagenicity test. *Mutat. Res.* **31**: 347–364.
39. Kier, L. E.; Brusick, D. J.; Auletta, A. E.; Von Halle, E. S.; Brown, M. M.; Simmon, V. F.; Dunkel, V.; McCann, J.; Mortelmans, K.; Prival, M.; Rao, T. K.; and Ray, V. 1986. The *Salmonella typhimurium*/mammalian microsomal assay. A report of the U.S. Environmental Protection Agency Gene-Tox program. *Mutat. Res.* **168**: 69–240.
40. Skopek, T. R.; Liber, H. L.; Krolewski, J. J.; and Thilly, W. G. 1978. Quantitative forward mutation assay in *Salmonella typhimurium* using 8-azaguanine resistance as a genetic marker. *Proc. Nat. Acad. Sci. USA* **75**: 410–444.
41. Skopek, T. R.; Liber, H. L.; Kaden, D. A.; and Thilly, W. G. 1978. Relative sensitivities of forward and reverse mutation assays in *Salmonella typhimurium*. *Proc. Nat. Acad. Sci. USA* **75**: 4465–4469.
42. Tennant, R. W.; Margolin, B. H.; Shelby, M. D.; Zeiger, E.; Haseman, J. K.; Spalding, J.; Caspary, W.; Resnick, M.; Stasiewicz, S.; Anderson, B.; and Minor, R. 1987. Prediction of chemical carcinogenicity in rodents from in vitro genetic toxicity assays. *Science* (U.S.A.) **236**: 933–941.
43. Tennant, R. W.; Stasiewicz, S.; and Spalding, J. W. 1986. Comparison of multiple parameters of rodent carcinogenicity and in vitro genetic toxicity. *Environ. Mutagen.* **8**: 205–227.
44. Adler, I. D.; Ashby, J.; and Wurgler, F. E. 1989. Screening for possible human carcinogens and mutagens: a symposium report. *Mutat. Res.* **213**: 27–39.
45. Williams, G. M.; and Weisburger, J. H. 1986. Chemical carcinogens. In *Casarett and Doull's Toxicology: The Basic Science of Poisons*, 3rd ed.; C. D. Klaassen, M. O. Amdur, and J. Doull (eds.) Macmillan, New York, pp. 99–173.
46. Frierson, M. R.; Klopman, G.; and Rosenkranz, H. S. 1986. Structure–activity relationships among mutagens and carcinogens: a review. *Environ. Mutagen.* **8**: 283–327.
47. Sunderman, F. W.; Jr. 1979. Mechanisms of metal carcinogenesis. *Biol. Trace Element Res.* **1**: 63–86.
48. Sigel, H. (ed.). 1980. *Metal Ions in Biological Systems,* Vol. 10: *Carcinogenicity and Metal Ions*, Marcel Dekker, New York.
49. Medinsky, M. A.; Popp, J. A.; Hamm, T. E.; and Dent, J. G. 1982. Development of hepatic lesions in male Fischer-344 rats fed AIN-76A purified diet. *Toxicol. Appl. Pharmacol.* **62**: 111–120.
50. Ames, B. N. 1983. Dietary carcinogens and anticarcinogens. *Science* (U.S.A.) **221**: 1256–1264.
51. Butterworth, B. E.; and Slaga, T. (eds.). 1991. *Chemically Induced Cell Proliferation: Implications for Risk Assessment,* Wiley-Liss, New York.
52. Yamasaki, E.; and Ames, B. N. 1977. Concentration of mutagens from urine by adsorption with the nonpolar resin XAD-2: cigarette smokers have mutagenic urine. *Proc. Nat. Acad. Sci. USA* **74**: 3555–3559.
53. Legator, M. S.; Connor, T. H.; and Stoeckel, M. 1975. Detection of mutagenic activity of metronidazole and niridazole in body fluids of humans and mice. *Science* **118**: 1118–1119.
54. Minnich, V.; Smith, M. E.; Thompson, D.; and Kornfeld, S. 1976. Detection of mutagenic activity in human urine using mutant strains of *Salmonella typhimurium*. *Cancer* **38**: 1253–1258.

55. Rorth, M.; Jorgenson, V.; Knudsen, I.; Larson, J. C.; and Munch, F. 1983. Mutagenicitet i urinen hos sygeplejersker pa onkologisk afdeling. *Ugeskr. Laeg.* **145**: 475–478.
56. Monteith, D. K.; Connor, T. H.; Benvenuto, J. A.; Fairchild, E. J.; and Theiss, J. C. 1987. Stability and inactivation of mutagenic drugs and their metabolites in the urine of patients administered antineoplastic therapy. *Environ. Molec. Mutagen.* **10**: 341–356.
57. Monteith, D. K.; Connor, T. H.; Benvenuto, J. A.; Fairchild, E. J.; and Thiess, J. C. 1988. The mutagenicity of urine fractions from patients administered antineoplastic therapy. *Toxicol. Lett.* **40**: 257–268.
58. Krepinsky, A.; Bryant, D. W.; Davison, L.; Young, B.; Heddle, J.; McCalla, D. R.; Douglas, G.; and Michalko, K. 1990. Comparison of three assays for genetic effects of antineoplastic drugs on cancer patients and their nurses. *Environ. Molec. Mutagen.* **15**: 83–92.
59. Newman, M. A.; Que Hee, S. S.; Schoeny, R. S.; and Lowry, L. 1990. Biological monitoring screening of patients provided antineoplastic drugs including adriamycin, cyclophosphamide, 5-fluorouracil, methotrexate and vincristine. *Cancer Res.* **50**: 3351–3366.
60. Newman, M. A.; Que Hee, S. S.; and Schoeny, R. S. 1990. Mutagenesis assays on urines produced by patients administered adriamycin and cyclophosphamide. *Environ. Molec. Mutagen.* **16**: 189–203.
61. Falck, K.; Grohn, M.; Sorsa, M.; Vainio, H.; Heinonen, E.; and Holsti, L. R. 1979. Mutagenicity in urine of nurses handling cytostatic drugs. *Lancet* **I** (8128): 1250–1251.
62. Nguyen, T. V.; Theiss, J. C.; and Matney, T. S. 1982. Exposure of pharmacy personnel to mutagenic antineoplastic drugs. *Cancer Res.* **42**: 4792–4796.
63. Bos, R. P.; Leenaars, A. O.; Theuws, J. L. G.; and Henderson, P. Th. 1982. Mutagenicity of urine from nurses handling cytostatic drugs, influence of smoking. *Int. Arch. Occup. Environ. Health* **50**: 359–369.
64. Anderson, R. W.; Puckett, W. H.; Dana, W. J.; Nguyen, T. V.; Theiss, J. C.; and Matney, T. S. 1982. Risk of handling injectable antineoplastic agents. *Am. J. Hosp. Pharm.* **39**: 1881–1887.
65. Kolmodin-Hedman, B.; Hartvig, P.; Sorsa, M.; and Falck, K. 1983. Occupational handling of cytostatic drugs. *Arch. Toxicol.* **54**: 25–33.
66. Venitt, S.; Crofton-Sleigh, C.; Hunt, J.; Speechley, V.; and Briggs, K. 1984. Monitoring exposure of nursing and pharmacy personnel to cytotoxic drugs: urinary mutation assays and urinary platinum as markers of absorption. *Lancet* **I**: 74–77.
67. Cloak, M. M.; Connor, T. H.; Stevens, K. R.; Theiss, J. C.; Alt, J. M.; Matney, T. S.; and Anderson, R. W. 1985. Occupational exposure of nursing personnel to antineoplastic agents. *Oncol. Nurs. Forum* **12**: 33–39.
68. Stucker, I.; Hirsch, A.; Doloy, T.; Bastie-Sigeac, I.; and Hemon, D. 1986. Urine mutagenicity, chromosomal abnormalities and sister chromatid exchanges in lymphocytes of nurses handling cytostatic drugs. *Int. Arch. Occup. Environ. Health* **57**: 195–205.
69. Putzrath, R. M.; Langley, D.; and Eisenstadt, E. 1981. Analysis of mutagenic activity in cigarette smokers' urine by high performance liquid chromatography. *Mutat. Res.* **85**: 97–108.
70. Aeschbacher, H. U.; and Chappuis, C. 1981. Non-mutagenicity of urine from coffee drinkers compared with that from cigarette smokers. *Mutat. Res.* **89**: 161–177.
71. Recio, L.; Enoch, H.; and Hannan, M. A. 1982. Parameters affecting the mutagenic activity of cigarette smokers' urine. *J. Appl. Toxicol.* **2**: 241–246.

72. Connor, T. H.; Ramanujam, V. M. S.; Ward, J. B.; Jr.; and Legator, M. S. 1983. The identification and characterization of a urinary mutagen resulting from cigarette smoking. *Mutat. Res.* **113**: 161–172.
73. Sorsa, M.; Falck, K.; Heinonen, T.; Vainio, H.; Norppa, H.; and Rimpelae, M. 1984. Detection of exposure to mutagenic compounds in low-tar and medium-tar cigarette smokers. *Environ. Res.* **33**: 312–321.
74. Menon, M. M.; and Bhide, S. V. 1984. Mutagenicity of urine of bidi and cigarette smokers and tobacco chewers. *Carcinogenesis* **5**: 1523–1524.
75. Kriebel, D.; Henry, J.; Gold, J. C.; Bronson, A.; and Commoner, B. 1985. The mutagenicity of cigarette smokers' urine. *J. Environ. Pathol. Toxicol. Oncol.* **6**: 157–169.
76. Mohtashamipur, E.; Norpoth, K.; and Lieder, F. 1987. Urinary excretion of mutagens in smokers of cigarettes with various tar and nicotine yields, black tobacco, and cigars. *Cancer Lett.* **34**: 103–112.
77. McCoy, E. C.; Hankel, R.; Rosenkranz, H. S.; Giuffrida, J. G.; and Bizzari, D. V. 1977. Detection of mutagenic activity in the urines of anesthiologists: a preliminary report. *Environ. Health Perspect.* **21**: 221–223.
78. Blum, A.; Gold, M. D.; Ames, B. N.; Kenyon, C.; Jones, J. F.; Hett, E. A.; Dougherty, R. C.; Horning, E. C.; Dzidic, I.; Carroll, D. I.; Stillwell, R. N.; and Thenot, J. P. 1978. Children absrob Tris-BP flame retardant from sleepwear: urine contains the mutagenic metabolite, 2,3-dibromopropanol. *Science* (U.S.A.) **201**: 1020–1023.
79. Falck, K.; Sorsa, M.; and Vainio, H. 1980. Mutagenicity in urine of workers in rubber industry. *Mutat. Res.* **79**: 45–52.
80. Dolara, P.; Mazzoli, S.; Rosi, D.; Buiatti, E.; Baccetti, S.; Turchi, A.; and Vannucci, V. 1981. Exposure to carcinogenic chemicals and smoking increases urinary excretion of mutagens in humans. *J. Toxicol. Environ. Health* **8**: 95–103.
81. Pasquini, R.; Monarca, S.; Sforzolini, G. S.; Conti, R.; and Fagioli, F. 1982. Mutagens in urine of carbon electrode workers. *Int. Arch. Occup. Environ. Health* **50**: 387–395.
82. Scarlett-Kranz, J. M.; Babish, J. G.; Stickland, D.; Goodrich, R. M.; and Lisk, D. J. 1986. Urinary mutagens in municipal sewage workers and water treatment workers. *Am. J. Epidemiol.* **124**: 884–893.
83. Whong, W. Z.; Long, R.; Ames, R. G.; and Ong, T. 1983. Role of nitrosation in the mutagenic activity of coal dust: a postulation for gastric carcinogenesis in coal miners. *Environ. Res.* **32**: 298–304.
84. Recio, L.; Enoch, H. G.; Hannan, M. A.; and Hill, R. H. 1984. Application of urine mutagenicity to monitor coal liquefaction workers. *Mutat. Res.* **136**: 201–207.
85. Wang, C. Y.; Benson, R. C.; Jr.; and Bryan, G. T. 1977. Mutagenicity for *Salmonella typhimurium* of urine obtained from humans receiving nitrofurantoin. *J. Nat. Cancer Inst.* **58**: 871–873.
86. Kilian, D. J.; Pullin, T. G.; Connor, T. H.; Legator, M. S.; and Edwards, H. N. 1978. Mutagenicity of epichlorhydrin in the bacterial assay system: evaluation by direct *in vitro* activity of urine from exposed humans and mice. *Mutat. Res.* **53**: 72, 1978.
87. Baker, R.; Arlauskas, A.; Bonin, A.; and Angus, D. 1982. Detection of mutagenic activity in human urine following fried pork or bacon meals. *Cancer Lett.* **16**: 81–89.
88. Dolara, P.; Caderni, G.; Salvatori, M.; Tringale, L.; and Lodovici, M. 1984. Urinary mutagens in humans after fried pork and bacon meals. *Cancer Lett.* **22**: 275–280.

89. Gelbart, S. M.; and Sontag, S. J. 1980. Mutagenic urine in cirrhosis. *Lancet* **I**: 894–896.
90. Garner, R. C.; Mould, A. J.; Lindsay-Smith, V.; Cartwright, R. A.; and Richards, B. 1982. Mutagenic urine from bladder cancer patients. *Lancet* **II**: 389.
91. Everson, R. B.; Gad-el-Mawla, N. M.; Attia, M. A. M.; Chevlen, E. M.; Thorgeirsson, S. S.; Alexander, L. A.; Flack, P. M.; Staiano, N.; and Ziegler, J. L. 1983. Analysis of human urine for mutagens associated with carcinoma of the bilharzial bladder by the Ames *Salmonella* plate assay. *Cancer* **51**: 371–377.
92. Working Group on Body Fluid Analysis. 1982. Body fluid analysis. *Mutat. Res.* **98**: 355–374.
93. Hirai, N.; Kingston, D. G. I.; Van Tassell, R. L.; and Wilkins, T. D. 1982. Structure elucidation of a potent mutagen from human feces. *J. Am. Chem. Soc.* **104**: 6149–6150.
94. Bruce, W. R.; Varghese, A. J.; Land, P. C.; and Krepinsky, J. J. F. 1981. Banbury Report 7. *Gastrointestinal Cancer: Endogenous Factors*, W. R. Bruce, P. Correa, M. Lipkin, S. R. Tannenbaum, and T. D. Wilkins (eds.), Cold Spring Harbor Laboratory, Cold Spring Harbor, New York, pp. 227–238.
95. Wilkins, T. D.; Lederman, M.; and van Tassel, R. L. 1982. Banbury Report 7. *Gastrointestinal Cancer: Endogenous Factors*, W. R. Bruce, P. Correa, M. Lipkin, S. R. Tannenbaum, T. D. Wilkins, (eds.), Cold Spring Harbor Laboratory, Cold Spring Harbor, New York, pp. 205–214.
96. Hagmar, L.; Bellander, T.; Persson, L.; Holmen, A.; Attewell, R.; Hogstedt, B.; and Skerfving, S. 1988. Biological effects in a chemical factory with mutagenic exposure. III Urinary mutagenicity and thioether excretion. *Int. Arch. Environ. Health* **60**: 453–456.
97. Vainio, H.; Sorsa, M.; Rantanen, J.; Hemminki, K.; and Aitio, A. 1981. Biological monitoring in the identification of the cancer risk of individuals exposed to chemical carcinogens. *Scand. J. Work Environ. Health* **7**: 241–251.
98. Vainio, H. 1985. Current trends in the biological monitoring of exposure to carcinogens. *Scand. J. Work Environ. Health* **11**: 1–6.
99. Krepinsky, A.; Bryant, D. W.; Davison, L.; Young, B.; Heddle, J.; McCalla, D. R.; Douglas, G.; and Michalko, K. 1990. Comparison of three assays for genetic effects of antineoplastic drugs on cancer patients and their nurses. *Environ. Molec. Mutagen.* **15**: 83–92.
100. Sorsa, M.; Pyy, L.; Salomaa, S.; Nylund, L.; and Yager, J. W. 1988. Biological and environmental monitoring of occupational exposure to cyclophosphamide in industry and hospitals. *Mutat. Res.* **204**: 465–479.
101. Stiller, A.; Obe, G.; Riedel, L.; Riehm, H.; and Kappes, C. 1982. Mutagens in human urine: test with human peripheral lymphocytes. *Mutat. Res.* **97**: 437–447.
102. Holmgren, J.; Lindholm, L.; Persson, B.; Lagergard, T.; Nilsson, O.; Svennerholm, L.; Rudenstam, C. M.; Unsgaard, F.; Yngvason, F.; Pettersson, S.; and Killander, A. F. 1984. Detection by monoclonal antibody of carbohydrate antigen CA-50 in serum of patients with carcinoma. *Br. Med. J.* **288**: 1479–1482.
103. Eastham, R. D. 1985. *Biochemical Values in Clinical Medicine*, 7th ed.; John Wright and Sons, Bristol, UK.
104. Marechal, F.; Berthiot, G.; and Deltour, G. 1988. Serum levels of CA-50, CA-19.9, CA-125, CA-15.3, enolase and carcinoembryonic antigen in non-neoplastic diseases of the lung. *Anticancer Res.* **8**: 677–680.
105. Hilkins, J. 1984. Monoclonal antibodies against human milk fat globule membrane detecting differentiation antigens of the mammary glands and its tumors. *Int. J. Cancer* **34**: 197–206.
106. Bast, R. C.; and Knapp, R. C. 1987. The emerging role of monoclonal antibodies in the clinical management of epithelial ovarian carcinoma. In *Important Advances*

in Oncology 1987, V. T. De Vita, S. Hellman, and S. A. Rosenberg (eds.), J. B. Lippincott, Philadelphia, PA, pp. 39–53.

107. Itzokowitz, S. H.; and Kim, Y. S. 1986. New carbohydrate tumor markers. *Gastroenterology* **190**: 491–493.
108. Laurence, D. J. R.; and Neville, A. M. 1981. Biochemical tests in diagnosis and monitoring of cancer. *Clin. Biochem. Rev.* **2**: 135–161.
109. Beatty, J. D.; and Terz, J. J. 1982. Value of carcinoembryonic antigen in clinical medicine. *Prog. Clin. Cancer* **8**: 9–29.
110. Kawahara, M.; Terasaki, P. I.; Chia, D.; Johnson, C.; Hermes, M.; and Tokita, K. 1986. Use of four monoclonal antibodies to detect tumor markers. *Cancer* **58**: 2008–2012.
111. Arteaga, C. L.; Hanauske, A. R.; Clark, G. M.; Osborne, C. K.; Hazarika, P.; Pardue, R. L.; Tio, F.; and Von Hoff, D. D. 1988. Immunoreactive alpha transforming growth factor activity in effusions from cancer patients as a marker of tumor burden and patient prognosis. *Cancer Res.* **48**: 5023–5028.
112. Dwivedi, C.; Dixit, M.; and Hardy, R. E.; 1988. Plasma sialyltransferase as a tumor marker. *Cancer Detect. Prevent.* **11**: 191–196.
113. Bucovaz, E. T. 1983. An assessment of serological testing for cancer and the B-protein assay. *IRCS Med. Sci.* **11**: 1–4.
114. Fischbach, F. 1988. *A Manual of Laboratory Diagnostic Tests*, 3rd ed.; J. B. Lippincott, Philadelphia, PA, pp. 514–517.
115. Gordon, S. G.; and Cross, B. A. 1990. An enzyme-linked immunosorbent assay for cancer procoagulant and its potential as a new tumor marker. *Cancer Res.* **50**: 6229–6234.
116. Lunt, R. 1984. Worldwide early detection of cervical cancer. *Obstet. Gynecol.* **63**: 708–713.
117. Schulte, P. A.; Halperin, W. E.; Ward, E. M.; and Ruder, A. M. 1990. Bladder cancer screening in high-risk groups. *J. Occup. Med.* **32**: 787–945.
118. Farrow G. M. 1990. Urine cytology in the detection of bladder cancer: a critical approach. *J. Occup. Med.* **32**: 817–821.
119. Melamed, M. R. 1990. Flow cytometry detection and evaluation of bladder tumors. *J. Occup. Med.* **32**: 829–833.
120. Guirguis, R.; Javadpour, N.; Sharareh, S.; Biswas, C.; El-Amin, W.; Mansur, I.; and Kim, J. S. 1990. A new method for evaluation of urinary autocrine motility factor and tumor cell collagenase stimulating factor as markers for urinary tract cancers. *J. Occup. Med.* **32**: 846–853.
121. Mason, T. J.; and Vogler, W. J. 1990. Bladder cancer screening at the du Pont Chambers works: a new initiative. *J. Occup. Med.* **32**: 874–877.
122. Hanke, J.; and Krajewska, B. 1990. Acetylation phenotypes and bladder cancer. *J. Occup. Med.* **32**: 917–918.
123. Smart, C. R. 1990. Bladder cancer survival statistics. *J. Occup. Med.* **32**: 926–928.
124. Fahey, R. C.; Newton, G. L.; Arrick, B.; Overdank-Bogart, T.; and Aley, S. B. 1984. *Entamoeba histolytica*: a eukaryote without glutathione metabolism. *Science* (U.S.A.) **224**: 68–72.
125. Arrick, B. A.; and Nathan, C. F. 1984. Glutathione metabolism as a determinant of therapeutic efficiency: a review. *Cancer Res.* **44**: 4224–4232.
126. Vina, J. 1990. *Glutathione: Metabolism and Physiological Functions*, CRC Press, Boca Raton, FL.
127. van Doorn, R.; Leijdekkers, Ch. M.; Bos, R. P.; Brouns, R. M. E.; and Henderson, P. Th. 1981. Detection of human exposure to electrophilic compounds by assay of thioether detoxication products in urine. *Ann. Occup. Hyg.* **24**: 77–92.
128. Kilpikari, I. 1981. Correlation of urinary thioethers with chemical exposure in a rubber plant. *Br. J. Ind. Med.* **38**: 98–100.

129. Kilpikari, I.; and Savolainen, H. 1982. Increased urinary excretion of thioether in new rubber workers. *Br. J. Ind. Med.*. **39**: 401–403.
130. Gonzalez, J., and Esteller, A. 1990. Glutathione and hepatobiliary transport of xenobiotics. In *Glutathione: Metabolism and Physiological Functions*, J. Vina (ed.), CRC Press, Boca Raton, FL.
131. Bakke, J. E.; and Gustafsson, J. A. 1986. Role of intestinal flora in metabolism of agrochemicals conjugated with glutathione. *Xenobiotica* **16**: 1047–1056.
132. Siegers, C. P.; Bose-Younes, H.; Thies, E.; Hoppenkamps, R.; and Younes, M. 1984. Glutathione and GSH-dependent enzymes in the tumorous and non-tumorous mucosa of the human colon and rectum. *J. Clin. Res. Clin. Oncol.* **107**: 238–241.
133. Jakoby, W. B.; Stevens, J.; Duffel, M. W.; and Weisiger, R. A. 1984. The terminal enzymes of mercapturate formation and the thiomethyl shunt. *Rev. Biochem. Toxicol.* **6**: 97–115.
134. Kodate, C.; Fukushi, A.; Narita, T.; Kudo, H.; Soma, Y.; and Sato, K. 1986. Human placental form of glutathione *S*-transferase (GST-pi) as a new immunohistochemical marker for human colonic carcinoma. *Jap. J. Cancer Res.*. **77**: 226–229.
135. Eimoto, H.; Tsutsumi, M.; Nakajima, A.; Yamamoto, K.; Takashima, Y.; Maruyama, H.; and Konishi, Y. 1988. Expression of the glutathione *S*-transferase placental form in human lung carcinomas. *Carcinogenesis* **9**: 2325–2327.
136. Meister, A. 1983. Selective modification of glutathione metabolism. *Science* (U.S.A.) **220**: 472–477.
137. van Doorn, R.; Bos, R. P.; Leijdekkers, Ch. M.; Wagenaas-Zegers, M. A. P.; Theuws, J. L. G.; and Henderson, P. Th. 1979. Thioether concentration and mutagenicity of urine from cigarette smokers. *Int. Arch. Occup. Environ. Health* **43**: 159–166.
138. Furuya, E. 1977. Effect of sodium sulfate on the hydrolysis of 17-hydroxy-corticosteroid- and *p*-nitrophenyl glucuronides with β-glucuronidase preparations from bovine liver. *Clin. Chem.* **23**: 982–985.
139. Sipes, I. G.; and Gandolfi, A. J. 1986. Biotransformation of toxicants. In *Casarett and Doull's Toxicology: The Basic Science of Poisons* 3rd ed.; C. D. Klaassen, M. O. Amdur, and J. Doull (eds.), Macmillan, New York, pp. 64–98.
140. Marsh, C. A. 1963. Metabolism of D-glucuronolactone in mammalian systems. Identification of D-glucaric acid as a normal constitutent of urine. *Biochem. J.* **86**: 77–86.
141. Colombi, A.; Maroni, M.; Antonini, C.; Cassina, T.; Gambini, A.; and Foa, V. 1983. Low-pH method for the enzymatic assay of D-glucaric acid in urine. *Clin. Chim. Acta* **128**: 337–347.
142. Colombi, A.; Maroni, M.; Antonini, C.; Fait, A.; Zoccheti, C.; and Foa, V. 1983. Influence of sex, age and smoking habits on the urinary excretion of D-glucaric acid. *Clin. Chim. Acta* **128**: 349–358.
143. Cunningham, J. L.; and Price Evans, D. A. 1974. Urinary D-glucaric acid excretion and acetanilide pharmacokinetics before and during diphenylhydantoin administration. *Eur. J. Clin. Pharmacol.* **7**: 387–391.
144. Latham, A. H.; 1974. D-Glucaric acid as an index of hepatic enzyme induction by anticonvulsant drugs in man. *J. Pharm. Pharmacol.* **26**: 284–286.
145. Hunter, J.; Maxwell, J. D.; Steward, D. A.; and Williams, R. 1972. Increased hepatic enzyme activity from occupational exposure to certain organochlorine pesticides. *Nature* (London) **237**: 399–401.
146. Lecamwasam, D. S.; Franklin, C.; and Turner, P. 1975. Effect of phenobarbitone on hepatic drug-metabolizing enzymes and urinary D-glucaric acid excretion in man. *Br. J. Clin. Pharmacol.* **2**: 257–262.

147. Ideo, G.; Bellati, G.; Bellobuono, A.; Mocarelli, P.; Marocchi, A.; and Brambella, P. 1982. Increased urinary D-glucaric acid excretion by children living in an area polluted with tetrachlorodibenzo-para-dioxin (TCDD). *Clin. Chim. Acta* **120**: 273–283.
148. Notten, W. R. F.; and Henderson, P. T. 1977. The interaction of chemical compounds with the functional state of the liver. II. Estimation of changes in D-glucaric acid synthesis as a method for diagnosing exposure to xenobiotics. *Int. Arch. Occup. Environ. Health* **38**: 209–220.
149. Ottevanger, C. F.; and van Sittert, N. J. 1979. Relation between *anti*-12-hydroxyendrin excretion and enzyme induction in workers involved in the manufacture of endrin. In *Chemical Porphyria in Man*, J. J. T. W. A. Strik and J. H. Koeman (eds.), Elsevier/North-Holland Biomedical Press, New York, pp. 123–129.
150. Vrij-Standhardt, W. G.; Strik, J. J. T. W. A.; Ottevanger, C. F.; and van Sittert, N. J. 1979. Urinary D-glucaric acid and urinary total porphyrin excretion in workers exposed to endrin. In *Chemical Porphyria in Man*, J. J. T. W. A. Strik and J. H. Koeman (eds.), Elsevier/North-Holland Biomedical Press, New York, pp. 113–121.
151. Maroni, M.; Colombi, A.; Antonini, C.; Cassina, T.; and Foa, V. 1981. D-Glucaric acid urinary excretion as a tool for biological monitoring in occupational medicine. *Organ Directed Toxicity: Chemical Indices and Mechanism*, S. S. Brown and D. S. Davies (eds.), Pergamon Press, Oxford, UK, pp. 161–168.
152. Brewster, M. A. 1988. Biomarkers of xenobiotic exposures. *Ann. Clin. Lab. Science* **18**: 306–317.
153. Pasquini, R.; Monarca, S.; Sforzoline, G. S.; Savino, A.; and Angeli, G. 1985. Mutagenicity studies and D-glucaric acid determinations in urine of workers exposed to mineral oil. *Int. Arch. Occup. Environ. Health* **56**: 275–284.
154. Walaszek, Z.; Hanausek-Walaszek, M.; Minton, J. P.; and Webb, T. E. 1986. Dietary glucarate as anti-promoter of 7,12-dimethylbenz(a)anthracene-induced mammary tumorigenesis. *Carcinogenesis* **7**: 1463–1466.
155. Walaszek, Z.; Hanausek-Walaszek, M.; and Webb, T. E. 1986. Dietary glucarate-mediated reduction of sensitivity of murine strains to chemical carcinogenesis. *Cancer Lett.* **33**: 25–32.
156. Strik, J. J. T. W. A.; and Koeman, J. H. (eds.). 1979. *Chemical Porphyria in Man*, Elsevier/North-Holland Biomedical Press, Amsterdam, The Netherlands.
157. Silbergeld, E. K., and Fowler, B. A., (eds.), 1987. *Mechanisms of chemical-induced porphyrinopathies. Ann. New York Acad. Sci.* Vol. 514, New York.
158. Centen, A. H. J.; Strik, J. J. T. W. A.; and Colombi, A. 1979. Coproporphyrinuria and chronic hepatic porphyria Type A found in people from Seveso (Italy) exposed to 2,3,7,8-tetrachloro-*p*-dioxin (TCDD). In reference 156, pp. 75–81.
159. Colombi, A. M. 1979. Subjective symptomatology prevalence as an additional criterion to define risk-groups exposed to TCDD in the Seveso area. In reference 156, pp. 83–106.
160. Strik, J. J. T. W. A.; Doss, M.; Schraa, G.; Robertson, L. W.; von Tiepermann, R.; and Hermson, E. G. M. 1979. Coproporphyrinuria and chronic hepatic porphyria Type A found in farm families from Michigan (U.S.A.) exposed to polybrominated biphenyls (PBB). In reference 156, pp. 29–54.
161. Strik, J. J. T. W. A.; Kip, H.; Yoshimura, T.; Masuda, Y.; and Hermsen, E. G. M. 1979. Porphyrins in the urine of Yusho patients. In reference 156, pp. 63–79.
162. Colombi, A.; Maroni, M.; Feriolo, A.; Castoldi, M.; Jun, L. K.; Valla, C.; and Foa, V. 1979. Increase in urinary porphyrin excretion in workers exposed to polychlorinated biphenyls. *J. Appl. Toxicol.* **2**: 117–121.

163. Strik, J. J. T. W. A. 1979. The occurrence of chronic hepatic porphyria in man caused by halogenated hydrocarbons. In reference 156, pp. 3–9.
164. Hoffman, R. E.; Stehr-Green, P. A.; Webb, K. B.; Evans, R. G.; Knutsen, A. P.; Schramm, W. R.; Staake, J. L.; Gibson, B. B.; and Steinberg, K. K. 1986. Health effects of long-term exposure to 2,3,7,8-tetrachlorodibenzo-*p*-dioxin. *J. Am. Med. Assoc.* **255**: 2031–2038.
165. Lange, C. E.; Block, H.; Veltman, G.; and Doss, M. 1976. Urinary porphyrins among PVC workers. In *Porphyrins in Human Diseases*, M. Doss (ed.), Karger, Basel, Switzerland.
166. Labbe, R. F.; Rettmer, R. L.; Shah, A. G.; and Turnlund, J. R. 1987. Zinc protoporphyrin: past, present and future. In reference 157, pp. 7–14.
167. Astrin, K. H.; Bishop, D. F.; Wetmur, J. G.; Kaul, B.; Davidow, B.; and Desnick, R. J. 1987. δ-aminolevulinic acid dehydratase isozymes and lead toxicity. In reference 157, pp. 23–29.
168. Woods, J. S., and Fowler, B. A. 1987. Metal alteration of uroporphyrinogen decarboxylase and coproporphyrinogen oxidase. In reference 157, pp. 55–64.
169. Fowler, B. A.; Oskarsson, A.; and Woods, J. S. 1987. Metal- and metalloid-induced porphyrinurias. In reference 157, pp. 172–182.
170. Doss, M. 1979. Normal ranges of porphyrins and precursors in human tissue, urine and feces. In reference 156, p. 221.
171. Vrij-Standhardt, W. G.; Strik, J. J. T. W. A.; Ottevanger, C. F.; and van Sittert, N. J. 1979. Urinary D-glucaric acid and urinary total porphyrin excretion in workers exposed to endrin. In reference 156, pp. 113–121,
172. Ottevanger, C. F.; and van Sittert, N. J. 1979. Relation between *anti*-12-hydroxy-endrin excretion and enzyme induction in workers involved in the manufacture of endrin. In reference 156, pp. 123–129.
173. Seutter-Berlage, F.; Wagenaars-Zegers, M. A. P.; Hoog Antink, J. M. T.; and Custers, H. A. F. M. 1979. Urinary thioether and D-glucaric acid excretion after industrial exposure to pesticides. In reference 156, pp. 131–135.
174. Kriebel, D.; Commoner, B.; Bollinger, D.; Bronsdon, A.; Gold, J.; and Henry, J. 1983. Detection of occupational exposure to genotoxic agents with a urinary mutagenicity assay. *Mutat. Res.* **108**: 67–79.
175. Pasquini, R.; Monarca, S.; Sforzolini, G. S.; Savino, A.; and Angeli, G. 1985. Mutagenicity studies and D-glucaric acid determination in urine of workers exposed to mineral oil. *Int. Arch. Occup. Environ. Health* **56**: 275–284.
176. Ahlborg, G.; Jr.; Bergstrom, B.; Hogstedt, C.; Einisto, P.; and Sorsa, M. 1985. Urinary screening for potentially genotoxic exposures in a chemical industry. *Br. J. Ind. Med.* **42**: 691–699.
177. Schwartz, J.; Landrigan, P. J.; Baker, E. L.; Jr.; Orenstein, W. A.; and von Lindern, I. H. 1990. Lead-induced anemia: dose–response relationships and evidence for a threshold. *Am. J. Public Health* **80**: 165–168.
178. Piomelli, S.; Seaman, C.; Zullow, D.; Curran, A.; and Davidow, B. 1982. Threshold for lead damage to heme synthesis in urban children. *Proc. Nat. Acad. Sci. USA* **79**: 3335–3339.
179. Hernberg, S. 1976. Biochemical, subclinical, and clinical responses to lead and their relation to different exposure levels. As indicated by the concentration of lead in blood. In *Effects and Dose–Response Relationships of Toxic Metals*, W. Nordberg (ed.), Elsevier, Amsterdam, The Netherlands.
180. Rosen, J. F.; Chesney, R. W.; Hamstra, A.; De Luca, H. F.; and Mahaffey, K. R. 1980. Reduction in 1,2,5-dihydroxyvitamin D in children with increased lead absorption. *New. Engl. J. Med.* **316**: 1037–1043.
181. Schwartz, J.; Landrigan, P. J.; Feldman, R. G.; Baker, E. L. Jr.; and von Lindern, I. H. 1988. Threshold effect in lead-induced peripheral neuropathy. *J. Pediatr.* **112**: 12–17.

182. Bellinger, D.; Leviton, A.; Waternaux, C.; Needleman, H.; and Rabinowitz, M. 1987. Longitudinal analysis of prenatal and postnatal lead exposure and early cognitive development. *New Engl. J. Med.* **316**: 1037–1043.
183. Baker, E. L.; Jr.; Landrigan, P. J.; Barbour, A. G.; Cox, D. H.; Folland, D. S.; Ligo, R. N.; and Throckmorton, J. 1979. Occupational lead poisoning in the United States: clinical and biochemical findings related to blood lead levels. *Br. J. Ind. Med.* **36**: 314–322.
184. Lofroth, G.; Osterman-Golkar, S.; and Wennerberg, R. 1974. Urinary excretion of methylated purines following inhalation of dimethyl sulfate. *Experientia* **30**: 641–642.
185. Shaikh, B.; Huang, S.-K. S.; and Pontzer, N. J. 1980. Urinary excretion of methylated purines and 1-methylnicotinamide following administration of methylating carcinogens. *Chem. Biol. Interact.* **30**: 253–256.
186. Thomale, J.; and Nass, G. 1982. Elevated urinary excretion of RNA catabolites as an early signal of tumor development in mice. *Cancer Lett.* **15**: 149–159.
187. Gehrke, C. W.; Kuo, K. C.; Davis, G. E.; Suits, R. D.; Waalkes, T. P.; and Borek, E. 1978. Quantitative high-performance liquid chromatography of nucleosides in biological materials. *J. Chromatogr.* **150**: 455–476.
188. Schoch, G.; and Heller-Schoch, G. 1977. Molekularbiologie und klinische Bedeutung des stoffwechsels normaler und modifizierter Nucleobasen. *Helv. Paediatr. Acta Suppl.* **38**: 7–171.
189. Waalkes, T. P.; Gehrke, C. W.; Zumwalt, R. W, Chang, S. Y.; Lakings, D. B.; Tormey, D. C.; Ahmann, D. L.; and Moertel, C. G. 1975. The urinary excretion of nucleosides of ribonucleic acid by patients with advanced cancer. *Cancer* **36**: 390–398.
190. Schoch, G.; Garbrecht, M.; Heller-Schoch, G.; Baisch, H.; and Leifer, W. 1979. Die Ausscheidung von normalen und modifizierten Nucleobasen im Urin bei chronischen meyloproliferativen Syndromen. *Blut* **38**: 391–396.
191. Tamura, S.; Amuro, Y.; Nakano, T.; Fujii, J.; Moriwaki, Y.; Yamamoto, T.; Hada, T.; and Higashino, K. 1986. Urinary excretion of pseudouridine in patients with hepatocellular carcinoma. *Cancer* **57**: 1571–1575.
192. Groopman, J. D.; Donahue, P. R.; Zhu, J.; Chen, J.; and Wogan, G. N. 1985. Aflatoxin metabolism in humans: detection of metabolites and nucleic acid adducts in urine by affinity chromatography. *Proc. Nat. Acad. Sci. USA* **82**: 6492–6496.
193. Autrup, H.; Seremet, T.; Wakhisi, J.; and Wasunna, A. 1987. Aflatoxin exposure measured by urinary excretion of aflatoxin B1-guanine adduct and hepatitis B virus infection in areas with different liver cancer incidence in Kenya. *Cancer Res.* **47**: 3430–3433.
194. Shuker, D. E. G.; Bailey, E.; Parry, A.; Lamb, J.; and Farmer, P. B. 1987. The determination of urinary 3-methyladenine in humans as a potential monitor of exposure to methylating agents. *Carcinogenicity* **8**: 959–962.
195. Cathcart, R.; Schweirs, E.; Saul, R. L.; and Ames, B. N. 1984. Thymine glycol and thymidine glycol in human and rat urine: a possible assay for oxidative DNA damage. *Proc. Nat. Acad. Sci. USA* **81**: 5633–5637.
196. Cerutti, P. A. 1985. Prooxidant states and promotion. *Science* (U.S.A.) **227**: 375–381.
197. Reddy, J. K.; and Lalwani, N. D. 1984. Carcinogenesis by hepatic peroxisome proliferators: evaluation of the risk of hypolipodemic drugs and industrial plasticizers to humans. *CRC Crit. Rev. Toxicol.* **12**: 1–58.
198. Boucher, R.; Livingston, G. K.; and Que Hee, S. S. 1992. In-vitro micronucleus assay with peripheral lymphocytes for detection of antineoplastic agents. Am. Ind. Hyg. Assoc. Cont. Expos.; May 30–June 5, 1992, Boston, MA. Abstract 311.
199. Snedecor, G. W.; and Cochran, W. G. 1989. *Statistical Methods*, 8th ed.; Iowa State University Press, Ames, IA, pp. 278–281.

PART 4

Adducts; Immunology; AIDS*

The next set of chapters introduces the concepts of adducts (Chapters 10–12), covalent binding (Chapter 10), immunoassays (Chapter 11), immunology (Chapter 13), and AIDS (Chapters 14–19), all of which are interlinked.

Xenobiotics can cause changes in host DNA and proteins through covalent binding. The altered DNA can produce abnormal proteins, which may trigger an immune system response, as can the appropriate protein adducts (Chapter 13). The same mechanisms also may be important after DNA mutation from other causes such as microorganisms and ionizing radiation. The protective immune mechanisms are subverted by such viral invaders as HIV-1 and HIV-2.

There are two basic mechanisms of protection in the body. One is prevention—skin, mucus, effect of pH, ciliary movement, tearing, salivating, defecating, urinating, sweating, and mechanical factors such as sneezing and coughing, all discussed in Chapters 3–6. Another preventive process is microorganism mutual competition, which we will not discuss here.

The other protective mechanism is chemical recognition by the body, leading to a chemical/cellular response (the immune response; *immunitas* is Latin meaning "freedom from"). There are two major parts to the immune response: the direct effect of soluble chemical factors and phagocytosis, which is the cellular component.

---

* Chapters 14–19 originated from a symposium that the author organized at Toronto, Canada on June 7, 1988 entitled "AIDS: Chemicals, Workplace Issues and Biological Monitoring" as part of the Third Chemical Congress of North America.

Sections 9.1.1 through 9.1.6 introduced the different types of white blood cells (leukocytes) involved in phagocytosis without elaborating on mechanisms. The point was also made there that WBC biological monitoring markers were nonspecific medical markers. The macrophage white blood cells have their counterparts in the alveolar macrophages of the lung, the Kupffer cells of the liver, mesangial cells in the kidney glomeruli, the brain microglia, connective tissue histiocytes, the bone osteoclasts, and macrophages in the lining of the spleen sinusoids, lymph node medullary sinuses, and synovial fluids. The macrophages defend mostly against bacteria, viruses, and protozoans, which can live within the cells of the host. In contrast, the neutrophils provide the major defense against pyrogenic bacteria. Both types of phagocytes can ingest inert or reactive particles as well as microorganisms, protozoans, and viruses after direct binding to the appropriate receptor sites on the phagocyte/foreign body pair by direct encounter or by chemotaxis (microorganisms may release chemicals or react with host soluble factors that allow the macrophage to home onto their membranes). An indirect chemical stimulation route is favored for small molecules such as industrial chemicals. The complement system is the analogous soluble factor entity of the body to protect against particles, protozoans, microorganisms, viruses, and specific chemicals.

Because immunological systems have evolved to protect the body against invasion of foreign molecules or molecules toxic to bodily functions, it is to be expected that markers associated with biological/medical monitoring of the immune system would assume great importance as markers and predictive markers of adverse effects. This has been shown by events during the Acquired Immune Deficiency Syndrome (AIDS) pandemic, where the T4-helper cell number is used as an index of integrity of the immune system (Chapter 14) and to help define AIDS or AIDS Related Complex (ARC; pre-AIDS).

The use of immunological tests as relatively specific and sensitive biological/medical monitoring markers is already known for some specific chemicals through utilization of their monoclonal and polyclonal antibodies. Chapters 10 to 12 introduce DNA and protein adducts as specific biological monitoring markers for specific chemicals. The way that these adducts interact to produce specific antigens and antibodies is discussed (in Chapter 13) before the AIDS chapters (Chapters 14–16), where viral invasion via foreign RNA attack will be addressed.

Chapters 15 and 16 are laboratory-based chapters concerning the use of analytical chemistry principles in the detection of HIV and other viruses, and in some approaches to therapy. The importance of this area is often understated in the literature; hence the inclusion of these two chapters, which give detailed insight into this specialized field. The techniques utilized are commonplace in immunology, and proficiency in them is essential before quantitative data can be deemed to be accurate.

Chapters 17 and 18 explore hygienic considerations involved with AIDS and HIV, while Chapter 19 addresses biological monitoring of volatile nitrites, once thought to be chemical depressants of the immune system.

10

Adducts: An Overview

10.0 INTRODUCTION

Adducts are the modified biomacromolecules produced when xenobiotics or their activated or stable metabolites bind covalently with biomacromolecules. Some investigators define adducts as any modified moiety including nucleotides, nucleosides, and amino acids; the modified macromolecular entities are "carcinogen–macromolecule adducts." We will not follow the latter definition here because then the initial Phase II conjugates and the initial complex formed at receptor sites would be called adducts.

Nucleic acids, proteins, lipids, and polysaccharide type biomacromolecules can be modified under the appropriate conditions. Nucleic acids may contain modified bases, sugars, or phosphate groups; proteins may contain modified amino acid residues or peptide links; lipids may contain modified fatty acids; phosphatidyl compounds may contain modified fatty acids, phosphate groups, or head-group moieties; and polysaccharides may contain modified sugars or carbohydrates, mostly at hydroxy groups.

Alkylation and hydroxyalkylation (up to a two-carbon chain length) are the most often observed modifications because such changes are generally not toxic enough to kill a cell (the most adverse acute effect), yet allow division until the tissue machinery eventually is affected (chronic effects). There is an endogenous methylation process also for both DNA bases and proteins, especially but for the histone proteins associated with DNA in the nucleus. Repair processes in the cell and tissue are also important, as is the balance between activation and detoxification/elimination of the key molecules, which are the attacking species. This balance is also dependent on diet, life-style, environmental influences, and genetic factors (Chapters 2 through 9).

The site of attack of a biomacromolecule by an attacking species obeys the rules of chemical reactions set forth in Chapter 1: the weakest available bond breaks first, and/or reaction occurs with any available nonbonded electrons on heteroatoms. The most reactive species often are charged. Extremely reactive species cause local tissue damage (for example, modified hemoglobin in blood), but the less reactive ones often are long-lived enough to be able to attack cellular DNA. For macromolecules, the availability for reaction is linked to geometrical considerations because all fundamental subunits are not equally available to be attacked; many may be buried in an inaccessible position because of their secondary, tertiary, and quaternary structure (Section 2.0). Thus the adducts formed for a linear sequence (as in heat-denatured protein) may differ from those formed by attack on the fully three-dimensional molecule. Adducts obtained with single-stranded DNA differ from those of double-helix DNA. Such factors may be important in evaluating any disparate results for *in vivo* and *in vitro* experiments.

There may be a geometrical constraint placed on the attacking species also because then species resembling a preferred substrate (as for enzymes) will have more chance of reaction than those of dissimilar structure. Stereospecificity considerations may often be very stringent, however; so Quantitative Structure Activity Relationships (QSAR) often require more than just knowing the primary structure of an attacking compound.

The order in which the xenobiotic encounters tissues and organelles after exposure also affects reaction yields. Thus, bloodstream macromolecules will be attacked more severely than most organs after the effects on the portal of absorption because the blood is the transfer system to the rest of the organs of the body. The white blood cells are the key blood cells in protecting the body (Sections 9.1.1–9.1.6), and xenobiotics must survive the chemotactic attacks of white cells to be able to muster an attack on target organs. The available molecules in the outer membranes of cells and organelles will be most severely affected by a xenobiotic. Conversely, if the attacking species is an activated intermediate produced by cytochrome P-450 reactions in the mitochondrial matrix, then the available molecules in the inner membranes or the matrix of the mitochondria may be most at risk. This would include mitochondrial DNA although no adducts have yet been reported for this DNA type, nor has the role of mitochondrial DNA been elucidated in the initiation of adverse cellular effects.

Immune system mechanisms (Sections 9.1.1–9.1.6 and Chapter 13) are important in determining how much of a xenobiotic is available for attack within tissues. The distribution between free and bound xenobiotic is another factor (Section 5.2.4). Other variables are discussed in Sections 5.2 and 5.3.

The analysis of adducts traditionally is approached in two ways. One procedure is the resolution/separation of the modified adduct itself from unmodified biomacromolecule (often by electrophoresis and gel filtration for proteins and DNA, or liquid or thin layer chromatography for DNA bases) by use of visualization techniques. The latter include tracer methods with ^{32}P (animal studies for high molecular weight xenobiotic–DNA adducts and certain phospholipids) or ^{14}C labels (for low molecular weight adducts), and with fluorescent labels.

The second analytical procedure is isolation and resolution of the modified fundamental subunits from unmodified fundamental subunits after degradation of the biomolecule polymer into its fundamental subunits, analyzable by standard techniques or by tracer methods. Thus the analysis of amino acids for proteins, purine/pyrimidine bases for nucleic acids, fatty acids for lipids, and sugars for carbohydrates often is also performed with ^{14}C or ^{32}P labels in animal experiments, and with modified subunit analyses in humans (Section 9.3.11).

Immunoassays are increasingly utilized techniques whereby host antibodies are selected for by an intruding molecule or the antigens of a microorganism. Adduct-specific polyclonal or monoclonal antibodies are increasingly used. The specificity of the antibody techniques is crucially dependent on the purity of the DNA adduct used to raise them. Immunoassays can be sensitive and specific (see Chapter 13). Direct-reading techniques based on fluorescence or luminescence probably will be important in the future. Antibodies to protein adducts are also possible.

The sensitivity of most DNA adduct methods is in the range of one adduct per 10^6 to 10^{10} nucleotides, or 1000 to 10,000 adducts per cell, about the levels of DNA adducts measured in humans [1]. For hemoglobin (Hb), the levels of human protein adducts (mostly in the globin portion) range from 0.02 to 13,000 fmol/mg Hb, the latter being 100-fold lower than the levels in exposed experimental animals [1]. Thus sensitivity is not a great problem for protein adduct detection. The concentrations quoted above are nevertheless near the detection limits of the present analytical biochemistry methods, a major reason why adduct determinations are not yet very practical for human biological monitoring.

Phase II conjugations (Sections 2.13 and Chapter 5) are special cases of adduct formation, with the initial conjugate being the small molecule analog of the modified biomacromolecule. Another analogous situation involves the lectin-type of receptor, which consists of carbohydrate or glycolipid polymer. The receptor–substrate complex is an adduct. The initial cytosolic receptor complexes for the polyhalogenated dibenzofurans, dibenzo-*p*-dioxins, and PCBs are also adducts. Membrane receptor sites of phospholipids and proteins similarly also facilitate initial adduct formation. If the receptor–substrate complex is subsequently modified (as for the initial conjugates of Type II processes), however, then the released modified small molecule products are metabolites. These metabolites, especially activated, can still be incorporated into macromolecules to form adducts. Overlaps in these classifications also occur. Thus the tripeptide glutathione forms an adduct in the first step of Phase II conjugation with a suitable xenobiotic in the same way that an amino acid exposed at the active site of an enzyme can be modified by reaction with the xenobiotic/metabolite or substrate. However, in the latter case the xenobiotic/metabolite must be activated in some manner.

We will consider DNA and protein adducts in Chapters 11 and 12, respectively. Carbohydrate and lipid adducts have not been reported, even in animal studies. Because adduct sampling usually involves invasive procedures such as blood sampling or surgery, adducts are not presently utilized in biological monitoring except for health surveillance research purposes. Most of the present data for adduct formation and significance have come from animal, not human, studies. Therefore, we will focus on human studies in Chapters 11 and 12.

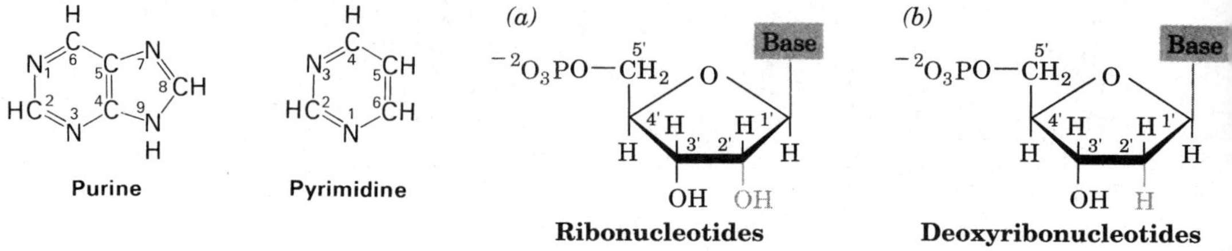

Names and Abbreviations of Nucleic Acid Bases, Nucleosides, and Nucleotides

Base Formula	Base X = H	Nucleoside X = ribose[a]	Nucleotide[b] X = ribose phosphate[a]
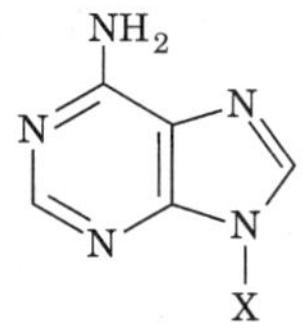	Adenine Ade A	Adenosine Ado A	Adenylic acid Adenosine monophosphate AMP
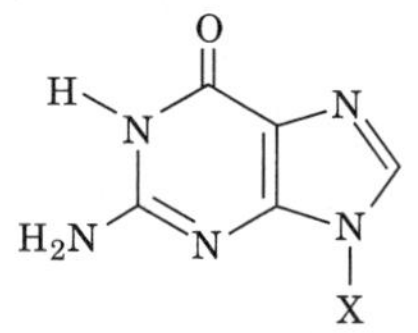	Guanine Gua G	Guanosine Guo G	Guanylic acid Guanosine monophosphate GMP
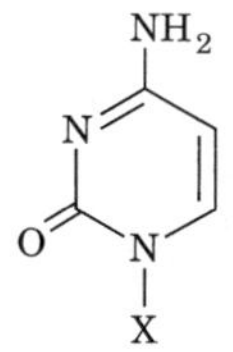	Cytosine Cyt C	Cytidine Cyd C	Cytidylic acid Cytosine monophosphate CMP
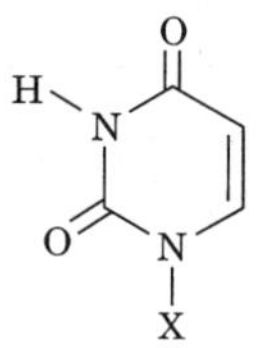	Uracil Ura U	Uridine Urd U	Uridylic acid Urdine monophosphate UMP
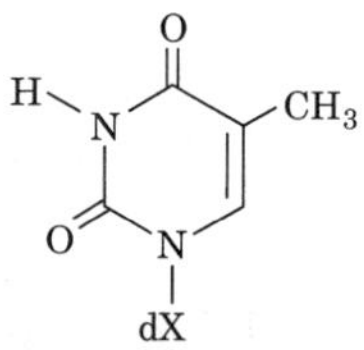	Thymine Thy T	Deoxythymidine dThd dT	Deoxythymidylic acid Deoxythymidine monophosphate dTMP

[a] The presence of a 2′-deoxyribose unit in place of ribose, as occurs in DNA, is implied by the prefixes "deoxy" or "d." For example, the deoxynucleoside of adenine is deoxyadenosine or dA. However, for thymine-containing residues, which rarely occur in RNA, the prefix is redundant and may be dropped. The presence of a ribose unit may be explicitly implied by the prefixes "ribo" or "r." Thus the ribonucleotide of thymine is ribothymidine or rT.

[b] The position of the phosphate group in a nucleotide may be explicitly specified as in, for example, 3′-AMP and 5′-GMP.

FIGURE 10.1. The basic subunits of DNA and RNA and their arrangements within these molecules. (Courtesy of *Biochemistry*. Voet/Voet, J. Wiley & Sons.)

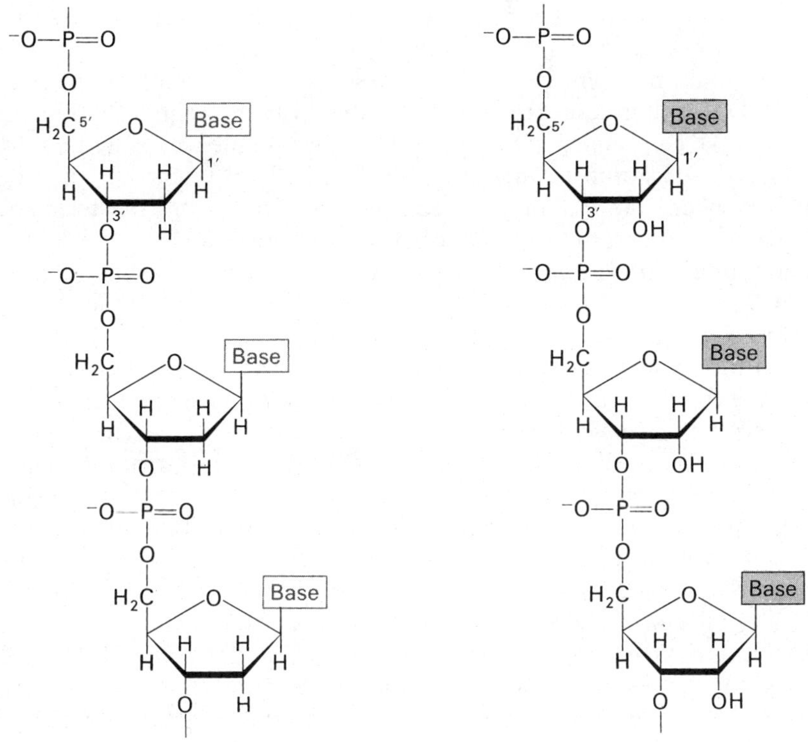

FIGURE 10.1 (*Continued*).

10.1 NUCLEIC ACIDS/PROTEIN SYNTHESIS IN HUMANS

10.1.1 DNA and RNA

DNA consists of deoxyribonucleotides (Section 2.11.7), each composed of a base, a deoxyribose sugar (which has one oxygen less than ribose, its analog in RNA, attached to the 2′-carbon atom), and at least one phosphate group. By convention, unprimed numbers designate the atoms of the ring bases, whereas primed numbers are utilized for the sugar atoms. The primary base sequence carries genetic information, and the sugar and phosphate groups are important for structural and geometric reasons. The bases in DNA are the purines adenine (A) and guanine (G) and the pyrimidines thymine (T) and cytosine (C). In RNA, the thymine is replaced with uracil (U). Figure 10.1 depicts these basic subunits.

In DNA, the C-1 (1′-) carbon atom of deoxyribose is bonded through a β linkage (above the plane of a Newman projection structure) to the N-1 of a pyrimidine or the N-9 of a purine. Two phosphate groups are bonded via phosphodiester links through the hydroxy groups on the 3′- and 5′-carbon atoms of the deoxyribose ring via two phosphodiester links to the 5′- and 3′-carbon atoms, respectively, of the adjacent deoxyribose sugars. Nucleosides do not contain phosphate groups. Because the sugars and the phosphates in a normal DNA molecule are invariant, the primary sequence of bases of a particular DNA defines the DNA. The base sequence is written from the terminal 5′-OH group to the terminal 3′-OH group (compare for proteins or peptides, where the amino acid sequence is written from the terminal amino group amino acid to the terminal carboxylate amino acid).

The primary DNA structure often has many repeating base sequences. More than 30% of human DNA consists of sequences repeated at least 20 times. Alu sequences of 300 base pairs of about 85% similarity occur nearly a million times in the human genome (about 7% of the DNA), and often also contain a target site for the Alu I restriction endonuclease. Alu sequences are similar to 7SL RNA, the small cytoplasmic RNA molecule in the signal recognition particle found in cell cytosol, which is used in protein targeting. This particle delivers membrane and secretory proteins to the endoplasmic reticulum for translocation. DNA fragments with repeating units are more buoyant than fragments with diverse bases, and are often concentrated in centromeric regions (Section 9.3.2).

Nearly all human DNA is used to encode proteins (about 2%), messenger RNAs (mRNAs), transfer RNAs (tRNAs), and ribosomal RNAs (rRNAs). mRNA constitutes only 5% of the total RNA, after rRNA and tRNA. Small nuclear RNA molecules participate in the joining together (splicing) of the pertinient parts of RNA molecules to create the active RNA template. Although the nucleus contains most of the DNA, the mitochondria have a small amount, which, however, is circular but still double helix. Human mitochondrial DNA contains 16,569 base pairs, which encode 13 proteins (60% for seven subunits of NADH-Q reductase), 22 tRNAs, and 2 rRNAs.

Nucleic acids were first discovered in 1869 by Miescher in the nuclei of pus cell leukocytes (white blood cells) from discarded surgical bandages. Before 1944, it was assumed that the chromosomal proteins carried genetic information because nucleic acids were not thought to have the base diversity needed to explain biological specificity. With the discoveries that DNA was the fundamental transforming principle of *Pneumococcus* Type III (in 1944 after a ten-year investigation by Avery, MacLeod, and McCarty) and that the T2 bacteriophage infection of *Escherichia coli* involved DNA (in 1951–52), the finding soon came that the DNA content of single cells of a given species was the same for all cells of the same ploidy. Chargaff in 1950 determined that the ratios of adenine to thymine and of guanine to cytosine were nearly 1.0 in the DNA of different species.

Watson and Crick in 1953, in competition with such other groups as Linus Pauling's, proposed the three-dimensional structure of pure dry DNA based on the X-ray diffraction patterns of Rosalind Franklin and Maurice Wilkins. Their model has the following features (Figure 10.2): two double helical polynucleotide chains are coiled around a common axis and run in opposite directions; the bases are on the inside of the helix (not the outside as in Pauling's model), perpendicular to the helix axis, with the phosphate and sugar groups on the outside; the helix diameter is 2 nm with adjacent bases separated by 0.34 nm along the helix axis and related by a rotation of 36 degrees so that

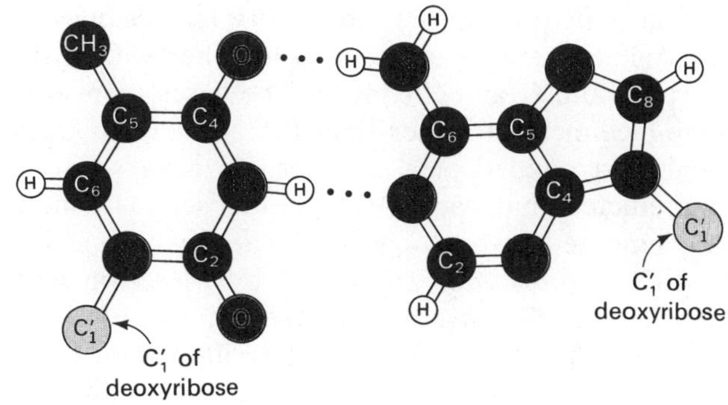

Model of an adenine-thymine base pair.

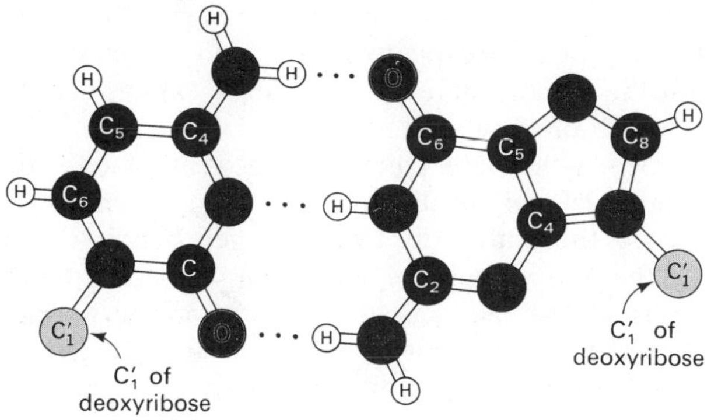

Model of a guanine-cytosine base pair.

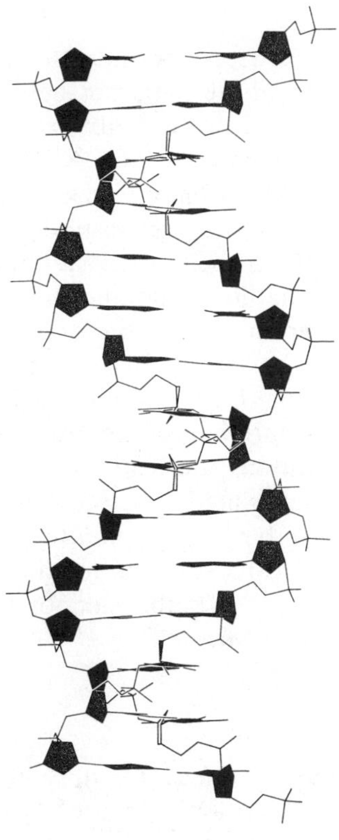

Skeletal model of double-helical DNA. The structure repeats at intervals of 34 Å, which corresponds to ten residues on each chain.

FIGURE 10.2. The Watson–Crick model of DNA. (Courtesy of Biochemistry. Third edition, Stryer, Freeman.)

the helical structure repeats after every ten residues or every 3.4 nm; and the two polynucleotide chains are held together with hydrogen bonds between A and T (two) and G and C (three). The bases themselves are predominantly in the keto/lactam form rather than the enol/lactim form. The glycosidic bonds attached to a bonded pair of bases are always 1.085 nm apart. Watson and Crick predicted that each DNA strand acts as a nonmodified template that is complemented in base pairing in a daughter DNA (this defines a "semi-conservative" process as confirmed by Meselson and Stahl in 1958). DNA changes its shape, depending on the amount of water and the ions present. The classic Watson–Crick form described above is now known as the B-conformation of DNA in the presence of sodium cation and 92% relative humidity. This form resembles that present in intact spermatozoa heads, a predominantly alkaline medium. Divalent cations such as Mg^{2+}, Mn^{2+}, Zn^{2+}, Co^{2+}, and Pb^{2+} bind avidly to the phosphate groups and affect the DNA structure. Human DNA for the haploid state (23 chromosomes) has nearly 3×10^9 base pairs and a total length of about one meter.

The hydrogen bonds between the base pairs are the weakest base bonds to disrupt, and subsequent attack on the heteroatoms through the exposed lone pairs can ensue. Because there are only two hydrogen bonds to disrupt between A and T, most of the nucleotide base adducts are generally modified adenine/thymine nucleotides. DNA adducts of guanine and cytosine are thought to be more important than those of A and T because G and C are more protected than A and T by three hydrogen bonds. The subsequent reversible unwinding of the double helix can be produced through denaturation by mild heating, by mild acid or alkali treatment, through ionic action, and through enzyme activity.

Double helical RNA does not resemble a B-DNA structure because the 2′-OH groups cause steric problems. Instead there are 11 base pairs per helical turn and a pitch of 3.0 nm, and its base pairs are inclined to the helix axis by about 14 degrees. This is the A-RNA or RNA-11 conformation. A-RNA resembles A-DNA (DNA at 75% relative humidity, which has 11 base pairs per helical turn, a pitch of 2.8 nm, and the planes of its base pairs tilted 20 degrees with respect to the helix axis). Many other RNAs such as transfer and ribosomal types contain complementary sequences that form double helical stems. Hybrid RNA/DNA has the A-DNA configuration. No studies have been concerned with RNA adducts with xenobiotics.

It is noteworthy that t-RNAs (there being at least one for each amino acid) contain many modified nucleotide bases such as dihydrouridine, pseudouridine, inosine, derivatives methylated at their ribose 2′ positions, derivatives where sulfur replaces oxygen, and many *N*-methylated, dimethylated, and acetylated bases. Many of these *N*-methylated bases in DNA have been detected after the attacks of xenobiotic alkylating agents. It is thought that most of the modifications to the normal bases in tRNA occur after translation. Whether xenobiotic alkylating agents cause tRNA base modification is unknown.

10.1.2 Chromosomes

Chromosomes were so named in the 1860s (*chromos*, color; *soma*, body) because they were strongly stained by specific dyes. The application of cytogenetics to biological monitoring is discussed in Section 9.3.2.

A human chromosome contains a single linear molecule of double helical DNA tightly bound to histones (basic proteins), the two together historically called chromatin. There are five types of histones (H1, H2A, H2B, H3, and H4, named in order for decreasing Lys/Arg ratios). Histones can be alkylated, acetylated, ADP-ribosylated, and phosphorylated. The amino acid sequences of H3 and H4 are nearly identical for different species. Kornberg in 1974 suggested that the chromatin is comprised of repeating units at a 10 nm repeating distance, each consisting of about 200 base pairs of DNA and two each of H2A, H2B, H3, and H4, the unit now called a nucleosome. The DNA content of nucleosomes from different organisms varies between 160 and 240 base pairs. Digestion with micrococcal nuclease yields a core particle of 140 DNA base pairs bound to the outside of a histone octamer in a supercoil (double helix chain becomes a fundamental subunit of a higher-order DNA structure), irrespective of vertebrate species. The core is a flat particle of dimensions $11 \times 11 \times 5.5$ nm, the DNA left-handed supercoil having a pitch of 2.8 nm with the H3 and H4 dimers being in the middle and one each of H2A and H2B being at either end of the center. One H1 unit is outside the central core near the linker DNA to the next nucleosome, near where the DNA interacts with the core H2A units. This keeps the DNA supercoil rigidly in place like a clasp. H1 is released when the DNA is trimmed from 160 to 140 bases. H1 is phosphorylated just before mitosis and is dephosphorylated after mitosis. DNA makes the most contact with the H3–H4 tetramer. The nucleosomes also may form a helical array, which may allow for greater DNA compaction and greater DNA supercoiling, especially when the cell is under chemical attack. The most compacted DNA is found in sperm heads where histones are replaced by protamines, arginine-rich proteins that assume an α-helix shape on binding to DNA.

10.1.3 DNA/RNA Replication

DNA replication is mediated by more than 20 proteins, many being template-directed polymerases that act in the presence of magnesium ion through step-by-step addition of activated deoxyribonucleotide triphosphate units to a primer DNA chain with a free 3′-OH group, with the subsequent release of free pyrophosphate, which is then hydrolyzed by pyrophosphatase. The latter step drives the process forward. Repair often is facilitated during these polymerase reactions by the rejection and the excision of aberrant bases. This mechanism makes the appearance of DNA adducts be a net effect rather than a cumulative effect of dose. Such a mechanism does not operate for protein adducts.

RNA molecules usually are single-stranded but can assume double helical regions by the chain folding back on itself. A similar enzyme synthesis system to DNA can exist for RNA templates in retro viruses such as HIV-1. RNA viruses synthesize complementary DNA in their hosts through the action of viral reverse transcriptase, which is an RNA-directed DNA polymerase. The primer DNA can be made in the next step by using the host's intrinsic DNA polymerases, but the utilization of RNA polymerases to create mRNA based on a DNA template is the normal process. In contrast, RNA polymerases do not require a primer, the DNA template is fully conserved, and they lack excision repair (nuclease) capability. In other respects, RNA polymerases act like, and have the same requirements as, DNA polymerases. Precursors to rRNA molecules may act as enzymes (ribozymes) and can self-splice, a reason why RNA polymerases do not need excision repair capability in ribosomes.

10.1.4 Expression

The flow of information from DNA to mRNA in cells is called transcription, and the resulting protein synthesis, based on the mRNA template aided and abetted by tRNA and rRNA, is called translation. The whole process is expression. The control of gene expression occurs mostly at the level of transcription. The transcriptionally active regions of the chromatin are sensitive to DNAse I. For alkylating attack, few cytosines suffer alkylation because there are three protective hydrogen bonds to break (Section 10.1.1). The transcription of genes for 5S RNA (S is the sedimentation coefficient in Svedbergs, a measure of the rate at which particles sediment at 20°C in a fluid with the density and viscosity of pure water) depends on the binding of a protein containing nine zinc-binding fingers (transcription factor IIIA) that lock into the DNA grooves in the internal control region of the gene. Transcription factors B and C serve to initiate transcription of tRNA genes. The glucocorticoid receptor also contains metal-binding finger domains. Most frequently the cellular regulation of transcription is at the level of initiation, usually by specific proteins.

The function of mRNA was set forth as a hypothesis by Jacob and Monod in 1961. The basic sequence of three contiguous bases in mRNA is called a codon and specifies one specific amino acid (proved first by Nirenberg in 1961 for phenylalanine which is encoded by UUU, for lysine which is encoded by AAA, and for proline which is encoded by CCC). The genetic code for amino acids is degenerate (more than one codon for a specific amino acid). Only tryptophan (UGG) and methionine (AUG) are specified by unique codons, whereas leucine, arginine, and serine are each specified by six codons. In most degenerate codons for amino acids, the first two bases are the same, thus negating the effects of mutation (Sections 9.3.1–9.3.5). Therefore alterations to the codons (mutations) specifying unique amino acids are more serious than mutations to degenerate codons.

Codons in mRNA are read sequentially by tRNAs through their complementary anticodons. The tRNAs then carry their specific amino acids in an activated form at the 3′-OH group of the terminal adenosine for sequential assembling of the amino acids on the ribosomes after facilitation of specific tRNA/rRNA interactions. This idea was advanced by Crick in 1958. The ribosomes are complex templates of rRNA and over 50 types of proteins. Nirenberg in 1964 discovered that a trinucleotide promotes the binding to rRNA of the particular tRNA molecule for which it is the code word.

DNA templates contain regions called promoter sites that specifically bind RNA polymerase and determine where transcription begins. Most eucaryotic genes have promoter sites with a TATAAA consensus sequence centered at about 25 bases on the 5′ side of the first base transcribed (written as "–25"). Many promoter sites also exhibit a CAAT consensus sequence centered at about –75. Enhancer sequences to stimulate transcription also are present, and discrete stop signals are encoded into the DNA template. Khorana in 1964 demonstrated that UAA, UAG, and UGA were codons to terminate chain lengthening. These codons are not read by tRNAs but by proteins called release factors. AUG or GUG closest to the 5′ end of a mRNA are usually part of the complex initiation signal, which includes a methionine-rich initiator tRNA.

In contrast, human mitochondria read UGA for tryptophan rather than termination; they read AGA and AGG as stop rather than for arginine; and AUA reads for methionine instead of isoleucine. Other differences in the genetic code of mitochondria relative to the cellular genetic code are also known. The genetic code in protozoa also differs from the multicellular genetic code. Thus the genetic code does not employ a universal encoding system, but it is relatively uniform in the nuclear DNA of vertebrates.

Although a continous array of sequential triplet codons encodes a specific protein in bacteria, this is not so in eucaryotes. In 1977, several genes were found to be discontinuous, as, for example, the β-globin gene of human hemoglobin, which contains three coding sequences (exons) separated by noncoding sequences (introns, which usually begin with GU and end a rich pyrimidine sequence with AG). The complementary mRNA freshly synthesized from the DNA then has its noncoding complementary base sequences excised and the relevant chains spliced by splicosomes (assemblies of proteins and small RNA molecules) to form the mature 9S mRNA. It has been postulated that there are fewer than 7000 fundamental exons in the proteins sequenced so far; this provides speed of assembly rather than the greatest possible diversity [2]. According to one view, introns are the fundamental ancient units with genes being assembled via intron-mediated recombination from exon modules that code for functional domains, folding regions, or structural elements. Another theory posits that introns are derived from eucaryotic genomes, being the results of bursts of parasitic elements invading early and continuous eucaryotic coding regions [2].

The genes encoding for rRNA are tandemly repeated with over 100 copies, and are located in specialized regions of chromosomes associated with nucleoli. The genes for 18S, 5.8S, and 28S rRNA are clustered, and are transcribed by RNAse polymerase I in nucleoli to give a 45S RNA precursor that is enzymatically modified and cleaved to yield the mature 18S, 5.8S, and 28S rRNAs. In addition, about 100 nucleotides are methylated, nearly all on the 2′-hydroxy groups of their ribose units. This structure is conserved across all vertebrate species. More than 100 uridines in the precursor RNA are isomerized to pseudouridines. Interactions also occur with many ribosomal proteins.

The genes for the histones are highly tandomly reiterated, with humans having 30 to 40 copies. The genes for the five histone types may also be highly clustered. Histone genes lack introns, and histone mRNAs do not have poly A tails.

Increased endogenous methylation of cytosines has been correlated with decreased gene activity. About 70% of CG sequences in mammalian DNA are methylated, and methylation may be used to regulate transcription (Section 10.1.5). The impact of xenobiotic alkylating agents on this process is not understood.

10.1.5 Cell Stability in the Face of Chemical Attack

The part of the expression process that is most prone to interference is translation. One way to prevent translation is to impede or prevent binding of guanine triphosphate because the energy source needed to drive translation is not available. Thus any agent capable of competitive binding will impede translation. Such an agent is cycloheximide, which binds to the 60S subunit of ribosomes in rat hepatocytes.

After a near-lethal dose to rats of cycloheximide, the uptakes of nutrients such as glucose and amino acids into hepatocytes are increased, and the intracellular circulation of proteins then is enhanced, probably through the accumulation of ATP not being used in the polysomes; and this is followed by direction of the existing protein constituents of ribosomes in the cytoplasm into the nucleolus of the nucleus. In this organelle, the proteins and ribosomal RNA combine, and the complexes are exported to the cytoplasm where they are assembled into ribosomes, or into polysomes in the presence of mRNA. In mild chemical stress, this production of new ribosomes and polysomes may allow protein synthesis to begin anew. At the same time that the protein–rRNA complexes are exported out of the nucleus, the proteins necessary for gene transcription (such as RNA polymerase II, which transcribes DNA into mRNA precursors) are imported into the nucleus, and the enhanced inflow of glucose and amino acids leads to more production of ATP by the mitochondria. In the nucleolus, initially the chromatin partially decondenses or uncoils to facilitate the fast transcription of the required genes. The whole process is over within 2 h.

At near-lethal concentrations of cycloheximide after the above 2-h initial period, the cell then enzymatically breaks down the polysomes into their constituent ribosomes. The polysomes that are degraded are those used to synthesize proteins to be exported to other cells. The 18S RNA (the rRNA) component in the 40S part then is enzymatically attacked to produce several basic fragments, which are reused. Thus 6 h after administration the cell can provide itself with many new functional polysomes and starts making protein again. These new polysomes usually are not connected to the endoplasmic reticulum, and they make only those proteins required for the cell's internal needs. The 60S components of the polysomes remain intact. In this period, the uncoiled chromatin in the nucleolus compacts more than is normal, in a process that lasts up to 12 h. The DNA geometry and the protein level normalize 18 to 24 h after administration, but protein production continues to increase. After 48 h, a new wave of synthesis of nuclear histones, proteins of the nuclear membrane, and DNA polymerases may occur. If this happens, at 60 h there is a burst of DNA replication, passing through one or more growth/division cycles until the export protein facility and the polysome attachment to the endoplasmic reticulum are normalized.

It is unclear whether the above description is a generalized or a unique response to chemical stress, but it is instructive relative to the close coupling of transcription and translation.

10.1.6 Polymerase Chain Reactions

The DNA base sequence is presently obtained in three steps: degradation of the pure DNA by restriction endonucleases (gene splicing) that cleave duplex (double helix) DNA at specific sequences; molecular cloning (recombinant DNA) in a suitable host microorganism to amplify the oligonucleotide fragments to detectable amounts; and subsequent base sequencing of the individual fragments (oligonucleotides) through use of exonucleases such as snake venom and spleen phosphodiesterases that cleave nucleotides from the 3′- and 5′-ends, respectively. Chemical cleavage methods and chain-termination methods also are used for sequencing. Oligonucleotide identity often is confirmed by direct synthesis of the suspected oligonucleotide.

The polymerase chain reaction (PCR) system first described in 1985 is a molecular cloning tool that amplifies a DNA oligonucleotide fragment of up to 6000 bases. It also allows definition of the distance between two oligonucleotide primers and the sequence in between them. A denatured DNA sample is incubated with DNA polymerase and two oligonucleotide primers that direct the enzyme to synthesize new complementary strands. After each synthesis cycle the two strands of duplex DNA are separated by heat denaturation (commonly at 90–100°C for 30–60 sec), the primers are annealed to their complementary segments on the DNA, and the next synthesis cycle is begun. The DNA polymerase of a thermophilic bacterium is utilized so that there is no need to add fresh enzyme after the heat treatment; thus the synthesis cycle is controlled by varying the temperature. Twenty-five cycles increase the original oligonucleotide concentration by about a factor of 10^6. The undenatured linear double helix is called the amplicon. The original DNA does not have to be pure; but if there are too many oligonucleotides, the polymerase becomes "anemic" and sometimes does not produce enough target oligonucleotide to be detected by the end of the standard 20 to 25 cycles. The latter situation also occurs when shorter oligonucleotides predominate, as they are amplified preferentially.

The DNA that is produced can be characterized by direct sequencing, by restriction-fragment-length polymorphisms or RFLPs (created by the oligonucleotides of different base lengths produced after restriction enzyme degradation), or by Southern blotting (binding by mechanical or electrophoretic means of single-stranded but not double-stranded DNA to nitrocellulose after 0.5 M NaOH DNA hydrolysis). The blotting techniques corresponding to the Southern for RNA and proteins are Northern and Western, respectively. Any RNA to be sequenced can be transcribed into its complementary DNA via reverse transcriptase, with the complementary DNA being then subjected to the above techniques. The error frequency in PCR per nucleotide varies between 0.06% and 0.28% over 20 to 33 cycles.

PCR amplification is a cell-free system that can produce large quantities of pure oligonucleotides in 3 to 4 h compared to days or weeks using other methods such as cellular cloning. It is an ideal technique to detect chromosomal translocations. If the key DNA sequence region associated with toxicity/pathogenicity/mutation is known, this region can easily be detected by PCR after the appropriate restriction enzyme treatment produces the key region oligonucleotide. The method is the basis of DNA identification in the forensic field and of the prenatal identification of sickle cell anemia, its first application. Thus PCRs have been used to diagnose diseases, detect pathogens, quantitate micro amounts of DNA, compare DNAs, and sequence genes.

An analogous reaction, the ligase chain reaction (LCR), is utilized both to amplify DNA and to discriminate a single base mutation. Allele-specific LCR employs four oligonucleotides: two adjacent ones that are hybridized to one strand of target DNA, and two other adjacent complementary sets, which hybridize to create the opposite strand. Thermostable ligase covalently links each set as long as there is complete complementarity at the junction. Amplification occurs on recycling, this being controlled as for PCR by temperature. Control of purity needs to be far more stringent for LCR than for PCR. If there is a single-base mismatch, amplification will not occur. Thus combined use of LCR and PCR allows definition and detection of mutant DNA species. Isothermal amplification has been developed for RNA amplification via a concerted three-enzyme reaction *in vitro* (3SR).

10.2 COVALENT BINDING AND ADDUCTS

The concept of covalent binding is used mostly in animal toxicology. The method consists of administering a tracer material (usually radiolabeled) so that any adducts can be tagged with the label. After a specified time the macromolecule is isolated after animal exsanguination, tissue processing, and biomacromolecule purification [3], a technique hardly applicable to humans except at autopsy, after surgery, for human tissue culture, or for easily accessible cell types in the mouth, skin, or white blood cells. However, there is no doubt that the process occurs in humans.

The first covalent binding experiment *in vitro* was performed in 1947 with 4-dimethylaminoazobenzene in rat liver [3]. The initial experiment on *in vivo* DNA binding occurred in 1957 for ^{14}C-methyl–labeled nitrogen mustard in rats and mice. Protein covalent binding was found usually to be more extensive than DNA binding for the same organ because of higher concentrations of protein, and proteins were mostly attacked before the DNA was reached.

The animal experiments also showed that the adduct or modified fundamental unit produced in greatest concentration was not necessarily related to carcinogenicity [3]. For biological monitoring for exposure purposes, a dose-effect must be obeyed, and to obtain the greatest sensitivity the most abundant adduct or modified fundamental subunit should be monitored. The marker is only that, and it may not be related to any observed toxic effects. A marker of adverse effect, however, must be related to the pathway causing toxicity in a dose-response manner or must be a by-product of the toxicity. For that the mechanism must be known.

The extent of adduct formation in animals may not be reflected in humans for many reasons. Differences in basal metabolic rates, metabolic pathways, and host susceptibility and resistance factors have already been alluded to (Section 5.1.7). The activities of DNA repair enzymes vary between animals and humans also. The activity of O^6-alkylguanine-DNA-alkyltransferase is usually tenfold higher in human tissues than in the corresponding rat tissue. All determinants of inbred animals such as rats used in research are always more consistent than those of outbred animals and humans. Human cells also divide more slowly than the corresponding cells in small animals such as rodents.

10.2.1 The CBI

The covalent binding index (CBI) to macromolecules is defined as the micromoles of chemical bound per mole of fundamental subunits in the macromolecule divided by the millimoles of chemical administered per kilogram of body weight. For radiolabeled materials, the CBI relative to DNA can be expressed as disintegrations per minute of the chemical bound per milligram of DNA divided by the disintegrations per minute of the chemical administered per kilogram of the animal, this quantity being then divided by 3.24×10^{-9}, assuming that one mole of nucleotides represents 309 g DNA [3]. For proteins, the fundamental subunits are amino acids; for lipids, fatty acids; for DNA, nucleotides; and for carbohydrates, sugar units.

Incorporation of any label into a macromolecule through biosynthesis must be corrected for. Thus the incorporation of labeled amino acids or nucleotides before they are assembled in the biomacromolecule is not regarded as covalent binding. Also, the label may be contained in the cleavage product from a biomacromolecule and subsequently incorporated biosynthetically. This is a big problem with a tritium label. Data from unexposed animals can address the tritium effect by providing tritiated water of comparable activity as a positive control. Biosynthetic incorporations are generally linear with time, the half-lives being variable and characteristic. Thus while the CBI for liver DNA for ^{14}C-benzene was 1.7, the apparent CBI for tritiated benzene was 2.4 [3].

All the label from ^{14}C-methyl from dichlorvos found in rat DNA is biosynthetically incorporated and does not come from DNA-methylation [3]. If the label is detected in the unmodified fundamental subunits, then this is a proof of biosynthetic incorporation. A knowledge of the biosynthetic pathways of the nucleotides (Section 2.11.7) and of whether metabolism of the xenobiotic can lead to incorporation of labels into nucleotide precursors is important for interpreting covalent binding data. The CBI values of ^{14}C-bicarbonate and 1-^{14}C-ethanol of 0.3 and 4.6, respectively, for mouse liver DNA indicate that only CBI values two or three times above these should be regarded as the lower CBI values for potential methylators and ethylators, respectively, in the mouse. These CBI values probably vary from species to species and from strain to strain.

Another subtle effect is that the fundamental subunits could be modified by reaction with xenobiotic/activated xenobiotic metabolite before biosynthesis. This will not be important for DNA because control is severe for such events, or for proteins down to the levels of mRNA and the tRNA adapter system. Modification during rRNA/tRNA interaction on the growing protein strand may be a likely point of origin for protein adducts.

Intercalation and physical adsorption effects also must be allowed for. These effects are most important for tritiated labels but must also be known for ^{14}C labels. The measurement of radioactivity on a biomacromolecule does not tell one whether the label is bound covalently or physically. Repetitive washings using incubation media at each step of biomacromolecule purification may remove the physically adsorbed label. Even if no label is detected, intercalation (adsorption to the inside of a three-dimensional structure rather than to a flat or two-dimensional surface) still may occur because such adsorbed moieties may not be available enough to be removed by repetitive washing. A way to produce an intercalation-free substrate is to disrupt the three-dimensional biomacromolecule structure without any degradation of fundamental subunits to produce a linear macromolecule that is then washed repetitively until no more label appears. The amounts of label in comparable amounts of one-dimensional and three-dimensional biomacromolecule samples then are compared to assess the degree of intercalation. Such considerations also are very important in the processing of human tissues for adduct formation.

The covalent binding information can be utilized in three ways. The first involves calculating the total amount of adducts of the macromolecule formed per organ or tissue or the adducts per gram of target organ (wet and dry weight), a staple of animal toxicology experiments using labeled materials. The second piece of information often desired is the detection of modified fundamental subunits or adducts. For radiolabeled compounds, this is accomplished by detection of the radiolabel. Tritium is not a good label because it can be lost through exchange with the hydrogens in water as well as those in macromolecules. The third parameter calculated is the calculation of the CBI in terms of mmol xenobiotic/kg body weight.

Although the CBI relative to DNA has been linked to carcinogenic potency, it is known that chemicals with high CBIs (for example, acrolein of rat liver DNA with CBI of 360 mmol/kg body weight) are not necessarily carcinogens [3]. CBI values also differ greatly for different organs and tissues. "Weak" hepatocarcinogens (*p*-aminoazobenzene, 4-dimethylaminoazobenzene, and ethionine) have rat liver DNA CBI values of 1 to 6 mmol chemical/kg body weight [3]; "moderate" hepatocarcinogens (2-acetylaminofluorene, Aflatoxin B2, *p*-aminoazotoluene, nitrosomorpholine, nitrosopiperidine, and nitrosopyrrolidine) have CBIs of 44 to 560; and "strong" hepatocarcinogens (Aflatoxin B1, Aflatoxin M1, and dimethylnitrosamine) possess CBI values $>$ 1600. An exception is the strong hepatocarcinogen diethylnitrosamine, which has a CBI in rat liver that varies between 42 and 430. Urethane is classed as a weak hepatocarcinogen with a CBI range of 29 to 90. The nonhepatocarcinogen saccharin has a CBI < 0.005.

The type of compound and the time of exposure influence the CBI also. Rat liver DNA CBI values at 2 to 4 h after intravenous or intraperitoneal injection for methyl methanesulfonate varied between 272 and 556 mmol/kg body weight. Vinyl chloride at 5 h after inhalation produced a liver DNA CBI of 525 mmol/kg body weight. In comparison, most of the aromatic hydrocarbons have rat liver DNA CBI values less than 68 [3].

The major problem with the above CBI concept is that it does not take into account that specific covalent binding sites may be more important than others. The specific binding sites can be interpreted as specific adducts or specific sites in the available fundamental subunits of these specific adducts.

Thus if all the adduct identities were known, as well as their biological potencies, it would be possible to weight the different adduct components to be able to obtain an index related to biological effect. This procedure (called the TCDD equivalent approach) has been done for the cytosolic receptor regulated by the AH locus for chlorinated dibenzofurans and chlorinated dibenzo-*p*-dioxins. This value is usually expressed in terms of aryl hydrocarbon hydroxylase or ethoxyresorufin *O*-deethylase molar EC_{50} enzyme induction potencies or molar EC_{50} receptor binding avidities [4, 5]. The EC_{50} values of the congeners of these two related chemical families are compared with the activity of 2,3,7,8-

tetrachlorodibenzo-*p*-dioxin, the reference compound. The net biological activity is the summation of these relative activities weighted by their mole fraction in the test medium to produce the TCDD equivalent values. The potential biological activity thus can be inferred from a knowledge of the concentrations of the congeners in environmental and biological media. However, as discussed in Sections 6.7.1 and 6.7.2, the more toxic dioxins and dibenzofurans (those substituted at three of four or all four of the vicinal ring carbon atoms, except the fully halogenated derivatives) are accumulated more in the liver than are the other congeners, the resulting autopsy concentrations in the fat and liver also reflecting the balance between incorporation and detoxification/elimination.

Further Reading

Section 10.1.

Schleif, R. 1988. DNA binding by proteins. *Science* (U.S.A.) **241**: 1182–1187.

Stryer, L. 1988. *Biochemistry*, 3rd ed., W. H. Freeman, New York, pp. 71–116, 823–850.

Section 10.1.5

Chih, J. J.; Duhl, D. M.; Faulkner, L. S.; and Devlin, T. M. 1979. Regulation of mammalian protein synthesis *in vivo*: stimulated transport of nuclear ribonucleoprotein complexes to the cytoplasm after cycloheximide treatment. *Biochemical J.* **178**: 643–649.

Todorov, I. N.; Smalko, P. Y.; and Galkin, A. P. 1978. State of the polyribosomes as a reflection of the functional interaction of the systems of translation and transcription during the restoration of protein biosynthesis inhibited by cycloheximide. *Biochemistry* **42**: 1693–1700.

Section 10.1.6

PCR: 1991. *Methods and Applications*, **1**: 1–75.

Voet, D., and Voet, J.G. 1990. *Biochemistry*, John Wiley and Sons, New York, pp. 824–846.

References

1. Perera, F. P. 1988. The significance of DNA and protein adducts in human biomonitoring studies. *Mutat. Res.* **205**: 255–269.
2. Dorit, R. L.; Schoenbach, L.; and Gilbert, W. 1990. How big is the universe of exons? *Science* (U.S.A.) **250**: 1377–1382.
3. Lutz, W. K. 1979. *In vivo* covalent binding of organic chemicals to DNA as a quantitative indicator in the process of chemical carcinogenesis. *Mutat. Res.* **65**: 289–356.
4. Bandiera, S.; Sawyer, T.; Romkes, M.; Zmudzka, B.; Safe, L.; Mason, G.; Keys, B. and Safe, S. 1984. Polychlorinated dibenzofurans (PCDFs): effects of structure on binding to the 2,3,7,8-TCDD cytosolic receptor protein, AHH induction and toxicity. *Toxicology* **32**: 131–144.
5. Mason, G.; Sawyer, T.; Keys, B; Bandiera, S.; Romkes, M.; Piskorska-Pliszczynska, J.; Zmudzka, B. and Safe, S. 1985. Polychlorinated dibenzofurans (PCDFs): correlation between *in vivo* and *in vitro* structure–activity relationships. *Toxicology* **37**: 1–12.

11

DNA Adducts

11.0 VARIABLES IN DNA ADDUCT FORMATION

Any factor that influences the reaction and concentration of the activated electrophilic form ("putative carcinogen") of the xenobiotic or metabolite with DNA or with other molecules important to division will affect the concentration of DNA adducts.

DNA adduct formation is the postulated initial event of the initiation stage of the multistage carcinogenesis model [1]. The multistages in chronological order include exposure, initiation, promotion, conversion, and progression (Section 9.3.3). The presence of host susceptibility factors, inducers of metabolic activation, inhibitors of metabolic deactivition, error-prone DNA repair, the stimulation of cell proliferation and viruses, and exposure to multiple carcinogens or co-carcinogens are thought to be enhancing factors for initiation, whereas the presence of host resistance factors, antioxidants, Phase II processes electrophile scavengers, inducers of metabolic deactivation, inhibitors of metabolic activation, error-free DNA repair, and terminal differentiation are inhibitory processes [1].

Promotion and conversion are enhanced by host susceptibility factors, hormones, the generation of superoxides, and promoting agents. Promotion and conversion are inhibited by host resistance factors, retinoids, protease inhibitors, anti-inflammatory steroids, and cyclic nucleotides [1]. The presence of repair factors for DNA signifies that biological monitoring markers associated with DNA adducts are more closely related to the biologically effective dose than to the total exposure dose, unlike hemoglobin adducts where there are no repair processes. Thus DNA adduct concentration may not be a good marker of cumulative exposure, whereas protein adducts are more likely to be.

On a cellular level, the initiated cell can form a preneoplastic ("benign") lesion through selective clonal expansion (one of the key events of the multistage model), and on genetic change through promotion or conversion it can be transformed to a malignant tumor (the second major event of the multistage model), which on progression produces detectable clinical cancers. In the first key event, a suppressed oncogene, called a proto-oncogene, is postulated to be activated directly or indirectly by the carcinogen by removal of its suppressor moiety to produce cell growth deregulation, and to provide gene amplification after the modification (mutation) of the primary, secondary, tertiary, or quaternary structure of the chromatin. The H-*ras* oncogene is thought to be implicated in the first key event. DNA–carcinogen adduct formation thus is linked to cancer appearance only for the direct-acting mutagen.

The loss of control of cell division after sufficient gene amplification is the second key event that produces the malignancy, an event thought to involve the activation/deactivation balance of tumor suppressor genes. The latter balance is postulated to be affected by promoters.

The phenotypic changes exhibited by preneoplastic lesions relative to normal cells include the presence of neoantigens, ectopic hormones, enzyme abnormalities, increased cell proliferation, altered differentiation, and endothelial stimulating factors. The phenotypic changes of malignant tumors include all those for preneoplastic cells, but also involve the presence of active tissue invasion, metastasis (malignancies distant from the initial site), altered cell surfaces, altered cytoskeleton, and chromosomal abnormalities (Sections 9.3.2–9.3.5) [1]. Micronucleus formation (Section 9.3.2) is thought to be an attempt to excise the tumor suppressor genes that must be inactivated for the cell to grow and divide normally. Thus cancer is the result of complex interactions between multiple environmental factors and multiple acquired and inherited host factors. From the above, DNA adduct formation does not have to lead to cancer.

DNA adduct concentrations are detectable with present techniques largely in the preneoplastic or malignant tumor stages, except for single cell studies, which are still research tools. Up to 150-fold variations between individuals in the same cultured human tissues from several chemical classes of procarcinogens (which require enzymatic activation to metabolites that bind covalently to DNA) have been observed although the natures of the dominant adducts themselves are similar whether in animals or humans. That similarity makes biological monitoring feasible, as the immunoassay techniques, the most sensitive of the available techniques to detect a DNA adduct presence, often involve the raising of monoclonal or polyclonal antibodies in animals. Well-known procarcinogen chemical classes are polynuclear aromatic hydrocarbons, *N*-nitrosamines, mycotoxins such as Aflatoxin B1 and T-2 toxin, hydrazines such as 1,2-dimethylhydrazine, and aromatic amines such as 2-acetylaminofluorene and 3-amino-1,4-dimethyl-5H-pyrido(4,3-b)indole, also called Tryp-P-1.

As expected from a knowledge of covalent binding in animal tissues (Section 10.2), the CBI varies among cultured human tissues exposed to procarcinogens [1]. As for the animal data, the CBI (Section 10.2.1) may not reflect carcinogenic potency because only specific adducts may be involved in the formation of specific cancers. The bulk of the DNA adducts may be implicated in noncarcinogenic pathways.

The large interindividual variations in DNA adduct formation in specific human tissues appear correlated with variations in rates of excision DNA repair [2] and in the activities of DNA-alkyltransferases, such as the one for O^6-alkylguanine-DNA alkyltransferase [3, 4], and of uracil-DNA glycosylase [4].

Another consideration barely touched on by researchers is the role of DNA adducts at the following levels and locations in tissues: tissue and cell relative to target tissue and cell, indicator cells, and the nucleus and mitochondria; the nucleus relative to the matrix, linker, and core of the nucleosome, and the replicon; and the DNA relative to the genome, repetitive sequences, introns, exons, gene, and intragene [1]. The advantages of developing immunoassays relative to specific cell types and carcinogenic agents make research on such techniques a "hot" area, for the present and in the future.

11.1 TECHNIQUES TO DETECT DNA ADDUCTS AND THEIR SIGNIFICANCE

This topic has been extensively reviewed [5–10], and only a summary is presented here.

Many of these techniques have also been utilized in animal studies. The general animal results indicate that [5]: (1) a dose-effect relationship does exist between a single carcinogen exposure and DNA adduct formation under acute exposure conditions; (2) the relationship between dose and adduct formation under conditions of chronic and intermittent exposure conditions (simulating human exposures) is not linear but shows increasing adduct levels with exposure duration, plateauing when the rate of removal equals the rate of formation—this varying from organ to organ of the same animal, from animal strain to animal strain, and from animal species to animal species; (3) adduct persistence may or may not reflect susceptibility and/or target tissue specificity; (4) more than one DNA adduct is invariably formed after exposure of a genotoxic agent, with the significance of each adduct unknown unless the mechanism of toxicity is known; (5) total DNA adduct concentration does not always correlate with carcinogenic potency except in cases where comparatively few DNA adducts are formed, or the concentration of one dominates; (6) the same DNA adduct can be produced by exposure to different compounds, implying nonspecificity of some DNA adducts and any assays based on such adducts; and (7) sampling time affects the concentration of DNA adducts, with the most being formed a few hours after the exposure. These considerations are in contrast to protein adducts where no repair processes are present, and where only a dose-effect is important so that hemoglobin adducts, for example, are markers of cumulative exposure over the lifetime of the red blood cell (3–4 months). It is unknown whether repair processes are fully operational in peripheral WBCs (they are certainly present in the activated WBCs in organs and tissues), or if stimulation into the division cycle is necessary for that. If the latter hypothesis is true, then DNA adducts in WBCs could be markers of cumulative exposure, especially for the long-lived types. There are very few human data to determine if these relationships hold for humans, as interindividual variation is great and the numbers of people utilized have been small. These studies are summarized in Section 11.2.

The methods used to determine DNA adducts require 10 to 100 μg of DNA, usually found in 200 to 1000 mg of human tissue or WBCs from 25 to 50 mL of human blood [5]. The enzyme immunoassay methods [10] are the most sensitive and specific because of the antibody–antigen reaction specificity, which is amplified by the linked enzyme. The major disadvantage of the immunoassay approach is the need to develop specific (non-cross-reactive) antibodies for each adduct of interest. It is not essential to know the primary structure of the DNA adduct, but only that it is pure so that the final monoclonal or polyclonal antibody reactions are specific. About 0.1% of the DNA must be modified to ensure sufficient antibody production. The modified DNA can be complexed physically to methylated bovine serum albumin before being mixed with an adjuvant for immunization of animals to raise the antibodies. The polyclonal antibodies thus produced may recognize not only the DNA adducts but also some of the surrounding DNA structure. Alternatively, the ribose form of the specific DNA adduct can be bound covalently to a protein, usually keyhole limpet hemocyanin, for similar immunization. The monoclonal antibodies resulting from this procedure are very specific, but generally less sensitive than the polyclonal equivalent. Modified deoxyribose nucleosides also can be coupled to protein before immunization. The antibodies raised in this way may be reactive to modified nucleoside, the DNA adduct, and the DNA surrounding the modification, leading to higher sensitivity but less specificity. Advantages for validated immunoassays include specificity, sensitivity, speed, low cost of the developed technique, and automatability. However, development costs are high.

11.1.1 Competitive Radioimmunoassay (RIA)

Competitive RIA involves the mixing of radiolabeled antigen with antibody sufficient to bind 50% of the tracer. On addition of "cold" (nonradioactive) antigen as inhibitor, some bound tracer is displaced. The antigen concentration in the biological sample is determined by comparing the value for inhibition of tracer–antibody binding with similar values from a standard curve generated by using the inhibition of known amounts of cold antigen. The bound tracer can also be determined by precipitation of antibody–antigen complexes with a second antibody or with ammonium sulfate. The principles are those of the classical isotope dilution technique.

11.1.2 Enzyme-Linked Immunosorbent Assay (ELISA)

In the ELISA, either the antibody or the antigen can be bound to an enzyme. This is done in the bottoms of optimally acid-etched wells of 96-microwell plastic plates coated with the antigen. The antibody binding usually is quantified with a second antibody conjugated to an enzyme such as alkaline phosphatase or peroxidase. Following a competition assay as described for competitive RIA (Section 11.1.1), quantitation of the product formed by reaction of the substrate with the enzyme is the analytical determinant. The product can be detected by luminescence, color, radioactivity, or another parameter. Ultrasensitive enzyme RIAs (USERIA) are also used in a hybrid technique utilizing radiolabeled substrate. ELISA techniques are generally more sensitive than competitive RIA because the enzyme amplifies the antigen–antibody reaction. To validate specificity, ELISA results should be confirmed by the appropriate blot tests (Section 10.1.6).

11.1.3 ^{32}P-Postlabeling

The pure DNA fraction is enzymatically digested to the constituent deoxyribonucleoside-3′-monophosphates by micrococcal endonuclease and spleen exonuclease in that order. These nucleotides are modified by the enzymatic incorporation of ^{32}P label in radiolabeled ATP, usually via polynucleotide kinase, to produce labeled deoxyribonucleoside-3′,5′-diphosphates. After separation of modified nucleotides from the unmodified ones by thin layer chromatography on PEI cellulose or by high performance liquid chromatography, the modified nucleotides are detected by measurement of the radioactivity of the digests via autoradiography, and are quantified by Cerenkov counting. The sensitivity may be enhanced by nuclease P1 digestion of the normal nucleotides before ^{32}P labeling, a procedure that must be validated for the particular DNA because some modified DNA nucleotides can be lost. The sensitivity is about one adduct in 10^{10} nucleotides. The technique is good for aromatic DNA adducts but not for small molecular weight aliphatic DNA adducts. The technique allows a fingerprint of all modified bases to be displayed and is not necessarily adduct-specific unless the specific DNA adduct can be separated before the enzymatic hydrolysis procedure. The nonspecific technique does not produce quantitative data unless the DNA adducts are known, or unless a pure DNA adduct was used originally.

11.1.4 Mass Spectrometry

Mass spectrometry is useful to the femtogram to picogram level in the selected ion monitoring mode following prior gas chromatography of a volatile derivative of the purine or pyrimidine (for example, a pentafluorobenzoyl chloride derivative [11]) liberated through further enzymatic digestion of the nucleotide end products, as described above for digestion of DNA in Section 11.1.3. HPLC/mass spectrometry is still sensitive only to the nanogram–microgram level and awaits further gain in sensitivity. The latter technique is potentially the most important of the mass spectrometry methods. Gas chromatography/electron capture detection is useful as a screening technique for the volatile pentafluorobenzoyl pyrimidine/purine derivatives, but GC/MS of apparently positive electron capture samples must be done because retention times are not unique identifiers of compounds.

11.1.5 Physical Methods

Fluorescence and luminescence methods can approach femtogram quantitation for suitable molecules. Thus, monoclonal antibody to O^6-ethyldeoxyguanosine coupled directly to a fluorescent probe detected 700 ethylations per cell (7 adducts/10^8 nucleotides) using computer-assisted imaging of amplified fluorescence images of single-cell preparations [12].

Aflatoxins and some polycyclic aromatic hydrocarbons (PAHs) have high fluorescence emission quantum yields, and their DNA adducts are thus tagged with a sensitive fluorescent label that can be released (for example, by acid hydrolysis) from the DNA adduct to be quantitated [13]. Fluorescence line-narrowing techniques using a laser as an excitation source at very low temperatures produce narrow-line fluorescence spectra on human samples [14]. The detection limit is about 1 adduct/10^6 nucleotides. Synchronous fluorescence spectrophotometry of benz[a]pyrene tetraols released from DNA adducts formed by activation of benz[a]pyrene has also been reported [15]. Both excitation and emission maxima are scanned, and a peak is registered only when the wavelength difference matches the wavelength gap between the two maxima. Simplified fluorescence spectra result with a sensitivity of 3 adducts/10^8 nucleotides. In practice, substantial background emissions may be observed, thus limiting sensitivity and specificity [15].

11.2 HUMAN STUDIES

DNA adducts have been utilized successfully for four major types of carcinogens: aflatoxins, PAHs, antineoplastic agents, and miscellaneous.

11.2.1 Aflatoxins

Aflatoxins are a family of naturally occurring mycotoxins produced by certain molds. Their occurrence is linked to primary hepatocellular carcinoma in Africa and Asia [16]. Human trials in Africa and Asia using monoclonal antibodies of the major DNA adduct of Aflatoxin B1 have occurred [16, 17], as well as detection of modified DNA bases in urine. These investigations led to the development of reusable monoclonal antibody chromatography affinity columns for the modified bases in urine.

11.2.2 PAHs

The PAHs are ubiquitous, as they are formed by incomplete combustion of fossil fuels, food, refuse, and vegetable matter. Benz[a]pyrene in particular has been much investigated. The benz[a]pyrene-7,8-diol-9,10-epoxide–DNA adduct has been detected by ELISA in tissue and peripheral blood samples of people exposed to PAHs [18, 19]. The adduct level in the lung was 0.14 to 0.18 pmol/mg DNA (5/27 subjects) [18]. Levels in the WBCs of roofers (7/28 subjects), foundry workers (7/20), and smokers (2/9) were between 40 and 4800 pmol/mg DNA using ELISA [19]. Few workers (1/30) and unexposed workers (0/10) in an aluminum-making facility had detectable DNA adducts greater than one adduct in 10^7 nucleotides via synchronous scanning fluorescence spectrophotometry [20]. The latter technique in conjunction with USERIA has confirmed DNA adduct presence at 0.1 to 34.3 pmol/mg DNA in the WBCs of coke oven workers (18/27, 13/38, and 4/38 workers) [15, 21]. Foundry workers (all 22) classified as zero, low, medium, and high exposure exhibited the following average DNA adduct levels in their WBCs: 0.06, 0.32, 0.53, and 1.2 pmol/mg DNA, respectively, as determined by ELISA [22]. DNA aducts of unidentified aromatic compounds were detected in the DNA of

WBCs of foundry workers (10/10) using ^{32}P-postlabeling although no DNA adducts characteristic of benz[a]pyrene exposure were evident [23]. Considerable interindividual variation was reported. The same research group found that DNA of the mononuclear and nonmononuclear cells from normal human bone marrow also contained aromatic DNA adducts of unknown origin (10/10), which were present in much lower concentrations in the peripheral WBCs [24].

Smokers exhibited variable adduct levels in their WBCs, some being five times those in nonsmokers but showing no difference from nonsmokers in others [25, 26]. Wide interindividual variations were observed, even for smokers who appeared to be exposed equally [26].

Defining truly unexposed populations is difficult for a xenobiotic as ubiquitous as benz[a]pyrene. Differentiating between life-style factors and occupational factors requires the measurement of personal baselines and the utilization of other distinctive markers.

11.2.3 Antineoplastic Agents

Many antineoplastic agents are themselves carcinogenic (usually causing acute nonlymphocytic leukemia). Huge known doses are administered via a defined route of exposure and duration, thus facilitating accuracy in the exposure dose estimate, the bane of most epidemiology studies. The patients under treatment have defined dosing intervals, and tumor progression and regression can be monitored. Such exposures are essentially acute because doses are administered at intervals > 3 half-times, so making dose-effect relationships more likely.

cis-Diamminedichloroplatinum (II) (cisplatin) modifies DNA by reacting to produce intrastrand bidentate N^7-*d* (GpG)- and N^7-*d* (GpA)-diammineplatinum adducts. Cisplatin is usually prescribed for testicular, ovarian, and lung cancers. ELISA detected these adducts in buffy coat DNA of WBCs in 99/231 test samples from 45 patients, whereas none was found in 18 unexposed people [27]. Another study on 55 chemotherapy patients [28, 29] showed that 88% of patients with at least one adduct determination over 160 fmol/mg DNA responded to chemotherapy, whereas 67% of those who did not showed no benefit from chemotherapy. The cisplatin adducts were also detected in another seven cancer patients receiving chemotherapy [30]. ELISA methodology using four antisera showed the adduct formed by intrastrand cross-links on pGpG sequences to be the most abundant DNA adduct but with much personal variation. The above studies show that not all patients administered cisplatin produce detectable DNA adducts, a situation that may change as techniques become more sensitive.

Nitrogen mustard, cyclophosphamide, busulfan, triethylenemelamine, cisplatin, BCNU, CCNU, streptozotocin, and dicarbazine all appear to react at the N-7 of guanine, and smaller amounts of cross-links between two N-7 guanines are produced by all but the last two antineoplastics [31].

Mitomycin C treatment of postoperative liver hepatoma caused DNA modifications as visualized by ^{32}P-postlabeling [32]. Four modified nucleotides were detected, the total DNA adducts in human livers 4 days after injection being 3×10^{-8} nucleotides, which decreased to 10^{-8} nucleotides from 2 to 8 weeks. The same adducts were detected in peripheral blood lymphocytes.

More human studies are urgently needed for these antineoplastics.

11.2.4 Miscellaneous

Monoclonal antibodies to 8-methoxypsoralen (antipsoriasis agent that appears to stimulate nonmelanoma skin cancer in the presence of ultraviolet light) are raised from adducts formed by covalent binding with DNA pyrimidines. The monoclonal assay does not correlate well with blood levels of 8-methoxypsoralen [33].

Everson et al. [34, 35] detected seven different types of DNA adducts in the placentas of smoking mothers by ELISA and ^{32}P-postlabeling (which provided results 100-fold different), many of which were not detectable in the WBCs of the mother. The concentration of the diol epoxide DNA adduct of benz[a]pyrene was much lower in lymphocytic DNA than in the placental DNA of smokers, and moreover was not significantly different in concentration relative to nonsmokers [36]. Adducts formed from endogenous *N*-nitrosation of the amines in cigarette smoke were significantly higher for smokers than nonsmokers in spite of an appreciable background in the nonsmokers [37].

Aromatic DNA adduct levels in the bronchus and larynx of smokers were easily detectable using ^{32}P-postlabeling and were about 0.1 to 0.18 pmol/mg DNA [38]. Similarly, five DNA adducts containing aromatic moieties were detected in exfoliated cells from the oral cavities of betel and tobacco chewers, inverted smokers, and nonsmokers, so that smokers and nonsmokers were not differentiated[39]. In the oral mucosa, smokers did have distinctive DNA adducts, but their identities were unknown [40]. The total DNA adducts for smokers (11/11) were 0.1 to 210 fmol/mg DNA, whereas the nonsmokers (2/8) had 0.4 to 1.7 fmol/mg DNA.

Reddy et al. [41] found nine DNA adducts (none with aromatic modifiers) in the placentas (4/4) but not the WBCs of women exposed to smoke from wood combustion. Both exposed and nonexposed women (5/5) had unidentified DNA adducts [41].

N-Nitrosamines are potent alkylating agents and known animal carcinogens. They also are found as products of incomplete combustion of nitrogenous compounds, including cigarette smoke. These compounds also are important in that they form O^6-alkylguanine DNA adducts, which are postulated to be related to the activation signal of the H-*ras* oncogene, which may in turn be related to either initiation activation or the conversion between the preneoplastic state and a malignant one, or both [9]. Such a unifying concept is always dear to the hearts of those molecular biologists who want to have a unique trigger for carcinogenicity.

O^6-methylguanine induces only G to A DNA mutations in circular bacterial DNA during transcription in *Escherichia coli* as directed through the virus M13mp8. The repair mechanism dependent on the methyl transferase can be saturated with sufficient *N*-methyl-*N′*-nitro-*N*-nitrosoguanidine (MNNG) at least in *E. coli* [42], implying a dose-effect above a critical lower level of MNNG.

An RIA using monoclonal antibodies against O^6-methyldeoxyguanosine has been employed in 37 human tissue specimens from patients undergoing surgery for esophageal cancer in China [43]. Detection was achieved for 27/37 patients in their esophageal mucosa, stomach mucosa, or the tumor itself, as opposed to low levels in 5/12 controls.

Vanderlaan et al. [44] have isolated five monoclonal antibodies that recognize tetra- and penta-polychlorinated dibenzo-*p*-dioxins and polychlorinated dibenzofurans. The ELISA detected these compounds at ppb concentrations. Monoclonal antibodies for the potent mutagens found in some cooked foods (2-amino-3-methylimidazo[4,5-f]quinoline, 2-amino-3,4-dimethylimidazo[4,5-f] quinoline, and 2-amino-1-methyl-6-phenylimidazo[4,5-b]pyridine) have also been utilized [32].

It might be noted here that 5-methylcytosine (less than 1% of the bases of human DNA) appears to act as an endogenous mutagen in the DNA of the human LDL receptor and p53 genes [45]. Methylated cytosines appear almost exclusively at CpG dinucleotides (they account for over 90%), which are the sites for more than 35% of all known disease-related point mutations. The mutations should be scored as transitions from 5-methylcytosine to thymine rather than the traditional cytosine to thymine. This transition is postulated to be implicated in the induction of mutations of tumor suppressor genes, the second key step in the multistage model for carcinogenesis. The methylated cytosines are visualized on Southern blotting (Section 10.1.6) on gel electrophoresis by their nonreaction with hydrazine, and therefore do not appear on the cytosine ladder of the sequencing gel. This technique will allow discrimination of indirect mutations produced by increased activity of endogenous methylation enzymes, relative to direct alkylation through DNA–carcinogen adduct formation.

It is clear that all human epidemiology studies with DNA adducts so far have been pilot explorations, and studies with large numbers of people are required to assess the DNA adduct technique further, in well-designed epidemiologic settings.

Further Reading

Anderson, M. W., and Reynolds, S. H. 1988. Activation of oncogenes by chemical carcinogens. In *The Pathology of Neoplasia,* A. E. Sirica (ed.), Plenum Press, New York, pp. 291–301.

Harris, C. C. 1985. Future directions in the use of DNA adducts as internal dosimeters for monitoring human exposure to environmental mutagens and carcinogens. *Environ. Health Perspect.* **62**: 185–191.

Klein, G. 1988. *Cellular Oncogene Activation,* Marcel Dekker, New York.

References

1. Harris, C. C. 1985. Future directions in the use of DNA adducts as internal dosimeters for monitoring human exposure to environmental mutagens and carcinogens. *Environ. Health Perspect.* **62**: 185–191.
2. Setlow, R. B. 1983. Variations in DNA repair among humans. In *Human Carcinogenesis*, C. C. Harris, and H. Autrup (eds.), Academic Press, New York, pp. 231–254.
3. Grafstrom, R. C.; Pegg, A. E.; Trump, B. F.; and Harris, C. C. 1984. O^6-alkylguanine-DNA alkyltransferase activity in normal human cells and tissues. *Cancer Res.* **44**: 2855–2857.
4. Myrnes, B.; Giercksky, K. E.; and Krokan, H. 1983. Interindividual variation in the activity of O^6-methylguanine-DNA methyltransferase and uracil-DNA glycosylase in human organs. *Carcinogenesis* **4**: 1565–1568.
5. Koh, H. K.; Prout, M. N.; and Groopman, J. D. 1989. Carcinogen monitoring by DNA adduct methodology in humans: clinical perspectives for the 1990s. *Adv. Intern. Med.* **34**: 243–264.

6. Adamkiewicz, J.; Nehls, P.; and Rajewsky, M. 1984. Immunological methods for detection of carcinogen–DNA adducts. In *Monitoring Human Exposure to Carcinogenic and Mutagenic Agents*, A. Berlin, M. Draper, K. Hemminki, et al. (eds.), International Agency for Research on Cancer, Lyon, France, *IARC Sci. Public.* **59**: 199–216.
7. Wogan, G., and Gorelick, N. 1985. Chemical and biochemical dosimetry of exposure to genotoxic chemicals. *Environ. Health Perspect.* **62**: 5–18.
8. Wogan, G. N. 1989. Markers of exposure to carcinogens. *Environ. Health Perspect.* **81**: 9–17.
9. Perera, F. P. 1988. The significance of DNA and protein adducts in human biomonitoring studies. *Mutat. Res.* **205**: 255–269.
10. Santella, R. M. 1988. Application of new techniques for the detection of carcinogen adducts to human population monitoring. *Mutat. Res.* **205**: 271–282.
11. Mohammed, G. B.; Nazaret, A.; Hayes, M. J.; Giese, R. W.; and Vouros, P. 1984. GC–MS characteristics of methylated perfluoroacyl derivatives of cytosine and 5-methyl cytosine. *J. Chromatogr.* **314:** 211–217.
12. Adamkiewicz, J.; Eberle, G.; Huh, N.; Nehls, P.; and Rajewsky, M. F. 1985. Quantitation and visualization of alkyl deoxynucleosides in the DNA of mammalian cells by monoclonal antibodies. *Environ. Health Perspect.* **62**: 49–55.
13. Jeffrey, A. M. 1985. DNA modification by chemical carcinogens. *Pharmacol. Ther.* **28**: 237–272.
14. Sanders, M. J.; Cooper, R. S.; Jankowiak, R.; Small, G. J.; Heisig, V.; and Jeffrey, A. M. 1986. Identification of polycyclic aromatic hydrocarbon metabolites and DNA adducts in mixtures using fluorescence line narrowing spectrometry. *Anal. Chem.* **58**: 816–820.
15. Haugen, A.; Becher, G.; Benestad, C.; Vahakangas, K.; Trivers, G. E.; Newman, M. J.; and Harris, C. C. 1986. Determination of polycyclic aromatic hydrocarbons in the urine, benzo[a]pyrene diol epoxide–DNA adducts in lymphocyte DNA, and antibodies to the adducts in sera from coke oven workers exposed to measured amounts of polycyclic aromatic hydrocarbons in work atmospheres. *Cancer Res.* **46**: 4178–4183.
16. Groopman, J.; Busby, W.; Donahue, P.; et al. 1986. Aflatoxins as risk factors for liver cancer; an application of monoclonal antibodies to monitor human exposure. In *Biochemical and Molecular Epidemiology of Cancer*, C. C. Harris (ed.) Alan R. Liss, New York, pp. 233–256.
17. Groopman, J.; Roebuck, B.; and Kensler, T. 1987. Application of monoclonal antibodies and dietary antioxidant-based animal models to define human exposure to Aflatoxin B1. *Prog. Exp. Tumor Res.* **31**: 52–62.
18. Perera, F. P.; Poirier, M. C.; Yuspa, S. H.; Nakayama, J.; Jaretzki, A.; Curnen, M. M.; Knowles, D. M.; and Weinstein, I. B. 1982. A pilot project in molecular cancer epidemiology: determination of benz[a]pyrene–DNA adducts in animal and human tissues by immunoassays. *Carcinogenesis* **3**: 1405–1410.
19. Shamsuddin, A. K. M.; Sinopoli, N. T.; Hemminki, K.; Boesch, R. R.; and Harris, C. C. 1985. Detection of benz[a]pyrene–DNA adducts in human white blood cells. *Cancer Res.* **45**: 66–68.
20. Vahakangas, K.; Haugen, A.; and Harris, C. C. 1985. An applied synchronous fluorescence spectrophotometric assay to study benzo[a]pyrene diol epoxide–DNA adducts. *Carcinogenesis* **6**: 1109–1116.
21. Harris, C. C.; Vahakangas, K.; Newman, M. J.; Trivers, G. E.; Shamsuddin, A.; Sinopoli, N.; Mann, D. L.; and Wright, W. E. 1985. Detection of benz[a]pyrene diol epoxide–DNA adducts in peripheral blood lymphocytes and antibodies to the adducts in serum from coke oven workers. *Proc. Nat. Acad. Sci. USA* **82**: 6672–6676.

22. Perera, F. P.; Hemminki, K. H.; Santella, R. M.; Brenner, D.; and Kelly, G. 1987. DNA adducts in white blood cells of foundry workers. *Proc. Am. Assoc. Cancer Res.* **28**: 94.
23. Phillips, D. H.; Hemminki, K.; Hewer, A.; and Grover, P. L. 1987. Postlabeling of white blood cell DNA from foundry workers. *Proc. Am. Assoc. Cancer Res.* **28**: 102.
24. Phillips, D. H.; Hewer, A.; and Grover, P. L. 1986. Aromatic DNA adducts in human bone marrow and peripheral blood leukocytes. *Carcinogenesis* **7**: 2071–2075.
25. Perera, F.; Santella, R.; and Poirier, M. 1986. Biomonitoring of workers exposed to carcinogens: immunoassays to benzo[a]pyrene–DNA adducts as a prototype. *J. Occup. Med.* **28**: 1117–1123.
26. Weston, A. S.; Trivers, G.; Vahakangas, K.; et al. 1987. Detection of carcinogen–DNA adducts in human cells and antibodies to these adducts in human sera. *Prog. Exp. Tumor Res.* **31**: 76–85.
27. Reed, E.; Yuspa, S.; and Zwelling, L. 1986. Quantitation of *cis*-diamminedichloroplatinum (II) (cisplatin)–DNA–intrastrand adducts in testicular and ovarian cancer patients receiving cisplatin chemotherapy. *J. Clin. Invest.* **77**: 545–550.
28. Reed, E.; Ozols, R.; Tarone, R.; Yuspa, S. H.; and Poirier, M. C. 1987. Platinum DNA adducts in leukocyte DNA correlate with disease response in ovarian cancer patients receiving platinum-based chemotherapy. *Proc. Nat. Acad. Sci. USA* **84**: 5024–5028.
29. Poirier, M.; Reed, E.; Ozols, R.; et al. 1987. DNA adducts of cisplatin in nucleated peripheral blood cells and tissues of cancer patients. *Prog. Exp. Tumor Res.* **31**: 104–113.
30. Fichtinger-Schepman, A. M.; van Oosterom, A. T.; Lohman, P. H. M.; and Berends, F. 1987. *Cis*-Diamminedichloroplatinum (II)-induced DNA adducts in peripheral leukocytes from seven cancer patients: quantitative immunochemical detection of the adduct induction and removal after a single dose of *cis*-diamminedichloroplatinum (II). *Cancer Res.* **47**: 3000–3004.
31. Sorsa, M.; Hemminki, K.; and Vainio, H. 1985. Occupational exposure to anticancer drugs—potential and real hazards. *Mutat. Res.* **154**: 135–149.
32. de Serres, F. J.; and Matsushima, T. 1988. Approaches for human population monitoring. *Mutat. Res.* **203**: 185–199.
33. Santella, R.; Gasparro, F.; and Hsieh, L. 1987. Quantitation of carcinogen–DNA adducts with monoclonal antibodies. *Prog. Exp. Tumor Res.* **31**: 63–75.
34. Everson, R.; Randerath, E.; and Santella, R.; et al. 1986. Detection of smoking-related covalent DNA adducts in human placenta. *Science* **231**: 54–57.
35. Everson, R.; Randerath, E.; and Avitts, T.; et al. 1987. Preliminary investigations of tissue specificity and strategies for identifying chemicals causing DNA adducts in human placenta. *Prog. Exp. Tumor Res.* **31**: 86–103.
36. Perera, F. P.; Santella, R. M.; Brenner, D.; Poirier, M. C.; Munshi, A. A.; Fischman, H. K.; and Vanryzin, J. 1987. DNA adducts, protein adducts and SCE in cigarette smokers and non-smokers. *J. Nat. Cancer Inst.* **79**: 449–456.
37. Hoffmann, D.; and Brunnemann, K. D. 1983. Endogenous formation of *N*-nitrosoproline in cigarette smokers. *Cancer Res.* **43**: 5570–5574.
38. Randerath, E.; Avitts, T. A.; Reddy, M. V.; Miller, R. H.; Everson, R. B.; and Randerath, K. 1986. Comparative ^{32}P-analysis of cigarette smoke-induced DNA damage in human tissues and mouse skin. *Cancer Res.* **46**: 5869–5877.
39. Dunn, B. P.; and Stich, H. F. 1986. ^{32}P-postlabeling analysis of aromatic DNA adducts in human oral mucosal cells. *Carcinogenesis* **7**: 1115–1120.

40. Chacko, M.; and Gupta, R. C. 1987. Evaluation of DNA damage in the oral mucosa of cigarette smokers and non-smokers by ^{32}P-adduct assay. *Proc. Am. Assoc. Cancer Res.* **28**: 101.
41. Reddy, M. V.; Kenny, P.C.; and Randerath, K. 1987. ^{32}P-assay of DNA adducts in white blood cells (WBC) and placentas of pregnant women exposed to residential wood combustion (RWC) smoke. *Proc. Am. Assoc. Cancer Res.* **28**: 97.
42. Essigmann, J. M.; Fowler, K. W.; Green, C. L.; and Loechler, E. L. 1985. Extrachromosomal probes for mutagenesis by carcinogens: studies on the mutagenic activity of O^6-methylguanine built into a unique site in a viral genome. *Environ. Health Perspect.* **62**: 171–176.
43. Umbenhauer, D.; Wild, C. P.; Montesano, R.; Saffhill, R.; Boyle, J. M.; Huh, N.; Kirstein, U.; Thomale, J.; Rajewsky, M. F.; and Lu, S. H. 1985. O^6-Methyldeoxyguanosine in esophageal DNA among individuals at high risk of oesophageal cancer. *Int. J. Cancer* **36**: 661–665.
44. Vanderlaan, M. 1988. As quoted in reference 32, p192.
45. Rideout, W. M.; III; Coetzee, G. A.; Olumi, A. F.; and Jones, P. A. 1990. 5-Methylcytosine as an endogenous mutagen in the human LDL receptor and p53 genes. *Science* **249**: 1288–1290.

12

Hemoglobin Binding as a Dose Monitor for Human Exposure to Carcinogens and Mutagens

by Michael A. Pereira*

12.0 INTRODUCTION

The estimation of the carcinogenic and mutagenic risk to humans resulting from exposure to a chemical carcinogen and/or mutagen requires knowledge of the dose and pharmacokinetics of the chemical in humans (Section 10.0). The mechanism of action of many carcinogens and mutagens involves their covalent binding to the DNA of the target cell (Chapter 11). Two types of assays are being developed and applied to estimate human exposure to these genotoxic hazards: biological indicators of exposure and biochemical dosimeters of exposure. Biological indicators of exposure most frequently use peripheral blood lymphocytes to measure genotoxic damage to chromosomes (Section 11.2). The damage to chromosomes can be determined by increases in sister chromatid exchanges, micronuclei, structural aberrations, and aneuploidy, as well as a mutagenic event (Sections 9.3.2–9.3.5).

Biochemical dosimeters of exposure being developed and applied include DNA adducts (Chapter 11), hemoglobin adducts, and urinary metabolites (Section 6.2), including excretion of degradation products of DNA adducts (Section 9.3.11). These biochemical dosimeters of exposure can provide quantitative data indicative of an individual's capacity for absorption, metabolism (including activation to the ultimate carcinogen), and excretion of the genotoxic agent. Hence, these dosimeters can provide many of the pharmacokinetic data required for risk assessment of the exposure to genotoxic agents.

12.0.1 Advantages of Hemoglobin Binding

The advantages of the hemoglobin binding assay as a dose monitor are: (1) ease and availability of sampling: blood is readily and repeatedly obtainable

* Environmental Health Research and Testing, Inc., Cincinnati, OH.

from people, (2) sensitivity: large quantities of hemoglobin are present in the blood (approx. 10–15% by weight), and (3) cumulative nature of the marker: the stability of circulating adducted hemoglobin is directly dependent upon red cell lifetime and is on the order of months. The stability of circulating carcinogens bound to hemoglobin allows the monitoring of an exposure months after it has ceased, and measurement of the accumulation of damage produced by low chronic exposures that by themselves would not be detected.

The binding of carcinogens to hemoglobin in circulating erythrocytes has been shown not to alter the life span of the red blood cell. The lifetime of carcinogen binding to hemoglobin has been shown to be approximately 40 days in mice [1, 2] and 70 days in rats [3], values corresponding to the lifetime of circulating erythrocytes in the respective species. Daily exposure of mice and rats to a carcinogen resulted in the accumulation of adducts in hemoglobin so that (1) a low level of exposure that was not detected as a single exposure was detected after 10 daily doses in rats [3], and (2) the extent of hemoglobin binding after chronic exposure approached $a(ter/2)$ where a is the degree of binding after a single exposure and ter is the average lifetime of circulating erythrocytes [2]. Therefore, in humans where the lifetime of circulating erythrocytes is approximately 120 days, it is expected that the half-life and the lifetime of hemoglobin adducts after a single exposure will be 60 and 120 days, respectively, and that the accumulation of the extent of hemoglobin adducts after a repeated chronic exposure (approaching or greater than 120 days) will be equal to 60 times the extent of binding found after a single exposure.

All carcinogens and mutagens so far evaluated have been demonstrated to bind hemoglobin in circulating erythrocytes. Pereira and Chang [4] reported the binding of different chemical classes of carcinogens to hemoglobin in rats. Direct-acting (binding) carcinogens after intragastric administration bound hemoglobin to a greater extent than those requiring metabolic activation. Even carcinogens that appear not to possess genotoxic activity and not to bind DNA, such as chloroform and carbon tetrachloride, bound hemoglobin, whereas noncarcinogens did not bind hemoglobin. The absolute binding level was not related to the carcinogenic potency of this broad spectrum of carcinogens. This lack of a relationship is not unexpected, as there is also a lack of a correlation between the DNA binding of this broad spectrum of carcinogenic potency in terms of CBI (Section 10.2.1).

The binding of carcinogens to hemoglobin was related to the dose of carcinogen and to the binding of the carcinogen to DNA in the target organ [2, 5, 6]. Once the mathematical relationship between hemoglobin binding and both dose and DNA binding was established, the binding of a carcinogen to hemoglobin was used to calculate both dose and DNA binding of carcinogen.

Chemical binding to hemoglobin has been used clinically as a dosimeter for exposure of diabetes to excess glucose [7, 8]. Glucose binds to the N-terminal valine and the ε amino group of lysine of the globin to yield glycosylated hemoglobin. The glycosylated hemoglobin is separated by cationic exchange chromatography and designated A_{Ic}. Acetylation of hemoglobin in alcoholics results in a species of hemoglobin that is separated by cationic exchange chromatography and that has been proposed as a dosimeter for alcohol exposure [9].

The amount of hemoglobin binding resulting from human exposure to carcinogens is below the detection limit of a new chromatographic species of hemoglobin; so isolation and quantitation of the carcinogen adduct are required. The rest of this chapter describes three procedures used to determine quantitatively the binding of carcinogens and mutagens to hemoglobin in humans.

12.1 METHODS OF MEASUREMENT AND APPLICATION AS DOSIMETER

12.1.1 Nucleophilic Binding Sites in Hemoglobin

There are four nucleophilic binding sites in hemoglobin: cysteine, histidine, lysine, and the α-NH_2 (N-terminal) of valine. The pK_a of lysine is about 10 so that at the pH of erythrocytes, pH = 7.4, the ε amino group of lysine is in the $-NH_3^+$ state and not acceptable for binding by the electrophilic species of the carcinogen. The pK_a of cysteine is about 8, that of histidine is 6 to 7, and that of the N-terminal valine is 7 to 8; therefore, at the pH of the erythrocytes these amino acids are expected to bind carcinogenic electrophiles. Carcinogens have been demonstrate to bind these three amino acids in hemoglobin, at the sulfhydryl group of cysteine, the N_1 and N_3 atoms of histidine, and the amino group of the N-terminal valine of both the α and the β chains.

12.1.2 Hemoglobin Hydrolysis and Adduct Isolation

Ehrenberg and his colleagues conducted the original research in the use of hemoglobin binding as a dosimeter [1, 10, 11]. The bindings to hemoglobin of ethylene oxide [12, 13], methyl methanesulfonate [2], and vinyl chloride [14] were begun by isolation of the hemoglobin from circulating erythrocytes. The globin was isolated by precipitation with 1% HCl in acetone to remove the heme [15]. The globin was hydrolyzed in 6 N HCl at 120° C, and the amino acids containing the carcinogen-derived adduct were isolated by ion exchange chromatography. Globin has also been broken down to amino acids by pronase with and without pepsin or trypsin digestion. Farmer et al. [16] modified the procedure by using gas chromatography–mass spectrometry (GC/MS) to identify and quantitate the binding to hemoglobin. Hutchins et al. [17] used high performance liquid chromatography (HPLC), UV spectrophotometry, and mass spectrometry to isolate and identify fluoranthene adducts in hemoglobin.

Application to Human Exposure

The hydrolysis of the globin followed by the separation and identification of the adduct has been used as a dosimeter in humans. *N*-(2-hydroxyethyl) histidine has been identified in the hemoglobin of humans occupationally exposed to ethylene oxide [13, 18]. The modified Edman degradation procedure (to be described later) for the determination of N-terminal adducts such as *N*-(2-hydroxyethyl) valine was more sensitive than the globin hydrolysis procedure to determine human exposure to ethylene oxide [18]. This was so because of the high background levels of the histidine adduct compared to the valine adduct. A high background level of *S*-methylcysteine has also been found in apparently unexposed humans, farm animals, and laboratory animals [19], which will decrease the sensitivity of the isolation of the *S*-methylcysteine adduct from hydrolyzed globin for the monitoring of human exposure to methylating agents. Propylene oxide exposure of humans has been monitored by the identification of *N*-(2-hydroxypropyl) histidine in globin hydrolysates [20], and acrylamide exposure by the identification of 2-carboxyethylcysteine [21].

12.1.3 N-Terminal Valine

The N-terminal amino acid of the two α and two β chains of human hemoglobin is valine, and the amino group has been shown to bind carcinogens and mutagens. The N-terminal valine of the globin is cleaved by the Edman sequencing reagent pentafluorophenyl isothiocyanate as described by Tornqvist et al. [22]. The released valine and alkylated valine are derivatized and analyzed by GC/MS. The advantage of this procedure is that (1) the alkylated valine does not have to be separated from the other amino acids of a globin hydrolyzate, and (2) unlike the released adduct procedure (to be described later) this one is suitable for monitoring exposure of carcinogens that bind hemoglobin to produce low molecular weight adducts such as methyl, hydroxyethyl, hydroxypropyl, etc. groups.

Application to Human Exposure

The Edman degradation procedure has been used to monitor human exposure to ethylene oxide in the workplace [18] and from cigarette smoke [23]. The presence of the ethylene oxide adduct, *N*-(2-hydroxyethyl) valine, was quantitated after Edman degradation. The N-terminal valine procedure used to monitor occupational exposure to ethylene oxide appeared more sensitive than the hydrolysis procedure for quantitating N^{6}-(2-hydroxyethyl) histidine [18].

12.1.4 Measurement of Released Adduct

The monitoring of high molecular weight and hydrophobic adducts in hemoglobin has been simplified and made more sensitive by release of the adduct from hemoglobin in the absence of globin hydrolysis. The adduct is released by either mild acid or base treatment. The adduct then can be separated from the globin by either (1) extraction with organic solvent (chloroform, hexane, or isoamyl alcohol), (2) passage through a C18 Sep-Pak cartridge, or (3) chromatography with Sephadex LH-20. The released adduct can be isolated and identified by the analytical procedures of HPLC [24, 25], HPLC combined with synchronous fluorescence spectroscopy [26], GC [27], and GC/MS [28].

Application to Human Exposure

The exposure of humans to cigarette smoke has been monitored by the binding of 4-aminobiphenyl to hemoglobin [28]. The 4-aminobiphenyl metabolite was released by base-catalyzed hydrolysis identified and quantitated by GC/MS analysis. The quantity of 4-aminobiphenyl adduct to hemoglobin has been related to both the quantity and the type of tobacco smoked, as well as to the acetylator phenotype of the smoker [29].

The benzo[a]pyrene-7,8,9,10-tetrahydrotetrol metabolite of benzo[a]pyrene was released by mild acid hydrolysis of hemoglobin from cigarette smokers [26]. HPLC combined with synchronous fluorescence spectroscopy (Section 11.1.5), used by Weston [26], appears to be a sensitive procedure for the detection of benzo[a]pyrene exposure of cigarette smokers. The *anti*-tetrahydrotetrol of benzo[a]pyrene has also been detected bound to fetal hemoglobin [30, 31]. The benzo[a]pyrene tetrol was released from the hemoglobin during enzymatic digestion, isolated by HPLC, and identified by capillary gas chromatography–mass spectrometery and fluorescence spectroscopy. The diol epoxide adduct of chrysene, *r*-1, *t*-2, *t*-3, *c*-4-tetrahydroxy-1,2,3,4-tetrahydrochrysene, has also been identified in fetal and in smoker's hemoglobin [31].

12.2 CONCLUSIONS

The binding of chemical carcinogens and mutagens to hemoglobin in circulating erythrocytes is a relatively new dosimeter for human exposure. The application of hemoglobin binding to clinical, occupational, and epidemiological investigations is at the stage of development that requires validation using pilot studies of known human exposure. The monitoring of human exposure to carcinogens that produce low molecular weight adducts including methyl, hydroxyethyl and hydroxypropyl, appears to be best done by use of the Edman degradation procedure for release of N-terminal valine–containing adducts. For carcinogens whose adducts are of high molecular weight and are hydrophobic, the procedure of mild acid or base release of the adduct followed by extraction and analytical analysis appears most promising.

References

1. Osterman-Golkar, S.; Ehrenberg, L.; Segerback, D.; and Hallstrom, I. 1976. Evaluation of genetic risks of alkylating agents. II. Haemoglobin as a dose monitor. *Mutat. Res.* **34**: 1–10.
2. Segerback, D.; Calleman, C. J.; Ehrenberg, L.; Lofroth, G.; and Osterman-Golkar, S. 1978. Evaluation of genetic risks of alkylating agents. IV. Quantitative determination of alkylated amino acids in haemoglobin as a measure of the dose after treatment of mice with methyl methansulfonate. *Mutat. Res.* **49**: 71–82.
3. Pereira, M. A., and Chang, L. W. 1982. Binding of chloroform to mouse and rat hemoglobin. *Chemi. Biol. Interactions* **39**: 89–99.
4. Pereira, M. A., and Chang, L. W. 1981. Binding of chemical carcinogens and mutagens to rat haemoglobin. *Chemi. Biol. Interactions* **33**: 301–305.
5. Pereira, M. A.; Lin, L. H. C.; and Chang, L. W. 1981. Dose-dependency of 2-acetylaminofluorene binding to liver DNA and hemoglobin in mice and rats. *Toxicol. Appl. Pharmacol.* **60**: 272–278.
6. Murthy, M. S. S.; Calleman, C. J.; Osterman-Golkar, S.; Segerback, D.; and Svensson, K. 1983. Relationships between ethylation of hemoglobin, ethylation of DNA and administered amount of ethyl methanesulfonate in the mouse. *Mutat. Res.* **127**: 1–8.
7. Bunn, H. F. 1981. Evaluation of glycosylated hemoglobin in diabetic patients. *Diabetes* **30**: 613–617.
8. Kaplan, L. A.; Cline, D.; and Gertside, P. 1982. Hemoglobin A_1 in hemolysates from healthy and insulin-dependent diabetic children, as determined with a temperature-controlled mini-column assay. *Clin. Chem.* **28**: 13–18.

9. Hoberman, H. D. 1983. Post-translation modification of hemoglobin in alcoholism. *Biochem. Biophys. Res. Commun.* **113**: 1004–1009.
10. Ehrenberg, L.; and Osterman-Golkar, S. 1980. Alkylation of macromolecules for detecting mutagenic agents. *Teratogen. Mutagen. Carcinogen.* **1**: 105–127.
11. Osterman-Golkar, S.; Farmer, P. B.; Segerback, D.; Bailey, E.; Calleman, C. J.; Svensson, K.; and Ehrenberg, L. 1983. Dosimetry of ethylene oxide in the rat by quanitification of alkylated histidine in hemoglobin. *Teratogen. Carcinogen. Mutagen.* **3**: 395–405.
12. Ehrenberg, L.; Hiesche, K. D.; Osterman-Gokar, S.; and Wennberg, I. 1974. Evaluation of genetic risks of alkyating agents: tissue doses in the mouse from air contaminated with ethylene oxide. *Mutat. Res.* **24**: 83–103.
13. Calleman, C.-J.; Ehrenberg, L.; Jansson, B.; Osterman-Golkar, S.; Segerback, D.; Svensson, K.; and Wachtmeiser, C. A. 1978. Monitoring and risk assessment by means of alkyl groups in hemoglobin in persons occupationally exposed to ethylene oxide. *J. Environ. Pathol. Toxicol.* **2**: 427–442.
14. Osterman-Golkar, S.; Hultmark, D.; Segerback, D.; Calleman, C. J.; Gothe, R.; Ehrenberg, L.; and Wachtmeister, C. A.; 1977. Alkylation of DNA and proteins in mice exposed to vinyl chloride. *Biochem. Biophys. Res. Commun.* **7**: 259–266.
15. Anson, M. L., and Mirsky, A. E. 1930. Protein coagulation and its reversal: the preparation of insoluble globin, soluble globin, and heme. *J. Gen. Physiol.* **13**: 469–476.
16. Farmer, P. B.; Bailey E.; Lamb J. H.; and Connors, T. A. 1980. Approach to the quantitation of alkylated amino acids in haemoglobin by gas chromatography–mass spectrometry. *Biomed. Mass Spectrom.* **7**: 41–46.
17. Hutchins, D. A.; Skipper, P. L.; Naylor, S.; and Tannenbaum, S. R. 1988. Isolation and characterization of the major fluoranthene–hemoglobin adducts formed *in vivo* in the rat. *Cancer Res.* **48**: 4756–4761.
18. Farmer, P. B.; Bailey, E.; Gorf, S. M.; Tornqvist, M.; Osterman-Golkar, S.; Kautiainen, A.; and Lewis-Enright, D. P. 1986. Monitoring human exposure to ethylene oxide by the determination of haemoglobin adducts using gas chromatography–mass spectrometry. *Carcinogenesis* **7**: 637–640.
19. Bailey, E.; Connors, T. A.; Farmer, P. B.; Gorf, S. M.; and Rickard, J. 1981. Methylation of cysteine in hemoglobin following exposure to methylating agents. *Cancer Res.* **41**: 2514–2517.
20. Osterman-Golkar, S.; Bailey, E.; Farmer, P. B.; Gorf, S. M. and Lamb J. H. 1984. Monitoring exposure to propylene oxide through the determination of hemoglobin alkylation. *Scand. J. Work. Environ. Health* **10**: 99–102.
21. Bailey, E.; Farmer, P. B.; Bird, I.; Lamb, J. H.; and Peal, J. A. 1986. Monitoring exposure to acrylamide by the determination of *S*-(2-carboxyethyl) cysteine in hydrolyzed haemoglobin by gas chromatography–mass spectrometry. *Anal. Biochem.* **157**: 241–248.
22. Tornqvist, M.; Mowrer, J.; Jensen, S.; and Ehrenberg, L. 1986. Monitoring of environmental cancer initiators through haemoglobin adducts by a modified Edman degradation method. *Anal. Biochem.* **154**: 255–266.
23. Tornqvist, M.; Osterman-Golkar, S.; Kautiainen, A.; Jensen, S.; Farmer, P. B.; and Ehrenberg, L. 1986. Tissue doses of ethylene oxide in cigarette smokers determined from adduct levels in hemoglobin. *Carcinogenesis* **7**: 1519–1521.
24. Shugart, L. 1985. Quantitating exposure to chemical carcinogens: *in vivo* alkylation of hemoglobin by benzo(a)pyrene. *Toxicology* **34**: 211–220.
25. Carmella, S. G.; and Hecht, S. S. 1987. Formation of hemoglobin adducts upon treatment of F344 rats with the tobacco-specific nitrosamines 4-(methylnitrosamino)-1-(3-pyridyl)-1-butanone and *N*-nitrosonornicotine. *Cancer Res.* **47**: 2626–2630.

26. Weston, A.; Rowe, M. L.; Manchester, D. K.; Farmer, P. B.; Mann, D. L.; and Harris, C. C. 1989. Fluorescence and mass spectral evidence for the formation of benzo(a)pyrene *anti*-diol-epoxide–DNA and –hemoglobin adducts in humans. *Carcinogenesis.* **10**: 251–257.
27. Green, L. C.; Skipper P. L.; Turesky, R. J.; Bryant, M. S.; and Tannenbaum, S. R. 1984. *In vivo* dosimetry of 4-aminobiphenyl in rats via a cysteine adduct in hemoglobin. *Cancer Res.* **44**: 4254–4259.
28. Bryant, M. S.; Skipper, P. L.; Tannenbaum, S. R.; and Maclure, M. 1987. Hemoglobin adducts of 4-aminobiphenyl in smokers and nonsmokers. *Cancer Res.* **47**: 601–608.
29. Vineis, P.; Caporaso, N.; Tannenbaum, S. R.; Skipper, P. L.; Glogowski, J.; Bartsch, H.; Coda, M.; Talaska, G.; and Kadlubar, F. 1990. Acetylation phenotype, carcinogen–hemoglobin adducts, and cigarette smoking. *Cancer Res.* **50**: 3002–3004.
30. Skipper, P. L.; Naylor, S.; Gan, L.-S.; Day, B. W.; Pastorelli, R.; and Tannenbaum, S. R. 1989. Origin of tetrahydrotetrols derived from human hemoglobin adducts of benzo[a]pyrene. *Chem. Res. Toxicol.* **2**: 280–281.
31. Day, B. W.; Skipper, P. L.; Wisnok, J. S.; Coghlin, J.; Hammond, S. K.; Gann P.; and Tannenbaum, S. R. 1990. Identification of an *in vivo* chrysene diol epoxide adduct in human hemoglobin. *Chem. Res. Toxicol.* **3**: 340–343.

13

Basic Immunology

This chapter is essentially an introduction to basic immunology. It stops short of a detailed biochemical description because much is still unknown about this aspect of immunology. The genetic aspects of immunology have been minimized here in the interests of clarity and space.

13.0 INNATE IMMUNITY

Innate immunity encompasses those immune responses that are not intrinsically affected by prior contact with a foreign agent. The markers associated with innate immunity thus are classical nonspecific medical monitoring markers.

13.0.1 Phagocytosis

Generally after attachment of a particle, microorganism, or protozoan to the membrane of a phagocytic cell by direct contact, an actin–myosin contracile system is activated that extends pseudopods around the foreign body. This process continues until the foreign object is completely enclosed in a vacuole called the phagosome. During this phase, the pentose phosphate pathway generating NADPH (Section 2.3) is markedly activated. The NADPH generated is used to reduce molecular oxygen bound to a unique plasma-membrane cytochrome b245. This series of events induces a burst of oxygen consumption and accumulations of superoxide ion, singlet oxygen (a reactive oxygen molecule in an excited state, with the excited electron paired relative to spin with its companion unexcited electron), hydrogen peroxide, and hydroxyl radicals, all highly reactive species. Chloride ions also are oxidized (Section 1.7) nonenzymically and enzymically (via myeloperoxidases) to hypochlorite ions, which are also microbicidal (analogous to those in water chlorination processes). These processes consume hydrogen ions, raising the pH (Section 1.6), they change intra- and extracellular Na/K/Ca ratios, and they affect membrane hydrophobicity, thus impelling the cytoplasmic granules of the macrophage to migrate to the phagosome. These granules then fuse with the phagosome and discharge their granular lysosomal packet agents (hydrolases, lysozyme, myeloperoxidases, lactoferrin, and cathepsins). These agents are concentrated around the foreign object in the small volume of the phagosome without killing the macrophage itself. Eventually the pH reaches a value that allows the cathepsin components to attack microorganism membranes directly or via their proteinase activity. While the oxygen-dependent process is occurring, anaerobic processes also flourish, characterized by low pH and lysozyme and lactoferrin participation and fueled by glycolysis (Section 2.1).

Digestion of the foreign body and hydrolysis of macromolecular degradation products occur until fragments useful for anabolic processes in the macrophage are produced. By this time, the ionic and osmotic strengths and enzyme hydrolase activities of the phagosome fluid reach critical limits. The thinnest portion of the membrane of the macrophage in contact with the phagosome is degraded, and the products from the digested particle are released into the surrounding medium.

The host macrophage and some invading microbes are protected by the action of their superoxide dismutase and catalase. Protozoa and viruses with these or other protective mechanisms prevent direct contact with the phagocyte, and/or prevent membrane activation to stimulate pseudopod formation. An alternative route of attack by the host is required for its own protection, this being the function of the complement system.

13.0.2 Complement

Complement is the name given to a complex series of about 20 proteins that, along with blood clotting and fibrinolysis (Section 9.1.15) as well as kinen formation, constitutes one of the triggered enzyme systems found in the blood. This means that a stimulus triggers an amplified "cascade" response where the product of a reaction is the enzymic catalyst of the next reaction. Each reaction is also regulated by inactivating factors so that runaway does not occur. The crucial initial step involves activation of a thioester bond in C3 (Complement 3) by Factor B in the presence of magnesium ions, and subsequent cleavage by Factor D to produce a "C3 convertase"–C3bBb complex with subsequent covalent binding (Section 10.2) of the reactive intermediate ($\overline{\text{C3bBb}}$) to the membrane of the foreign microorganism, protozoan, or virus to produce membrane-bound C3b with the splitting off of a much smaller biologically active peptide C3a. This step is repeated many times, leading to a large endogenous CBI (Section 10.2.1). This has been termed the "alternative pathway" of complement activation. Reaction of the membrane-bound complex C3b then occurs in order with C5, C6, C7, C8, and C9 (each step splitting off smaller biologically active "a" peptide entities, and with "b" large molecular weight residues remaining in the microorganism membrane, each being autocatalytic relative to the next step), eventually producing insertion of C9b into the lipid bilayer of the membrane and polymerization into an annular membrane attack complex (MAC). The MAC forms a cylindrical transmembrane channel permeable to water and electrolytes. This causes efflux of K^+ and influx of Na^+ and Ca^{2+}, leading to eventual foreign cell lysis from osmotic shock.

Complement produces adherence of C3b-coated entities to specific receptors on the phagocyte membrane. C3a and C5a act directly on phagocytes [especially neutrophils (Section 9.1.2)] to stimulate oxygen consumption; both trigger mediator release from mast cells (essentially noncirculating basophils in the connective tissues that often line the arterial walls) and blood basophils (Section 9.1.4). Mediators released include preformed agents such as histamine (vasodilator), heparin (anticoagulant), tryptase (which activates C3), β-glucosaminidase (which splits off glucosamine), ECF (eosinophil chemotactic factor), NCF (neutrophil chemotactic factor), and PAF [platelet activating factor (Section 9.1.15)].

Some other mediators are newly synthesized by the cyclooxygenase pathway, such as leukotrienes C4, D4, and B4 [vasoactive bronchoconstrictors that also produce chemotaxis and chemokinesis (randomly increased motility)], as well as prostaglandins and thromboxanes that influence bronchial muscles and platelets. The key event for the lipoxygenase and cyclooxygenase pathways is arachidonic acid production mediated by the phospholipase A2 associated with the mast cell membrane.

C5a is a potent neutrophil chemotactic agent and produces vasodilatation (redness) and increased permeability of capillary endothelial cells, an effect prolonged by leukotriene B4 (from the lipoxygenase pathway) released by mast cells and activated basophils. Thus neutrophils are recruited to the site where the foreign agent is located, amplifying the phagocyte response. The arteriolar walls become relaxed, allowing increased blood flow and dilatation of arterioles, while contraction of capillary endothelial cells causes exudation of plasma proteins and of fluid (edema); this causes the neutrophils to slow down and hug the capillary walls, increasing their concentration, the whole process being termed the "acute inflammatory response." The greater numbers of neutrophils increase the likelihood of their encountering a C3b-coated foreign agent or being able to respond chemotactically, leading to adherence via the neutrophil C3b receptors, activation of neutrophil respiration by C3a and C5a, and then phagocytosis. MAC synthesis also may lyse the foreign cell but does not appear to lyse host cells (i.e., to cause autolysis).

Many of these markers have been utilized as nonspecific medical monitoring markers. Appendix A contains reference ranges for some of them.

13.0.3 Soluble Factors

These factors, sometimes called humoral factors, are primarily those enzymes released through tissue injury that activate the clotting mechanism (Section 9.1.15). The most important of these factors probably is lysozyme, a muramidase that digests the exposed peptidoglycan wall of susceptible bacteria. The acute-phase proteins such as C-reactive protein (CRP), amyloid A protein, α_1-antitrypsin, α_2-macroglobulin, fibrinogen, ceruloplasmin, C9, and Factor B (see Section 9.0.2 for all these globulins) also increase dramatically (up to 1000-fold) in the plasma. CRP binds in a calcium-dependent manner to microorganisms with phosphorylcholine in their membranes. The complex then can activate complement mechanisms to cause C3b formation on the membrane surface, with subsequent adherence to phagocytes. An animal protein closely related to CRP is horseshoe crab limulin, the basis of the *Limulus* amoebocyte assay for endotoxins, a medical monitoring test based on clotting time for the presence of gram-negative bacteria in the plasma. In another example during gram-negative bacterial infection, bacterial endotoxins stimulate release of host interleukin-1, an endogenous pyrogen that can raise body temperature and stimulates liver secretion of CRP.

Another broad class of soluble chemical factors is the interferons. These are antiviral agents present in reptiles, birds, fishes, and mammals with at least 14 different α-interferons produced by lymphocytes and β-interferons produced by all cell types, especially fibroblasts (connective tissue cell that is flat and elongated with cytoplasmic processes at each end in addition to a flat, oval, vesicular nucleus; fibroblasts differentiate into chondroblasts, collagenoblasts, and osteoblasts). The third type of interferon, γ-interferons, is not induced by viruses. Cells synthesize α- and β- interferons when infected by a virus. After secretion into the extracellular fluid, the interferon binds to uninfected cells. This causes a protein kinase to catalyze phosphorylation of a specific ribosomal protein and one of the initiation factors for protein synthesis, so as to reduce mRNA translation. Another enzyme induces a short polymer of adenylic acid that activates an endonuclease, which then degrades both viral and host mRNA. This results in the infected cell's being surrounded by uninfectable cells, thus stopping viral spread. Certain viruses cannot be stopped by this mechanism, however, and others may take a long time to overcome this defense pathway, sometimes a large contributory factor to the lag period needed to detect a virus's presence via antibody-based assays. An increased plasma interferon level may have many possible causes, typical of a medical monitoring marker.

Interferons also help recovery from viral infections and may modulate natural killer (NK) cell activity. It may be important to know the time course of the interferon concentrations to make judgments about viral infection at time zero.

13.0.4 Extracellular Killing

As viruses are unable to self-replicate, they must take over the genetic machinery of some cells of the host to survive and proliferate. The function of NK cells is to kill infected host cells before they have time to help viruses reproduce. The NK cells are large granular lymphocytes that recognize specific glycoproteins on the surface of infected cells to aid in distinguishing infected cells from uninfected cells. After contact of the two cells, the activation of the NK cell causes extracellular release of the NK granule contents, including a C9-type molecule, into the space between the two cells, with the resultant formation of a MAC-type structure that kills infected cells. The amount of circulating antibodies against the C9-type molecule modulates the killing rate. Autolysis of the NK cell itself is prevented by other factors also released by the granules. The various interferons (Section 13.0.3) then enhance NK cytotoxicity in a feedback defense system.

Large parasites such as helminths cannot be phagocytosed because of their size, and they are resistant to C9 attack. Extracellular killing by eosinophils (Section 9.1.3) is thought to occur after helminth covering by C3b, which facilitates eosinophil attachment and resultant release of granule factors that damage the membrane of the parasite, leading to lysis and parasite death.

Some enzymic activities identified in these granules include those for aryl-sulfatase B, peroxidase, phospholipase D, and histaminase. Most successful parasites, however, can be tagged by C3b, but adhering eosinophils are not activated. Most successful bacterial invaders also prevent activation of any adhering macrophages. Very successful invaders may cause inhibition of phagocytic cell synthesis so that the entire immune system is weakened, as occurs in AIDS.

13.1 SPECIFIC ACQUIRED IMMUNITY

This is the term used to describe an immune response based on prior contact with a toxicant or a microrganism. Antibody molecules are utilized by the host to recognize a specific invader, to determine if it and/or its concentration is harmful to the host, and, if so, to activate the innate immunity mechanisms of phagocyte adherence, complement activity, and phagocytosis.

Human antibodies are γ-globulins (Section 9.0.2) of five main types: IgG, IgA, IgM, IgD, and IgE. The small lymphocyte (T- and B-cells) is essential for the production of antibody. The route whereby complement is activated by antibody is termed the "classical complement sequence."

13.1.1 Classical Complement Sequence

When bound to a microbe, antibody links to and activates C1q. The latter has a central collagen-like stem with six peptide chain branches, each tipped by an antibody-binding subunit. C1q is associated with C1r and C1s subunits in a complex (C1qrs) stabilized by calcium ion, both being activated sequentially. The C1s subunit, when activated ($\overline{\text{C1qrs}}$), has the proteolytic activity necessary to activate C4 repeatedly, to cleave out many C4a fragments and leave residual

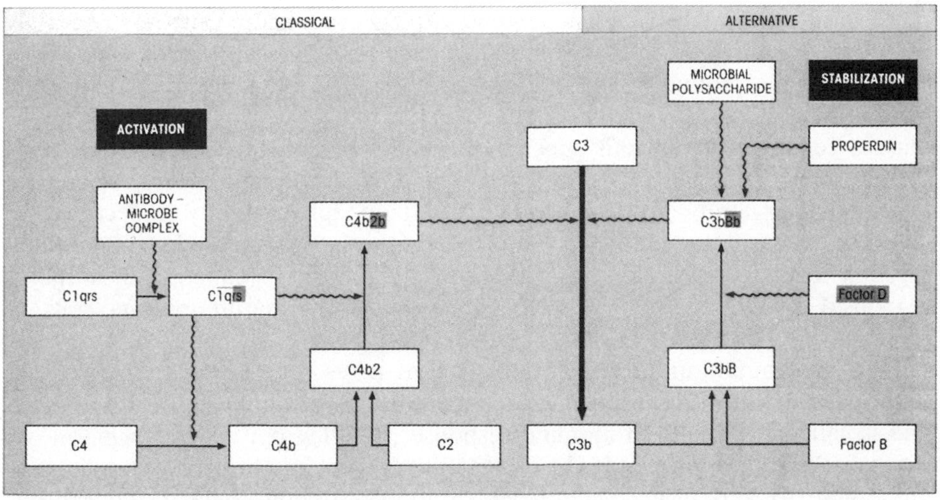

FIGURE 13.1. Comparison of the alternative and classical complement pathways. The classical pathway, with odd exceptions such as C-reactive protein, is antibody-dependent; the alternative pathway is not. The C3b common product eventually forms a membrane attack complex (MAC) that results in foreign cell death by osmotic shock.

C4b, which can bind covalently via its internal thioester bond to the antibody–C1 complex (Section 13.2.1) or to the surface of the microbe.

In the presence of magnesium cation, C2 can complex with C4b to become a new substrate (C4b2) for $\overline{\text{C1qrs}}$ the complex $\overline{\text{C4b2b}}$ having the convertase activity required to activate C3 with the same specificity as generated by the alternative pathway (Section 13.0.1). The degradation of the activity of the complex is effected through a C4 binding protein or a cell surface C3b receptor in the presence of Factor I. Events of the post-C3 pathway continue as in Section 13.0.1 until a MAC appears. Both the classical and the alternative complement pathways are shown in Figure 13.1.

13.1.2 Antibody-Stimulated Phagocytosis without Complement Activation

Many C3b-coated microorganisms adhere to phagocytic cells without provoking phagocytosis. In the presence of antibody, however, phagocytosis can be stimulated. A critical number of antibody molecules must be bound to specialized receptors on the phagocyte surface and also to the surface receptors of the bacterium to cause a critical amount of cross-linking of the phagocyte receptors before activation of the latter can occur.

13.1.3 Antigen Selection of B-Lymphocytes to Make Antibody

The molecules in microorganisms that evoke and react with antibodies are called antigens. Confusingly, the designation antigen is also used for any molecule that generates an immune response (also called an immunogen). Already existing antibodies are selected for by antigen. Each B-lymphocyte (Section 9.1.5) is programmed to make only one antibody. Each carries the antibody (about 10^5 molecules) on its outer membrane surface to act as receptor. Antigen binding only occurs at those antibody sites that allow physical fit and thus close physical binding. This recognition process generally is for foreign antigens and large modified "foreign" host molecules such as the macromolecular adducts discussed in Chapters 10 through 12 or the abnormal protein made after mutagenic events. This activates the lymphocyte to form a plasma cell that secrets this specific antibody, which then can combine with the appropriate antigen, thus protecting the host. Antibody synthesis decreases as antigen–antibody reaction slows. If not enough antibody is secreted to combine with all the antigen, antibody synthesis is increased exponentially through cell division of the stimulated lymphocyte (called the humoral response) to eventually produce antibody-secreting mature plasma cells, a process called clonal selection.

This division/maturation/secretion process takes several days after contact with antigen to produce detectable concentrations of antibodies in the blood, and is called the acquired immune response; the "lag period" or "window" is the time required for antibody detectability. The humoral response is very vulnerable to antimitotic agents. Peak blood antibody concentrations occur about 3 weeks after exposure. The time when no antibodies can be detected cannot be interpreted as a true negative test of exposure to the antigen source unless subsequent antibody testing at regular monthly time intervals is also negative. Such testing is very relevant to the interpretation of all antibody-based tests, including HIV antibody tests.

13.1.4 Acquired Memory through Antibodies

Once activated, the acquired immune response leaves behind a residual memory system that facilitates much greater responsiveness relative to antibody concentration and synthesis rate when subsequent invasion by the same antigen occurs. A state of immunity is then said to exist. The more efficient response is caused by the presence of more than one resting B-lymphocyte capable of recognizing the same antigen and by these cells' storage of essential precursors of cell division and key gene activators for specific antibody synthesis (Figure 13.2). Such a mechanism is much more specific than the innate immunity responses (Section 13.0). This response is also the basis of the effectiveness and specificity of vaccination. Vaccination usually involves injection of an innocuous form of an infective microorganism or its toxins together with the antigens responsible for inducing an enhanced population of B-lymphocytes, which can be stimulated to produce the specific protective antibody when subsequent invasion by antigen occurs. At the other extreme, hypersensitivity can occur if too many B-lymphocytes carry memory for antigen.

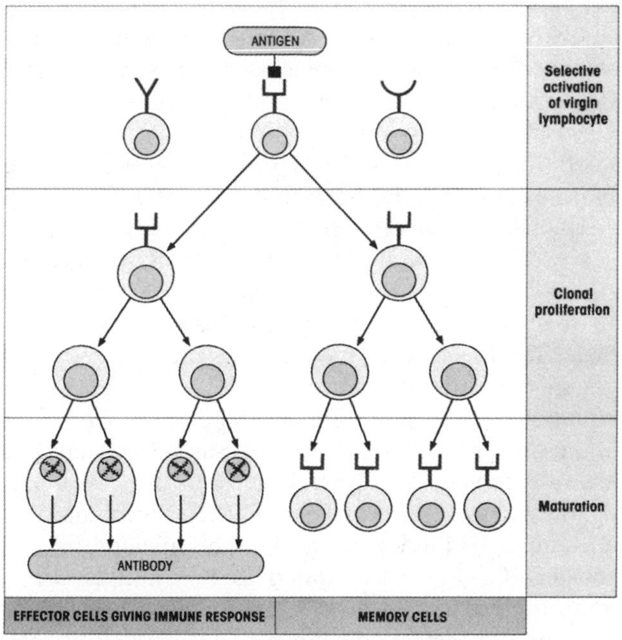

FIGURE 13.2. The cellular basis for the generation of effector and memory cells after primary contact with antigen. A fraction of the progeny of the original antigen-reactive lymphocytes become nondividing memory cells and others the effector cells of humoral or, as we shall see subsequently, cell-mediated immunity. Memory cells require fewer cycles before they develop into effectors, and this shortens the reaction time for the secondary response. The expanded clone of cells with memory for the original antigen provides the basis for the greater secondary relative to the primary immune response. Priming with low doses of antigen can often stimulate effective memory without producing very adequate antibody synthesis. The blocks on the antigen surface represent binding sites for antibody; the goalpost on the phagocyte surface represents antibody site. Note that the memory cells are smaller than the effector cells.

This may bring about a massive response that inflicts damage on the host's own tissues (Sections 13.1.6 and 13.3).

13.1.5 Protection against Intracellular Attack

Microorganisms such as viruses (both DNA and RNA) must replicate inside cells; mycobacteria and leishmania can replicate inside cells but do not have to. The intracellular parasites survive by subverting the intrinsic host cell processes for their own purposes. Such microorganisms cannot be reached by humoral antibody. T-lymphocytes (Section 9.1.5) recognize foreign antigen on the surfaces of infected host cells, leading to adherence, activation, and phagocytosis. The host cell is recognized through a specific major histocompatibility complex (MHC) on the cell surface. The recognition of the MHC is a key step to successful tissue and organ transplants. Nonrecognition of the correct MHC causes activation of humoral responses directed toward the "foreign" cell, called rejection in unsuccessful transplants. The presence of an intracellular parasite can be signaled by the host cell's displaying on its surface small antigenic peptide fragments ("antigen processing") derived from the cytoplasmic protein of the parasite, as a small amount of degradation of the parasite does occur. The degradation is achieved through action of the low-molecular-mass polypeptide complex in the cytoplasm. The peptide fragments (9 to 12 amino acids) migrate to the endoplasmic reticulum and are carried by transport proteins through the endoplasmic reticulum membranes to bind to the Class I MHC proteins inside the membrane. This complex then migrates to the cell surface so that the peptide is finally pointed outward on the membrane surface. Without the peptide the MHC is not stable on the cell membrane surface and migrates back inside the membrane.

Another mechanism of antigen processing, discovered by Hunt et al. in 1992, involves a specialized part of the Class I MHC molecule, the HLA.A21 portion. The latter bears specific "signal sequence" peptides at the membrane surface rather than peptides from specific parasite antigens. These signal sequence peptides do not need to have carrier proteins for transport from the cytoplasm through the endoplasmic reticulum as in the first mechanism. This finding could imply that the signal sequence peptide is a key recognition factor for humoral immunity in addition to a "lock-and-key" physical fit model for the Class I MHC receptor. This pathway could also be a backup pathway. Whether this pathway is present for Class II MHC molecules is unknown.

Macrophages and B-lymphocytes can also be invaded by parasites without activation. T-helper ($CD4^+$) cells primed to that antigen will recognize and bind to both the antigen and the host Class II MHC molecule on the surface of an infected (but not activated) macrophage or B-cell. Binding releases from the T-helper cell soluble factors called lymphokines, including γ-interferon and other macrophage activating factors. These trigger the previously subverted microorganicidal mechanisms of the macrophage, resulting in death of the parasite.

Another way to kill a virus is to kill virally infected cells before the virus can replicate. NK cells can perform this function (Section 13.0.4) but have a limited range of operation. Cytotoxic T-cells, each being specific for one antigen, bind to a wide range of surface antigens in addition to host Class I

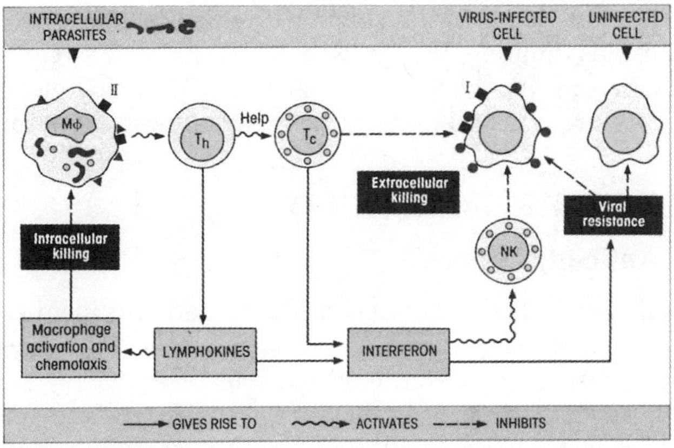

FIGURE 13.3. T-cells link with the innate immune system to resist intracellular infection. Class I and class II major histocompatibility molecules (■) are important for T-cell recognition of surface antigen. The T-helper cells (T_h) cooperate in the development of cytotoxic T-cells (T_c) from precursors. The macrophage ($M_\emptyset$) microbicidal mechanisms are switched on by macrophage activating lymphokines. γ-interferon inhibits viral replication and stimulates NK cells, which together with T_c kill virus-infected cells.

MHC molecules, killing infected cells. On activation, T-helper cells release γ-interferon, which reduces viral spread to adjacent cells. The rest of the process is analogous to that described for humoral immunity, involving clonal selection, proliferation, and memory effects (Section 13.1.3). The killing pathways for intracellular parasites are summarized in Figure 13.3.

Class I and II MHC molecules are transmembrane glycoproteins with a characteristic amino acid sequence for each haplotype individual, implying a slow mutation of the genes that give rise to these molecules. All nucleated cells carry Class I MHC molecules, especially on lymphoid cells, but less so in liver, lung, and kidney, and sparsely on brain and skeletal tissue. Class II molecules are more restricted in distribution and are mostly associated with B-cells, antigen-presenting cells, and macrophages. Once activated by agents such as γ-interferon, capillary endothelia and many epithelial cells stain for Surface MHC Class II.

13.1.6 Immunopathology

When an immune response is persistent or if there is chronic exposure to foreign antigens, damage to tissue and/or hypersensitivity may result. Some examples are allergies to pollens and microorganisms and chemical and drug hypersensitivities. The ability to discriminate between foreign and nonforeign cells may eventually be lost, causing autoimmune effects such as those encountered in thyrotoxicosis, myasthenia gravis, and some rheumatological disorders. Rejection mechanisms in transplants may cause autoimmune sequelae. Autoimmune processes are thought to be important in AIDS during the subversion of the immune system.

Immunodeficiency is a pathological state characterized by persistent infection of microorganisms, usually found in low concentrations in healthy people. A good example is the appearance of microorganism infections seen for cases of full-blown AIDS. Inadequate functioning of the immune system upsets the control mechanisms limiting the growth of these microorganisms. (This is considered further in the chapters on AIDS.) The biological markers for immunodeficiency are classical nonspecific medical monitoring markers.

13.2 MOLECULAR IMMUNOLOGY

13.2.1 The Antibody Molecule

The antibody molecule has two identical heavy and two identical light chains held together by interchain disulfide bonds (Figure 13.4). The antigen combining sites are between the N-terminal portions of the heavy and light chains at the ends opposite to the disulfide linkages. The antigen binding sites of both chains show much amino acid sequence variability. Thus the amino acid sequence in three segments on both light and heavy chains in the binding regions is related to antigen binding specificity. The nonbinding portions of the four chains are relatively constant in amino acid sequence. These portions of the antibodies that code for virally coded surface antigens displayed on infected host cells can cause binding of NK cells (Section 13.1.5).

Intra-disulfide links bend part of the protein to form loops in the protein chains. The loops are compactly folded to constitute tertiary structure (Section 2.0) in the shape of globular domains that have a β-pleated sheet protein structure. Such domains also are often stabilized by interchain hydrogen bonds between amide carbonyl and amide amino groups (secondary structure—

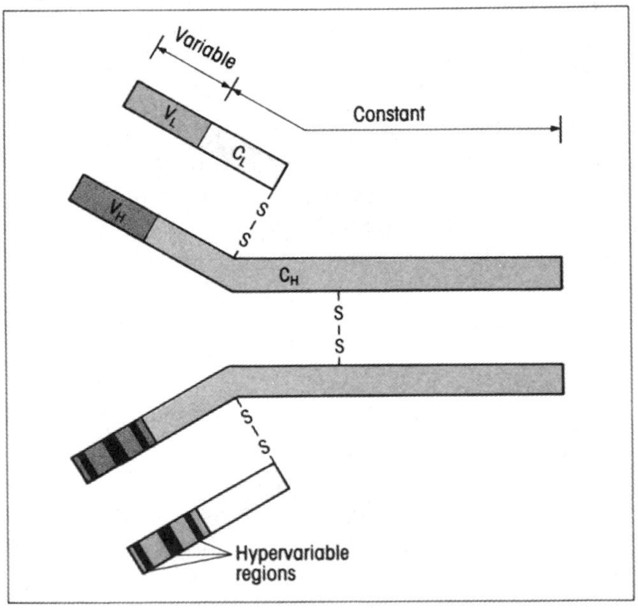

FIGURE 13.4. Amino acid sequence variability in the antibody molecule. ■ hypervariable; ■ variable; □ relatively constant. The terms "V region" and "C region" are used to designate the variable and constant regions respectively, "V_L" and "C_L" are generic terms for these regions on the light chain, and "V_H" and "C_H" specify variable and constant regions on the heavy chain. As stressed previously, the pairs of heavy chains are identical, as are the pairs of light chains.

Section 2.0). The variable amino acid sequences are parts of the β-turn loops, and are clustered close to one another in space. Thus the secondary and tertiary structures are important in antigen–antibody recognition and binding. In fact, the binding is by spatial complementarity and not by covalent binding. This implies that many types of molecules may act as antigens. The reversibility of the interaction has been shown by dialysis.

The amino acid residues of the antibody in close physical contact (to within their Van der Waals radii as characteristic of the physical adsorption process) with antigen are called the paratope. The part of the antigen in contact with the paratope is the epitope. Each antigen has several distinct contact areas, each with its own specific antibody (monoclonal; mAb). Therefore several antibodies (polyclonal; pAb) may arise from just one antigen, depending on the number of contact areas.

For example, in multiple myeloma, one cell type makes one specific immunoglobulin by dividing repeatedly in an uncontrolled manner just as a cancer does, and a large clone of identical cells arises that all secrete predominantly the myeloma or M protein mAb, which is detectable in the blood as a relatively specific medical monitoring marker for multiple myeloma. If instead several antibody proteins are secreted in moderate to high amounts, the secretion is called a pAb. Fusing mAb-secreting cells with a B-cell tumor allows production of mAb by the tumor. A specific antiserum can be raised by injecting pure human antibody protein into an animal such as the rabbit. The animal manufactures pAbs to the foreign binding portions, and the antibodies then are harvested. Monoclonal antiserum, for example, for human M protein is produced by injection of the polyclonal antiserum into an animal with myelomas other than the one to be combated in humans so that the common antibodies are absorbed, leaving the desired mAb to be harvested. Such a synthesis process is expensive and time-consuming.

The most specific antiserum raised that recognizes individual antibody molecules and that discriminates between different mAbs is also a specific and very sensitive tool for detecting the mAb for a key toxic antigen, whether this be from chemical exposure or from microorganism invasion. Such a marker will be a predictive one of adverse effect because no macroscopic damage has yet occurred. To achieve this, the mechanism of action must be known.

Thus for a new epidemic where mechanistic data are unavailable, a pAb may be utilized initially that may not be specific, by raising antibodies to a mixture of undefined antigens from an affected population. Problems with specificity are thus expected in the early developmental stages for most new antibody kits, as experienced in the early HIV antibody kits (Chapter 15).

The immunoglobulins that have heavy and light chain portions where the amino acid content is relatively constant are termed "isotypes." The constant-region domains mediate secondary biological functions for relatively nonspecific reactions by the host. Such known functions include C4b binding (Section 13.1.1), C1q fixation to control catabolic rate, and binding to cell surface receptors. There are five isotypic classes of immunoglobulin in humans based on heavy chains: IgG, IgA, IgM, IgD, and IgE (Section 9.0.2). There are two light chain isotypes (κ or λ) for each class of heavy chain isotype.

IgG is the major immunoglobulin synthesized during the acquired immune response, and it can cross the placenta, unlike other immunoglobulins. It defends the extravascular body spaces from germs and is very low in germ-free animals. IgA defends the exposed external surfaces of the body against attack by microorganisms, as it is present in all aqueous secretions of the body and inhibits adherence of coated microorganisms to the surfaces of mucosal cells. Aggregated IgA binds to polymorphs and activates the alternative complement pathway. IgM appears early in the response to infection and is mostly localized in the bloodstream. IgM appears to be important in multiple binding mechanisms of antigen to antibody. Nearly all blood IgD is present along with IgM on the surface of certain blood lymphocytes and may interact to modulate lymphocyte activation and suppression. IgE appears to be important in hypersensitivity and allergic responses. The main physiological role of IgE appears to be protection of external mucosal surfaces of the body via local recruitment of plasma factors and effector cells through the triggering of an acute inflammatory reaction. It is the backup to the primary IgA defense because it is bound to mast cells.

Alternative immunoglobulins encoded by alleles or alternative genes at a single locus also can be produced. These allotypes are related to interindividual genetic variation as reflected, for example, in different blood type antigens A, B, O and in different Ig heavy chains. Such genetic variation may also cause hyper- and hyposensitivity.

The characteristics of the antibody that are specific are called the idiotype. Most of the idiotypic determinants are located in the hypervariable regions of the amino acid primary sequence, but they are also determined by secondary and tertiary structure so that nonadjacent amino acids also must be considered. Specific antisera that react with one antibody and no other are termed "private," whereas those that share idiotypes are "public" or "cross-reacting" idiotypes. The body can also make autoanti-idiotypic sera.

13.2.2 The T-Cell Receptor

Like the B-lymphocyte, the T-cell has a specific receptor for antigen recognition on its surface. The B-cell receptor is a membrane-bound IgM monomer. The T-cell receptor is a heterodimer composed of an α and a β chain each of about 40,000 to 50,000 amu. Each chain is folded into two domains, one being relatively invariant and the other exhibiting much greater amino acid sequence variability. The latter is probably the area of binding of antigen and cell surface MHC molecules. In all immunocompetent T-cells, the antigen receptor is noncovalently associated with T3, a molecule consisting of three peptide chains that transduces the antigen recognition signal from the antigen receptor to the inside of the cell. The α and β chains of the T3 complex are those missing in patients with severe immunodeficiency. The γ chain is retained in the latter state.

The MHC Class I surface molecule is the key recognition element for cytotoxic T-cells, and the MHC Class II surface molecule is necessary for antigen presentation to helper T-cells. Both cells also require some surface fragment spliced out from, or related to, the intracellular parasitic microorganism or foreign antigen, or perhaps in addition some "signal sequence" antigen (Section 13.1.5). The α and β T-cell receptor genes carry the information to recognize both antigen and MHC.

13.2.3 Hapten Antibody Formation

A hapten is a well-defined chemical grouping or functional group (for example, a benzene ring) of the antigen that can select out its specific antibody. Small molecules such as benzene or metal ions are not immunogenic by themselves, but they can become immunogenic by covalent binding of the small molecule or ion to a "carrier" molecule that is itself immunogenic, to create the geometrical requirements for antibody selection. The carrier molecules may be specific proteins/polypeptides (protein adducts are discussed in Chapter 12) or carbohydrate and lipid adducts, or may be created indirectly by DNA/RNA adducts (discussed in Chapter 11) via their expressed "abnormal" proteins. The hapten-combining site on an antibody usually accommodates five to six amino acids or hexose units for linear peptides or carbohydrates, respectively. For globular proteins, up to 16 amino acids may be in contact with an antibody. Clearly, for macromolecules, the exposed portions of haptens must satisfy exacting geometrical requirements to evoke an immune response. It is also apparent that not all macromolecular adducts will be immunogenic.

With such a process, absolute specificity is not expected and is not observed experimentally. Thus *ortho, meta,* and *para* isomers of aminobenzene sulfonate will cross-react *in vivo* with each of their antibodies, but the original molecule always binds best. Changing sulfonate to arsonate leads to weaker binding; the amino carboxylates show even less affinity. The point is that *some* activity is observed—the interaction is not 100% specific. This also indicates that the binding (affinity) constant must be measured to identify which compound is binding with the antibody. This is usually done by dialysis. Thus there are degrees of cross-reactivity for haptens of closely related electronic/geometric structure. The overall geometrical configuration is more important to the interaction than is the specific chemical nature. Denatured antibody samples usually do not evoke an immunogenic response, showing that the secondary and tertiary structures are important even though the primary amino acid sequence has not changed.

The presence of mAb binding usually is confirmed by the occurrence of linear Scatchard plots (Section 4.3). The presence of pAb causes nonlinear Scatchard plots. In addition, the presence of pAbs can be recognized by the synergistic binding of the antigens when exposed together to antibody, relative to the binding of each separately. Paradoxically, the spectrum of induced pAbs may be more specific than the mAb antibody assay in the case of exposure to unknown chemicals because the cross-reactivity of monoclonals means that specificity and hence interpretation are not absolute. On the other hand, if exposures to known chemicals occur, the mAb concentration is directly related to its hapten content and is extremely specific. However, the exposure/dietary history of the persons examined must be known, something that is often unknown (and/or not measured) in epidemiologic studies.

As the genes controlling the variable amino acid region of antibodies have a high rate of spontaneous mutation, and as immunoglobulin variability is achieved by a multigenic system, there must be another mechanism that is inherently much more specific than hapten binding for specific antigen recognition purposes. This is thought to be the T-cell receptor (Section 13.2.2), whose genes do not mutate. Thus primed cytotoxic T-cells with their Type I

MHC and primed T-helper cells with their Type II MHC are postulated to be the means by which specific fragments of antigens are presented to select their specific antibody. Antibodies to Type I and II MHC block this selection process. Blocking the low pH phase of phagocytosis with chloroquine, leading to spillage of lysosomal and endosomal enzymes, prevents fragment presentation. Transfection of the appropriate MHC genes so that cells of the wrong haplotype can present antigen to the T-effector cells restricted to the haplotype of the transfected genes also confirms that MHC participation is essential for antigen presentation.

The ability of haptens covalently bound to specific "carrier" immunogens to constitute antigen to evoke antibodies can now be understood, as only fragments of the antigens are actually displayed for T-cell antibody selection purposes, and these may include fragments with haptens. Fragments of host cell proteins probably are also presented but do not evoke a T-cell response, as these fragments are not "foreign." In this regard, B-cells tend to react with natively folded antigen but not polypeptide fragments, whereas T-cells can recognize unfolded peptide chains as well as native antigen. Thus while there is no protein repair mechanism, selective splicing of invading protein occurs to feed the presentation process so that lymphocytes can recognize foreign invaders.

The use of immunoassays in biological monitoring has just begun because of their sensitivity and relative specificity. The quantitative aspects of antibody-based methods for xenobiotics are summarized in Sections 11.1.1 and 11.1.2.

13.3 HYPERSENSITIVITY

Once a person has been immunologically primed, another contact with antigen leads to boosting of the immune response (called the secondary response). If the boosting is excessive, gross tissue damage (hypersensitivity) may occur if the antigen concentration is large (toxic effect of excess exposure) or if the humoral (B-cell–based) and cellular (T-cell–based) immune systems over-respond even at low subsequent antigen concentrations. This susceptibility is highly variable from individual to individual. There are five types of hypersensitivity (Table 13.1) depending on the interaction with humoral antibody, with one, Type IV, involving receptors bound to lymphocyte surfaces of longer time course ("delayed sensitivity").

13.3.1 Type I Hypersensitivity

This is also called anaphylactic hypersensitivity because of the symptoms of the occurrence of generalized anaphylaxis: intense contraction of smooth muscle, dilatation of capillaries, and wheezing with eventual asphyxia in terminal cases. Such symptoms have been observed after bee and wasp stings, penicillin injections, and exposure to specific chemicals in sensitive individuals. About 10% of the population suffer from allergies involving localized anaphylactic reactions to extrinsic allergens such as grass pollens, animal danders, mite feces in house dust, food components, and so on, to produce the symptoms of chemical asthma or hay fever. Food allergens may also produce nausea, vomiting, and diarrhea as well as bone or skin problems. There is a strong genetic inheritance factor associated with this hypersensitivity type.

TABLE 13.1 Comparison of different types of hypersensitivity.

	I Anaphylactic	II Cytotoxic	III Complex-mediated	IV Cell-mediated	V Stimulatory
Antibody mediating reaction	Homocytotropic Ab Mast-cell binding	Humoral Ab ± CF*	Humoral Ab ± CF	Receptor on T-lymphocyte	Humoral Ab Non-CF
Antigen	Usually exogenous (e.g. grass pollen)	Cell surface	Extracellular	Associated with MHC antigens on macrophage or target cell	Cell surface
Response to intra-dermal antigen: Max. reaction	30 min (+ late reaction)	—	3–8 hours	24–48 hours	—
Appearance	Wheal and flare	—	Erythema and oedema	Erythema and induration	—
Histology	Degranulated mast cells; oedema; (late reaction cellular incl. eosinophils)	—	Acute inflammatory reaction; predominant polymorphs	Perivascular inflammation: polymorphs migrate out leaving predominantly mononuclear cells	—
Transfer sensitivity to normal subject	← Serum antibody →			Lymphoid cells Transfer factor	Serum antibody
Examples:	Atopic allergy, e.g. hay fever	Haemolytic disease of newborn (Rh)	Complex glomerulonephritis Farmer's lung	Mantoux reaction to TB Granulomatous reaction to schistosome eggs Contact sensitivity	Thyrotoxicosis

* CF = Complement fixation

The response is caused by a massive secretion of histamine from explosive degranulation of the two types of mast cells (Section 13.0.3) evoked by massive cross-linking mainly of the IgE receptors in response to anti-IgE or antigen challenge—which, if not countered by adrenaline injection, may lead to death. The cross-linking of the antigen receptors is followed by breakdown of outer membrane phosphatidyl inositol through induction of phospholipase c activation (Section 2.8.1), by the generation of diacylglycerol (Section 2.8.2), by protein kinase c activation, and by a large increase in intracellular calcium ion, the latter peaking before protein kinase c and diacylglycerol. The peaking of the latter markers is correlated to exponential secretion of histamine and the activation of the arachidonic acid metabolites formed by the cyclooxygenase and lipoxygenase pathways (Section 13.0.1).

A predictive marker for this type of hypersensitivity is higher than reference range IgE in the blood. The best-known markers of anaphylaxis are skin prick tests to the suspected sensitizer. The wheal and flare reactions usually are completed within 30 minutes, but a late phase reaction mediated by a neutrophil chemotactic factor from the mast cell may take up to a day for visualization. This factor also has been implicated in the onset of chronic chemical asthma. Sputum analysis of asthma patients reveals large amounts of the major basic protein of the eosinophil granule, which thus is a medical monitoring marker of adverse effect. This protein damages bronchial epithelia and must be coughed up to prevent further damage, especially where the usual clearance mechanisms are overloaded. The correlation between skin prick test responses and the radioallergosorbent test for IgE is good. However, intranasal challenge with the suspected sensitizer is recommended, as this test is often positive when the other two tests are negative. Avoidance of exposure to allergen as much as possible is also necessary. Controlled treatment with small amounts of allergen to build up immunity is not effective if T-lymphocyte cooperation is important for IgE synthesis. Another mode of treatment uses agents such as isoprenaline and sodium cromoglycate, which inhibit mast cell triggering. Steroids must be used for late-phase allergy treatment.

13.3.2 Type II Hypersensitivity

Another name for this is antibody-dependent cytotoxic hypersensitivity. It occurs when an antigenic complex forms with the surface of a formed element of the blood, with subsequent induction of antibodies that are cytotoxic for the cell–antigen complex. Cell death then occurs, which can be brought about by several mechanisms. Those already discussed include phagocytosis (Section 13.0) or the activation of the full complement system (alternative and classical systems) up to C8 and C9 to overcome any repair processes. Cells coated with IgG antibody also can be killed nonspecifically *in vitro* by nonsensitized lymphoreticular cells that bind via their IgG receptors. Phagocytic and nonphagocytic myeloid cells as well as large granulated lymphocytes with surface receptors for IgG (K cells) also possess this capability after direct contact. It is assumed that the mechanism also occurs *in vivo*. Transfusion and tissue incompatibility are thought to occur by this mechanism. Autoantibodies to the host red blood cells can also be caused by red cell adherence to phagocytic cells with parallel anemia (autoimmune hemolytic anemia). Drugs and absorbed chemicals after adduct formation may stimulate conversion from a hapten to a full antigen, which then causes hypersensitivity in certain individuals. If IgE antibodies also are induced, Type I hypersensitivity can be observed. If binding to serum proteins occurs, Type II complex-mediated reactions also may be observed. The Type II process for chemicals and drugs is thought to be reversible after withdrawal of exposure; for example, after chlorpromazine, phenacetin, amidopyrine, quinidine, and Sedormid treatments.

13.3.3 Type III Hypersensitivity

This is the hypersensitivity associated with the union of antibody and antigen at fixed sites within the body. The intensity of the reaction depends on the concentrations of antibody and antigen as well as their ratio to each other. Between antibody excess and mild antigen excess, precipitation of complexes >19S is observed (particles and large organisms will be phagocytosed), whereas soluble complexes are formed in moderate to gross antigen excess. C3 complement inhibits the formation of insoluble complexes during the antibody–antigen reaction. The hypersensitivity is associated with antibody–antigen complex precipitation in the joints, kidneys, and skin, and the degree of activation of the classical complement pathway. A Type I response often is observed simultaneously. The best-known examples of inflammatory lesions due to locally formed complexes at the skin and lung are caused by: thermophilic actinomycetes of moldy hay ("farmer's lung"); dried feces in respirable dusts from mites, birds ("pigeon fancier's disease"), and animals; antigenic proteins of urine; exposure to microorganisms ("cheese washer's disease," "maple bark stripper's disease," and aspergillosis); dander proteins ("furrier's lung"); drug interactions; and dead filarial worms causing elephantiasis.

Diseases resulting from circulating complexes include: serum sickness from deposition of soluble complexes formed in antigen excess about a week after injection of large doses of foreign serum, which induces increases in body temperature, swollen lymph nodes, a general urticarial rash, painful swollen joints, low serum complement, and transient albuminuria; immune complex glomerulonephritis from chronic exposure to antigens as in chronic infections and to haptens in polluted areas, and in autoimmune diseases (the mechanism involves stepwise release of vasoactive mediators from basophils and platelets, separation of endothelial cells, attachment of large complexes to the exposed basement membrane of kidney glomeruli, platelet aggregation, chemotactic attraction of neutrophils which release granule contents in ever larger amounts so damaging the basement membrane, and finally deposition in glomerular capillaries); central nervous disorders after deposition at the choroid plexus in systemic lupus and subacute sclerosing panencephalitis; vasculitic skin rashes due to deposition of Ig and C3 at the basement membrane of the dermal–epidermal junction; polyarteritis nodosa where the HBs antigen of the hepatitis B virus is a component; and hemorrhagic shock syndrome associated with dengue virus.

13.3.4 Type IV Hypersensitivity

This is also called cell-mediated (delayed-type) hypersensitivity. It is a very common allergic reaction: to bacteria, viruses, and fungi; in contact dermatitis after exposure to chemicals; and during the rejection of transplanted tissue.

There is an interaction of primed T-cells with antigen rather than the antibody–antigen reaction characteristic of the other hypersensitivity processes. The mechanism of the enhanced interaction is still largely unknown but involves T-helper cells, cytotoxic T-cells, MHC Type II surface molecules, and lymphokine release (Section 13.1.5) in addition to a low molecular weight transducer molecule in viable white blood cells, called Lawrence's transfer factor. Another subpopulation of T-cells is activated by Class I MHC antigens to become directly cytotoxic to target cells bearing the appropriate antigen.

Bacterial allergic reactions often are seen in human tuberculosis and in borderline leprosy. When bacterial factors overwhelm the body defenses, the T-lymphocytes continually release lymphokines, which attract and accumulate large numbers of macrophages, many giving rise to arrays of epithelioid cells or to giant cells. This is an attempt by the body to isolate a persistent infection by enclosure. Killer T-cells then may destroy macrophages that display bacterial antigen on their surfaces. The mass of proliferating lymphocytes and fibroblasts, together with the areas of fibrosis and necrosis, is called a chronic granuloma. Nonimmunological granulomas can arise from persistent indigestible antigen–antibody complexes or inorganic materials such as talc, silica, or short asbestos fibers inside macrophages. Such a phenomenon occurs also in chronic beryllium disease.

The skin rashes in smallpox, measles, and herpes simplex are largely caused by damage to virally infected cells by cytotoxic T-lymphocytes. Reactions against soluble enzymes released by the eggs of parasites that lodge in the liver capillaries in leishmaniasis and schistosomiasis, and against factors released by fungi in candidiasis, dermatomycosis, coccidioidomycosis, and histoplasmosis are well known, many appearing with the adventitious diseases of AIDS. Type IV hypersensitivity is thought to be implicated with the onset of sarcoidosis in the lymphoid tissue, involving chronic granuloma formation there. Chronic beryllium disease appears to have many features of sarcoidosis. Contact dermatitis is thought to occur through a T-cell response by the presentation of antigen by Ia-rich dendritic Langerhans cells that migrate from the pancreas to the lymph nodes. Specific protein and DNA adducts of xenobiotics can induce the response. Some chemicals known to cause such contact sensitivity are picryl chloride, chromates, urushiol (from poison ivy), *p*-phenylenediamine, neomycin, and nickel salts. The venoms from insect bites and wasp and bee stings induce a substantial delayed hypersensitivity component.

13.3.5 Type V Hypersensitivity

Alternatively called stimulatory hypersensitivity, this process is controlled by hormones that interact with surface receptors to cause changes in configuration at a distance ("allosteric"), thus activating transducers to the cell interior. For example, thyroid stimulating hormone from the pituitary gland when bound to the thyroid cell receptors activates adenyl cyclase in the membrane, which then causes ATP to degrade to cyclic-AMP, the latter stimulating activity in the thyroid cell. The same type of process occurs after antigen or immunoglobin antibody binding with the immunoglobin receptors of B-lymphocytes. T-lymphocytes are transformed by monoclonal antibodies to the T3 antigen. Thyroid cells divide after binding with "growth" autoantibodies.

13.3.6 Innate Hypersensitivity

Overactivation of the alternative complement pathway causes such tissue-damaging hypersensitivity reactions as disseminated intravascular coagulation. Endotoxin from bacteria also appears to induce the latter condition during gram-negative septicemia, as do viral factors released during dengue hemorrhagic shock after massive viremia. Erythrocytes also lyse during paroxysomal nocturnal hemoglobinuria following red cell surface C3b deficiency. High C3 consumption is correlated with mesangiocapillary glomerulonephritis in individuals with the C3 nephritic factor, which may be an IgG autoantibody that activates the alternative complement pathway.

Further Reading

Bona, C. A. (ed). *Molecular Basis of the Immune Response*, New York Academy of Sciences, Vol. 546, 1988.

Henderson, R. A.; Michel, H.; Sakaguchi, K.; Shabanowitz, J.; Appella, E.; Hunt, D.; and Engelhard, V. H. 1992. HLA-A2.1-associated peptides from a mutant cell line: a second pathway of antigen presentation. *Science* **255**: 1264–1267.

Hunt, D. F.; Henderson, R. A.; Shabanowitz, J.; Sakaguchi, K.; Michel, H.; Sevilir, N.; Cox, A. L.; Appella, E.; and Engelhard, V. H. 1992. Characterization of peptides bound to the class I MHC molecule HLA-A2.1 by mass spectrometry. *Science* **255**: 1261–1263.

Langman, R. E. 1989. *The Immune System*, Academic Press, New York.

Roitt, I. M. 1992. *Essential Immunology*, 7th ed., Blackwell Scientific Publications, Boston, MA.

14

AIDS and HIV

The reader should review Sections 9.1.1 through 9.1.6, Sections 9.1.15 through 9.1.21, Section 11.1, and Chapter 13 before beginning the chapters on AIDS. AIDS, HIV infection, and HIV detection are regarded in the context of the immune system and immunoassays in general, with the HIV example being the best-known one. Chapter 14 introduces the molecular aspects of AIDS and HIV without dwelling on clinical matters. Chapters 15 and 16 describe the different tests used to detect HIV-1. Chapter 17 considers individual protection with condoms. Chapter 18 is a general hygienic guideline for the protection of laboratory workers to minimize exposure to blood and tissue including medical wastes with HIV, AIDS, or viral/infectious materials. Chapter 19 is concerned with the role of volatile nitrites ("poppers," now banned in the United States) in immunosuppression and their biological monitoring markers.

Biological monitoring is used to assess whether exposure to HIV has occurred. It is equally important to consider how biological monitoring can be used to determine how effective protective measures are as individual and workplace hygienic aspects of the AIDS prevention problem, much as blood lead is used to assess the effectiveness of a respirator program in a nonferrous foundry, or as urinary metabolite concentrations are utilized to define the protectiveness of gloves and other garments to solvents in a personal protection program.

14.0 DEFINING HIV AND AIDS

Human Immunodeficiency Viruses (HIV) are the RNA viruses (retroviruses) thought to be responsible for the depletion of the human immune system to such an extent (immunodeficiency) that adverse health effects occur [1]. This latter clinical stage has been called Acquired Immune Deficiency Syndrome (AIDS) until the new definition for AIDS can be agreed upon. AIDS was originally called Gay Related Immune Disorder (GRID) and Gay Compromise Syndrome in 1981 because gay men were the first afflicted group to be detected in the United States.

People with (full-blown) AIDS (PWAs) often exhibited severe weight loss; sharply decreased T4-helper (CD4 or $CD4^+$) lymphocyte cell numbers (not always for Kaposi's sarcoma); opportunistic infections related to uncontrolled growth of usually symbiotic microbes (*Mycobacterium avium*), fungi (*Cryptococcus neoformans*), protozoa (for example, *Pneumocystis carinii* and *Toxoplasma gondii*), other viruses (*Cytomegaloviruses*, herpes, Epstein-Barr, hepatitis B), and invertebrates (spirochetes, for example, as in increased incidence of tuberculosis); Kaposi's sarcoma; and B-lymphocyte cell lymphomas. The T4-helper lymphocyte is essential to activate macrophages; to stimulate induction of cytotoxic T-cell function, of natural killer (NK) cell function, of suppressor cell function, and of B-cell function; and to enhance the secretions of growth and differentiation factors for lymphoid cells, of hematopoietic colony stimulating factors, and of factors that induce non-lymphoid cell function. The immunologic factors are discussed in Sections 13.0, 13.1, 13.2.2, 13.2.3, and 13.3.4. The stage before full-blown AIDS symptoms is often characterized by significantly lowered T4-helper lymphocyte cell counts [below their reference range of 800 to 1200 cells/mm^3 (Section 9.1.5)], weight loss, fever, rash, swollen lymph glands, diarrhea, thrush, shingles, severe athlete's foot, oral hairy leukoplakia, appetite loss, lack of resistance to infection, persistent night-sweating, persistent fatigue, and persistent coughing/lung problems. This stage has been called AIDS Related Complex (ARC), often seen at a helper T-cell count of 200 to 400/mm^3. Individuals infected with HIV with no overt external symptoms are called asymptomatics. HIV viruses are transmitted among humans by sexual contact, from mother to child in utero and through breast milk, by infected blood products and body fluids, or by nonsterile needles contaminated by residual infected blood or body fluid products. AIDS can be thought of as a venereal disease like syphilis or hepatitis-B.

The original definition of AIDS in 1981 in the United States by the Centers for Disease Control (CDC) required the following: any young male under 40, with Kaposi's sarcoma and/or *Pneumocystis carinii* pneumonia, and with no apparent reason to have immunosuppression. In 1983, the criteria were expanded to include "any opportunistic infection" for any age or gender. In 1985, AIDS could be diagnosed for any infection, any pneumonia, and any lymph gland involvement. A positive HIV test also was introduced as a criterion in addition to the clinical symptoms for AIDS, pre-AIDS, and ARC [2]. In 1987, the definition of AIDS was again extended, to include 31 other chronic diseases and ten lymphomas [3]. Up to 1993, the CDC reported data in terms of HIV seroprevalence (40% of AIDS patients in 1987) and placement in high-risk groups (homosexuals, bisexuals, intravenous drug users, hemophiliacs, babies of parents with AIDS or parents infected with HIV).

The CDC proposed two different definitions in 1992. The first used the following criterion: a blood T-helper lymphocyte count $<200/mm^3$ [4] in HIV-infected persons plus the defining medical conditions formulated in 1987. This definition would swell the number of PWAs at least threefold in the United States. The major problem was that the roll of opportunistic diseases still did not include women's or intravenous drug users' unique immune-compromised diseases, HIV-related or not. Another problem was the poor reproducibility of counting T-helper cells by different clinical laboratories at low T-cell <1000. Also the reference ranges differ for women and different ethnicities relative to white males. The influence of circadian rhythms relative to blood sampling has not been addressed, and there is no standardized blood sampling protocol that is mandatory. CDC also recommended that antiretroviral therapy be begun for all persons with a CD4-lymphocyte count $<500/mm^3$, and prophylaxis against *Pneumocystis carinii* pneumonia be begun at $<200/mm^3$. On Oct 27 1992, the CDC added invasive cervical cancer, pulmonary tuberculosis, and recurrent pneumonia to the list of defining medical conditions. In addition, those who are asymptomatic but who are HIV-positive and whose CD4-lymphocyte count is less than $200/mm^3$ would be considered to have AIDS. This latest definition is now official (Jan, 1993). In the author's opinion, the HIV requirement should be dropped. The World Health Organization (WHO), which uses a different definition of AIDS (Section 14.2.1), estimated that about 1.5 million people had AIDS, and 9 to 11 million were HIV-infected in 1991. WHO guesstimates that 40 million will be infected by the year 2000, using its present definition of AIDS.

There are two HIVs, 1 and 2 [1]. In terms of the pre-1992 definitions, they should not be called "AIDS viruses," a term widely used in the news media and some physicians, because not all people infected with HIV develop or have symptoms of full-blown AIDS. Some cases have been reported of persons with the defining medical conditions in whom HIV-infection has not ever been detected. HIV infection alone is still not enough to define the AIDS condition—another reason to discontinue the use of the term "AIDS virus." If AIDS is defined as the clinical condition represented by a immune system that is so weakened that it cannot control symbionts, then HIV may not be the sole cause of such a condition.

The HIV-1 [formerly called the Human T-cell Lymphotropic Virus-III (HTLV-III), Lymphadenopathy Virus-I (LAV-I), and AIDS-associated retrovirus (ARV)] is present in most (but not all) subjects before the onset of full-blown AIDS, but is less frequently detected for PWAs with full-blown AIDS symptoms. The HIV-2 virus (also formerly called LAV-II) incidence is high in west-coastal tropical countries of Africa, and as of the end of 1992 about 500 cases of HIV-2 infection had been reported in the United States. Some antibody tests for HIV-1 may not detect ("cross-react" with) HIV-2 antigens [1]. Over 160,000 persons were known to have died of AIDS in the United States by early 1993, with 70,000 alive under the 1987 CDC definition and about 220,000 alive under the 1992 CDC definitions [4]. The number of deaths before 1993 according to the new 1993 CDC definitions is unknown. Before 1993, over one-third of PWAs in the United States had been residents or visitors in New York City or San Francisco. Since 1985, fewer than 7% of people in these cities have had HIV tests, compared with >60% in most other areas.

The oldest sera that have responded to the HIV-1 antibody test date back to 1959 (a British sailor who died in Manchester, England of *Pneumocystis carinii*; and a case from Zaire, Africa); the next earliest case outside of Africa appears to have been in Norway, in a sailor who probably became infected in 1966 and whose wife, daughter and himself died in 1976 [5, 6]. The serum of a 15-year-old black male in St. Louis, Missouri admitted to a hospital in 1968 also tested positive for HIV-1; he died of Kaposi's sarcoma and progressive cachexia less than a year after hospital admission [6]. Thus sporadic cases of full-blown AIDS occurred in developed countries a few decades before AIDS was formally recognized in the United States in June 1981. Kaposi's sarcoma has been known since 1872, and occurred in elderly men of Ashkenazi Jewish or Mediterranean origin [7, 8], in young and old men of sub-Saharan Africa [8], and in patients receiving immunosuppressive therapy after kidney transplants [8]. Approximately 15% of PWAs had Kaposi's sarcoma in 1990, a steady decline in proportionality since 1981. A current hypothesis is that HIV fosters the development of growth-stimulating factors that initiate and maintain the sarcoma as an outgrowth of endothelial (blood vessel) tissue [9]. HTLV-II also appears to be able to activate these growth factors in T-cells [9]. The *tat* gene of HIV appears to be a growth factor for Kaposi cells [9], but other cofactors, presently unknown, are essential for Kaposi tumor growth, as HIV infection is not necessary.

HIV-1 has been detected in blood, semen, "precum", cervical secretions, saliva, tears, cerebrospinal fluid, urine, breast milk, and plasma, as well as most tissues [1]. The latency period (the median time from infection to full-blown disease development) for full-blown AIDS is currently about 8 years [1]. The maximum latency period has changed with time, and has generally been set as the number of years since 1981.

AIDS is widespread in central Africa where even some monkey species (for example, the sooty mangabey monkey) contain lentiviruses [simian immunodeficiency virus (SIV)] related to HIV-1 and HIV-2. The RNA nucleotide base sequences in the two HIV viruses agree only to the extent of 40%, whereas the HIV-2 and monkey viruses agree 75%, leading to the suggestion of an ultimate monkey source [1]. Both HIV viruses exhibit extreme base sequence variability, thought to result from the absence of proofreading 3′–5′ exonuclease activity in the viral RNA-dependent polymerase (Section 10.1). The reverse transcriptase enzymes of HIV are not very accurate; so the virus genome can vary from one infected person to the next, making a vaccine impractical unless common sequences relating to the immunosuppressive actions of the various viral strains can be known for vaccine production—still a clear research need.

HIV can mutate with time, even in the same infected person [10]. As of the end of 1990, at least 1000 different sequences had been deciphered from over a hundred HIV-1 viral isolates [11]. HIV-1 samples with different base sequences have been isolated from the same person at the same point in time [10]. About 40% of the children of HIV-positive mothers may also test positive at birth; and about half of the infected children lose the antibodies around 6 months of age for unknown reasons [10]. This is an instance where HIV infection does not necessarily lead to full-blown AIDS. In Africa, most seropositive babies die in their second or third year, but 14 Rwandan children were found to have survived beyond 4 years of infection and even as long as 14 years with a blood CD4 cell count of 200 to 400/mm^3 [12]. These long-lived children were much shorter in height than their uninfected age-group peers. Their blood contained elevated somostatin, a neuropeptide that inhibits the growth hormone somatropin. Another Rwanda study [13], involving the development of infants born to 212 mothers who were seronegative at delivery, showed that after an average of 16.6 months, 16/212 (7.55%) of the mothers became seropositive for HIV-1. Of their 16 infants, 9 became seropositive, a seroconversion rate of 4.7 to 6.3% per year. All were breast-fed. A review of the role of sexual contact patterns relative to AIDS demographics in Africa has been published [14]. An epidemiological analysis for the United States is also available [15].

To complicate matters, there also are HIV-related viruses. The Adult T-cell Leukemia Virus (ATLV/HTLV-I) is prevalent in Japan, and early HIV-1 antibody kits cross-reacted with sera infected with HTLV-I because of the heterogeneity of the early isolates used to raise the antibodies (Section 13.1.3). The HTLV-I virus contains genes coding for the gag (core), pol (enzymes), and env (envelope) structural proteins found in HIV-1, but fewer than 1% of infections progress to leukemia, indicative of the need for additional cofactors [16]. HIV-type viruses including HTLV-II have been postulated to be implicated in chronic fatigue syndrome (the CDC definition requires at least 6 months of fatigue that reduces normal activities more than 50% in the absence of other known diseases). One of the surface antigens of the helminth worm *Schistosoma mansoni* has an epitope (base sequence) identical to the *vif*, which codes for the protein factor necessary for entry of the HIV-1 into T-cells [18]. There is an association between seropositivities for hepatitis B virus surface antigen and HIV-1 core antibody [19]. Hepatitis B virus can infect lymphocytes and produce a protein that activates HIV-1 [20]. Approximately 30% of patients with Sjogren's syndrome (an autoimmune disease causing dryness of the mouth and eyes, one of the symptoms of ARC) produce serum antibodies that react with the major capsid protein of HIV-1 and sometimes with the *gag* protein p17; similar percentages of patients with systemic lupus erythematosus, scleroderma, and juvenille rheumatoid arthritis also produce HIV-1 *gag*-reactive serum antibodies [21]. An intracisternal A-type retroviral particle antigenically related to but distinguishable from HIV-1 has been detected in lymphoblastoid cells exposed to homogenates of salivary tissue from patients with Sjogren's syndrome [21].

The advent of full-blown AIDS is also postulated to require more than HIV infection, and mycoplasmas (a prokaryote without a cell wall) may be necessary to complete T-cell lysis [22]. The lysis of T-cells contributes to lack of immunocompetence and hence enhances AIDS onset. Cytomegalovirus, adenovirus, herpes simplex virus, and hepatitis B virus can all potentiate T-cell lysis ability [22] indicative of a complex number of alternatives. The case for HIV as the sole cause of AIDS is still being debated [23–26]. The argument revolves around whether HIV meets the 1840 and 1890 postulates of Koch and Henle as well as the "six cardinal rules of virology" [23]. Most HIV proponents counter with epidemiological evidence [24, 25]. Life-style cofactors are also thought to be important, with any parameters leading to depletion of the immune system being adverse (Section 9.1.5).

The association of AIDS with HIV infection was made in 1984 after isolation of HIV-1 in 1983—priority in this discovery still being much argued [27–30]. An animal model for AIDS is the induction of AIDS in rhesus monkeys by molecularly cloned simian immunodeficiency virus. HIV-1 infection of monkeys does not lead to full-blown AIDS [31, 32], although *Macaca nemestrina*, the most susceptible to SIV, can be infected with HIV-1 [93].

Rhesus monkeys provided with a live SIV vaccine with a deletion in the *nef* gene have been protected from full SIV attack [94]. SIV-infected rhesus monkeys show neurobehavioral impairments similar to those observed in PWAs. HIV-1 infection of human-PBL-SCID mice has been reported as a small animal model for studies of the pathogenesis and treatment of AIDS [33].

14.1 MECHANISM OF HIV INFECTION

HIV has [34] a spherical membrane ("coat") consisting of glycoprotein (gp), gp120 (coded for by the viral *gag* gene via translation to gp160, which is itself cleaved to form gp120 and transmembrane gp 41). The membrane encloses a cylindrical core containing two strands of viral RNA [34]. The HIV proviral genome is about 10 kilobases in length and comprises the flanking long terminal repeat (LTR) sequences that contain regulatory segments for HIV replication as well as the *gag*, *pol*, and *env* genes coding for the core proteins, the reverse transcriptase/protease/endonuclease and integrase, and the internal and external envelope glycoproteins, respectively. The *env*, *gag*, and *pol* RNA genes are also present in all known retroviruses. HIV-1 has also at least five additional genes, *tat*, *trs/art*, *nef*, *R*, and *sor*. The *tat* gene encodes a protein that activates transcription of the provirus DNA. The *rev* gene encodes a protein that regulates the splicing of viral messenger RNA (mRNA). The *nef* gene may encode proteins that inhibit virus replication in infected cells and/or encode proteins that increase virulence. The functions of *vif*, *vpr*, *vpx*, and *vpu* regulatory genes are still unknown.

HIV appears to home in on the CD4 molecule on the surface of T-cells. CD4 is a glycoprotein expressed on most thymocytes and on the subset of peripheral T lymphocytes that includes T-helper cells and Class II major histocompatibility complex (MHC) specific cytotoxic T-cells [34]. Such cells are also termed $CD4^+$ or CD4 cells, CD being the abbreviation for "cluster of differentiation." (See Chapter 13 for an introduction to T-cells and MHC molecules.) HIV can also infect macrophages. CD4 is normally a receptor for the MHC Class II antigens, an accessory to the T-cell receptor (Section 13.2.2), and a receptor for $p56_{lck}$, a cellular tyrosine kinase [34, 35]. CD4 can also associate with other CD4-containing cells. HIV-1 binding does not lead to tyrosine protein kinase signaling or calcium mobilization, although this is disputed [36].

The MHC Class I antigen receptor of T-cells (to which CD8 but not CD4 binds) recognizes [37] specific peptide fragments from all the proteins that any nucleated cell (including infected ones) is making (Section 13.1.5). These are displayed on the cell's surface ("antigen presentation"; see Section 13.1.5). The diagnostic peptides, which vary according to an individual's genetic makeup, are transported to the cell surface by a transport protein [37]. β_2-microglobulin ensures the correct folding of MHC Class I antigens and their transport to cell surfaces and also participates in the selection of MHC Class I molecule-associated peptides [38].

The CD8 bearing T-cells from asymptomatic patients suppress virus production in infected CD4 cells without killing the HIV-1 or -2 infected CD4 cells. The key inhibitory factor is an identified soluble molecule which is not [39] a known cytokine (Section 13.0.3), but appears to inhibit HIV RNA synthesis.

CD8 T-cells from donors who have developed ARC or pre-AIDS are much less effective than this, and CD8 T-cells from PWAs virtually do not produce the factor [39].

The mechanism of the Class II antigen MHC receptor (Section 13.2.2) is still unknown, and there is some evidence for binding to specific parts ("domains") of CD4 [40]. MHC Class II antigens are known to play a role in the multistage carcinogenesis associated with papillomaviruses [41]. It is known that the peptides presented at the surface on the Class II MHC receptor (13–17 amino acids in length) come from proteins degraded in cellular vesicles rather than the cytoplasm as for Class I MHC sites, and can be self or non-self peptides [42].

The viral envelope glycoprotein gp120 binds to CD4 (facilitated by a physical interaction also with gp41). This leads to fusion of viral and T-cell membranes via breakdown of the host cell's phosphatidyl inositol moieties, and facilitates entry of the HIV into the helper T-cell [34]. Inhibition of this initial event by binding antibodies to the "principal neutralizing determinant" of HIV-1 is currently the object of much research [34]. The V3 loop area (consisting of about 35 amino acids) not only serves as a target of the host immune response but also is implicated in determining HIV-1 tissue tropism, though it is not necessary for CD4 binding to viral gp120 [43].

The retroviral RNA is next reverse-transcribed by RNAse H/polymerase into double-stranded DNA, also called provirus DNA (the polymerase process is slowed by 3′-azido-3′-deoxythymidine, commonly called AZT or zidovudine), which is then incorporated via an HIV integrase into the host cell chromosome, where it is then called a provirus [34, 40]. The reverse transcriptase has been found to contain a third enzymic activity, that of ribonuclease D, where HIV RNA is cleaved in a complex with tRNA for lysine [44].

The integrase (encoded by the viral *pol* gene) cleaves the host cell DNA, and its resulting 5′ ends are joined to the 3′ ends of viral DNA. This process is reversible *in vitro* [45]. Peripheral blood lymphocytes from HIV-infected asymptomatic individuals contain predominantly unintegrated proviral DNA, that is, not integrated into the host DNA [39]. In contrast, PWA peripheral lymphocytes contain mostly DNA where the proviral DNA has been integrated into host DNA [39].

On antigenic stimulation of the T-cell, the host RNA polymerase II transcribes the provirus (regulated by Tat, Nef, and Rev proteins) to produce viral RNA. There is evidence of the need for an inducible transcription factor from the host cell to make viral transcription a high-efficiency process. The factor binds to the regulatory sites in the HIV enhancer sequence after T-cell activation.

The viral RNA is then packaged into retroviral particles (virions) consisting of two retroviral RNA molecules that are eventually released by budding [46]. These virions, which also contain HIV-1 protease and a small amount of viral DNA tightly complexed with reverse transcriptase [39], can infect other T-cells. Some of the viral RNA in the nucleus is also translated into viral proteins, the Tat, Nef and Rev proteins being used to regulate continuing transcription of the integrated host/viral DNA in the nucleus, with continuing unanswered replication leading to T-helper cell death [39]. Other viral protein products, for example, HIV-1 protease and reverse transcriptase, are incorporated into the virion particles for virion maturation. When HIV-1 buds from the surface of an infected T-cell, its heavy sugar coat shields it from immune system detection and any direct exposure to antibody [39].

The crystal structure of CD4 was elucidated toward the end of 1990 [47]. Evidence exists that CD4 may modulate CD3 (but not CD2)-induced membrane-signaling, and that HIV-1-infected T cells cannot respond to CD3 stimulation [48].

The present anti-AIDS drug research is focused [49] on inhibitors of reverse transcriptase [AZT (approved by the FDA), ddI (approved by the FDA), ddC (approved by the FDA), fluorothymidine, 4′-azidothymidine, L-drugs, Bl-RG-587, hypericin from the St-John's-wort, and TIBO] and of HIV-1 protease. The use of ddI and AZT in combination shows some promise [50], as does AZT/acyclovir [51], both showing characteristic variability in effectiveness. Zn^{2+} has been found to inhibit HIV-1 protease, and prophylaxis has been successful on some zinc-deficient patients [52]. HIV-1 protease breaks down a protein made by HIV-1 into subunits crucial for assembling a mature viral particle [49]. Blocking of the protease inhibits viral infectivity even if the virus gains entrance into the T-cell. Several clinical trials are under way with anti-protease agents. Protein integration blockers include myrisoylation inhibitors. Uniroyal Jr blocks an unknown critical stage of viral entry into the host cell, and CD4-PE40 conjugates with the soluble receptor better than does HIV. RO 24-7429 inhibits *tat* function or its expression toward HIV RNA [53]. *N*-(*n*-Butyl)-deoxynojirimycin alters the local conformation of gp120, preventing fusion of host cells and viral membranes. Although most of the drugs mentioned above are effective inhibitors of HIV-1 in a test tube, this does not mean they will be clinically effective—hence the many ongoing clinical trials with these agents.

Only a small proportion of blood T-cells is actually infected (1 in 10^4 or 10^5 T-cells) [39]. PWAs have HIV-1–derived DNA in their CD4 T-cells at a frequency of about 1/100 cells. HIV-1–infected patients not having full-blown AIDS contain HIV-1–derived DNA in about 1/1000 cells. Asymptomatic patients infected with HIV-1 show HIV-1–derived DNA in about 1/10,000 cells [35]. These data answer one of Duesberg's persistent criticisms that HIV-1–derived DNA in the host often is not found in PWAs [23], as the incidence of HIV-infection is better correlated with ARC/pre-AIDS symptoms than those of full-blown AIDS. Because full-blown AIDS is characterized by a very low peripheral T-cell count in general, the absolute number of these cells infected with HIV will be much smaller than in ARC/pre-AIDS, but the proportion infected is greater.

However, there are still many unknowns. Brain neurons that can be infected by HIV (dementia and neurobehavioral changes are shown by some PWAs) do not contain CD4 molecules; so there must be other mechanisms of infection. Some investigators favor brain infection via monocytes, in which most of the HIV accumulates in cytoplasmic vacuoles associated with the Golgi apparatus rather than being budded as virions, as occurs for T-cells [53]. HIV-1 infection by other means could also involve neurons and glial cells [54]. There is some evidence for a role of a galactocerebroside or similar receptor for HIV-1 entry into neural cells [55]. It is also known that virally infected neurons do not have enough MHC Class I to allow cytotoxic T-cell lymphocytes to detect their presence via the "antigen presentation" process [56]. Thus once infected viruses are inside neurons, the infected cells cannot be effectively neutralized by cytotoxic T-cells. Langerhans cells in mucous membranes have been shown to contain the highest concentrations of HIV-1 [39]. These cells process foreign antigens that they encounter, and, once activated, migrate to lymph nodes where they transform into dendritic cells, which present antigens to and "nurture" CD4 T-cells. Langerhans cells are more sensitive to HIV-1 infection than T-helper cells, and produce much greater amounts of virions (80% of the amount produced in the body). They are not killed by HIV-1 infection because their CD4 antigen concentration is low. It has been postulated that AIDS could be an infection of the dendritic cells that kills off the CD4 cells that try to interact with the infected dendritic cell [39]. This mechanism has much in common with Type IV hypersensitivity (Section 13.3.4).

Another proven alternative route of HIV-1 entry is through co-infection of host cells with another retrovirus ("phenotypic mixing") without the requirement of CD4-containing cells, for example, B cells and CD8/CD4$^-$ T-lymphocytes [57]. Thus mycoplasmas, viruses, protozoans, and microbes may be important co-infection vectors, and this possibility supports one of Duesberg's objections to HIV-1 as the sole cause of AIDS. HIV infection may also make host cells more susceptible to these vectors, or vice versa. Certainly the increased occurrence of tuberculosis, syphilis, gonorrhea, leprosy, chancroid, chlamydia, herpes, and B-cell lymphomas in PWAs relative to non-AIDS controls supports this idea, no matter what the actual mechanism is.

The *tat*, *nef*, and *rev* parts of HIV are essential for viral replication and internal regulation [34], but how these viral segments interplay in the mechanism of viral multiplication and subversion of host-cell machinery is still unclear. It is known that *tat*-mediated transactivation requires the transactivation response RNA sequences located at the 5′ end of the untranslated leader region of all viral mRNAs, the first 57 nucleotides of which form a stable stem-loop structure *in vitro*, with nucleotides spanning positions +19 to +42 being required for an *in vivo* response. A direct interaction between *tat* and these transactivation response RNA sequences occurs [58]. The *rev* portion reaction with RNA is determined through HIV-1 secondary structure interaction with *env* [59]. The Rev protein enhances the accumulation of viral large genomic and virion structural RNAs at the expense of the short, spliced viral mRNAs that code for many viral accessory or regulatory proteins; *rev* therefore regulates viral protein expression by regulating RNA transport from the nucleus [60]. The inhibition of RNA transport by suitable drugs may be a basis for inhibiting viral proliferation. Whereas *rev* and *tat* are positive regulators of HIV-1 replication, the function of *nef* appears to be as a negative regulator of HIV-1 replication [39] by encoding p27 protein, which binds GTP, has GTPase activity, autophosphorylates, and down-modulates the CD4 receptor molecule, thereby determining pathogenesis in the host [61]. There is still some controversy over whether *nef* is a negative regulator of HIV-1 replication or not [62]. The effect may be related to the duration and stage of the infection. Concentrations of Nef protein in HIV-infected brain astrocytes have been correlated with rapidly progressing central nervous system disease [39]. The *nef* gene is essential for SIV replication and progression to AIDS in the rhesus monkey, a phenomenon shown *in vivo* but not *in vitro* [63].

What happens after daughter virion production is still uncertain except that the peripheral T-lymphocytes are not fully activated until used in organs and tissues to combat some other foreign invader. It has been reported that about 70% of individuals exhibit acute influenza-like symptoms shortly after infection with HIV-1 [39]. HIV can circulate dormant for a long time or be stored until the host cells are activated by interaction with some antigen. The latter route is similar to a chemical promoter mechanism, and this may account for the variable lag periods before expression of adverse symptoms. The HIV-1 concentration in blood (as reflected by antibody ELISA testing) can cycle around low values for some time before an exponential HIV increase, the median time from infection to full-blown AIDS onset being 8 years. Full-blown AIDS after the initial HIV-1 infection appears in <1% of those persons infected within 3 years, and in 6% per year after the third year, with 50% having developed AIDS by the tenth year [39].

Attempts to explain the initial control of HIV and the eventual breakdown of the immune system in terms of simple immunological mechanisms have not been successful because the population dynamics of cells and the virus are complex, and the sequence diversity of propagating HIV is too complicated because continuous mutation occurs [64], which may exhaust the $CD4^+$ population [65]. Another theory is that mutation allows the HIV-1 to escape cytotoxic T-cells [66]. Other suggestions involve autoimmune processes and the presence of HIV superantigens, fusion with uninfected cells to form clumps of nonfunctional cells called syncytia, and cofactors [67].

In addition, knowledge of immunological mechanisms is still not advanced enough to be of much help. Instead, through AIDS research much is being learned about basic mechanisms of the immune system. Many books and reviews have been published on AIDS [1, 34, 39, 65, 68–74].

14.2 TESTS FOR PRESENCE OF AIDS AND HIV

14.2.1 AIDS

The major 1992/3 CDC definition of AIDS [4] was that the T-helper cell number for blood infected with HIV is <200 cells/mm^3. The laboratory categories were in $CD4^+$ lymphocyte cells/mm^3: 1, >499 cells; 2, 200 to 499; and 3, <200 for HIV-infected people >13 years of age via HIV-1 antibody testing confirmed for HIV presence by another test. The respective ranges based on $CD4^+$ percent of total lymphocytes were: 1, >29; 2, 14 to 28; and 3, <14.

Clinical categories have been proposed for the same age group, as follows. Category A includes at least one of the following in HIV-infected individuals in the absence of conditions in Categories B and C: (i) asymptomatic HIV infection, (ii) persistent generalized lymphadenopathy, and (iii) acute primary HIV infection with accompanying illness or history of acute HIV infection. Category B includes symptomatic conditions not included in Category C (severe immunodeficiency) meeting at least one of the following criteria: (i) the conditions are attributed to HIV infection and/or are indicative of a defect in cell-mediated immunity; (ii) physicians consider the conditions to have a clinical course or management that is complicated by HIV infection. Category

C includes any condition associated with severe immunodeficiency that is of frequent occurrence in HIV-infected individuals and causes serious morbidity or mortality, and that is also listed in the 1987 surveillance case definition for AIDS. The 1993 CDC definition added invasive cervical cancer, pulmonary tuberculosis, and recurrent pneumonia to the 1987 medical conditions.

The CDC surveillance case definition was proposed for persons in the same age and HIV-infected group as above who have laboratory evidence of severe immunosuppression, that is, <200 $CD4^+$ cells/mm^3 or a $CD4^+$ percent of total lymphocytes <14 if the absolute count is not available. The new case definition also includes persons with clinical conditions listed in the 1987 CDC case definition. The second 1992 definition became effective on Jan 1 1993.

To show the diversity of the adventitious diseases linked with AIDS, it is instructive to discuss the 1987 CDC definition [75]. The definition was classified into three sections depending on whether HIV infection had been detected or not [76].

AIDS was defined as present in the absence of HIV infection and the presence of any other cause of immunodeficiency. The latter conditions included: long-term or high-dose corticosteroid or other immunosuppressive/cytotoxic therapy, for a period less than or equal to 3 months after diagnosis of Hodgkin's disease, non-Hodgkin's lymphoma (not primary brain lymphoma), lymphocytic leukemia, multiple myeloma, any other cancer of the lymphoreticular/histiocytic tissue, and angioimmunoblastic lymphadenopathy; and the presence of genetic (congenital) immunodeficiency syndrome or an acquired immunodeficiency syndrome atypical of HIV infection such as hypogammaglobulinemia. It might noted that some of these conditions may cause lowering of blood T-helper cell number to <200 cells/mm^3, the threshold for the 1993 CDC AIDS definition. The following indicator diseases then had to be present: candidiasis of the esophagus, trachea, bronchi, or lungs; cryptococcus (outside of the lung); cryptosporidiosis with diarrhea persisting >1 month; cytomegalovirus disease other than of the liver, spleen, or lymph nodes in a patient >1 month of age; herpes simplex infection causing a mucocutaneous ulcer persisting >1 month; bronchitis, pneumonitis, or esophagitis for any duration for a patient >1 month of age; Kaposi's sarcoma for a patient <60 years of age; lymphoma (primary) of the brain for a patient <60 years of age; lymphoid interstitial pneumonia and or pulmonary lymphoid hyperplasia (LIP/PLH complex) affecting a patient <13 years of age; *Mycobacterium avenium/kansasii* complex/disease at a site other than or in addition to ("disseminated") lungs, skin, or cervical or hilar lymph nodes; *Pneumocystis carinii* pneumonia; progressive multifocal leukoencephalopathy; and toxoplasmosis of the brain affecting a patient >1 month of age. In addition, if the patient had either *Pneumocystis carinii* pneumonia or the diseases diagnosed presumptively just below in the presence of a T-helper/inducer or CD4-T-cell lymphocyte count <400/mm^3, the person had AIDS in the absence of HIV presence.

When there was evidence of HIV infection by any means (regardless of the presence of other causes of immunodeficiency), any disease listed above indicated AIDS, as did the following: bacterial infections, multiple or recurrent within a period of at least 2 years; for children <13 years of age, septicemia, pneumonia, meningitis, bone/joint infections, and abscess of an internal organ/body cavity except otitis media or surface skin/mucosal abscesses caused by *Haemophilus, Streptococcus, Pneumonococcus*, or other pyrogenic bacteria;

coccidioidomycosis, histoplasmosis and any disseminated mycobacterial disease other than *Mycobacterium tuberculosis* in the lungs, the skin, and the cervical or hilar lymph nodes; encephalopathy; disease outside the lungs caused by *M. tuberculosis*; isosporiasis with diarrhea persisting >1 month; Kaposi's sarcoma at any age; primary lymphoma of the brain at any age; other non-Hodgkin's lymphoma of B-cell (not T-cell) or unknown immunologic phenotype plus Burkitt/non-Burkitt–type lymphomas, immunoblastic sarcoma such as immunoblastic lymphoma, large-cell lymphoma, diffuse histiocytic lymphoma, diffuse undifferentiated lymphoma, or high-grade lymphoma; recurrent *Salmonella* non-typhoid septicemia; and wasting syndrome.

The following diseases indicated AIDS presumptively in the presence of HIV infection (about 10–15% of PWAs before 1993): candidiasis of the esophagus; cytomegalovirus retinitis with loss of vision; Kaposi's sarcoma; lymphoid interstitial pneumonia and/or pulmonary lymphoid hyperplasia affecting children <13 years of age; disseminated mycobacterial disease (acid-fast bacilli with unidentified species except as above); *Pneumocystis carinii* pneumonia; and toxoplasmosis of the brain for patients >1 month of age.

Patients who were not HIV-positive or had none of the listed diseases above in the presence of HIV infection were diagnosed as having HIV disease on exhibiting clinical/laboratory characteristics of AIDS or having a known history of exposure to HIV. The HIV test did not have to be confirmed with another test (unlike the criteria for the 1992 definitions).

The CDC had also developed a staging system for PWAs in 1987 [77]: Group I, acute infection (mononucleosis-like syndrome associated with HIV seroconversion); II, asymptomatic infection; III, persistent generalized lymphadenopathy; IV, other disease—(A) constitutional, (B) neurological, (C) secondary infectious diseases [subdivided into C-1 (specified secondary infectious diseases listed by CDC) and C-2 (other specified secondary infectious diseases)], (D) secondary cancers, and (E) other conditions. Subcategories A3, B3, C1, C2, and C3 are defined as Category C cases in the first 1992 AIDS definition. Similarly, category B comprises B1, B2, and B3 subcategories from the 1987 case definition. This remains true for the 1993 definition.

The present WHO definition for AIDS is in terms of at least two major signs and at least one minor sign in the absence of known causes of immunosuppression including cancer and malnutrition [78]. The major signs are: weight loss greater than or equal to 10% of body weight; chronic diarrhea >1 month; Kaposi's sarcoma (no minor signs are necessary); cryptococcal meningitis (no minor signs are necessary); and prolonged intermittent or constant fever >1 month. The minor signs are: persistent cough >1 month; generalized pruritic dermatitis; recurrent herpes zoster; oropharyngeal candidiasis; chronic progressive and disseminated herpes simplex infection; and generalized lymphadenopathy. HIV infection and T-helper cell number are not used as markers. In 1990 the WHO proposed the addition of $CD4^+$ and total lymphocyte counts to its clinical symptom classification above [79].

AIDS in children is defined by the WHO to occur [78] when at least two of the following major signs are exhibited with at least two of the following minor signs in the absence of known causes of immunosuppression. The major signs are: weight loss or abnormally slow growth; chronic diarrhea >1 month; and prolonged fever >1 month. The minor signs are: generalized lymphadenopathy; oropharyngeal candidiasis; repeated common infections such as otitis and pharyngitis; persistent cough; generalized dermatitis; and confirmed maternal HIV infection.

The U.S. military has proposed its Walter Reed (WR) classification based on a Kinsey-type scale in terms of HIV status, chronic lymphadenopathy signs, delayed hypersensitivity reactions, thrush, opportunistic infections presence, and T-helper cells/mm^3 blood [80]. The critical concentration for the last parameter is 400, with WR stages 0, 1, and 2 being above and WR stages 3, 4, 5, and 6 being below. The WR0 stage has no detectable HIV, chronic lymphadenopathy, thrush, or opportunistic infection, and exhibits normal delayed hypersensitivity. WR1 is HIV-positive but shows no other differences from WR0. The rest of the stages all must be HIV-positive, with or without chronic lymphadenopathy. WR4 marks the appearance of partial delayed hypersensitivity, with WR stages 5 and 6 showing partial or complete characteristics. Thrush distinguishes the WR5 stage, as do opportunistic infections for WR6. How this system will be affected by the 1993 CDC definition is unknown.

It may be noted that 12 PWAs exposed to aggressive preventive therapy against opportunistic infections were found to have survived between 3 months and 2 years with a T-helper cell count <10 cells/mm^3 [81]. Most PWAs die of opportunistic infections within one year after their T-helper cell counts fall below 50 cells/mm^3. Thus prevention of opportunistic infections even after T-helper cell depletion is still possible.

14.2.2 HIV

Host antibody production can be detected by ELISA (Section 11.1.2) at least 6 to 8 weeks after infection, this being a matter of exceeding the detection limit of the analytical technique and defensive factors associated with the host's immune system [82]. This means that there is a time window (Section 13.1.3) where a person who is infected tests negative, giving a false negative for methods based on host antibodies. These antibodies are protective and merely indicate that an immune response of the body to HIV infection has occurred over the detection limit of the analytical method used. Analytical methods based on HIV antigens do not have this time window defect of antibody-based tests, but even there the detection limit of the analytical technique must be exceeded, so that enough HIV multiplication must occur for adequate detection. Unfortunately, these antigen-based tests are much more cumbersome and expensive than the ELISA-based antibody tests. A positive HIV-1 antibody screening test must be confirmed by another technique commonly a Western blot assay using p24 (CDC-recommended), p31, gp41, gp160, and pr 53 gag proteins (see Section 10.1.6) on polyacrylamide electrophoresis after some means of visualization such as reaction with biotin–avidin or strip radioimmunoassay (Section 11.1.1). Another confirmation technique often used is immunofluorescence.

Tests to detect antibody to HIV-1 were first licensed by the U.S. FDA in 1985. As with most other forms of biological monitoring, at least two samples separated in time are necessary for interpretation. Thus two samples a few months apart should be taken, especially where the first produces indeterminate results, to allow antibody production to increase above the detection limit of the technique. Some people who tested positive for HIV but did not have full-blown AIDS stopped [83] making detectable levels of antibody against HIV (0.4% of people with antibodies) even if three different assays were used for confirmation (ELISA and two Western blot tests). However, most of these patients still contained DNA encoded in the host by HIV as detected by the polymerase chain reaction (PCR; Section 10.1.6), but HIV could not be cultured from their tissues. One person eventually became HIV-negative even in the PCR test, and another ultimately became antibody-positive but lost reactivity on the PCR test. The interpretation of the above results is still unknown, but may involve the sequence against which the antibodies for the ELISA and Western blot were raised, the type of PCR, disappearance of the HIV from the blood but not necessarily the body, or a successful defense by the body resulting in HIV elimination/deactivation. The other two major periods in an adult where an HIV-infected person may not have detectable antibodies are soon after infection (sometimes up to 42 months after infection [71]) and when the immune system is so suppressed that PWAs cannot make detectable levels of antibodies, as discussed in Section 13.1. About half of the children testing HIV-positive at birth may lose their positivity by six months [10]. HIV infection risk from the mother has been reported to be higher for the first-born twin [84]. Selective transmission of HIV viral sequences occurred from mother to child because the child's viral sequences were less diverse than the mother's [85]. Also the relative abundances in the mother of proviral DNA was not observed in the infant.

HIV antibody tests for saliva now are available [86]. Similar noninvasive tests for urine are being developed [87] and are available. An autologous red cell agglutination assay for HIV-1 antibodies to gp41 with whole blood has been published [88].

In 1988, there were seven ELISAs (Abbott, Du Pont, Electro-Nucleonics, Genetic System, Ortho Diagnostics, Travenol, and Wellcome) and one Western blot kit (Biotech/Du Pont) licensed by the U.S. FDA [89]. All of these kits use HIV antigens derived from disruption of whole virus cultured in human-derived cell lines (H9 or CEM). Once antibodies from a test sample bind with the antigen in the ELISAs, the Abbott, Du Pont, Genetic Systems, and Ortho kits then employ a wash step to remove all material except the bound antibody/antigen. A third immunoreactant, an enzyme-labeled antihuman immunoglobulin E-antihuman Ig, then is added and binds to the human HIV antibody bound to the immobilized HIV antigen. A wash procedure removes all unbound material, leaving the HIV antigen–HIV antibody–antihuman antigen–enzyme complex. A chromogen such as biotin–avidin then is added to produce a color, which is read by spectrophotometry; the greater is the amount bound, the more intense the color. The Wellcome kit uses a competitive assay. The present sensitivity and specificity of these kits exceed 99.0%. ELISA incubation times range from 1.3 to 3.5 h. All of the ELISAs apart from the Abbott kit (bead) are microwell. The College of American Pathologists, in conjunction with the American Association of Blood Banks, conducts an open proficiency testing program for laboratories performing HIV tests.

The Western blot assay begins with purification of HIV from culture materials, followed by dissociation of the concentrated HIV with detergent (sodium dodecyl sulfonate), usually involving loss of gp120 and gp160 [75]. The material then is resolved by polyacrylamide gel electrophoresis on the basis of molecular weight and is electrophoretically transferred to a support medium such as nitrocellulose paper. Individual strips are reacted with test or control sera and developed to reveal bands where the serum antibodies have bound to the resolved viral proteins. The development process (about 2.5 h) involves using photographic plates to reveal radioactivity (strip radioactivity) or, more commonly, colorimetry by chemical incubation (such as biotin–avidin). The latter method is fast and does not use radioactive materials.

Tests with ELISAs reveal that p24 and gp41 serum antigen increase first from 2 to 5 weeks after infection, stay constant between 5 and 10 weeks, and decline between 10 and 12 weeks. At week 6 anti-envelope gp41 begins to increase, increasing to week 12 and staying constant thereafter. Anti-core p24 increases between weeks 7 and 13, and may stay constant for years before decreasing during full-blown AIDS. Serum antigen p24 increases at the end of ARC and into full-blown AIDS. The significance of these events is still unknown. Most of the commercial kits detect p24 antigen (Abbott, Du Pont Biotechnology). Detection of antibodies thus must be interpreted in terms of which antigens the antibodies were raised against (see Chapters 15 and 16). Such assay results do not provide any information on whether HIV has been inactivated because of treatment, and thus constitute possible false positives relative to HIV infectivity.

Such techniques as light and electron microscopy can confirm the presence of HIV in CD4–T-lymphocytes, but are not very sensitive, cost-effective, or convenient. Immunofluorescence assays are used to locate HIV-1 antigen in infected cells using mono-/polyclonal antibodies, usually raised against p17 or p24 [75]. Immunohistochemical staining combines the advantages of immunofluorescence and Giemsa staining without the disadvantages of the former, as preparations can be stored for months. HIV antigen ELISA assays have been most used on core antigen and are more sensitive than the nonspecific reverse transcriptase–based tests. Solid phase and liquid phase radioimmunoassays are specific but utilize ^{125}I-labeled IgG anti-HIV-1. Gene probe assays are advantageous when the production of HIV is low or where the virus may be latent, and, in spite of using radioactive labeled materials (^{32}P), provide the most sensitive technique. Such assays are expensive and time-consuming, involve radioactive material, and require skill. HIV-2 reactivity with HIV-1 gp120/gp41 recombinant antibody ELISA is about 62% although the reactivity can vary between 0 to 90%, depending on what antigens the antibodies are raised against [90].

PCR technology (Section 10.1.6) has been applied to HIV situations since 1986 because its enormous amplification power allows detection of viral RNA in the few infected host cells [91]. Thus new mRNAs and rare messenger RNAs can be detected that cannot be found by other techniques. PCR facilitates the investigation of the RNA sequence over time in the same and in different individuals, and the critical sequences required for infection of host cells. Many PCR applications thus lie more in the research realm than in routine monitoring. However, PCR helps identify those children of HIV-positive mothers who will become infected by their mothers' infection (approximately 30% of pregnant infected mothers). Recognition of susceptibility then can lead to prophylaxis. The PCR test thus acts as a predictive biological monitoring marker bioassay of future adverse effect.

A nonspecific marker for early HIV exposure presence (usable up to a year before the conventional antibody tests) has been reported to be blood interleukin-2 [92], a soluble factor protein (Section 13.0.3) released by T-helper cells when they come into contact with foreign antigen.

References

1. Piot, P.; Plummer, F. A.; Mhalu, F. S.; Lamboray, J. L.; Chin, J.; and Mann, J. M. 1988. AIDS: an international perspective. *Science* **239**: 573–579.
2. Centers for Disease Control. 1985. Revision of the case definition of acquired immunodeficiency syndrome for national reporting—United States. *Morbid. Mortal. Weekly Rep.* **34**: 373.
3. Centers for Disease Control. 1987. Revision of the surveillance case definition for acquired immunodeficiency syndrome. *Morbid. Mortal. Weekly Rep.* **36**, Suppl. 1S.
4. Centers for Disease Control. 1991. 1992 Revised classification system for HIV infection and expanded AIDS surveillance case definition for adolescents and adults: draft, Nov. 15, 1991.
5. Karpas, A. 1990. Origin and spread of AIDS. *Nature* (London) **348**: 578.
6. Garry, R. F. 1990. Early case of AIDS in the USA. *Nature* (London) **347**: 509.
7. Kaposi, M. 1872. Idiopathisches multiples pigmentsarkom der haut. *Arch. Derm. Syph.* **4**: 265–273.
8. Safai, B., and Good, R. A. 1980. Kaposi's sarcoma: a review and recent developments. *Clin. Bull.* **10**: 62–69.
9. Mark, J. 1990. Kaposi's sarcoma puzzle begins to yield. *Science* **248**: 442–443.
10. Marx, J. L. 1988. The AIDS virus can take on many guises. *Science* **241**: 1039–1040.
11. Wain-Hobson, D. S., and Myers, G. 1990. Too close for comfort. *Nature* (London) **347**: 18.
12. Anderson, C. 1991. Small wonders in Africa. *Nature* (London) **353**: 4.
13. Anonymous. 1991. The transmission of AIDS. *Nature* (London) **353**: 2.
14. Anderson, R. M.; May, R. M.; Boily, M. C.; Garnett, G. P.; and Rowley, J. T. 1991. The spread of HIV-1 in Africa: sexual contact patterns and the predicted demographic impact of AIDS. *Nature* (London) **352**: 581–589.
15. Brookmeyer, R. 1991. Reconstruction and future trends of the AIDS epidemic in the United States. *Science* **253**: 37–42.
16. Jeang, K. T.; Widen, S. G.; Semmes, O. J., IV; and Wilson, S. H. 1990. HTLV-I trans-activator protein, Tax, is a trans-repressor of the human β-polymerase gene. *Science* **247**: 1082–1084.
17. Palca, J. 1990. Does a retrovirus explain fatigue syndrome puzzle? *Science* **249**: 1240–1241.
18. Cox, F. E. G. 1990. The worm and the virus. *Nature* (London) **347**: 618.
19. Solomon, R. E.; VanRaden, M.; Kaslow, R. A.; Lyter, D.; Visscher, B.; Farzadegan, H.; and Phair, J. 1990. Association of hepatitis B surface antigen and core antibody with acquisition and manifestations of human immunodeficiency virus type 1 (HIV-1) infection. *Am. J. Public Health* **80**: 1475–1478.
20. Twu, J. S.; Chu, K.; and Robinson, W. S. 1989. Hepatitis B virus X gene activates KB-like enhancer sequences in the long terminal repeat of human immunodeficiency virus 1. *Proc. Nat. Acad. Sci. USA* **86**: 5168–5172.
21. Garry, R. F.; Fermin, C. D.; Hart, D. J.; Alexander, S. S.; Donehower, L. A., and Luo-Zhang, H. 1990. Detection of a human intracisternal A-type retroviral particle antigenically related to HIV. *Science* **250**: 1127–1129.
22. Wright, K. 1990. Mycoplasmas in the AIDS spotlight. *Science* **248**: 682–683.
23. Duesberg, P. 1988. HIV is not the cause of AIDS. *Science* **241**: 514. Also Blattner et al. reply, *Science* **241**: 514–517.
24. Blattner, W.; Gallo, R. C., and Temin, H. M. 1988. HIV causes AIDS. *Science* **241**: 515. Also Duesberg reply, *Science* **241**: 515–516.
25. Moss, A. R.; Osmond, D., and Bacchetti, P. 1988. The cause of AIDS. *Science* **242**: 997–998 Also Trachtenberg, A. I., and Winter, S. L., also Duesberg, P., reply.
26. Duesberg, P. H. Duesberg replies. 1990. *Nature* (London) **346**: 788.

27. Culliton, B. J. 1990. Deja vu in AIDS priority fight. *Science* **247**: 1532–1533.
28. Culliton, B. J. 1990. Inside the Gallo probe. *Science* **248**: 1494–1498.
29. Rubenstein, E. 1990. The untold story of HUT78. *Science* **248**: 1499–1507. Responses by Sabin, A. B., and Shields, J. W., in *Science* **249**: 465–466.
30. Anderson, C.; Concar, D., and Anderson, A. 1990. NIH launches surprise Gallo investigation. *Nature* (London) **347**: 502.
31. Kestler, H.; Kodama, T.; Ringler, D.; Marthas, M.; Pedersen, N.; Lackner, A.; Regier, D.; Sehgal, P.; Daniel, M.; King, N., and Desrosiers, R. 1990. Inductions of AIDS in rhesus monkeys by molecularly cloned simian immunodeficiency virus. *Science* **248**: 1109–1112.
32. Palca, J. 1990. A reliable animal model for AIDS. *Science* **248**: 1078.
33. Mosier, D. E.; Gulizia, R. J.; Baird, S. M.; Wilson, D. B.; Spector, D. H., and Spector, S. A. 1991. Human immunodeficiency virus infection of human-PBL-SCID mice. *Science* **251**: 791–794.
34. Fauci, A. S. 1988. The human immunodeficiency virus: infectivity and mechanisms of pathogenesis. *Science* **239**: 617–622.
35. Schnittman, S. M.; Psallidopoulos, M. C.; Lane, H. C.; Thompson, L.; Baseler, M.; Massari, F.; Fox, C. H.; Salzman, N. P., and Fauci, A. S. 1989. The reservoir for HIV-1 in human peripheral blood is a T-cell that maintains expression of CD4. *Science* **245**: 305–308.
36. Horak, I. D.; Popovic, M.; Horak, E. M.; Lucas, P. J.; Gress, R. E.; June, C. H., and Bolen, J. B. 1990. No T-cell tyrosine protein kinase signalling or calcium mobilization after CD4 association with HIV-1 or HIV-1 gp120. *Nature* (London) **348**: 557–560.
37. Baringa, M. 1990. Immune mystery revealed: how MHC meets antigen. *Science* **250**: 1657–1658.
38. Perarnau, B.; Siegrist, C. A.; Gillet, A.; Vincent, C.; Kimura, S., and Lemonnier, F. A. 1990. β 2-microglobulin restriction of antigen presentation. *Nature* (London) **346**: 751–754.
39. Baum, R. M. 1991. Florence meeting focusses on latest insights into the AIDS puzzle. *Chem. Eng. News*, July 15, pp. 9–17.
40. Lamarre, D.; Ashkenazi, A.; Fleury, S.; Smith, D. H.; Sekaly, R. P., and Capon, D. J. 1989. The MHC-binding and gp120-binding functions of CD4 are separable. *Science* **245**: 743–746.
41. Han, R.; Breitburd, F.; Marche, P. N., and Orth, G. 1992. Linkage of regression and malignant conversion of rabbit viral papillomas to MHC class genes. *Nature* (London) **356**: 66–68.
42. Rudensky, A. Y.; Preston-Hurlburt, P.; Hong, S. C.; Barlow, A., and Janeway, C. A., Jr. 1991. Sequence analysis of peptides bound to MHC class II molecules. *Nature* (London) **353**: 622–627.
43. Hwang, S. S.; Boyle, T. J.; Lyerly, H. K., and Cullen, B. R. 1991. Identification of the envelope V3 loop as the primary determinant of cell tropism in HIV-1. *Science* **253**: 71–74.
44. Thayer, Ann. 1991. HIV enzyme finding sparks new program at Bio-Technology General. *Chem. Eng. News*, Dec. 16, pp. 9–10.
45. Chow, S. A.; Vincent, K. A.; Ellison, V., and Brown, P. O. 1992. Reversal of integration and DNA splicing mediated by integrase of human immunodeficiency virus. *Science* **255**: 723–726.
46. Hu, W. S., and Temin, H. M. 1990. Retroviral recombination and reverse transcription. *Science* **250**: 1227–1233.
47. Ryu, S. E.; Kwong, P. D.; Truneh. A.; Porter, T. G.; Arthos, J.; Rosenberg, M.; Dai, X.; Xuong, N.; Axel, R.; Sweet, R. W., and Hendrickson, W. A. 1990. *Nature* (London) **348**: 419–425.

48. Linette, G. P.; Hartzman, R. J.; Ledbetter, J. A., and June, C. H. 1988. HIV-1-infected T cells show a selective signalling defect after perturbation of CD3/antigen receptor. *Science* **241**: 573–576.
49. Palca, P. 1991. The growing anti-HIV armamentarium. *Science* **253**: 263.
50. St. Clair, M. H.; Martin, J. L.; Tudor-Williams, G.; Bach, M. C.; Vavro, C. L.; King, D. M.; Kellam, P.; Kemp, S. D., and Larder, B. A. 1991. Resistance to ddI and sensitivity to AZT induced by a mutation in HIV-1 reverse transcriptase. *Science* **253**: 1557–1559.
51. Aldhous, P. 1992. Confusion over therapy. *Nature* (London) **355**: 102.
52. Anon. 1991. Zn^{2+} found to inhibit HIV-1 protease. *Chem. Eng. News*, Sept. 23, p. 16.
53. Palca, J. 1991. Promising AIDS drug looking for sponsor. *Science* **253**: 262–263.
54. Barinaga, M. 1990. New HIV infection mechanism? *Science* **250**: 758.
55. Harouse, J. M.; Bhat, S.; Spitalnik, S. L.; Laighlin, M.; Stefano, K.; Silberberg, D. H., and Gonzalez-Scarano, F. 1991. Inhibition of entry of HIV-1 in neural cell lines by antibodies against galactosyl ceramide. *Science* **253**: 320–323.
56. Joly, E.; Muckc, L., and Oldstone, M. B. A. 1991. Viral persistence in neurons explained by lack of major histocompatibility class I expression. *Science* **253**: 1283–1285.
57. Lusso, P.; Veronese, F. D. M.; Ensoli, B.; Franchini, G.; Jemma, C.; DeRocco, S. E.; Kalyanaraman, V. S., and Gallo, R. C. 1990. Expanded HIV-1 cellular tropism by phenotypic mixing with murine endogeneous retroviruses. *Science* **247**: 848–852.
58. Weeks, K. M.; Ampe, C.; Schultz, S. C.; Steitz, T. A., and Crothers, D. M. 1990. Fragments of the HIV-1 tat protein specifically bind *tar* RNA. *Science* **249**: 1281–1285.
59. Olsen, H. S.; Nelbock, P.; Cochrane, A. W., and Rosen, C. A. 1990. Secondary structure is the major determinant for interaction of HIV rev protein with RNA. *Science* **247**: 845–848.
60. Dayton, E. T.; Powell, D. M., and Dayton, A. I. 1989. Functional analysis of CAR, the target sequence for the rev protein of HIV-1. *Science* **246**: 1625–1629.
61. Cheng-Mayer, C.; Iannello, P.; Shaw, K.; Luciw, P. A., and Levy, J. A. 1989. Differential effects of *nef* on HIV replication: implications for viral pathogenesis in the host. *Science* **246**: 1629–1632.
62. Barinaga, M. 1990. AIDS meeting: unexpected progress. *Science* **248**: 1596–1597.
63. Cullen, B. R. 1991. The positive effect of the negative factor. *Nature* (London) **351**: 698–699.
64. Bangham, R. M., and McMichael, A. J. 1990. Why the long latent period? *Nature* (London) **348**: 388.
65. Nowak, M. A.; Anderson, R. M.; McLean, A. R.; Wolfs, T. F. W.; Goudsmit, J., and May, R. M. 1991. Antigenic diversity thresholds and the development of AIDS. *Science* **254**: 963–969.
66. Philips, R. E.; Rowland-Jones, S.; Nixon, D. F.; Gotch, F. M.; Edwards, J. P.; Ogunlesi, A. O.; Elvin, J. G.; Rothbard, J. A.; Bangham, C. R. M.; Rizza, C. R., and McMichael, A. J. 1991. Human immunodeficiency virus genetic variation that can escape cytotoxic T cell recognition. *Nature* (London) **354**: 453–459.
67. Marx, J. 1991. Clue found to T cell loss in AIDS. *Science* **254**: 798–800.
68. Wormser, G. P.; Stahl, R. E., and Bottone, E. J. (eds.). 1987. *AIDS: Acquired Immune Deficiency Syndrome and Other Manifestations of HIV Infection*, Noyes Publications, Park Ridge, NJ.
69. Kelly, J. A., and St. Lawrence, J. S. 1988. *The AIDS Health Crisis: Psychosocial and Social Interventions*, Plenum Press, New York.
70. Brown, K. C., and Turner, J. G. 1989. *AIDS: Policies and Programs for the Workplace*, Van Nostrand Reinhold, New York.

71. Gong, V., and Rudnick, N. (eds.). 1987. *AIDS: Facts and Issues*, Rutgers University Press, New Brunswick, NJ.
72. Am. Assoc. Advanc. Sci. 1986. *AIDS: Papers from Science, 1982–1985*, R. Kulstad (ed.), Am. Assoc. Advanc. Sci., Washington, DC.
73. Am. Assoc. Advanc. Sci. 1988. *AIDS 1988 AAAS Symposia Papers*, R. Kulstad (ed.), Am. Assoc. Advanc. Sci., Washington, DC.
74. Surgeon General. 1986. *Surgeon General's Report on Acquired Immune Deficiency Syndrome*, U.S. Department of Health and Human Services.
75. Weiss, S. H. 1987. Laboratory detection of human immunodeficiency viruses. In *AIDS: Acquired Immune Deficiency Syndrome and other Manifestations of HIV Infection*, G. P. Wormser (ed.), Noyes Publications, Park Ridge, NJ, pp. 270–293.
76. Kulstad, R. (ed.). 1988. AIDS case definitions—1. National reporting. In *AIDS 1988*, Am. Assoc. Advanc. Sci., Washington, DC, pp. 427–432.
77. Kulstad, R. (ed.). 1988. Staging systems—2. CDC classification. In *AIDS 1988*, Am. Assoc. Advanc. Sci., Washington, DC, p. 436.
78. Kulstad, R. (ed.). 1988. AIDS case definitions—2. Reporting where diagnostic resources are limited. In *AIDS 1988*, Am. Assoc. Advanc. Sci., Washington, DC, pp. 433–434.
79. WHO. 1990. Interim proposal for a WHO staging system for HIV infection and diseases. *Weekly Epidemiol. Record* **65**: 221–224.
80. Kulstad, R. (ed.). 1988. Staging systems—1. Walter Reed Classification. In *AIDS 1988*, Am. Assoc. Advanc. Sci., Washington, DC, pp. 435.
81. Nowak, R. 1991. Conditional approval touted. *Science* **352**: 464.
82. Barnes, D. M. 1988. Losing AIDS antibodies. *Science* **240**: 1407.
83. Crawford, M. H. 1989. AIDS tests fail. *Science* **246**: 1564.
84. Palca, J. 1991. HIV risk higher for first-born twins. *Science* **254**: 1729.
85. Wolinsky, S. M.; Wike, C. M.; Korber, B. T. M.; Hutto, C.; Parks, W. P.; Rosenblum, L. L.; Kunstman, K. J.; Furtado, M. R., and Munoz, J. L. 1992. Selective transmission of human immunodeficiency virus type-1 variants from mothers to infants. *Science* **255**: 1134–1137.
86. Schaefer, E. 1990. AIDS Testing: trial approved for saliva test. *Nature* (London) **346**: 687.
87. Holden, C. 1990. Testing for HIV in urine. *Science* **249**: 121.
88. Kemp, B. E.; Rylatt, D. B.; Bundesen, P. G.; Doherty, R. R.; McPhee, D. A.; Stapleton, D.; Cottis, L. E.; Wilson, K.; John, M. A.; Khan, J. M.; Dinh, D. P.; Miles, S., and Hillyard, C. J. 1988. Autologous red cell agglutination assay for HIV-1 antibodies: simplified test with whole blood. *Science* **241**: 1352–1354.
89. Kulstad, R. (ed.). 1988. Serologic testing for antibody to HIV-1: enzyme immunoassays, the Western blot procedure, and other tests for the presence of antibodies in human blood. In *AIDS 1988*, Am. Assoc. Advanc. Sci., Washington, DC, pp. 422–426.
90. Neumann, J. 1990. New, synthetic HIV-2 ELISA offers excellent sensitivity, specificity, and speed. *Du Pont Biotech Update* **5**(1): 2.
91. Keeler, R. 1991. Uses for PCR are multiplying in gene-related research. *Research and Development*, Aug., pp. 30–34.
92. Dagani, R. 1991. New test detects early exposure to AIDS virus. *Chem. Eng. News*, July 8, p. 35.
93. Agy, M. B.; Frumkin, L. R.; Corey, L.; Coombs, R. W.; Wolinsky, S. M.; Koehler, J.; Morton, W. R., and Katze, M. G. 1992. Infection of *Macaca nemestrina* by human immunodeficiency virus type-1. *Science* **257**: 103–106.
94. Daniel, M. D.; Kirchhoff, F.; Czajak, S. C.; Sehgal, P. K., and Desrosiers, R. C. 1992. Protective effects of a live attenuated SIV vaccine with a deletion in the *nef* gene. *Science* **258**: 1938–1941.

15

Some Analytical Chemistry Approaches to Virus Detection

by John P. McCue*

15.0 ABSTRACT

First-generation licensed immunosorbent assay kits to detect the presence of antibodies to human immunodeficiency virus type 1 (HIV-1) use HIV-1 grown in cell cultures as the source of surface immobilized antigens. Various enzyme-linked immunosorbent assay (ELISA) kits were evaluated quantitatively. Those kits utilizing purified virus allowed reliable antibody detection at 40 ng/mL. False test results were obtained in those kits where the virus was not separated from cell culture debris, and where fewer than three replicate wells were utilized. Improvements in the sensitivity of HIV-1 detection by immunosorbent antigen capture assays can be achieved by increasing the amount of surface covered by antibody, by increasing the binding of this antibody to virus antigens, and by decreasing the ability of antibodies in the blood sample to bind antigens. Use of such techniques has resulted in improved detection of cytomegalovirus (CMV) antigens using ELISA antigen capture, by several orders of magnitude. Such techniques can be used to enhance any immunosorbent assay, including those for HIV-1.

15.1 HIV ANTIBODY DETECTION

15.1.1 Introduction

Different assay methods exist to detect HIV-1 [1] (Section 14.2.2). The cell-based methods measure the amount of infectious agent in a sample. However,

*Chapters 15 and 16 are dedicated to Professor John L. Engelke, whose understanding and support made Dr. McCue's work possible. Dr. Engelke was chairman of Dr. McCue's Department until his death in Paris on August 16, 1989. He will be missed!

relatively large amounts of virus must be cultured to achieve a detectable level of infection (50–100 intact virions per cell). Quality control problems common to all cell culture systems also must be solved.

Antigen capture assays detect antigenic components of HIV-1. Because the antigen concentration is greater than that for virions, such assays are more sensitive than infectivity techniques. If the antigens are viral proteins, the latter reflect active HIV-1 infection except when antibodies are also present in the blood sample. If the antigens are viral RNA, it is, in addition, a sign of active HIV-1 infection. However, the viral RNA is several orders of magnitude lower in concentration than the viral protein antigens.

The detection of virus-induced DNA in host cells by the polymerase chain reaction (PCR; Sections 10.1.6 and 14.2.2) has also been accomplished [2]. It is unclear whether the PCR assay results mean that an active HIV-1 infection is present, or mean that exposure to HIV-1 occurred in the past but HIV-1 is not active at present; thus this test has an interpretation similar to that of an antibody biological monitoring marker.

Most commercial techniques for HIV-1 exposure use detection of host antibodies. A positive test reveals only that there has been exposure in the past to HIV-1, not that HIV-1 is actively depleting the immune system. As thousands of antibody molecules are synthesized in response to each antigen molecule (Sections 13.1.5 and 13.3.4), these techniques have high sensitivity. These assays were designed to screen blood samples, but also have exhibited false test results [3–6].

In response to this problem, kits from various manufacturers were compared by determination of the detection limits of the kits. Two types of kits were evaluated, those using purified HIV-1 extract and those utilizing crude virus extracts from tissue cultures.

15.1.2 Materials and Methods

Antibodies for evaluation of the ELISA kits were isolated as polyclonal immunoglobulin G (IgG) from pooled human plasma of 3000 donors using Cohn/Oncley Method 9 [7, 8]. The rationale for choosing IgG is discussed in Section 13.2.1. Three antibody preparations were made, two from pools seropositive to HIV-1 and one from a pool seronegative to HIV-1. The antibody preparations when assayed by radial immune diffusion (RID) were >99.9% IgG, and contained the same relative amounts of IgG subclasses found in plasma. In radial immune diffusion, the suitably diluted antiserum is incorporated into agar gel, and antigen is allowed to diffuse into it. Precipitation of antigen–antibody complexes in a circle with the antigen well as its center occurs when optimal proportions are reached after sufficient diffusion/dilution of the antigen into the gel. The higher the concentration of antigen is, the greater the ring diameter. Thus calibration curves can be constructed by the external standards method, and unknown concentrations of antigen found.

On Western blot analysis (Sections 10.1.6 and 14.2.2), one preparation, denoted as (++), was found to contain antibodies to HIV-1 proteins p15, p24, p31, gp41, p53, and p64. The second preparation, denoted as (+), contained antibodies only to p24, the CDC-recommended criterion (Section 14.2.2). The third preparation, denoted as (−), was free of detectable antibodies to HIV-1 proteins.

ELISA kit evaluations were performed by applying dilutions (0.01–0.32 mg/mL) of the three IgG preparations in eightfold replicates to antigen-coated plates obtained with the kits from DuPont, Electro Nucleonics (ENI), and Travenol. The IgG dilutions were made with the dilluent buffers supplied with the kits. Color development on the plates was read at 414 nm with a 540 nm background correction (to account for nonspecific absorption), using a Titertek Multiskan MCC/340 plate reader (Flow Laboratory, Inc.). Determination of the maximum dilution at which the various kits could distinguish among the three IgG samples was carried out by comparing each set of experimental points along the response curves using a paired, two-tailed Student *t*-test [9].

Determination of the amount of antibody to HIV-1 that the kits were able to detect was obtained by allowing dilutions (100–100,000 ng/mL) of the (++) preparation to adsorb for 2 days on the surface of the wells of blank microtiter plates. After the 2-day absorption period, the plating solutions were removed and analyzed for protein by the Lowry method [10]. The wells also were soaked once with water for 1 h, and the soak solutions were analyzed for protein. The amount of IgG adsorbed on the surfaces was calculated by summing the protein content of the plating and soak solutions. The plates then were developed with alkaline phosphatase conjugated antihuman IgG supplied with and in a manner identical to that used with the DuPont HIV plates. The color developed at 414 nm after correction for the 540 nm background was compared with the IgG calibration curve to obtain the amount of HIV-specific antibodies detected.

15.1.3 Results

The responses of the HIV-1 antibody test kits of the IgG preparations are shown in Table 15.1. The intersection of the dilution curves of purified IgG occurred at 10 μg/mL of diluent for all kits. This is caused by nonspecific binding of IgG to the assay plate surfaces. The minimum dilution at which the kits could distinguish the three IgG preparations at $p < 0.01$ (in other words, their practical detection limit) was 40 μg/mL for the DuPont kit and 160 μg/mL for the other kits. The latter two kits did not distinguish between IgG preparations (+) and (−) based on antibody content. They also showed greater binding of the seronegative IgG sample to the virus coatings on their plates than for the IgG sample containing antibody to HIV-1 p24 antigen. The Du Pont kit was able to make the correct relative assignments for all three IgG preparations according to their HIV-1 antibody composition.

The principal difference among the three kits is the degree of virus purification for the antigen coats on the plates. The DuPont plates use HIV-1 purified from H-9 cell tissue culture by a two-stage density gradient procedure after glycine precipitation. The other two kits use virus obtained from glycine precipitation alone. This point is also demonstrated in Table 15.2, depicting binding of seropositive and seronegative IgG preparations to ELISA plates coated with uninfected H-9 cell tissue culture glycine extract. The binding observed in the ENI and Travenol kits is caused by nonspecific binding to cell

TABLE 15.1. Comparison of the Electro Nucleonics (ENI), Travenol, and DuPont ELISA kits for antibodies to HIV-1 in purified human IgG preparations. The Western blot absorbances at 414 nm are corrected for background at 540 nm.

IgG concentration (mg/mL)	Kit Mean Corrected Absorbances								
	ENI			Travenol			DuPont		
	A	B	C	A	B	C	A	B	C
0.008	0.056	0.025	0.013	0.080	0.028	0.010	0.100	—	0.022
0.019	0.072	0.030	0.016	0.092	0.070	0.020	0.222	0.033	0.044
0.032	0.122	0.035	0.018	0.105	0.052	0.025	0.300	0.025	0.056
0.039	0.144	0.035	0.022	0.130	0.057	0.038	0.333	0.033	0.067
0.063	0.211	0.056	0.025	0.195	0.092	0.058	0.500	0.033	0.067
0.080	0.256	0.060	0.033	0.252	0.105	0.084	0.555	0.078	0.100
0.159	0.391	0.099	0.067	0.659	0.278	0.188	0.866	0.091	0.291
0.316	0.556	0.188	0.131	0.833	0.498	0.389	1.360	0.167	0.266

A: Positive for antibodies to p15, p31, gp41, p53, and p64.
B: Negative for antibodies to HIV-1.
C: Positive for antibodies to p24.

debris on the plate surfaces. When the HIV-1 antibody concentration is small relative to the concentration of antibodies reactive to the tissue culture cell debris, false negative results occur.

The purified polyclonal IgG preparations were also used to estimate the detection limits of kits in terms of absolute amount of specific antibody against HIV-1. Because the detection limit for the DuPont kit was 40 μg IgG/mL for preparation (++), the mass of specific antibody in a 40 μg IgG/mL sample bound to the plate was the detection limit for specific antibody. This was determined by making calibration plates from IgG preparation (++) adsorbed on antigen-free plates. Because identical assay conditions and IgG preparations were utilized for the calibration and assay plates, a simple comparison of absorbance revealed that approximately 1 μg of antibodies to HIV-1 was present in each mg of IgG in preparation (++). Thus the detection limit achievable with ELISA plates prepared with purified virus was approximately 40 ng of HIV-1–specific antibody/mL of diluent.

15.1.4 Discussion

The above results demonstrate that the limiting factor for ELISAs is the amount of nonspecific binding of IgG to the support surface on which the antigens have been immobilized. This determines the practical detection limit of the assays and will not be changed by the use of genetically engineered antigens. The situation is much worse when nonpurified antigen is used because false negative results ensue when the amount of antibody specific to HIV-1 in the sample is less than the total amount of antibody "reacting" with nonviral proteins on the plate, whether this is specific or nonspecific in nature. The ENI and Travenol kits attempt to deal with this problem by specifying a low positive response threshold, which actually leads to inclusion of samples with no antibody to HIV-1.

The limiting amount of antibody to HIV-1 detectable by the DuPont assay is 800 ng/mL plasma, taking into account the 1:20 dilution of plasma before analysis. Because an individual produces 1 to 10 μg antibody/mL plasma in response to an antigenic episode such as immunization with attenuated virus, the DuPont assay should detect anyone capable of a normal antibody response.

The data in Tables 15.1 and 15.2 were obtained from eightfold replicates of each sample dilution of the three IgG preparations to allow statistical differences at the 99% confidence level ($p < 0.01$) to be demonstrated. Commonly, even the best assay kits are used with only one or two assay wells allocated to each sample. The confidence level for two replicates is only 90%. This is an unacceptable margin of error for screening blood for transfusion.

This work has shown that the performance of test kits for detection of antibodies to HIV-1 is significantly compromised by the use of nonpurified virus and by the use of fewer than eight replicate assay wells per sample. The first finding has its analogy in traditional analytical chemistry when impure materials are used for quantitation in spectrophotometry, leading to underestimation of the true concentration of a test sample from the incorrect calibration curve—assuming that the impurities also absorb at the wavelength selected. Another analytical chemistry analogy occurs when two or more detected compounds used for calibration purposes have the same retention time/volume on chromatography. A sample containing just one of the compounds will yield data that underestimate the true concentration of the unknown compound if the response factors are different. A third analogy from the field of HIV-1 virology is the initial culture on established cell lines of the original HIV-1 by Robert C. Gallo's research group in 1984, from a contaminated isolate containing LAV-I originating from the laboratory of Luc Montagnier and his research group of the Pasteur Institute in 1983 [11–13]. In the latter case, the LAV-I competed successfully against the other viruses, and was grown by Gallo's group and was so enriched that it could be sequenced (Section 14.0).

TABLE 15.2. Comparison of ELISA responses (absorbance at 414 nm with background correction at 540 nm) to purified human IgG preparations assayed on microtiter plates coated with tissue culture extract free of HIV-1 or HIV-2 antigens. The IgG preparations are the same as those defined in Table 15.1.

IgG concentration (mg/mL)	Corrected Mean Absorbance for		
	A	B	C
0.032	0.044	0.033	0.011
0.039	0.061	0.044	0.022
0.063	0.092	0.063	0.033
0.080	0.125	0.067	0.039
0.159	0.200	0.094	0.056
0.316	0.211	0.168	0.111

A: Western blot positive for antibodies to p15, p24, p31, gp41, p53, and p64.
B: Western blot negative for antibodies to HIV-1.
C: Western blot positive for antibodies to p24.

The use of eight replicate wells has its analogy in statistical power calculations of how many replicates are necessary to achieve a stated statistical confidence level. Thus the current procedure of using one or two wells should be replaced by one utilizing at least eight wells if 99% confidence is desired, or at least three wells if 95% confidence is deemed sufficient. The dependence of the statistical power of replicates on the square root of the number of replicates is well known [9]. The FDA should mandate a standard protocol involving these recommendations.

15.2 IMPROVEMENTS IN ANTIGEN CAPTURE ASSAYS FOR DETECTION OF VIRUSES

15.2.1 Introduction

Viruses that are hidden from detection in blood and tissues after infecting an individual present special problems for clinical evaluation and management of patients. For example, quiescent $CD4^+$ T-lymphocytes may be a major and inducible HIV reservoir [14]. Asymptomatic infected individuals harbor full-length, unintegrated complementary proviral DNA in their T-lymphocytes, whereas in PWAs (pre-1992 definition) the ratio of integrated proviral DNA to unintegrated extrachromosomal proviral DNA is increased [14].

Another virus that shows similar powers is cytomegalovirus (CMV). CMV is capable of chronic latent phase infections. It can alter cellular immune response [for example, it can potentiate T-cell lysis in the presence of HIV-1 (Section 14.0)], and it can proliferate in tissues in immune-compromised patients but not in non-immune-compromised patients (Sections 14.0 and 14.2.1). Much about the clinical problems associated with CMV has been learned from organ transplant patients, where CMV is a common cause of postoperative complications and is the leading reason for their morbidity and mortality. Testing for antibodies to CMV before transplant helps identify those persons at risk of complications. There is a high rate of seropositivity, but many seropositives do not develop CMV infections when immunosuppressed [15–17]. Thus there is a great need to develop assays for the level of active virus. Such assays would better identify those at risk of potential viral activation, and would help to assess the effectiveness of antiviral therapy.

The development of appropriate assays for the detection of latent phase viral infections is also important to the study and management of AIDS. Like patients who are immunosuppressed by chemotherapy and radiation, PWAs experience complications from CMV, and the clinical progression of their HIV infection may be influenced by a potentiative interaction with CMV [18–20]. The current dogma is that nearly all individuals antibody-positive for HIV will develop AIDS. Although this is supported by the current epidemiologic evidence [21], the representativeness of the populations studied is unknown. Thus, the scenario may be different for such other groups as infected hemophiliacs [22].

Direct testing for HIV antibodies has its drawbacks in terms of interpretation of the data (Section 15.1). Another approach involves virus antigen capture assays using monoclonal and affinity purified polyclonal antibodies

(Sections 11.0 and 11.1). However a patient's own antibodies to viruses compete for binding sites on the appropriate antigens and thus mask the presence of virus antigens. This problem is especially severe during latent phase infection when the amount of virus antigen is small compared to the amount of circulating antibody against the virus.

Enhancing the ability of the immobilized antibodies used to assay plates to compete for binding of the antigens of interest is a logical next step in improving virus antigen capture assays. This is the theme of the following sections.

15.2.2 Materials and Methods

IgG for use in coating microtiter plates was isolated from CMV seropositive human plasma as Cohn Effluent III at pH 5.2 [7, 8]. The final manipulation of this pure but dilute ethanol-containing IgG fraction was carried out by two different methods.

The first technique was the pH 7 method. The IgG from an aliquot of Cohn Effluent III was concentrated by the conventional method of precipitating the proteins near their isoelectric point (pH 7.4) in 25% ethanol at 8°C and then removing the residual alcohol by freeze-drying. The IgG was then solubilized in 50 mM phosphate buffer at pH 7.2 and stored at 5°C until needed.

The second technique was the pH 4 method. An aliquot of the Cohn Effluent III was adjusted to pH 4.5 with acetic acid and ultrafiltered (30,000 molecular weight cutoff membrane) at 5°C to concentrate the protein. The alcohol was removed by diafiltration (7 volume replacement) with water. The resultant IgG solution was then buffered at pH 4.6 with 50 mM phosphate buffer and stored at 5°C until needed. These two methods yielded preparations with identical IgG content based on protein measurements at 280 nm. Similarly, both were shown to contain >99% of the protein in the starting aliquots of Cohn Effluent III.

Another IgG preparation for use in coating microtiter plates was isolated from the plasma of CMV immunized goats. The plasma was diluted 1:10 in 50 mM phosphate buffer at pH 6.8 and loaded on a *Staphylococcus aureae* protein G affinity column (Genex Corp., Gaithersburg, MD). The column was washed with 7 column volumes of loading buffer to remove non-IgG proteins. The IgG was then eluted with 5 mM acetic acid. Immediately after collection of the IgG fraction, its pH was adjusted to 4.2 with 5 mM sodium acetate buffer, and it was stored at 5°C until needed.

For the ELISAs, each antigen capture experiment was confined to an individual microtiter plate to minimize plate variability and eliminate solution variabilities. Polystyrene plates with 96 wells were used throughout. The requisite wells for the experiment at hand were filled with 200 μL of the appropriate IgG plating solutions and allowed to sit at least 2 days before the plates were used in ELISA experiments.

At the start of each ELISA experiment, the wells of the plate to be used were washed six times with 300 μL of sterile filtered distilled water and allowed to soak in sterile distilled water for 1 h. The wells then were washed again six times with 300 μL of sterile filtered distilled water to remove unbound IgG. Comparison of the relative amounts of IgG that remained attached to a plate was made by reacting IgG-coated wells with alkaline phosphatase–conjugated antihuman or antigoat IgG (Sigma Chemical Co., St. Louis, MO) at a 1:2000 dilution in 100 mM carbonate buffer at pH 8.2 with 0.1% bovine serum albumin (BSA) (Sigma Chemical Co., St. Louis, MO) for 2 h at room temperature. The wells were then washed six times with sterile filtered distilled water, and the amount of retained alkaline phosphatase activity was measured by adding to these wells 1 mg/mL of *p*-nitrophenyl phosphate (pNPP) (Sigma Chemical Co., St. Louis, MO) in 100 mM glycine at pH 10.4 with 1 mM magnesium chloride and zinc chloride. Measurement of the conversion of pNPP by the retained enzyme was made at 414 nm with 540 nm background correction using a Titertek Multiskan MCC/340 (Flow Laboratories, Ayrshire, Scotland) plate reader.

CMV antigen for the antigen capture experiments was a crude glycine precipitated extract from the supernatant of virus (strain AD-169) grown in human foreskin fibroblast cells. The virus fraction was inactivated by ultraviolet irradiation with a deuterium lamp. The stock virus was diluted to various concentrations in 50 mM TRIS at various pH values to determine a pH at which all coated IgG surfaces captured the antigen in a dose-response fashion. The final reaction conditions used for quantitative analysis were CMV antigen diluted in TRIS at pH 6.5 with dilutions of CMV reacting with IgG-coated plates for 2 h at room temperature with gentle mixing on a plate rocker. Unbound antigen was then removed by washing the plates three times with sterile filtered distilled water. The amount of antigen captured was visualized by allowing it to react with anti-CMV IgG conjugated to alkaline phosphatase. Before addition of the alkaline phosphatase substrate (pNPP), the plates were washed six times with distilled water.

For the analysis of data, the average of eight replicate assay well responses at each concentration of CMV was compared to the average of well responses for the diluent matrix without CMV (that is, the background response). Statistical comparison of the average response at each CMV concentration was made relative to the background response using an unpaired, two-tailed Student t-test [9]. The concentration range in which an assay system was judged capable of detecting CMV was the range in which these was dose-response and a $p < 0.05$ relative to background response.

15.2.3 Results and Discussion

The conventional wisdom is that purified antibodies for use in antigen capture assays are most stable in physiological buffers [23], and that adsorption on surfaces is best accomplished from solutions in or slightly above the physiological pH range [24, 25]. However, purified IgG is unstable in and above the physiological pH range, and the antibodies contained in such preparations lose binding affinity for virus antigens [26]. By comparing purified IgG prepared and formulated under different pHs, it was found that these materials behave differently when used to coat surfaces for antigen capture assays.

Table 15.3 contains background-corrected absorbance results comparing a surface covered by pure IgG purified and formulated near pH 4 with one covered by IgG prepared and formulated near pH 7. The results for the pH 7

TABLE 15.3. Effect of pH on adsorption of IgG onto polystyrene microtiter plate surfaces, on CMV capture by IgG-coated microtiter plate surfaces, and on CMV capture from seropositive plasma by IgG-coated microtiter plate surfaces. The concentrations of the IgG solutions and the CMV antigen protein were obtained by measuring the absorbance at 414 nm and correcting for background at 540 nm.

Challenge condition	Challenge concentration (ng/mL)	Average Corrected Absorbance at	
		pH 4 IgG	pH 7 IgG
IgG	100	0.010	0.011
	1,000	0.041	0.210
	10,000	0.800	0.686
	100,000	0.870	0.654
	1,000,000	0.919	0.595
Pure CMV antigen	50	0.094	0.011
	500	0.147	0.017
	5,000	0.634	0.322
CMV antigen captured from serum	50	0.093	0.011
	500	0.143	0.019
	5,000	0.638	0.325

IgG preparation are similar to those reported in the literature, with optimum adsorption occurring near 10 μg IgG/mL. The optimum is a result of competition between concentration effects on surface adsorption and intermolecular IgG association in solution. The latter effect does not occur at >10 μg/mL at pH 4, the assay showing the expected saturation of binding sites at high concentrations. The dose-effect range for both assays is between 100 and 10,000 ng/mL.

Table 15.3 also depicts the relative ability of surfaces coated with pH 4 and pH 7 IgG preparations to capture purified CMV antigens. The pH 4 data are the result of adsorption from a 50 mM phosphate solution at pH 4.6 at 5 μg IgG/mL. The pH 7 data were collected after adsorption from a 50 mM phosphate solution at pH 7.2 at 15 μg IgG/mL. Under these conditions, the surface coverages of IgG are not statistically different at the two pH conditions. The ability of the pH 4 IgG-coated surfaces to capture purified CMV antigen is clearly better than that of the pH 7 IgG-coated surfaces. This does not necessarily mean that CMV in seropositive plasma would be captured better by pH 4 IgG-coated surfaces. The results for the latter experiment also are provided in Table 15.3. Freshly collected seropositive plasma to CMV was diluted 1:100 in TRIS, and this was then diluted further for analysis. Though the presence of plasma antibodies dramatically reduced the ability of the ELISA plates to capture the antigens, the surfaces covered with pH 4 IgG were still able to detect the presence of the antigen at 50 ng/mL at $p < 0.05$, unlike the surfaces covered with pH 7 IgG. Even at 500 ng/mL, the pH 7 IgG-coated surfaces did not detect CMV antigen at $p \gg 0.10$.

The sensitivity of these comparisons was limited by the relative amount of CMV specific antibodies (that is, the CMV antibody titer of 1:50) in the human IgG preparations. When IgG at a CMV antibody titer of 1:5000 isolated from the plasma of immunized goats was used to coat plates, detection limits of CMV antigen down to 100 pg/mL were achieved.

15.2.4 Conclusions

Antibodies are large complex molecules (Section 13.2.1) whose physical and functional behavior is influenced by the chemical conditions to which they have been exposed [27]. The present work has demonstrated that even the functional properties of surface immobilized antibodies are sensitive to such conditions. These experimental results show that IgG antibodies isolated, formulated, and plated near pH 4 yield superior results compared with pH 7 conditions in terms of surface coverage, purified CMV antigen binding, and the capture of CMV antigen from seropositive plasma. Further pH optimization studies need to be done.

Nevertheless, the improvements described here coupled with the greater sensitivity obtainable with monoclonal or affinity purified polyclonal antibodies will allow low levels of virus antigens to be detected in the presence of the patient's own antibodies to the virus. These results may also be applicable to HIV-1 antigen capture assays.

References

1. Khan, N. C.; and Hunter, E. 1988. Detection of human immunodeficiency virus type 1. *Am. Clin. Prod. Rev.*, May, pp. 20–25.
2. Erlich, H. In press 1993. *PCR Technology: Principles and Application for DNA Amplification*, Stockton Press, New York.
3. Fang, C. T.; Darr, F.; Kleinman, S.; Wehling, R. H.; and Dodd, R. Y. 1986. Relative specificity of enzyme linked immunosorbent assays for antibodies to human T cell lymphotropic virus type III and their relationship to Western blotting. *Transfusion* **26**: 208–209.
4. Epstein, J. S. 1987. Use of multiple immunoassay systems to determine antibodies directed against the human immunodeficiency virus. *Transfusion* **27**: 1.
5. Wartick, M. G.; McCarroll, D. R.; and Wittbank, T. R. 1987. A second discriminator for biological false positive results in enzyme linked immunosorbent assays for antibodies to human immunodeficiency virus (HTLV-III). *Transfusion* **27**: 109–111.
6. Kleinman, S.; Fitzpatrick, L.; Secord, K.; and Wilke, D. 1988. Follow up testing and notification of anti-HIV Western blot atypical donors. *Transfusion* **28**: 280–282.
7. Cohn, E. J.; Strong, L. E.; Hughes, W. L.; Mulford, D. J.; Ashworth, J. N.; Melin, M.; and Taylor, H. L. 1946. Preparation and properties of serum and plasma proteins IV. A system for the separation into fractions of the proteins and lipoprotein components of biological tissues and fluids. *J. Am. Chem. Soc.* **68**: 459–475.
8. Oncley, J. L.; Melin, M.; Richert, D. A.; Cameron, J. W.; and Gross, P. M. 1949. The separation of antibodies, isoagglutinins, prothrombin, plasminogen and β-lipoprotein into subfractions of human plasma. *J. Am. Chem. Soc.* **71**: 541–550.
9. Colton, T. 1974. *Statistics in Medicine*, Little, Brown, Boston, MA.
10. Sigma Chemical Co. Procedure P 5656, Sigma Chemical Co.; St. Louis, MO.
11. Gallo, R. C. 1991. . . . and his response. *Lett. Nature* **351**: 358.
12. Wain-Hobson, S.; Vartanian, J. P.; Henry M.; Chenciner, N.; Cheynier, R.; Delassus, S.; Martins, L. P.; Sala, M.; Nugeyre, M. T.; Guetard, D.; Klatzmann,

D.; Gluckman, J. C.; Rozenbaum, W.; Barre-Sinoussi, F.; and Montagnier, L. 1991. LAV revisited: origins of the early HIV-1 isolates from Institut Pasteur. *Science* **252**: 961–965.
13. Palca, J. 1991. The true source of HIV? *Science* **252**: 771.
14. Bukrinsky, M. I.; Stanwick, T. L.; Dempsey, M. P.; and Stevenson, M. 1991. Quiescent T lymphocytes as an inducible virus reservoir in HIV-1 infection. *Science* **254**: 423–427.
15. Meyers, J. D. 1984. Cytomegalovirus infection following marrow transplantation: risk, treatment and prevention. *Birth Defects* **20**: 101–117.
16. Kaden, J.; Scholz, D.; Eichler, C.; and May, G. 1985. Frequency of cytomegalovirus infection after kidney transplantation and first experiences with prophylactic CMV gammaglobulin. *Immunitat. Infekt.* **13**: 290–295.
17. Fassbinder, W.; Bechstein, P. B.; Scheuermann, E. H.; and Schoeppe, W. 1985. Incidence of cytomegalovirus infection after renal transplantation and first experiences with prophylactic hyperimmunoglobulin. *Scand. J. Urol. Nephrol.* (Suppl.) **92**: 23–28.
18. Berris, B. 1985. Chronic viral diseases. *Can. Med. Assoc. J.* **135**: 1260–1268.
19. Gluckman, J. C. 1986. Physiopathologie du SIDA et epidemiologie de l'infection par le virus LAV. *Rev. Epidemiol. Sante Publique.* **34**: 112–117.
20. Blazer, M. J.; and Cohn, D. L. 1986. Opportunistic infections in patients with AIDS: clues to the epidemiology of AIDS and the relative virulence of pathogens. *Rev. Infect. Dis.* **8**: 21–30.
21. Curran, J. W.; Jaffe, H. W.; Hardy, A. M.; Morgan, W. M.; Selik, R. M.; and Dondero, T. J. 1988. Epidemiology of HIV infection and AIDS in the United States. *Science* **239**: 610–616.
22. Andes, W. A.; Daul, C. B.; de Shazo, R. D.; and Palmer, C. H. 1988. Seroconversion to human immunodeficiency virus (HIV) in hemophiliacs. Relation to lymphadenopathy. *Transfusion* **28**: 98–102.
23. Tijssen, P. 1985. *Practice and Theory of Enzyme Immunoassays*, Elsevier, Amsterdam, The Netherlands.
24. Oreskes, I.; and Singer, J. M. 1961. The mechanism of particulate carrier reactions. I Adsorption of human gammaglobulin to polystyrene latex particles. *J. Immunol.* **86**: 338–344.
25. Catt, K.; and Tregear, G. W. 1967. Solid phase radioimmunoassay in antibody coated tubes. *Science* **158**: 1570–1572.
26. McCue, J. P.; Sasagawa, P. K.; and Hein, R. H. 1988. Changes induced in antibodies by isolation methods. *Biotechnol. Appl. Biochem.* **10**: 63–71.
27. McCue, J. P.; Hein, R. H.; and Tenold, R. 1986. Three generations of immunoglobulin G preparations for clinical use. *Rev. Infect. Dis.* **8**(Suppl. 4): S374–381.

16

AIDS Therapy: Functional Changes in Immune Regulating Proteins Caused by Preparation Techniques

by John P. McCue

16.0 ABSTRACT

Various proteins isolated from human plasma or their biotechnology-based counterparts isolated from tissue culture may be useful therapeutic agents for managing the clinical status of immune-compromised patients. However, laboratory and clinical experience with these biologicals is variable in nature compared with pharmaceuticals, and this variability is often overlooked during clinical trials. Much care is needed in characterizing and standardizing biologicals. Without it, product variability will result in conflicting clinical experiences. Now that a number of immune regulating proteins are being studied in clinical trials with PWAs, it is important to understand how clinical effectiveness can be influenced by the methods used to prepare the proteins. This chapter presents some data on how preparative methods influence the behavior of immunoglobulin G type antibodies. It was found that formulation pH changes affect the toxicity of the preparations to humans, and these changes appeared to be correlated with the presence of high molecular weight aggregates.

16.1 INTRODUCTION

A complete road map of the cellular and humoral events leading to AIDS is not yet available, but Chapter 14 details the major events on this map. It is clear from the progressive imbalance of helper and suppressor T-lymphocytes and the abnormal B-lymphocyte production of antibodies that loss of homeostatic control of the acquired and innate immune responses to infection (Sections 13.0 and 13.1) underlies the terminal events. Important factors in this control are the immune modulators called interferons (Section 13.0.3), interleukins (Section 13.0.1), colony stimulating factors (the factors responsible for differentiating and propagating stem cells in the bone marrow and thymus), and immunoglobulins (Section 13.2.1). It is not surprising that clinical trials of purified preparations of these materials are under way to test their therapeutic value in PWAs.

The best studied of these materials are the interferons and the immunoglobulins, though research results for both classes of compounds are contradictory and are not very reproducible [1]. In particular, adverse reactions and clinical efficacy have varied from study to study. This variation usually is attributed to differences in clinical setting and individual differences in the patients (Chapter 8). However, results with the immunoglobulins (Sections 15.1 and 15.2) have demonstrated that differences can arise from variability in the protein preparations because of different isolation techniques and varying formulations.

This chapter reviews experiences with purified immunoglobulin G (IgG) products as a model system for understanding the problems that can arise during the development of biological products for clinical use, as for patients with human immunodeficiency virus (HIV) infection.

16.2 EXPERIMENTAL SECTION

16.2.1 Immunoglobulin Preparations

The preparations of purified IgG for intramuscular administration (ISG), chemically modified IgG for intravenous administration (IGIV pH 6.8), and nonmodified IgG for intravenous administration (IGIV pH 4.2) have been described elsewhere [1]. In brief, these materials were isolated from pooled human plasma by the Cohn/Oncley method [2, 3] using cold ethanol precipitation. At the Cohn Effluent III stage, the process was modified to allow alternative methods for concentrating the purified IgG and removing the alcohol.

The ISG preparation was obtained by precipitating the IgG from Cohn Effluent III at pH 7.4 with 25% ethanol at 8°C to give Cohn Precipitate II. The alcohol was then removed by freeze-drying the precipitate. The ISG was formulated as a 16.5% IgG solution in water with 0.32 M glycine and 0.45% sodium chloride at pH 6.8 to 7.4.

The IGIV pH 6.8 preparation was obtained from Cohn Precipitate II by removing the alcohol with diafiltration and then reducing and alkylating the disulfide links in the hinge region of the IgG molecules [4]. IGIV pH 6.8 was formulated as a 5% IgG solution in water with 0.2 M glycine and 10% maltose at pH 6.4 to 7.2. A later version of this material involved formulation at pH 5.0 to 5.5 (IGIV pH 5.2) after it was realized that formulation changes were necessary.

The IGIV pH 4.2 preparation was obtained from Cohn Effluent III by concentrating the protein with ultrafiltration and removing the alcohol with diafiltration at pH 3.9 to 4.5, according to the method of Tenold [5]. This nonmodified IgG preparation was then formulated as a 5% IgG solution in water with 10% maltose at pH 4.0 to 4.5.

16.2.2 Clinical Evaluation of IgG Preparations

Clinical evaluation of IGIV pH 6.8 preparations was carried out in a retrospective analysis of adverse reactions of primary immunodeficiency patients to

18 experimental lots of this material [6]. Each lot was received on average twice by 22 patients. Each infusion was 100 to 200 mg IgG/kg body weight given intravenously once a month.

Six experimental lots of the IGIV pH 4.2 preparation were evaluated in 39 immunodeficient and 22 immune thrombocytopenic purpura (ITP) patients, who received intravenous infusions monthly for 3 months.

16.2.3 Laboratory Characterization of IgG Preparations

IgG aggregation was measured [1] by ultracentrifuge (UC), gel permeation chromatography (GPC), and high performance liquid chromatography (HPLC). The UC analysis was carried out on a model E ultracentrifuge with Schlieren optics (Beckman Instruments, Fullerton, CA) at 56,000 rpm with a 12 mm centerpiece and a phase plate angle of 70 degrees. GPC analysis utilized a Bio Gel A equilibrated and eluted with 100 mM phosphate buffer at pH 6.5 containing 150 mM sodium chloride and 0.05% sodium azide. Elution occurred at 20 mL/hr at 20°C. Detection of eluting protein was at 280 nm. HPLC analysis was done on a TSK 3000 size exclusion column (Toyo Soda TSK, Japan) eluted isocratically with the above phosphate-buffered saline at 0.5 mL/min and detected at 280 nm.

IgG anticomplement activity was measured by the ability of the IgG preparations to inhibit complement-mediated lysis of sheep red cells [1]. The anticomplement activity was calculated as the mg/mL concentration of IgG product that produced a 50% reduction in complement-mediated lysis of the sheep red cells.

IgG thermal stability was measured nephelometrically with a Hatch nephelometer (Loveland, CO) using wide band visible radiation from a tungsten lamp, and by crossed immunoelectrophoresis after the IgG preparations had been heated at 60°C. Crossed immunoelectrophoresis was performed on 1% agarose gel in 75 mM veronal buffer at pH 8.6. The first phase was run at 50 to 60 mA and 300 V; the second phase was run at 20 mA and 100 V with 1 mL of rabbit antisera to human serum (Daakopatts, Copenhagen, Denmark) per 15 mL of agarose gel. Coomassie blue was used to stain immunoprecipitant bands, and destaining was accomplished in methanol, acetic acid, and water [7].

IgG binding to antigens was carried out by enzyme-linked immunosorbent assay (ELISA) techniques [8]. In brief, these studies utilized assay kits from Behring Diagnostics of La Jolla, CA, for binding of antibodies to cytomegalovirus (CMV), herpes simplex virus type 1 (HSV), and rubella virus. An ELISA kit from DuPont (Wilmington, DE) was used for binding studies of antibodies to HIV-1 (see Section 15.1 for the rationale for the selection of this kit). All IgG samples for analysis were serially diluted in the buffers supplied with the kits over a range of 1:40 to 1:3600. Quantitative comparison of antibody binding to assay plate antigens was carried out for all IgG samples assayed side by side on the same plates. Alkaline phosphatase conjugated to antihuman IgG supplied with the kits was used to detect the amount of antibody captured. Enzyme conversion of *p*-nitrophenyl phosphate substrate was measured at 405 nm with a 620 nm background absorbance correction using a Flow Laboratories MCC/340 plate reader. Results were summarized as the relative percent binding of each IgG preparation to the viruses on the plates after correction for nonspecific IgG binding to uncoated plate surfaces (see Section 15.1). A two-tailed Student's t-test was used to evaluate the statistical differences among the mean values for the dilutions of IgG samples. A paired Student t-test was also performed among IgG preparations [9] for $p < 0.05$.

16.3 RESULTS

Since the 1950s, ISG has been known to cause life-threatening clinical reactions if given intravenously [10, 11]. The underlying causes are physical changes in the proteins due to the preparation technique [11]. In the present experiments, ISG suitable for intravenous administration was produced by chemically modifying the proteins [4] so that the adverse effects were not elicited [12]. However, chemically modified ISG preparations with variable clinical behavior also were encountered (Table 16.1). Some lots elicited adverse reactions consisting of chills, nausea, and pain in 50 to 70% of the patients (lots 12, 16, and 17), whereas others (lots 1, 3, 13, and 14) produced such symptoms in <10% of the patients. All lots were prepared in accordance with the same manufacturing protocol and tested in accordance with accepted standards [13]. Inspection of production records revealed no differences in the preparative procedures for the lots. Supporting test data, which included measurements of purity, potency, aggregation, fragmentation, anticomplement activity, and animal response, did not correlate with the human clinical results. When storage and followup test data were evaluated, there appeared to be smaller amounts of high molecular weight (HMW) aggregates in the administered material than at the factory. In fact, four lots that showed adverse reactions in >25% of the patients also had HMW aggregate contents >2% of the total IgG. Seven of the lots eliciting adverse reactions in <20% of the patients had HMW aggregate contents of <1% of the total IgG. The anticompliment activity associated with IgG aggregation of the IGIV pH 6.8 preparation was only 10 to 15% of that of ISG over the IgG concentration range 2 to 10 mg/mL.

Of the various approaches tried in eliminating HMW aggregates from the IGIV pH 6.8 products, only change in formulation pH resulted in significant change. pH values of 7 to 11 caused aggregation, with an optimum at pH 8.0 as measured by nephelometry after heating for 15 minutes at 60°C. Below a pH of 5.5 very little aggregation occurred. These conclusions were also supported by the HPLC/280 nm detection data for native IgG solutions formulated at dif-

TABLE 16.1. Percentage of patients showing adverse clinical reactions to intravenous administration of 18 lots of IGIV pH 6.8 prepared and tested according to the same protocols.

	Lot Number																	
	1	2	3	4	5	6	7	8	9	10	11	12	13	14	15	16	17	18
*	3.0	12	8.0	24	32	29	31	11	10	20	11	50	7.0	4.0	17	55	74	21

* signifies the percentage of patients in each group of 18 showing adverse clinical reactions

TABLE 16.2. ISG and IGIV pH 4.2 binding in relative percent to some virus antigens.

Product	HIV-1	CMV	HSV-1	Rubella
ISG	52	64	68	60
IGIV pH 4.2	100	100	100	100

ferent pH values. No aggregates were detected at pH 3.5 and few at pH 4.5, but appreciable amounts were observed at pH 5.5 and above. When the formulation pH was lowered to 5.2, clinical reactions on average were reduced to <10% of the patients. In addition, the new IGIV pH 5.2 product showed improved ability to promote dependent opsonic activity of bacteria [14].

Lowering the pH still further to 4.2 resulted in even fewer adverse reactions (<5% of all infusions). The IGIV pH 4.2 preparation also showed further improvement of activity against bacterial pathogens [12]. The improved biological activity of this preparation was contrary to the long-standing belief that exposure of IgG to pH 4 conditions would result in denaturation [11].

After crossed immunoelectrophoresis of the various IgG preparations, it was found that IGIV pH 4.2 resembled IgG in plasma in terms of its gross physical properties [1, 7, 8, 15]. However, ISG and IGIV pH 6.8 did not resemble IgG in its native milieu. For example, in plasma, IgG moves in a cathodic direction when complexed with antisera to it; so does IGIV pH 4.2. In contrast, both ISG and IGIH pH 6.8 had a large anodic moving component. This component was increased by heating IgG at 60°C for 1 h.

The physical changes in IgG produced by pH changes also altered the ability of specific antibodies to bind their antigens (Table 16.2). Antibodies to HIV-1 lost 50% of their binding capacity for the virus when prepared as ISG rather than as IGIV pH 4.2. This change has been shown to result from exposure of the antibodies to the denaturing effects of pH and freeze-drying encountered in ISG preparation [8].

16.4 DISCUSSION

The above experience shows that each step of production of a clinical agent has to be monitored minutely; for example, for appropriateness of isolation methods, of standards of molecular integrity and function, and of suitability of formulation. "Cookbook"-style preparations generally will succeed only if the method is extremely rugged—a statement also true for the standard analytical chemistry methods of the U.S. EPA and NIOSH.

IgG preparations for clinical use are subject to some degree of conformity with respect to the isolation methods utilized for licensed products [14]. Most product variation thus results from the preparative steps after purification. This is not the case for other immune regulating proteins, where no degree of conformity of the isolation technique is agreed upon. A good example is the isolation of α-interferons, where >50 individual isolation methods have been reported, many employing extreme physical and chemical conditions.

There is little wonder that the clinical performance of interferons has been varied and even conflicting [15–17].

Given the nature of the damage that HIV-1 can do to the immune system, and that no drugs are known that reverse this damage, it is important that the promise of purified immune regulating proteins in restoring the balance of the immune system be judged in terms of defined procedures and physical and chemical properties, so that contradictions and artifacts can be detected and resolved. However, it is in the interests of PWAs to require comparative testing of such preparations. This is a major departure from the way that biologicals are developed and licensed in the United States, and will require leadership from the clinical groups using these materials and the Food and Drug Administration.

References

1. McCue, J. P.; Hein, R. H.; and Tenold, R. 1986. Three generations of immunoglobulin G preparations for clinical use. *Rev. Infect. Dis.* **8**(Suppl. 4): S374–381.
2. Cohn, E. J.; Strong, L. E.; Hughes, W. L.; Mulford, D. J.; Ashworth, J. N.; Melin, M.; and Taylor, H. L. 1946. Preparation and properties of serum and plasma proteins. IV. A system for the separation into fractions of the proteins and lipoprotein components of biological tissues and fluids. *J. Am. Chem. Soc.* **68**: 459–475.
3. Oncley, J. L.; Melin, M.; Richert, D. S.; Cameron, J. W.; and Gross, P. M. 1949. The separation of antibodies, isoagglutinins, prothrombin, plasminogen and β lipoprotein into subfractions of human plasma. *J. Am. Chem. Soc.* **71**: 541–550.
4. Pappenhagen, A.; Lundblad, J. L.; and Schroeder, D. D. 1975. Pharmaceutical compositions comprising intravenously injectable modified serum globulin, its production and use. U.S. Patent 3,903,262.
5. Tenold, R. 1983. Intravenously injectable immune serum globulin. U.S. Patent 4,396,608.
6. McCue, J. P. 1989. Changes in therapeutic proteins caused by preparation techniques. *Ann. Intern. Med.* **111**: 2–3.
7. McCue, J. P.; and Johnson, S. 1986. Noncomparability among IgG products. *Transfusion* **26**: 489–490.
8. McCue, J. P.; Sasagawa, P. K.; and Hein, R. H. 1988. Changes induced in antibodies by isolation methods. *Biotechnol. Appl. Biochem.* **10**: 63–71.
9. Colton, T. 1974. *Statistics in Medicine*, Little, Brown, Boston, MA.
10. Janeway, C. A., and Rosen, F. S. 1966. The gamma globulins. IV Therapeutic uses of gamma globulin. *New Engl. J. Med.* **275**: 826–831.
11. Barandum, S.; Kistler, P.; Jennet, F.; and Isliker, H. 1962. Intravenous administration of human gamma globulin. *Vox Sanguinis* **3**: 157–174.
12. Pirofsky, B. 1984. Intravenous immune globulin therapy in hypogammaglobulinemia. A review. *Am. J. Med.* **76**(Suppl 3A): 53–60.
13. Jamieson, G. A. 1972. The development of plasma derivatives for clinical use. *Vox Sanguinis* **23**: 1–150.
14. Hill, H. R.; Augustine, N. H.; and Shigeoka, A. O. 1984. Comparative opsonic activity of intravenous gamma globulin preparations for common bacterial pathogens. *Am. J. Med.* **76**(Suppl 3A): 61–66.
15. Hill, H. R., and Bathras, J. M. 1986. Protective and opsonic activities of a native, pH 4.25 intravenous immunoglobulin G preparation against common bacterial pathogens. *Rev. Infect. Dis.* **8**(Suppl. 4): S396–400.

16. Hein, R.H.; McCue, J. P.; and Hink, J. 1985. Non A, Non B hepatitis from intravenous immunoglobulin. *Lancet* **2**: 405.
17. Came, P. E., and Carter, W. A. 1987. Clinical use of interferons in the treatment of viral infections. In *Mechanisms of Interferon Actions*, Vol. II, L. M. Pfeffer (ed.), CRC Press, Boca Raton, FL, pp. 129–141.

17

Effectiveness of Condoms as Barriers to HIV-1

by A. S. Chawla and I. Hinberg

17.0 ABSTRACT

Three brands of latex condoms and one brand of animal membrane condoms were tested for leakage of iodine-125 and bovine albumin-I-125. The condoms were filled with the radioactive material and suspended in a container of distilled water. The water was monitored for the appearance of the radioactivity, for 65 h. A very small amount (0.0015% to 0.0030%) of the iodine-125 passed through the latex condoms. However, no albumin-I-125 was detected passing through. Because HIV-1 is about 50 times larger than the albumin molecule, these results suggest that intact latex condoms are an effective barrier to the virus. A small but significant amount of albumin-I-125 passed through the animal membrane condoms. It thus can not be concluded that these condoms are effective barriers to HIV-1. Latex condoms that failed the water-leakage test of Schedule I of the Canadian Medical Devices Regulations were examined by scanning electron microscopy. Tears, holes, and other types of defects were observed on these condoms, and most of these defects would readily allow the transmission of HIV-1.

17.1 INTRODUCTION

Condoms are widely promoted as a means of preventing the transmission of HIV-1 among sexual partners. Several investigators have studied the effectiveness of condoms as a barrier to HIV-1 (HTLV-III/LAV) virus by testing the permeability of the condoms to a variety of disease-causing viruses and other molecules. Conant et al. [1] found that both latex and natural membrane

Bureau of Radiation and Medical Devices, Health Protection Branch, Health and Welfare Canada, Environmental Health Centre, Ottawa, Ontario.

condoms were impermeable to herpes simplex virus (HSV-2). Katznelson et al. [2] tested five brands of latex condoms and found them to be impermeable to cytomegalovirus (CMV). Experiments with mouse retrovirus and AIDS-associated retrovirus (ARV-2) by Conant et al. [3] indicated that both latex and animal membrane condoms were impermeable to viruses.

Minuk et al. [4] demonstrated that hepatitis B surface antigen (HB_sAg) labeled with iodine-125 did not pass through latex condoms, but leaked through condoms made of animal membranes. Minuk's positive results with the animal membranes differed from Katznelson's and Conant's findings [2, 3], possibly because Minuk's radioactive tracer method was more sensitive than the tissue culture method used to detect the viruses by the other investigators.

In addition to serving as a mechanical barrier, condoms treated with spermicide may destroy HIV-1. Studies by Hicks et al. [5] and Reitmeijer et al. [6] showed that nonoxynol-9, an ingredient in many spermicides, inactivates HIV-1. However, the virus can escape the inactivation process through holes that may be present in the condoms.

In the present study, the leakage of radioactive molecules through intact condoms membranes was measured. Latex condoms that failed the water-leakage test of Schedule I of the Canadian *Medical Devices Regulations* [7] were analyzed by scanning electron microscopy to determine the nature and extent of the defects.

17.2 MATERIALS AND PROCEDURES

17.2.1 Materials

The following condoms, believed to be the most frequently used brands in Canada, were tested: Shields Conceptrol (lubricated) from Ortho Pharmaceutical (Canada), Ltd., Don Mills, Ontario, M5C 1L9; and Ramses Regular (nonlubricated) and Fetherlite, both from Julius Schmid of Canada Ltd., Scarborough, Ontario, MIR 2T8. Naturalamb condoms from Comforts Products Ltd., Downsview, Ontario, M3J 2S5, also were tested as a representative of natural membrane condoms.

Seven condoms that failed the water-leakage test of Schedule I of the Canadian *Medical Devices Regulations* [7] were used in the scanning electron microscopy (SEM) investigations. These condoms will be referred to in this paper as "leaky condoms." Table 17.1 describes the condoms. Albumin-I-125

TABLE 17.1. Leaky condoms analyzed by scanning electron microscopy.

Sample	Brand	Approximate distance of leak from tip of condom (cm)
58–01	Ramses	4
58–02	Ramses	5
58–03	Ramses	2
78–00	Shiek	13
78–00	Shiek	0.5
78–06	Shiek	14
78–07	Shiek	7

was purchased from New England Nuclear, Montreal. The scanning electron microscope used was a Joel, Model JSM 35 CF.

17.2.2 Procedures

The undialyzed albumin-I-125 solution, which contained about 3% of unbound iodine, was used to test the leakage of iodine through the condoms. Shields and Fetherlite condoms were used for this study. Twenty-five milliliters of water containing 16.1 μCi of albumin-I-125 was added to each condom. The condoms were knotted at the open end and were placed in separate beakers, each containing 150 mL of water. The leakage of radioactive material was monitored by sampling 1 mL of water from the beakers at different time intervals over a 65-h period. The radioactivity of the samples was measured on a gamma counter (LKB, Fisher Scientific). Standards were used for background corrections and for correlating counts per minute (CPM) to concentration of albumin.

To measure the albumin passing through the condoms, unbound iodine was removed from the albumin-I-125 solution by dialysis: the albumin-I-125 was placed in dialysis tubing immersed in a beaker containing 4 L of normal saline. After 24 h of dialysis, 2 mL of solution was recovered from the dialysis tubing. This dialyzed albumin solution was diluted with normal saline to produce a solution with 0.64 μCi activity/mL. This solution was used for the leakage tests described below.

Three condoms were tested from each of the following brands: Shields, Ramses, and Naturalamb. Twenty-five milliliters of the diluted albumin-I-125 solution (a total of 16.1 μCi activity) was added to each condom. The condoms were placed in beakers containing 100 mL of water. The leakage of albumin was monitored by measuring the radioactivity in the outside water over a 30-h period.

17.2.3 Scanning Electron Microscopy (SEM)

Samples of the condoms were examined under a scanning electron microscope. Surfaces on the inside and the outside and in the wall cross-sections were examined. For studies of the wall cross-sections, the samples were prepared from condoms fractured under liquid nitrogen or cut with scissors. The liquid nitrogen–cooled condom membranes were in a glassy state, well below the glass transition temperature (T_g) of 165°K for latex rubber. Therefore, the cooled membranes fractured without any tears or producing artifacts. The samples were mounted edgewise for SEM examinations.

The leaky areas of the condoms described in Table 17.1, were cut out with scissors so that the defects were approximately it the middle of the excised pieces. The pieces were washed in a laboratory detergent (Sparkleen, Fisher Scientific) to remove lubricants and other surface coatings. The washed pieces were mounted on SEM sample holders for analysis of the outside surfaces. The mounted samples also were examined under a light microscope. The samples were then sputter-coated with gold and analyzed by SEM. After the analysis of the outside surfaces, some of these samples were turned over, mounted, and again coated with gold so that the inner surfaces also could be examined.

17.3 RESULTS

Figure 17.1 shows the results obtained with the unpurified albumin-I-125 solution containing free I-125. A very small percent of the radioactive material passed through both latex condoms. After 65 h, 0.003% of the radioactive material in the Shields condom and 0.0015% of the radioactive material in the Fetherlite condom had leaked out.

The results obtained with the purified albumin-I-125 solution (Figure 17.2) show that a small but significant amount of radioactive material passed through the Naturalamb animal membrane condoms. After 3 h, the water surrounding the Naturalamb condoms contained 0.7% of the radioactivity. However, very

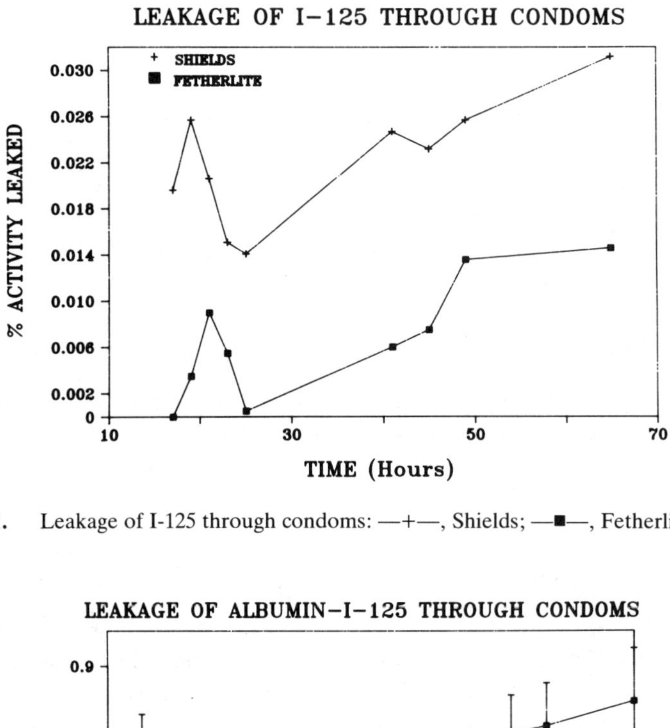

FIGURE 17.1. Leakage of I-125 through condoms: —+—, Shields; —■—, Fetherlite.

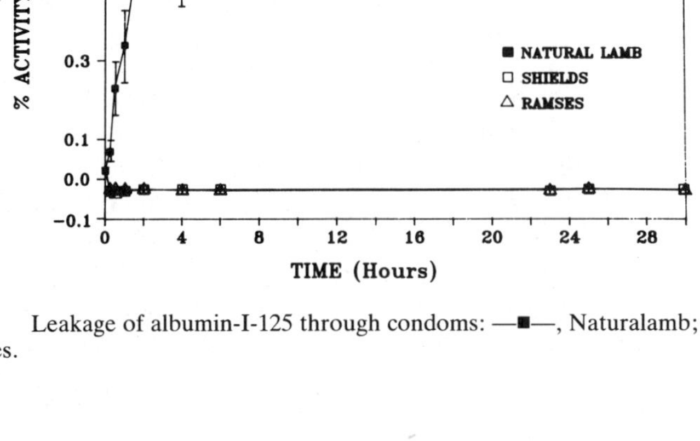

FIGURE 17.2. Leakage of albumin-I-125 through condoms: —■—, Naturalamb; —□—, Shields; —△—, Ramses.

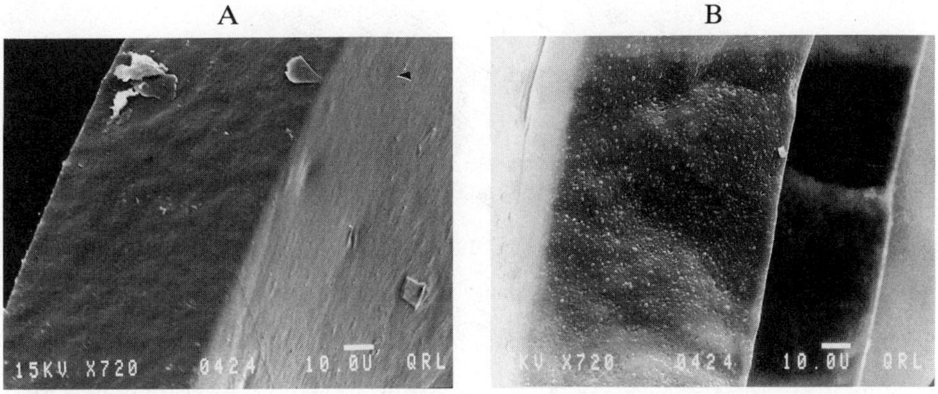

FIGURE 17.3. SEM photomicrographs of latex condom material. Arrows show wall thickness. (A) Shields; (B) Fetherlite. The thickness is about 70 μm. The AIDS virus is about 0.1 μm in diameter.

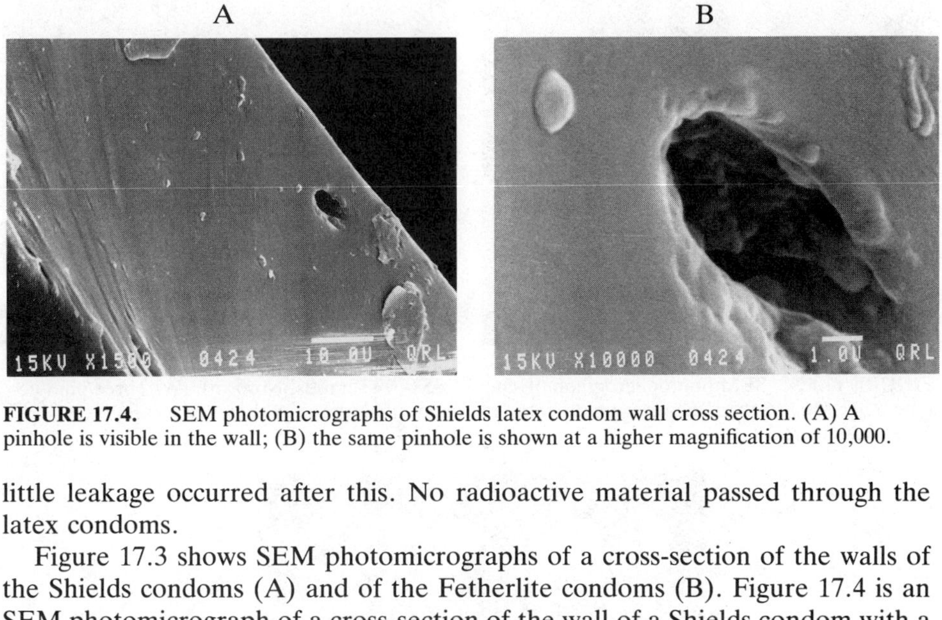

FIGURE 17.4. SEM photomicrographs of Shields latex condom wall cross section. (A) A pinhole is visible in the wall; (B) the same pinhole is shown at a higher magnification of 10,000.

little leakage occurred after this. No radioactive material passed through the latex condoms.

Figure 17.3 shows SEM photomicrographs of a cross-section of the walls of the Shields condoms (A) and of the Fetherlite condoms (B). Figure 17.4 is an SEM photomicrograph of a cross-section of the wall of a Shields condom with a pinhole-type defect in the wall. The defect appears to run almost parallel to the length of the condom. The elliptical hole has major and minor axes of about 7 and 3 μm, respectively.

Figure 17.5 shows a surface defect on sample #58-01 (Table 17.1), which does not appear to penetrate deep enough to be of potential harm or cause a leak. The morphology of the defect suggests that it was produced by the eruption of a small air bubble left entrapped in the latex rubber.

A scan of the sample revealed seven pinholes. Three of these are shown in Figure 17.6A. Figure 17.6B, a higher magnification (3600X) of the middle hole in Figure 17.6A, shows that the hole is about 2 μm across.

There were no holes or other defects on the inside surface of the samples. This finding suggests that the holes observed in the walls did not traverse the entire wall thickness of the condom.

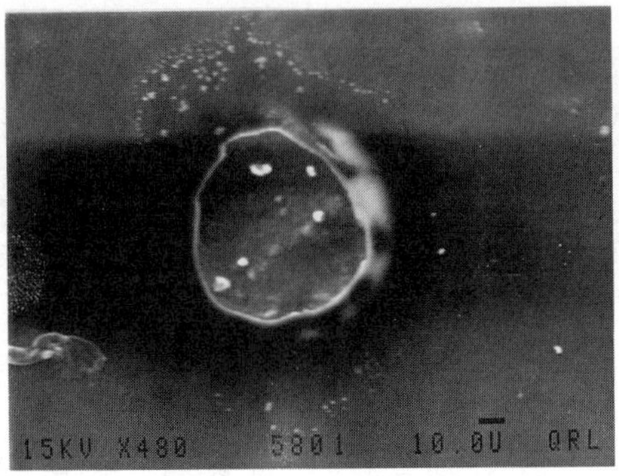

FIGURE 17.5. SEM photomicrograph of sample #58-01 (Ramses, Nuform) latex condom. The defect appears to have resulted when a small air bubble entrapped in the wall ruptured.

A B

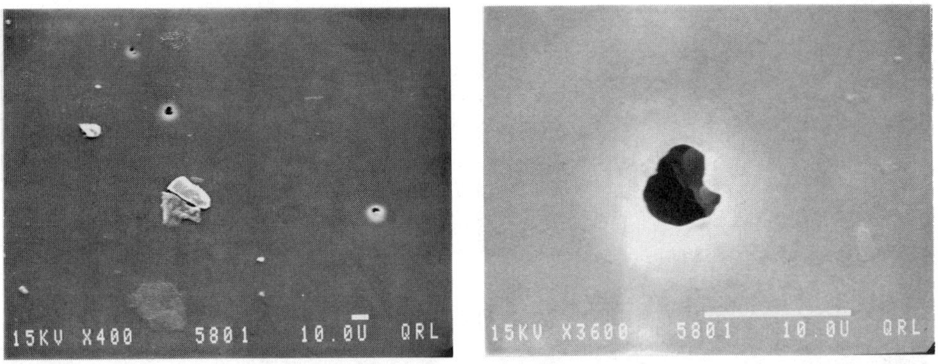

FIGURE 17.6. SEM photomicrograph of sample #58-01 (Ramses, Nuform). (A) Three pinhole-type defects are visible; (B) the pinhole in the middle of photograph A shown at a higher magnification of 3600.

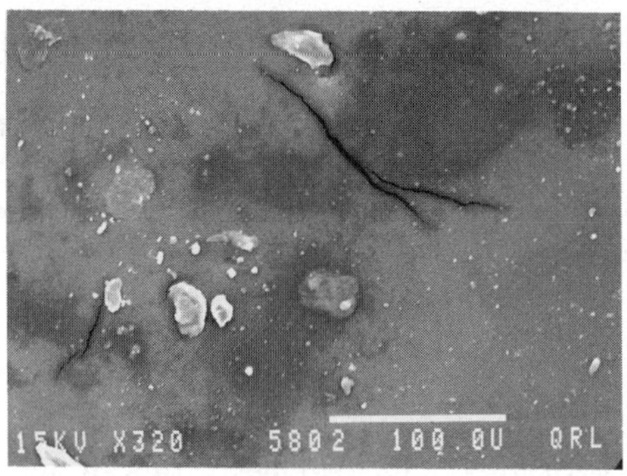

FIGURE 17.7. SEM photomicrograph of sample #58-02 (Ramses, Nuform). A superficial fissure is visible.

Figure 17.7 shows fissures on the outside surface of sample #58-02 (Table 17.1). However, closer examination and analysis of the inside surfaces showed that the defects did not cross the entire wall thickness.

Sample #58-03 (Figure 17.8) had a number of small elongated fissures on

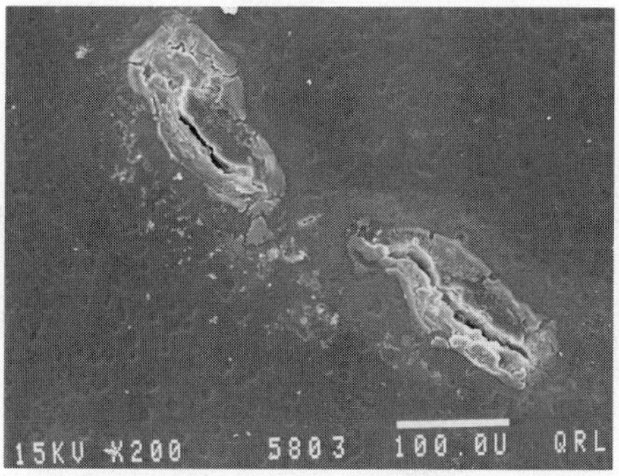

FIGURE 17.8. SEM photomicrograph of sample #58-03 (Ramses, Nuform). Two fissures are clearly visible.

A B

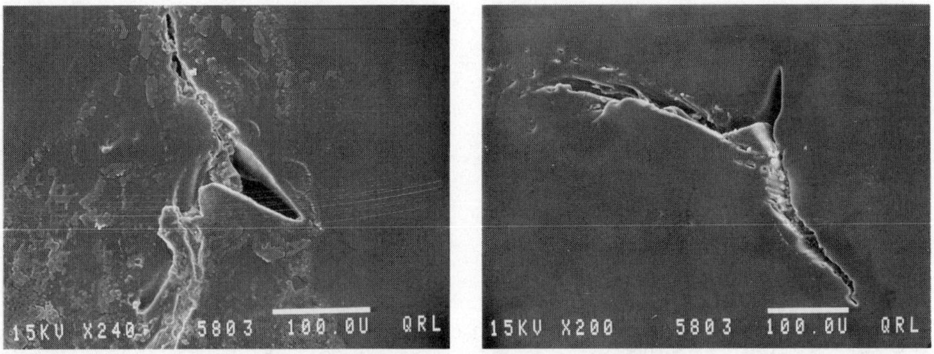

FIGURE 17.9. SEM photomicrograph of sample #58-03 (Ramses, Nuform). (A) Outside surface showing a fissure; (B) the same fissure as in (A) from the inside surface.

A B

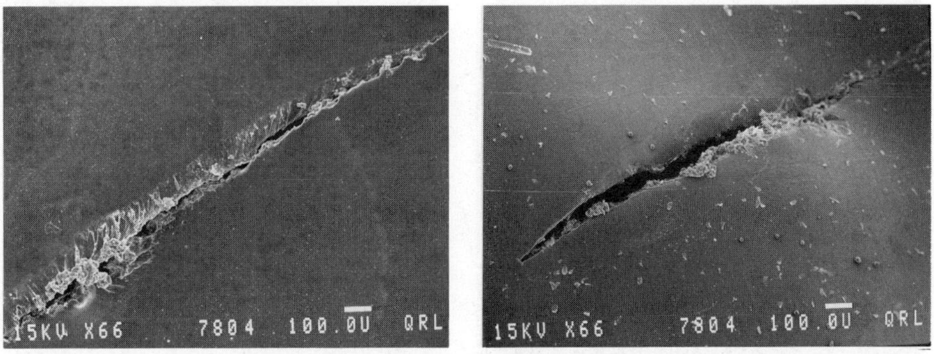

FIGURE 17.10. SEM photomicrograph of sample #78-04 (Sheik). (A) Outside surface, X66; (B) inside surface, X66. The fissure appears to traverse the entire wall thickness of the condoms.

the surface, two of which are shown in the figure. Figure 17.9A shows an additional fissure. The inner surface of the sample is shown in Figure 17.9B. A fissure is again visible. Thus, fissures shown in Figures 17.9A and 17.9B were essentially of the same shape and size but viewed from outside and inside surfaces, respectively. These results suggest that the fissures traverse the entire

A B

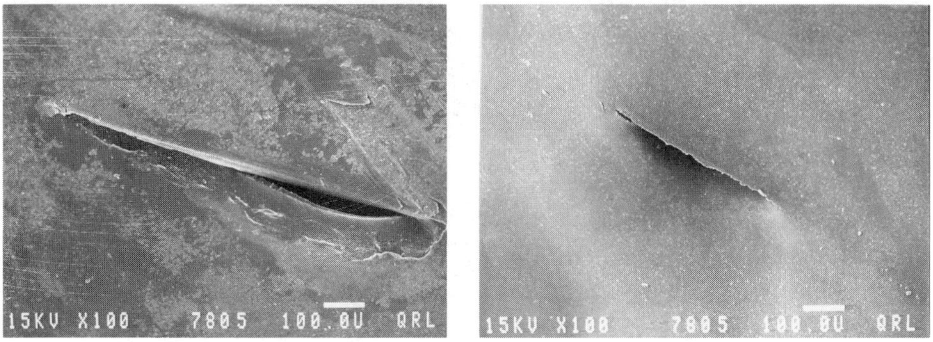

FIGURE 17.11. SEM photomicrograph of sample #78-05 (Sheik). (A) Outside surface showing a split; (B) inside surface showing the split visible in (A).

A B

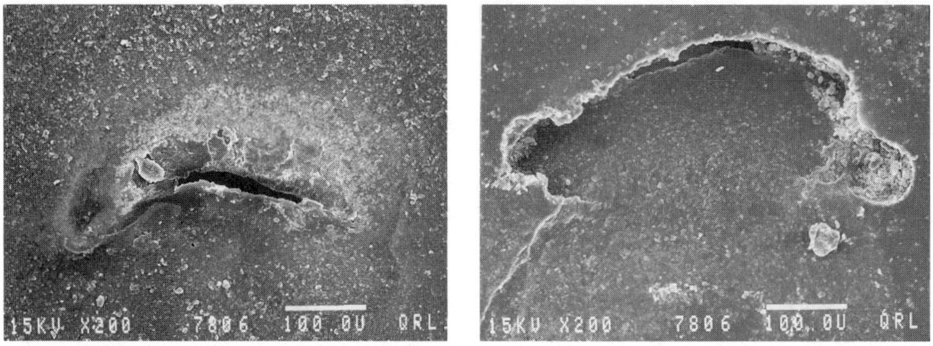

FIGURE 17.12. SEM photomicrograph of sample #78-06 (Sheik). (A) Outside surface showing void; (B) the same void seen on the inside surface.

A B

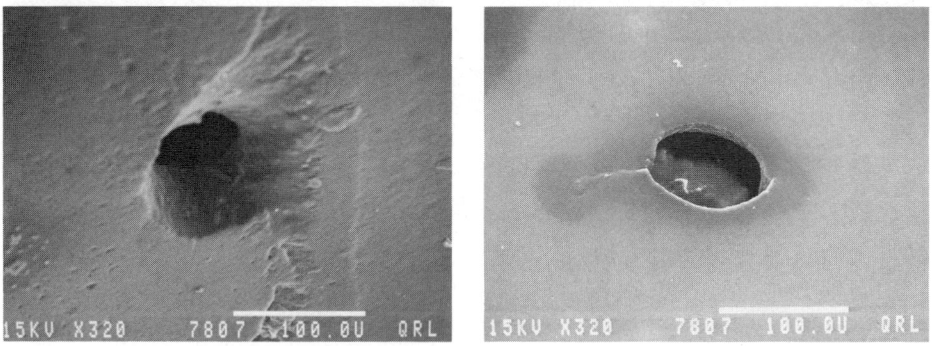

FIGURE 17.13. SEM photomicrograph of sample #78-07 (Sheik). (A) Outside surface showing a pinhole-type void; (B) inside surface showing the same void visible in (A).

wall thickness of the condom. The fissures are large enough to allow HIV-1 to pass through.

Figure 17.10A shows a rupture on the outside surface of sample #78-04. Figure 17.10B, a photomicrograph of the inside surface, suggests that the rupture extends through the entire thickness of the condom wall.

Figure 17.11A shows a split on the outside surface of sample #78-05. This split is located at the tip of the condom (Table 17.1), where it could be most damaging. The appearance of a similar split on the inside surface (Figure 17.11B) suggests that the split traverses the entire wall thickness of the condom.

Figure 17.12A shows a breach in the outside surface of sample #78-06. A photomicrograph of the inside surface (Figure 17.12B) suggests that the breach extended through the entire thickness of the condom wall.

Figure 17.13A and 17.13B show a pinhole that extends through the entire wall thickness of sample #78-07. The diameter of the hole is about 60 μm—large enough for HIV-1 easily to pass through.

17.4 DISCUSSION

In the experiments with the undialyzed albumin-I-125 solution, which contained some free iodine-125, a very small amount (0.0015–0.0030%) of radioactive material passed through the latex condoms. However, when the dialyzed albumin-I-125 solution was used, no radioactivity was detected passing through. These findings indicate that free iodine can leak through latex condoms, but albumin cannot. Because HIV-1 is about 50 times larger than the albumin molecule [8], these results suggest that intact latex condoms are an effective barrier to the virus. This conclusion is supported by the observation (Figure 17.3) that the wall thicknesses of the Shields and the Fetherlite condoms are about 700 times the size of HIV-1. Thus, it is highly unlikely that HIV-1 will be able to diffuse through the condoms.

A small but significant amount of albumin passed through the animal membrane condoms; so it can not be concluded that these condoms are effective barriers to HIV-1. However, the data do not prove that HIV-1, which is about 50 times larger than the albumin molecule, will pass through animal membrane condoms.

Electron scanning microscopy of latex condoms that failed the water-leakage test revealed a variety of defects, such as tears, cuts, fissures, and pinholes. Most of these defects would allow HIV-1 readily to pass through the condoms. There are a number of possible explanations for the occurrence of these defects, including (a) air bubble entrapment and impurities in the latex; (b) contaminants of, or resulting from additives; (c) the use of improperly cleaned or defective condom formers; and (d) mishandling during manufacturing, packaging, and transportation.

References

1. Conant, M.; Spicer, D.; and Smith, C. 1984. Herpes simplex virus transmission: condom studies. *J. Sexually Transmitted Dis.* **11**: 94–95.
2. Katznelson, S.; Drew, W.; and Mintz, L. 1984. Efficacy of the condom as a barrier to the transmission of cytomegalovirus. *J. Infect. Dis.* **150**: 155–157.
3. Conant, M.; Hardy, D.; Sernatinger, J.; Spicer, D.; and Levy, J. 1986. Condoms prevent transmission of AIDS-associated retrovirus. *J. Am. Med. Assoc.* **255**: 1706.
4. Minuk, G.; Bohme, C.; and Bowen T. 1986. Letter to the editor. *J. Am Med. Assoc.* **256**: 1443.
5. Hicks, D.; Martin, L.; and Getchell J. 1985. Inactivation of HTLV-III/LAV infected cultures of normal human lymphocytes by nonoxynol-9 in vitro. *Lancet* **II**: 1422–1423.

6. Reitmeijer, C. A. M.; Krebs, J. M.; Feorino, P. M.; and Judson, F. N. 1988. Condoms as physical and chemical barriers against human immunodeficiency virus. *J. Am. Med. Assoc.* **259**: 1851.
7. Health and Welfare Canada, *Medical Devices Regulations*, Ottawa, Canada K1A 0L2.
8. Braude, A. I.; Davis, C. E.; and Fierer, J. 1982. *Microbiology*, W. B. Saunders, Philadelphia, PA.

18

Guideline for the Protection of Laboratory Workers from Infectious Disease Transmitted by Blood and Tissue

by Stanley Bauer*

18.0 ABSTRACT

The increasing prevalence of human retroviral infections has been noted with concern by those health-care workers who must treat infected patients or handle blood, body fluids, and tissues of infected individuals. The acquired immunodeficiency syndrome and the postulated etiologic agent, human immunodeficiency virus-1, have attracted the most attention. However, related agents, human immunodeficiency virus-2 and human T-cell leukemia virus, are now recognized as hazards to laboratory and other health-care workers. The attention paid to retroviruses has served to reemphasize the hazards associated with hepatitis viruses and has refocused interest in preventing nosocomial hepatitis B infection through the use of recombinant hepatitis B vaccine.

The National Committee for Clinical Laboratory Standards (NCCLS) has published a tentative guideline entitled *Protection of Laboratory Workers from Infectious Disease Transmitted by Blood, Body Fluids, and Tissue*. The guideline was intended to provide a procedure manual for laboratory workers and was commissioned to address the growing concern over the potential exposure of laboratory personnel to bloodborne infections. The guideline gives specific and detailed recommendations in the areas of personal protection, decontamination of *in vitro* medical devices, decontamination of the workplace, the safe performance of clinical laboratory procedures, and the management of laboratory accidents.

18.1 INTRODUCTION

The epidemic of acquired immunodeficiency syndrome (AIDS) in the United States has been growing exponentially since it was first recognized in 1981 [1,

* Department of Pathology, The Bronx-Lebanon Hospital Center, Bronx, NY.

2]. A number of guidelines for the protection of laboratory workers from nosocomial infection with human immunodeficiency virus (HIV) have been published [3–5].

The National Committee for Clinical Laboratory Standards (NCCLS), a voluntary consensus standards organization, published a tentative guideline entitled *Protection of Laboratory Workers from Infectious Disease Transmitted by Blood, Body Fluids, and Tissue* in 1989 [6]. The guideline is the product of the NCCLS Task Force on Protection of Laboratory Workers and the Subcommittee on Laboratory Workers. These groups were composed of representatives of many professional organizations, manufacturers of *in vitro* diagnostic products, and governmental agencies. Although many diseases are transmissible by blood and tissue, the guideline focuses on HIV and hepatitis B virus (HBV) because they pose a risk of infection that is both common and grave. The guideline is in the form of a laboratory procedure manual. It gives authoritative and current recommendations that are intended to provide a rational system of protective measures to be used by laboratory workers. The guideline addresses many issues, including those that are summarized herein, and is consistent with, and supplemental to, the general recommendations of the Centers for Disease Control (CDC), which are being enforced by the Occupational Safety and Health Administration (OSHA).

In keeping with the policy of the NCCLS, the guideline was revised and reissued in 1990 with a companion guideline for the safe handling of *in vitro* diagnostic instrument systems by service personnel.

18.2 DEFINING THE RISK

18.2.1 The Nature of the Risk

The source of the risk of nosocomial HIV or HBV infection to the laboratory worker is the routine exposure to blood, body fluids, and tissues of patients. The risk of nosocomial infection cannot be avoided because the infectious agents are integral to the specimens being analyzed and the tissues being studied. This exposure may take place in the laboratory, at the bedside (phlebotomy), in the morgue, and in the research laboratory. Laboratories not directly involved in patient care may process human blood or body fluids as source materials in pharmaceutical preparations and in field trials of new drugs. If currently recommended safety precautions [5–7] are followed, there should be no occupational hazard to the laboratory worker, barring any accidental exposure. It is the potential for accidents, and the certainty that they will occur, that must be considered in implementing a protection program. It is necessary to examine each individual procedure practised in the laboratory setting to detect potential areas for contamination of workers. Once these areas are identified, standard operating procedures (SOPs) should be developed, and are required by OSHA, to minimize the probability and magnitude of potential exposure [8].

The SOPs will require equipment and supplies that may add substantially to the cost of operating the laboratory. There will be a need to develop an in-depth educational program to train workers in safe practices, to reinforce consistently this education, to monitor the implementation of the program, and to counsel and retrain workers if infractions are detected.

18.2.2 The Magnitude of the Risk

HIV has been found to be transmitted by routes similar to HBV [5]; so the precautions used to prevent nosocomial infection with HBV serve well as a model for HIV [8]. HIV has been isolated from blood, semen, vaginal secretions, saliva, tears, breast milk, cerebrospinal fluid, amniotic fluid, alveolar fluid, and urine [5, 7, 9]. However, only blood, semen, vaginal secretions, and breast milk have been implicated in transmission [5, 7]. HIV appears to be less easily transmitted through laboratory accidents, such as accidental needlesticks, than HBV [5, 7]. The risk of HBV infection after accidental needlestick has been reported to be between 6% and 30% whereas the seroconversion rate after needlestick exposure to HIV infective blood is estimated to be less than 1% (average 0.5%) [8, 12, 13]. Long-term follow-up of large numbers of HIV-exposed workers is needed to refine this estimate.

The magnitude of the risk is determined by the nature of the procedure being carried out, the frequency of the procedure, the route of inoculation in any accident, the volume of the inoculum, and the concentration of virus in the inoculum. For hepatitis B (HB), the immune status of the exposed worker and the promptness and appropriateness of postexposure prophylaxis are important [14].

The seroprevalence of hepatitis B surface antigen (HBsAg) and of HIV antibodies varies widely in differing patient groups. The prevalence of Western blot–positive HIV antibodies in the United States was reported to be 0.042% for first-time voluntary blood donors during the period 1985 through 1988 [2], 0.14% for civilian applicants for military service from 1985 to 1988 [2], 0 to 4.3% in childbearing women in 1986 through 1988 [2], 14 to 50% in homosexual men in 1988 [2], 1 to 57% in intravenous drug abusers from 1985 to 1988 [2], 0 to 50% in the long-term sexual partners of HIV-infected patients from 1982 through 1988 [2], and 33% to 92% in hemophiliacs in 1987 [15]. The U.S. prevalence of HBsAg in adults was reported to be 0.1 to 0.3% in the general population in 1989 [2], and in 1989 it was reported to be 5 to 15% in groups at high risk for HBV infection including homosexual men and intravenous drug abusers [2].

18.2.3 HIV Infection in Health-Care Workers

In April 1988 the CDC reported [16] that there had been 26 HIV infections in health-care workers who denied other risk factors and who had parenteral, nonintact skin, or mucous membrane exposures to HIV-infected blood or concentrated virus. The exposures were: from needlesticks or cuts, 19; of nonintact skin, 4; of mucous membrane, 2; and cutaneous, 1. The occupations involved were: nurse, 4; phlebotomist, 1; technologist/technician/lab worker, 3; dentist, 1; research lab worker, 2; home health-care provider, 2; and not specified, 13. Two of the above had AIDS.

18.2.4 Avoiding the Risk

The route of accidental exposure is important; percutaneous exposure is more effective than mucosal or conjunctival exposure in transmitting HIV [12, 13]. Because it is impossible to know with certainty which patient is infected with HIV or HBV, the NCCLS, following the CDC guidelines, recommends that all patients be treated as if they were known to be infectious for HIV and HBV [6, 7]. It has been recommended [5] that HIV antibody screening be done on all admissions to the hospital or on patients admitted for surgery. Whereas an assay for HBsAg and HB e antigen might identify those patients with the highest potential of transmitting HB [17], these assays are costly and time-consuming. Routine admission testing for HIV antibodies is problematical, as HIV antibody assays may not be effective in detecting HIV-infected persons in the latent period [18], and HIV antigen capture assays, HIV genetic probe virus assays, and virus culture are not readily available, are costly, and will not necessarily detect all infected individuals [19–21]. Therefore, HIV testing on admission may be deceptive, may lower the level of sensitivity to the risk, and may be counterproductive [22].

All discussions of routine testing are important to the laboratory community because laboratory workers would have to test all specimens for antibody, antigen, or virus for detection purposes, and thus could be exposed to infectious bloods. In any case, it is important that all specimens be treated as if they are capable of transmitting serious disease.

18.2.5 Minimizing the Risk

To protect against nosocomial infection with HIV and HBV the NCCLS recommends that blood and body fluid precautions be used with all patients, referred to as universal precautions [5]. These universal precautions include practical and familiar procedures for protecting the laboratory worker: (1) use barrier protection as the first line of defense; (2) wear gloves when touching blood, body fluids, and tissue; (3) change gloves after patient contact or physical damage to the gloves; (4) use facial protection if spattering is likely; (5) use protective clothing; (6) wash your hands if they become contaminated and after removing gloves; (7) take extraordinary precautions with needles, etc. (sharps); (8) dispose of sharps properly; (9) minimize spatters and spills; (10) clean contaminated surfaces with a tuberculocidal hospital disinfectant; and (11) minimize mouth-to-mouth resuscitation. Detailed instructions are given in the guideline for implementing these recommendations. Additionally, the guideline lists types of effective barrier protection for many special circumstances and gives sources of recommended protective devices.

18.3 LABORATORY PRACTICES

18.3.1 Decontamination

Decontamination of spills is important in the laboratory. The guideline gives explicit directions for such decontamination, including a list of sources of Environmental Protection Agency (EPA)–registered tuberculocidal and virucidal hospital disinfectants to be used in the decontamination procedure. Decontamination SOPs for spills [6] include: (1) wear barrier protection; (2) absorb the spilled material; (3) clean the site with a detergent solution; (4) clean the site with an appropriate hospital disinfectant; and (5) dispose of all contaminated materials appropriately. The chemical composition and concentrations of recommended hospital disinfectants are given in the guideline.

Among the recommended disinfectants is a 1:10 aqueous dilution of liquid household bleach (5.25% sodium hypochlorite).

18.3.2 Specimen Collection and Handling

The guideline gives specific recommendations for phlebotomy, arteriotomy, and skin puncture, all of which pose special hazards to the laboratory worker. Special precautions are spelled out for the processing of specimens, including transportation, centrifugation, preparation of smears, and the use of instrumentation. The use of a secondary container for the transportation of all specimens is recommended to contain any spills or broken containers.

18.3.3 Accidental Inoculation

Detailed instructions for the postexposure immunoprophylaxis of HBV infection as recommended by the Immunization Practices Advisory Committee [14] are given in the guideline. This prophylaxis includes the selected use of hepatitis B immune globulin and hepatitis B vaccine. Instructions are given for the counseling and testing of workers after exposure to HIV infectious material. Recommendations for the prevention of transmission of HIV by exposed laboratory workers, who are potentially infected, are detailed in the guideline and are in agreement with those of the CDC [23].

The guideline calls attention to the potential use of zidovudine (AZT) as a chemo-prophylactic agent to prevent HIV infection of health-care workers after accidental inoculation with HIV infective specimens. The prophylactic use of AZT is currently being utilized and evaluated by several institutions [24, 25]. Other FDA-approved agents like ddI and ddC will doubtless be added to updates.

18.3.4 Autopsy and Surgical Specimens

The performance of postmortem examinations poses a greater risk to pathologists and their assistants than does the routine processing of clinical laboratory specimens. During the autopsy the pathologist is exposed to large quantities of blood over long periods of time. The guideline contains an extensive set of recommendations addressed to the hazards of the autopsy as well as the hazards associated with the handling of surgical specimens. Discussion of some of the special considerations follows.

It is common for latex gloves to be broken accidentally or to develop leaks with no observed physical damage to the glove. The use of two pairs of gloves is recommended (double gloving). Double gloving does not provide puncture resistance, but if the outer glove develops a leak, the inner glove will prevent skin contamination. It is improbable that both gloves will develop a spontaneous leak in the same location simultaneously. The inner glove may be made of plastic for increased durability, and the outer glove may be latex for increased slip resistance. Heavy-duty gloves that offer puncture resistance are recommended for procedures where the loss of tactile sensitivity will not impair the performance of the autopsy. Stainless steel mesh gloves are recommended for use during an autopsy, especially when saws, chisels, and so on, are used. Sources of these special protective devices are given in the guideline.

The morgue should be considered a biohazard area, and entry should be limited. Recommended morgue practices include the participation of an assistant (circulator) who remains uncontaminated during the autopsy. The circulator assists in the collection of fluid and tissue specimens, the photography of organs, and the recording of data.

Barrier protection should include coverage of the hair (bonnet), a face shield, a neck-to-wrist-and-ankle water-repellent garment (jumpsuit), a waterproof apron, gloves, and shoe covers. Modification of the classical Rokitansky or Virchow evisceration and dissection is recommended to minimize blind dissection in the removal of the larynx, rectum, and genito-urinary tract. Consideration of omitting portions of the autopsy that pose an increased risk of accidents is discussed (e.g., not examining the larynx, but transecting the trachea at a lower level).

Recommendations for reducing hazardous procedures during the dissection of the organs include: the limitation of personnel at the autopsy table; the use of only one scalpel, which only the prosector is permitted to handle; the discontinuance of the practice of hand-to-hand passing of instruments; and the discontinuance of frozen sections on unfixed autopsy tissues. All organs and tissues should be retained on the autopsy table until properly fixed or placed into appropriate containers. Decontamination procedures for instruments, the autopsy table, the photographic apparatus, and the morgue are given in the guideline.

18.4 TRAINING OF PERSONNEL

The guideline stresses the need for a coherent biosafety program in the laboratory. Implementation of a training program with an assigned trainer and written SOPs is stressed. This program should include complete training of new personnel plus the ongoing training and retraining of current workers. Documentation and auditing of the biosafety program are emphasized.

18.5 COMMENT

The recommendations in the guideline may seem burdensome and costly, but omitting these practices may create a risk to the laboratory worker that cannot be justified by any consideration of the effort or dollars expended.

The guideline was distributed to all members of the NCCLS and selected national organizations. The NCCLS, as part of its voluntary consensus standards-setting process, was to receive comments and to revise the guideline in an effort to obtain consensus on this important issue. The guideline is expected to answer many questions of a practical nature that have caused confusion and apprehension in the laboratory community. The guideline may be obtained from the National Committee for Clinical Laboratory Standards,

771 East Lancaster Ave., Villanova, PA 19085, (215) 525-2435, for a cost of $30.00 (U.S.).

Further Reading

National Committee for Clinical Laboratory Standards. 1990. *Protection of Laboratory Workers from Infectious Disease Transmitted by Blood, Body Fluid, and Tissue: Tentative Guideline.* NCCLS Document M29-T, Villanova, PA, NCCLS.

References

1. CDC. 1981. *Pneumocystis* pneumonia—Los Angeles. *MMWR* **30**: 250–252.
2. CDC. 1989. AIDS and human immunodeficiency virus infection in the United States: 1988 update. *MMWR* **38**(Suppl. S-4): 1–38.
3. CDC. 1982. Acquired immune deficiency syndrome (AIDS): precautions for clinical and laboratory staffs. *MMWR* **31**: 577–580.
4. CDC. 1983. Acquired immunodeficiency syndrome (AIDS): precautions for health-care workers and allied professionals. *MMWR* **32**: 450–451.
5. CDC. 1987. Recommendations for the prevention of HIV transmission in health-care settings. *MMWR* **36**(Suppl. 2S): 3s.
6. National Committee for Clinical Laboratory Standards. 1989. *Protection of Laboratory Workers from Infectious Disease Transmitted by Blood, Body Fluid, and Tissue; Tentative Guideline*, NCCLS Document M29-T, Villanova, PA, NCCLS, pp. 1–141.
7. CDC. 1988. Update: universal precautions for prevention of transmission of human immunodeficiency virus, hepatitis B virus, and other bloodborne pathogens in health-care settings. *MMWR* **37**: 377–382, 387–388.
8. DOL-OSHA. 1989. Occupational exposure to bloodborne pathogens; proposed rule and notice of hearing. 29 CFR Part 1910. *Fed. Reg.* **54**: 23042–23139.
9. Ziza, J. M.; Brun-Vezinet, F.; Venet, A.; et al. 1985. Lymphadenopathy-associated virus isolated from bronchoalveolar lavage fluid in AIDS-related complex with lymphoid interstitial pneumonitis. *N. Engl. J. Med.* **313**: 183.
10. Goady, G. F.; Lee, V. A.; et al. 1978. Hepatitis B immune globulin for accidental exposures among medical personnel: final report of a multicenter controlled trial. *J. Infect. Dis.* **138**: 625–638.
11. Seeff, L. B.; Wright, E. C.; Zimmerman, H. J.; et al. 1978. Type B hepatitis after needlestick exposure: prevention with hepatitis B immune globulin. *Ann. Intern. Med.* **88**: 285–293.
12. Vlahov, D.; and Polk, B. F. 1987. Transmission of human immunodeficiency virus within the health care setting. *Occup. Med: State of the Art Rev.* **2**: 429–450.
13. Gerberding, J. L.; Bryant-LeBlanc, C. E.; Nelson, K.; et al. 1987. Risk of transmitting the human immunodeficiency virus, cytomegalovirus, and hepatitis B virus to health care workers exposed to patients with AIDS and AIDS-related conditions. *J. Infect. Dis.* **156**: 1–8.
14. CDC. 1984. Adult immunization: recommendations of the immunization practices advisory committee (ACIP). *MMWR* **33**(Suppl. 1S): 5s–6s.
15. CDC. 1987. HIV infection and pregnancies in sexual partners of HIV-seropositive hemophilic men—United States. *MMWR* **36**: 593–595.
16. CDC. 1988. Update: Acquired immunodeficiency syndrome and human immunodeficiency virus infection among health-care workers. *MMWR* **37**: 229–234.
17. Favero, M. S.; Petersen, J. P.; and Bond, W. W. 1986. Transmission and control of laboratory-acquired hepatitis infection, in *Laboratory Safety: Principles and Practices*, B. M. Miller et al. (eds.), American Socicty for Microbiology, Washington, DC, p. 49.

18. Ranki, A.; Valle, S. L.; Krohn, M.; et al. 1987. Long latency precedes overt seroconversion in sexually transmitted human-immunodeficiency-virus infection. *Lancet* **II**: 589–593.
19. Casareale, D.; Dewhurst, S.; Sonnabend, J.; et al. 1984–85. Prevalence of AIDS-associated retrovirus and antibodies among male homosexuals at risk for AIDS in Greenwich Village. *AIDS Res. Hum. Retroviruses* **1**: 407–421.
20. Feorino, P.; Forrester, B.; Schable, C.; et al. 1987. Comparison of antigen assay and reverse transcriptase assay for detecting human immunodeficiency virus in culture. *J. Clin. Microbiol* **25**: 2344–2346.
21. Ou, C. Y.; Kwok, S.; Mitchell, S. W.; et al. 1988. DNA amplification for direct detection of HIV-1 in DNA of peripheral blood mononuclear cells. *Science* **239**: 295–297.
22. Gerberding, J. L. 1986. The University of California–San Francisco Task Force on AIDS: recommended infection-control policies for patients with human immunodeficiency virus infection. *N. Engl. J. Med.* **315**: 1562–1563.
23. CDC. 1985. Provisional public health service inter-agency recommendations for screening donated blood and plasma for antibody to the virus causing acquired immunodeficiency syndrome. *MMWR* **34**: 1–5.
24. Bauer, S. 1989. Trial of chemo-prophylaxis of HIV infection and health-care workers right-to-know vis-à-vis the patient's right to confidentiality. *Abstracts of the V Int. Conf. on AIDS*, Montreal, Canada, p. 960.
25. Booth, W. 1989. NIH offers AZT to exposed workers. *Science* **243**: 1137 (news).

19

Volatile Nitrites: A Valid Health Concern

by J. Thomas Pierce* and Evelyn R. Waring**

19.0 ABSTRACT

Volatile nitrites have acquired widespread use as inhalants of abuse, having been used at times by over five million Americans [1]. Owing to a rather peculiar designation of these compounds as industrial chemicals, they have been sold under this guise while being widely abused. Few precedents exist in the United States for such unrestricted access to an abusable substance.

Conflicting epidemiologic and toxicologic data exist regarding their significance as cofactors in the development of AIDS. However, a compelling body of information exists regarding their potential for fatalities and cardiovascular and neural damage.

Proper choice of a sampling and analytical methodology is a critical issue in both human exposure monitoring and toxicology experiments. Although methods thought to be suitable to broad classes of nitrite compounds may be adapted to the volatile nitrites, investigations of the optimal means for the quantification are limited. Except for a proposed biological monitoring method, references to the interpretation of sampling and analysis data are nonexistent.

19.1 BACKGROUND

19.1.1 Pharmacology

Even though amyl nitrite has been in clinical use for over one hundred years, a clear picture of its toxic features has yet to evolve. The primary medical use of

*Center for Environmental and Occupational Health, the University of Kansas Medical Center, Kansas City, Kansas.

amyl nitrite is in the relief of angina pectoris. Its effects are transient, and it has been largely replaced by nitroglycerin and longer-acting nitrates. Amyl nitrite has been shown to decrease arterial pressure and forearm vascular resistance while it increases venous tone and cardiac output [2].

In his review of the medical literature, Mayer [3] noted that many of the immediate physiologic responses to inhaled nitrites are well known; the primary mode of action relies upon the relaxation of vascular smooth muscle by the nitrite ion. The subsequent acute preload reduction (e.g., vascular dilatation) results in a compensatory tachycardia, allowing a stable cardiac output.

Amyl nitrite and possibly other volatile nitrites have been used in the treatment of cyanide and sulfide poisoning. The toxicity of amyl nitrite in converting hemoglobin to methemoglobin is viewed as far less important than the interruption of oxidative phosphorylation caused by cyanide or sulfide [4].

In general the aliphatic nitrites exert a pronounced vasodilator effect although exceptions have been noted [5]. Certain of the volatile nitrites' effects are attributable to available nitrite ions. The effects of organic nitrates are identical to the effects of corresponding nitrites to the extent that reduction takes place.

The mechanism of vascular smooth muscle relaxation for organic nitrites and other compounds (organic nitrates, nitroprusside, and nitric oxide) may well proceed through *S*-nitrosothiols. Such nitrosothiols may activate guanylate cyclase, elevating cyclic GMP levels [6].

19.1.2 Toxicology

Certain basic features of the acute inhalation toxicity of aliphatic (C_1-C_5) nitrites have only recently been revealed. The slopes for the dose–mortality curves for C_1-C_5 aliphatic nitrites are extremely high. To properly assess inhalation hazard, both the LC_{50} values and the slopes of the dose mortality curves must be considered [7]. These results stand in sharp contrast to the generally perceived belief that aliphatic nitrites are relatively benign substances.

Except for the C_1 compound, the LC_{50} values increase with increasing molecular weight: methyl nitrite, 176 ppm; ethyl nitrite, 160 ppm; *n*-propyl nitrite, 300 ppm; *n*-butyl nitrite, 420 ppm. For a given carbon number, branching tends to decrease toxicity, leading to higher LC_{50} values. For the series of normal methyl, ethyl, propyl, and butyl compounds, the slopes of the LC_{50} curves ranged from 18 to 47. The hazards associated with acute inhalation may be greater than the LC_{50} values alone indicate.

The work of Klonne et al. [7] appears to indicate that cardiovascular effects are the major determinant of acute toxicity, despite the more observable methemoglobinemia. Rats initially showed increased activity and blanching of the ears and feet, gradually becoming cyanotic and later developing respiratory difficulties (possibly pulmonary hemorrhage). Animals that survived the actual exposures later improved, even if they appeared close to death at the time of cessation of exposure.

Rees et al. [8] examined mice for effects on lethality and motor performance following inhalation exposures to the series of isoamyl, *n*-butyl, and isobutyl nitrite. All three nitrites produced concentration-related effects on both measures, with median effective concentrations for motor performance at approximately one-half of the median lethal concentrations (LC_{50}'s) for lethality [8]. A human fatality from ingestion of volatile nitrite recently was reported in which methemoglobinemia (Section 21.4.13) was observed [9].

Organic nitrites, including amyl, butyl, and isobutyl compounds, are known to react with biological amines and amides to produce *N*-nitrosamines and *N*-nitrosamides [10]. According to numerous *in vivo* and *in vitro* methodologies, the nitrosamines have been shown to be mutagenic, carcinogenic, and teratogenic. It is feasible that the *N*-nitroso compounds are produced in physiologic media, given the reaction of nitrite-containing compounds with various amines [11].

Various *in vivo* and *in vitro* studies have shown some degree of depression of host defense mechanisms due to exposure to street-variety butyl nitrite compounds [12–14]. Haverkos [15] suggests that a potentially definitive experiment in this area would be to challenge retrovirus-infected animals with large quantitites of alkyl nitrites and look for skin changes consistent with Kaposi's sarcoma.

19.1.3 Epidemiology

Because of the clandestine nature of the industry that supports repackaging and ultimate sale of small bottles containing butyl nitrites in drug paraphernalia stores, adult novelty shops, and other locations, little is known about the seriousness of exposures. Exposures could be occupational, as in repackaging, or they may be recreational, as in sniffing packaged products. Data from poison control centers have been checked to determine any pertinent trend analysis (Table 19.1) [16].

Nationally, these data show a steady increase in the reported incidence of volatile nitrite exposure. Interpretation of the data must reflect the increases reported for all toxic exposures. It is unclear whether this increase reflects an actual increase in incidence, as opposed to improved public utilization of poison center services. Given various bans on these substances that are spottily enforced on a local or a state basis, it is surprising to note an increase in reporting. Federal regulation of abused substances includes the volatile nitrites in a schedule that allows state and local initiatives or lack thereof.

The role of potential HIV cofactors such as the volatile nitrites needs additional investigation and explanation. Lifson [17] has indicated that there may be no one universal cofactor, but combinations of infectious or environmental agents that cause immune stimulation and reactivation of latent HIV.

TABLE 19.1. Reported exposures to volatile nitrites in the U.S. [16].

Year	Reported exposures
1983	29
1984	87
1985	142
1986	185
1987	164
1988	166
1989	191
1990	164
1991	86

From an objective viewpoint, it is fair to say that toxicology experiments and epidemiology studies to date are inconclusive regarding the role of volatile nitrite compounds as important cofactors in the development of HIV-diseases. However, from a public health viewpoint, it is necessary to advise persons at risk for exposure to HIV infection that they should refrain from using volatile nitrites.

19.2 EXPOSURE MONITORING

Given the status of these substances as prescription-controlled medicinal compounds and industrial chemicals, it is not surprising that no data exist regarding occupational and recreational exposure concentrations. Not only are exposure monitoring data nonexistent, but the methods needed to perform such analyses have not been field-tested. Additionally, occupational exposure limits do not exist for these compounds.

19.2.1 Biological Monitoring

Biological analysis of the aliphatic nitrites consists of methemoglobin measurements and agent-specific analyses. Volatile nitrites and many other compounds may be responsible for the production of methemoglobinemia. If fact, the mechanisms for the oxidation of hemoglobin to methemoglobin are not well understood.

Differences do exist when exposures are to the organic nitrites as opposed to inorganic species. Methemoglobin reductase and possibly other systems maintain a low level of (met)hemoglobin in the higher oxidation state. Typically, methemoglobin levels should be below 2% [18]. Correlations for methemoglobin levels as a function of concentration–time exposure relationships are not available for the volatile nitrites.

Methemoglobin measurements typically rely upon colorimetric changes induced by the addition of cyanide ion. Addition of cyanide to a blood specimen eliminates the analytical peak in the range of 630 to 635 nm [19].

Sunshine [20] indicates the basis for qualitative analysis of methemoglobin as complex ion formation occurring between the ferric heme of methemoglobin and potassium cyanide. Aliphatic nitrites have been analyzed using a nitrometric method or diazotization with α-naphthylamine (or dimethyl-α-naphthylamine). The spectrophotometric determination has been applied to blood, urine, gastric juices, and saliva [5].

19.2.2 Air Sampling and Analysis

Although not specifically demonstrated for aliphatic nitrite compounds, sampling methods intended for trinitrotoluene (TNT), cyclotrimethylenetrinitramine (RDX), and nitroglycerin are potentially useful for volatile nitrite compounds [21, 22]. Traditionally, much of the analysis of chamber concentrations used in animal toxicology has been done by using infrared instruments [7, 8]. Although this method is convenient for chamber applications, interference and calibration difficulties may prevent its effective use in field industrial applications.

19.2.3 Exposure Limits

The only occupational exposure limits pertinent to the volatile nitrites are biological monitoring standards, namely the Biological Exposure Index (BEI) for methemoglobin (Section 21.4.13), which is currently set at 1.5% [23]. Although this value may be useful for occupational scenarios, it obviously is not intended for monitoring recreational use. Additionally, three notations are included in the BEI, indicating that methemoglobin usually is present in a significant amount in biological specimens collected from subjects who have not been occupationally exposed, that the determination of methemoglobin is nonspecific, and that it is an indicator of exposure to the chemical; but the quantitative interpretation of the measurement is ambiguous.

19.3 REGULATORY AND POLICY CONSIDERATIONS

Perhaps because of the peculiar categorization of butyl nitrites as industrial chemicals, no federal agency has stepped forward to effectively control their distribution and abuse. Point-of-sale warnings and prohibition of sales have been employed in California. The degree of enforcement, and thus the effectiveness, of these measures is subject to question.

Given the nature of the butyl nitrite repackaging and distribution industry, no data are available concerning exposures to workers. Numerous information shortfalls would need to be addressed before such a preliminary evaluation could be conducted. Given that the recreational exposures are surreptitious, they obviously have not been monitored. Simulation of such exposures is a possibility.

Warning pamphlets from the National Institute of Drug Abuse have been reformatted and used by municipalities in drug abuse education seminars, health fairs, and schools. Given that few precedents exist for such unrestricted access to an abusable substance, education is critical to a greater public awareness of the risks.

References

1. Johnson, L.; Bachman, J.; and O'Malley, P. 1979. *Highlights: Drugs and the Nation's High School Students; Five-Year National Trend*, National Institute on Drug Abuse, Rockville, MD, pp. 1–235.
2. Chrysant, S. G.; Dunn, F. G.; DeCarvalho, J. G. R.; et al. 1977. Action of nitroglycerin and amyl nitrite in labile and essential hypertension. *Arch. Intern. Med.* **137**: 1702–1705.
3. Mayer, Kenneth H. 1986. Medical consequences of the inhalation of volatile nitrites. In *Sexually Transmitted Diseases in Homosexual Men*, Ostrow et al. (eds.), Plenum Medical Book Co., New York, pp. 237–242.
4. EllenHorn, M. J.; and Barceloux, D. G. 1988. *Medical Toxicology: Diagnosis and Treatment of Human Poisoning*, Elsevier Science Publishing Co., New York, pp. 548–552.

   nitrites. *Clin. Toxicol.* **16**: 317–329.
6. Ignarro, L. J.; Lippton, H.; and Edwards, J. C. 1981. *J. Pharmacol. Exp. Ther.* **218**: 739–742.
7. Klonne, D. R.; Ulrich, C. E.; Weissmann, J.; and Morgan, A. K. 1987. Acute inhalation toxicity of aliphatic nitrites in rats. *Fund. Appl. Toxicol.* **8**: 101–106.

8. Rees, D. C.; Coggeshall, E. M.; Dragan, Y.; Breen, T. J.; and Balster, R. L. 1986. Acute effects of some volatile nitrites on motor performance and lethality in mice. *Neurobehav. Toxicol. Teratol.* **8**: 139–142.
9. O'Toole, J. B.; Robbins, G. B.; and Dixon, D. S. 1987. Ingestion of isobutyl nitrite, a recreational chemical of abuse, causing fatal methemoglobinemia. *J. Forensic Sci.* **32**: 1811–12.
10. Jorgensen, K. A.; and Lawesson, S. 1982. Amyl nitrite and Kaposi's sarcoma in homosexual men (letter). *N. Engl. J. Med.* **307**: 893–894.
11. Quinto, I. 1980. Mutagenicity of alkyl nitrites in the *Salmonella* test. *Soc. Ital. Biol. Sper.* **56**: 816–20.
12. Goedert, J. J. 1982. Amyl nitrite may alter T-lymphocytes in homosexual men. *Lancet* **1982**: 412.
13. Jacobs, R. F.; Marmer, D. J.; Steele, R. W.; and Hogue, T. R. 1983. Cellular immunotoxicity of amyl nitrite. *J. Toxicol. Clin. Toxicol.* **20**: 421–449.
14. Lewis, D. M.; Koller W. A.; Lynch D. A.; and Spira, T. J. 1985. Subchronic inhalation toxicity of isobutyl nitrite in BALB/c Mice. II. Immunotoxicity studies. *J. Toxicol. Environ. Health* **15**: 835–846.
15. Haverkos, H. W. 1988. Kaposi's sarcoma and nitrite inhalants. In *Psychological, Neuropsychiatric, and Substance Abuse Aspects of AIDS*, Bridge et al. (eds.), Raven Press, New York, pp. 165–172.
16. American Association of Poison Control Centers Annual Reports. 1984–88. *Am. J. Emerg. Med.* **2–6, 9, 10**: 420; 423; 427; 405; 479; 494; and 487.
17. Lifson, A. R. 1988. The natural history of human immunodeficiency virus infection. *J. Infect. Dis.* **158**: 1360–1367.
18. Smith, R. 1986. Toxic responses of the blood. In *Toxicology*, Curtis D. Klaassen, Mary O. Amdur, and John Doull (eds.), Macmillan, New York, pp. 223–244.
19. Fairbanks, V. F., and Klee, G. G. 1986. Biochemical aspects of hematology. In *Textbook of Clinical Chemistry*, N. Tietz (ed.), W. B. Saunders, Philadelphia, PA., pp. 1495–1588.
20. Sunshine, I. 1978. *Analytical Toxicology*, CRC Press, Boca Raton, FL.
21. Lodge, J. P., Jr. (ed.). 1989. *Methods of Air Sampling and Analysis*, 3rd ed., Intersociety Committee, Lewis Publishers, Boca Raton, FL, p. 82 and 177.
22. Bishop, R. W.; Ayers, T. A.; and Rinehart, D. S. 1981. The use of a solid sorbent as a collection medium for TNT and RDX vapors. *Am. Ind. Hyg. Assoc. J.* **42**: 586–588.
23. American Conference of Governmental Industrial Hygienists. 1990. *Documentation of the TLVs and BELs*, ACGIH, Cincinnati, OH.

PART 5

Special Topics

20

Quantitative Posturography as an Early Monitoring Tool for Chemical Toxicity

by Amit Bhattacharya*

20.0 ABSTRACT

The study of postural stability (body sway) characteristics is used as an indirect measure of the health status of the nervous system of individuals with a history of low-level exposure to industrial and/or environmental chemicals. Noninvasive quantitative posturography provides a real-time measure of the movement pattern of the body's center of pressure associated with postural sway. This technique is accurate and sensitive, and can be administered in about 2 minutes. The results from our ongoing study on 5-year-old children with a known history of blood lead (mean value for 5 years of life 20.7 μg/dL) show significant impairment in their postural stability. In particular, results indicate a significant association of the second year of blood lead (mean value of second year: 21.8 μg/dL) with postural sway measures at age 5 years. Results from a clinical case study of a 15-year-old boy lead-poisoned at age 2 years showed significantly impaired postural stability compared to that of a nonexposed 14-year-old boy, as well as results obtained from a group of young adults (26 years old). These results further suggest that a residual lead effect on body balance was carried over into the later years of life. The applications of posturography in studying the effect of industrial chemicals on workers also have been addressed. The long-term significance of this noninvasive technique needs to be further evaluated for use as a preclinical (early) screening/monitoring tool for workers and/or the general public exposed to a variety of neurotoxic chemicals.

20.1 INTRODUCTION

Many chemicals have been reported to produce both central and peripheral neurological disorders. For example, solvents such as xylene and styrene have

* University of Cincinnati Medical Center, Department of Environmental Health, Cincinnati, OH.

been shown to be associated with neurological disorders at acute exposure levels higher than the Threshold Limit Values (TLV), as well as at chronic low-level values. Therefore, it can be postulated that exposures to specific solvents at levels below recommended TLVs for a long-term period may be cumulative and may result in detectable health effects. Like those of solvents, the neurological/neurobehavioral effects of industrial and environmental lead exposure have been well documented in the literature. Most of the health effects of low-level exposure are not detectable at a preclinical stage; therefore, an effective preventive measure can not be instituted before the chemical has caused significant and often irreparable damage to the body. Hence, there is need for a measurement tool or test that can be used as an "early warning" or monitoring indicator of health impairment due to occupational and/or environmental exposure to chemicals. Such a technique should be reliable, valid, sensitive, nonivasive, and quick and easy to administer. Furthermore, the test procedure should allow the evaluation of a body function that is indirectly controlled by central as well as peripheral nervous systems. One such body function is human postural stability (sway), which receives controlling signals from both the central and the peripheral nervous systems. The study of postural balance or sway provides indirect insight into the gross health status of the nervous system, which controls the functioning of simple and complex behaviors ranging from basic neuromuscular and cognitive functioning to the performance of highly skilled tasks.

In the following discussion, examples of neurotoxicity and neurobehavioral effects of solvents in industrial workers and neurobehavioral effects of environmental lead in children are presented. This brief review of the literature will summarize the scope of the problem at hand, and will set the stage for discussion of the use of posturography as an early monitoring tool for detecting chemical toxicity.

20.2 NEUROBEHAVIORAL ASPECTS OF INDUSTRIAL SOLVENT EXPOSURE

Previous studies [1] have shown that exposures to various benzene homologs such as toluene, xylene, and styrene are common at workplaces. For example, workers in boat building and printing ink industries and painters are exposed to a variety of solvents such as styrene and xylene. Acute high-dose exposure to these solvents can produce a transient narcotic effect on the central nervous system (CNS). Acute effects have been reported following the inhalation of jet fuels and exposures to toluene, styrene, and methylene chloride [2, 3]. Common symptoms are intoxication, fatigue, poor endurance, dizziness, slight depression, tremor, and balance impairment [4]. Persons exposed to solvents often have a lower than normal tolerance to alcohol. Generally, these symptoms disappear over a weekend. However, if exposure continues for a longer period, recovery may be increasingly prolonged [5]. With such subchronic exposures, the symptoms may persist for weeks or months following exposure, possibly because the solvent or its metabolites have accumulated in the body and have been eliminated slowly. The data on subchronic exposures have been far from comprehensive.

Chronic exposures to solvents have produced impairment of both the central and the peripheral nervous systems [1]. For example, Gregerson et al. [6] have found occurrences of brain atrophy in painters, and solvent-induced peripheral neuropathy has been reported by other investigators [7, 8]. Typical clinical characteristics of solvent peripheral neuropathy are unstable motor coordination including unsteady body balance and gait, muscle cramps, pain in the extremities, lack of sensation in the lower extremities, and modest slowing of motor and sensory conduction [9, 10]. Arlien-Şoberg [11] found vestibular impairment in house and car painters. Lindstrom [12], in a follow-up test performed 5 or more years after removal from solvent exposure, found persistent functional impairment of visual/motor performance. This work and epidemiological studies by other investigators [13] have led to the conclusion that solvent-exposed workers run almost twice the risk of neurological and/or psychiatric diagnosis for disability when compared to unexposed workers.

20.3 NEUROBEHAVIORAL ASPECTS OF ENVIRONMENTAL LEAD EXPOSURE

In the industrialized world, the use of lead has increased significantly since 1940. Although acute, high-level lead toxicity in children, as well as in lead workers, has been well documented in the literature, very few studies have investigated the effects of long-term, low-level exposures to lead. Some neurobehavioral studies in lead workers [14] have shown that chronic exposure to lead causes impairment of the central as well as the peripheral nervous system. Earlier studies have well documented lead toxicity, not only in lead workers but also in their wives and their offspring [15]. With gradual improvement in industrial hygiene standards, overt congenital lead poisoning has decreased. Although young children residing in older inner-city slums remain at a relatively high risk, the problem of undue exposure to lead has penetrated far beyond the "lead belt" and the lower socioecomomic population. The lead sources in children's environments include lead paint, plaster, and airborne lead. Studies by Lin-Fu [16], Sayre et al. [17], Charney et al. [18], and Bornschein et al. [19] have indicated that in a polluted environment (lead in house dust) even normal hand-to-mouth activities can introduce a toxic amount of lead into a child's body. Studies by Landrigan et al. [20] found undue exposure to lead in children living close to lead smelters and processing plants. It is generally accepted that children represent the population at high risk to lead exposure because of hand-to-mouth activity, a relatively high rate of intestinal absorption and retention, and a high sensitivity of the heme biosynthetic pathways and nervous system to lead exposure [21, 22]. During the 1960s Pentschew [23] and Pentschew and Garro [24] and in the 1970s others [25, 26] showed morphological changes in the CNS of neonatal rats similar to those in children with lead encephalopathy. Several studies [27–31] have found that lead exposure interferes with a variety of biochemical processes (mitochondrial respiration, enzyme activity, neurotransmitter release, and competitive inhibition of calcium) that are essential for the normal nervous system.

From autopsy studies in children exposed to lead, it was found that there are two types of morphologic effects on the CNS. First, there is a cerebral edema, which may be reversible [32]. Second, there is a direct loss of neurons in certain areas of the brain (such as gray matter, hypothalamus, and basal ganglia) where neurons are most concentrated. Previous follow-up studies with children who survived the lead exposure episode have shown that the above-mentioned CNS effect are irreversible in nature. Some of these children have seizures, mental retardation, and behavioral changes.

A considerable amount of research has been performed to investigate the effect of low-level lead exposure on the cognitive performance of preschool children [33–35]. For example, Hawk et al. [36] have found a statistically significant inverse relationship between blood lead levels and scores on the Stanford Binet IQ test in 3- to 7-year-old children with a mean blood level of 20.8 μg/dL. In younger children (3–6 months old), the mental developmental status has been found to be associated with prenatal exposure to lead. Dietrich et al. [35] found significant association between prenatal blood lead level and the 3 and 6 months' Bailey Mental Developmental Index. For this study, the mean prenatal blood lead level was 8.0 μg/dL.

So far, only a few studies have attempted to document the effects of lead on neuromotor function in children. Most of these studies have reported some kind of gross motor function impairment at relatively high blood lead levels exceeding 40 μg/dL [37, 38]. This lack of evidence of low-level lead effect on neuromotor function can be partly due to lack of a sensitive measurement tool/technique. In our laboratory, with the help of a microprocessor-based force platform system, we were able to show a significant inverse relationship between blood lead level and performance on the postural stability test [39, 40] in a group of 5-year-old children with a mean blood lead level of 20.7 μg/dL. The results of low-level lead effects on neurocognitive and neuromotor performance support the current Centers for Disease Control (CDC) standard of 10 μg/dL for postnatal lead exposure in children.

20.4 POSTURAL BALANCE

The ability to maintain postural balance is controlled primarily by the balance of continual afferent and cerebellar input to motor pathways. The afferent system, which provides information regarding the position of the body in space, consists of vision [56], proprioceptors [55], vestibular apparatus [55], and cutaneous receptors [55]. The signals from these biological receptors are processed [41, 42] at both spinal and supraspinal levels (Figure 20.1). In response to these afferent signals the postural muscle reflexes are elicited by the efferent signals from the cerebellum as well as the motor cortex [41]. The major purpose of this afferent–efferent loop is to keep the body's center of pressure within the boundary of the supporting base provided by the feet. As long as the person's center of pressure movement pattern stays within the boundary of the supporting feet, he or she will not fall. Because the human stature is considerably larger than its base of support, it becomes a challenging task for the nervous system continually to assess the location of the body's center of pressure and, accordingly, to send efferent commands to the postural muscles to keep the body balanced in the upright position. This continuous process of feedback control causes the body to "sway" in the anterior–posterior as well as the lateral directions. This phenomenon of postural sway is normal, and generally the frequency of sway is less than 2 Hz. However, exposure

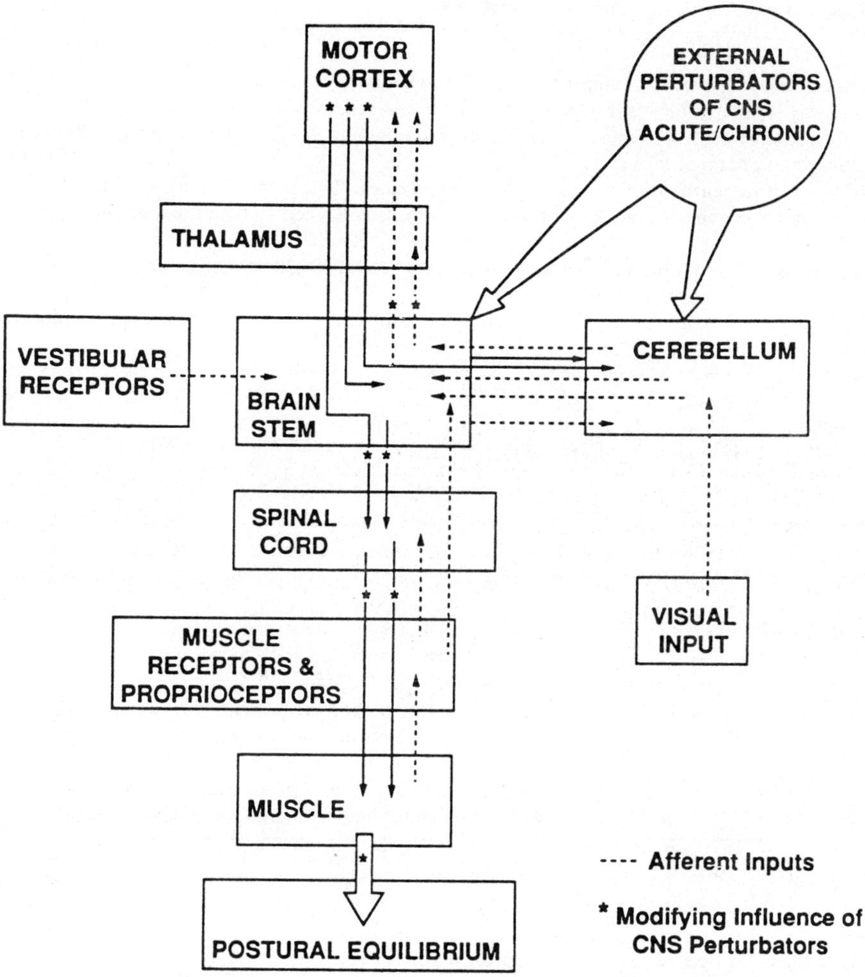

FIGURE 20.1. Possible physiological pathways affected by external perturbators of the central nervous system, such as drugs, toxic chemicals, and disease.

to drugs or chemicals, certain nervous diseases, and fatigue can modify the postural sway significantly. These external perturbators may affect the postural balance mechanism, at both the central and the peripheral levels of the nervous systems. A brief summary of the features of normal postural sway and that in certain nervous disorders is presented in Tables 20.1 and 20.2. Table 20.3 gives a brief description of the postural sway effect of acute exposure to various chemicals.

20.5 POSTURAL SWAY TEST FOR DETECTING CHEMICAL TOXICITY

The essential physiological criteria for the design of the postural sway test must address the following issues. The test should be sufficiently difficult to selectively challenge the relevant afferent systems critical for the maintenance

TABLE 20.1. Features of normal postural sway.

- A–P sway > lateral sway.
- Postural sway frequency contents lie within 0–1 Hz range.
- The sway is independent of body height, weight, and sex, in adults.
- Proprioceptive control loop is characterized by medium latency (80–120 msec) stretch reflexes. Its frequency content falls above 1 Hz range.
- Removal or impairment of proprioceptive control causes longer latency reflexes (200–400 msec) of vestibular system to come into play. This produces enhanced sway in low-frequency range: up to 0.5 Hz.
- The visual control loop also has a longer latency period (200–300 msec) similar to that of vestibular system (0.1–0.5 Hz).
- Closing eyes increases the sway, but standing is maintained as long as either proprioceptive or vestibular afferents are available.

TABLE 20.2. Features of postural sway in disease.

Affected area	Sway response
Degeneration of dorsal column (tabes dorsalis and polyneuropathy)	(A) Very high eyes closed/eyes open ratio. (B) Increased sway in 0–1 Hz range; subdued sway and tremor above 1 Hz [48].
Labyrinthine disorders	(A) Least pronounced eyes closed/eyes open ratio. (B) Shows increase in sway of excessive low frequency and high amplitude [49]. (C) With eyes open increase in sway in the <1 Hz range (visual control) and with eyes closed sway in the high-frequency range imply extensor hypertonicity.
Cerebellar defect	Increase in sway plus a pronounced tremor at 2–3 Hz.
Brain stem	Predominance and augmentation of lower-frequency sway.

TABLE 20.3. Effect of chemicals on postural sway.

Chemical	Dose	Exposure period	Effect
Xylene	64–400 ppm (2.6–16.4 μmol/L)	6 h/day	Initial increase in eyes closed/eyes open response implying effect on the vestibular reflexes [50].
Xylene + trichloroethane	8.2 μmol/L	4 h	Decrease in eyes closed/eyes open response [51].
Trichloroethane	>8.2 μmol/L	4 h	Increase in eyes closed/eyes open response [51].
Toluene	100–300 ppm range	8 h	Dizziness, muscular weakness, incoordination [52].
Toluene	60–100 ppm range	Chronic (3–4 months)	Increase in tendon reflexes, muscular weakness [53].

of upright posture. Generally, this is accomplished by designing tests that can modify by enhancing, weakening, or excluding the afferent system(s) relevant for postural maintenance. Over the years, a variety of techniques have been used for measuring the postural balance phenomenon. Some techniques have used measurement of body acceleration, whereas others used electromyography for recording the postural muscle contraction patterns associated with body sway. More recently, some investigators have used a force platform system for locating and documenting the movement pattern of the center of pressure associated with body sway [42, 43]. The following paragraphs present a brief summary of the results from our ongoing study dealing with the use of the force platform technique for characterizing the lead effect.

20.5.1 Postural Sway and Environmental Lead Exposure

The postural sway effect of chronic lead exposure was studied in the Cincinnati Lead Program Project cohort children. So far, 63 out of 300 children of mean age 5.74 years ± 0.51 SD have been given the postural sway test [39, 40]. The average maximum blood lead (PbB) of these children during the first 5 years of life was 20.7 µg/dL (range 9.2 to 32.5). The mothers of these children were recruited into this study at the prenatal stage, provided they met the rigorous and stringent exclusion criteria. In particular, mothers with disorders such as diabetes, alcoholism, confirmed drug use, and psychotic or mental retardation were not included in this study. A detailed description of exclusion criteria can be found in Dietrich et al. [35].

The postural sway was measured using a multicomponent force platform system (Advanced Mechanical Technology Inc., Newton, MA), which can measure forces and moments along three orthogonal axes. In our previous study [44], the validity and the accuracy of the force platform system's measurement of time-dependent changes in the location of the center of pressure was documented. The force platform used in our study can locate the center of pressure with an error of about 2.0%. In our previous study the sensitivity of this technique was established by documenting changes in postural sway produced by acute ingestion of small amounts of ethanol. It was shown that, with this technique, we can detect statistically significant changes in postural sway with a blood alcohol level as low as 0.015%.

On the test day, each child's middle ear pressure was measured. This information was useful for determining the presence or absence of acute ear infection, which might affect the sway data. For the postural sway test, each child performed the following four tasks: EO, stand on the force platform with eyes open; EC, stand on the force platform with eyes closed; FO, stand on a 3-inch-high foam pad placed on the force platform with eyes open; and FC, stand on a 3-inch-high foam pad placed on the force platform with eyes closed. Each of these tests was performed for a 30-sec period. The data were collected with a custom-developed software (Body Balance Software, copyright University of Cincinnati, All rights reserved, 1988) and a Zenith 241 microcomputer. The above-metioned four postural tests are designed to indirectly challenge some of the afferent systems relevant to the maintenance of upright balance. For example, the EO and EC tests are specifically suited to evaluate the role of vision (without any modification of the standing surface) in postural balance. On the other hand, in FO and FC tests, where the standing surface is modified by the foam pad, the proprioception cues are misleading, thereby placing more reliance on the vestibular system than in the tests of EO and EC. As the subject progresses through the four tests (EO, EC, FO, and FC), the reliance on the vestibular system and on the higher centers progressively increases [43, 44]. In particular, for the FO and FC tests where the CNS has to synthesize conflicting signals from proprioception and vision, the maintenance of balance becomes a relatively challenging task. In general, if the CNS is provided with no input or with conflicting inputs from the afferent system(s), the task of maintaining balance becomes difficult. Therefore, the four tests used in our study are designed to provide an increasing level of difficulty as the testing progresses through EO, EC, FO, and FC. In Figures 20.2 and 20.3, it is shown that as the testing conditions become difficult, the movement pattern of the center of pressure of the body becomes more erratic and tends to deviate from the center of the *X-Y* plot. The *X-Y* plot (in the horizontal plane) of movement pattern of the center of pressure is traditionally known as a stabilogram. Our Body Balance Software allows quantitation of the stabilogram patterns by calculating a variety of sway parameters such as area, mean radius, velocity, length, direction, fast Fourier transform parameters, and so on. A detailed description of these parameters has been published [39, 40, 44, 54].

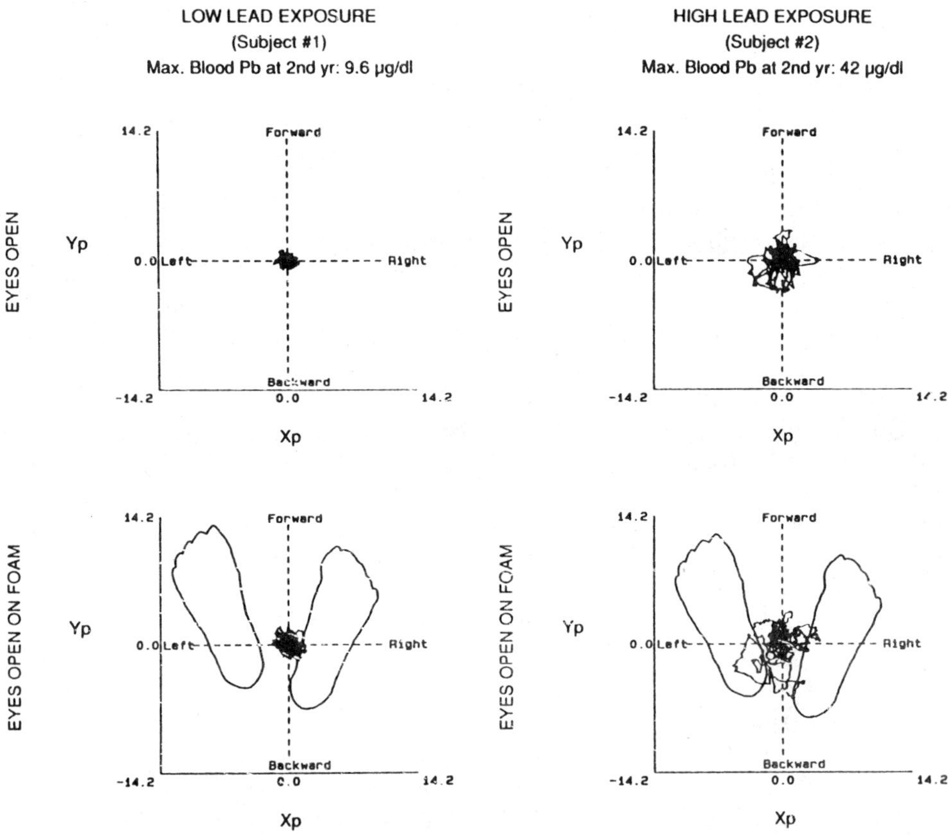

FIGURE 20.2. Stabilograms obtained during postural sway tests of eyes open on firm and compliant surfaces. Footprints are shown in two of the four stabilograms to illustrate the relative size of the sway patterns. (Adapted from Bhattacharya et al., Postural disequilibrium quantification in children with chronic lead exposure, *Neurotoxicology* **9**(3): 327–340, 1988.)

In Figures 20.2 and 20.3, typical stabilograms from two children (one with a higher PbB level than the other) are presented [39]. A qualitative comparison of these two sets of stabilograms clearly shows that the high-lead child had major difficulty in maintaining balance during all four tests, as compared to the low-lead child. A quantitative analysis of these stabilograms also showed that the postural sway areas were about two to seven times larger for the high-lead child than for the low-lead child for all test conditions [39].

For the 63 children, a stepwise regression analysis with backward elimination of nonsignificant variables indicated that the only statistically significant PbB parameter was maximum second-year PbB [40]. Also, this finding was significant only for the eyes closed, no foam pad condition (EC). Data from an additional 39 lead-exposed children recently have been analyzed, and the relationship between PbB and the postural sway is still significant for the total of 102 subjects. This finding implies that PbB has caused some level of impairment in the functional capacities of the vestibular and/or proprioception systems at 2 years of age, and that the detrimental effects on postural balance were persisting even at age 5 years. Although the issue of the long-term effect of childhood Pb exposure needs further investigation, the findings from a

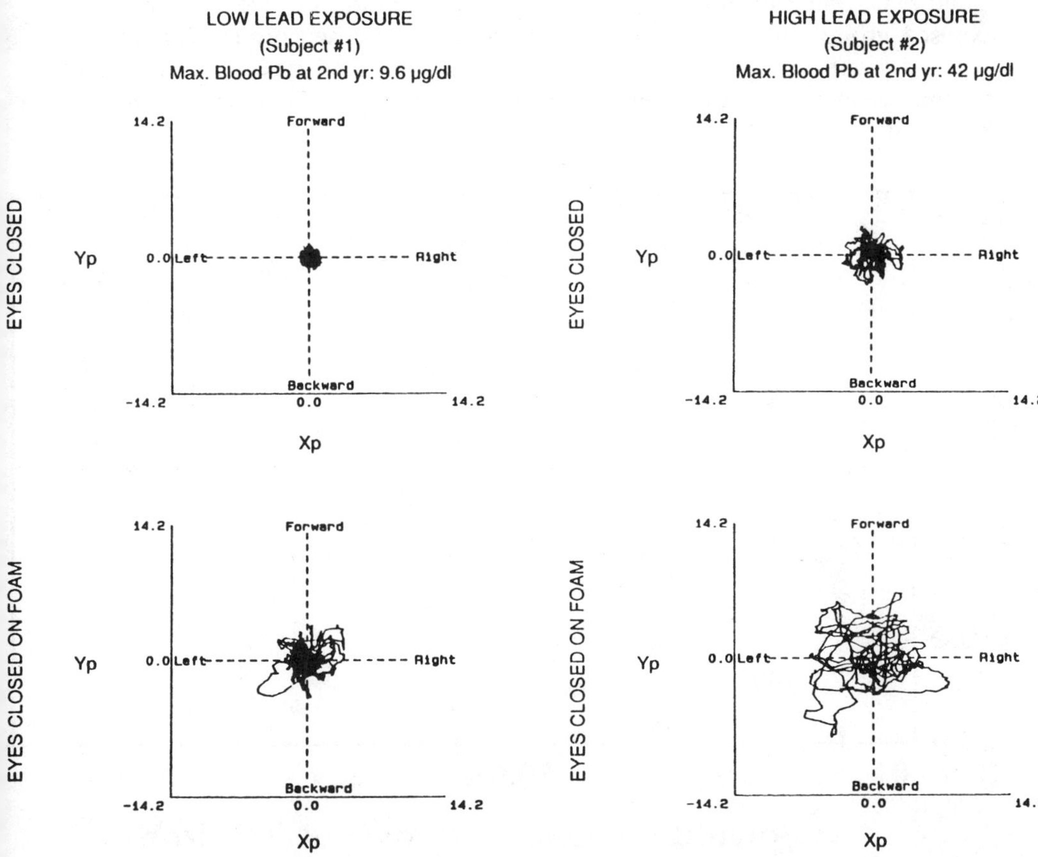

FIGURE 20.3. Stabilograms obtained during postural sway tests of eyes closed on firm and compliant surfaces. (Adapted from Bhattacharya et al., Postural disequilibrium quantification in children with chronic lead exposure, *Neurotoxicology* **9**(3): 327–340, 1988.)

clinical case study [45] from our laboratory provide suggestive evidence that early childhood Pb insult may have a detrimental effect on the maturation of postural balance. Results [45] from this clinical case study of a 15-year-old boy lead-poisoned at age 2 years showed significantly impaired postural stability compared to that of a nonexposed 14-year-old boy as well as those obtained from a group of young adults (26 years old). Therefore, the results further suggest that a residual effect on balance was carried over from the second year into the fifth year when the postural balance was measured. This study is ongoing, and some of these issues are being further investigated.

20.5.2 Postural Sway and Occupational Chemical Exposure

Recently, the force platform technique has been used to detect the postural balance effects of occupational exposure to chemicals. Two pilot studies have been initiated. One deals with the effect of chronic exposure of pesticides on the postural balance in organophosphate pesticide applicators. The second one is focused on investigating the effect of chronic exposure of solvents on the postural stability of painters. In the pesticide study of 37 applicators, it was found that significant differences in sway area and radius existed between the exposed group and an age- and sex-matched nonexposed group [46]. In the exposed group, the parameters of pesticide exposure and recent exposure and plasma cholinesterase level were significantly associated with increased postural sway [46].

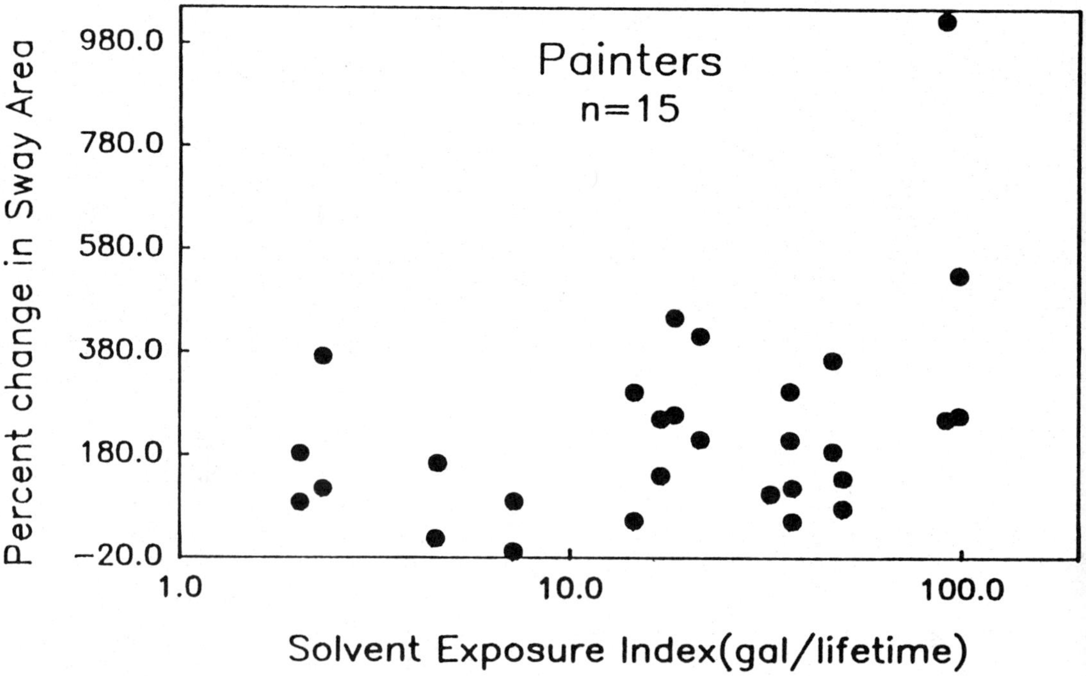

FIGURE 20.4. Results of preliminary study on the effects of paint solvent exposure on postural sway. The arithmetic mean ± standard deviation was (55.1 ± 12) years. The r^2 was 0.25 for $p < 0.01$.

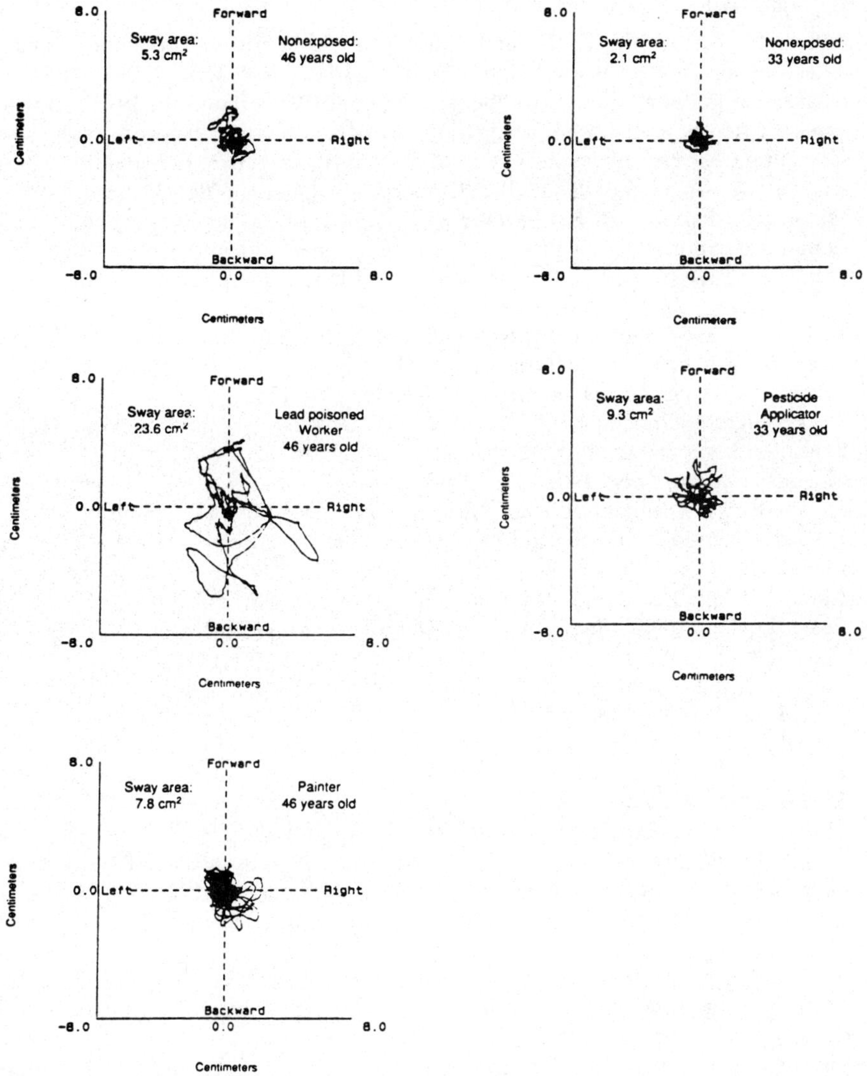

FIGURE 20.5. Examples of body sway patterns (stabilograms) for workers exposed to different kinds of environmental and/or industrial toxicants. A larger body sway implies difficulty in maintaining upright balance.

In the painters study [47], the preliminary analysis of data from 15 subjects tested twice shows a significant association between the solvent exposure index and the percent change in postural sway for the FC condition compared to that of the FO test. In Figure 20.4, a scatter plot of the percent change in postural sway versus solvent exposure index is presented. Figure 20.5 gives illustrative examples of stabilograms from a lead-poisoned worker, a pesticide applicator, and a painter. In comparison to respective nonexposed workers' stabilograms, the exposed workers' stabilograms are relatively larger and erratic in nature, a finding indicative of lack of postural control. Data from more subjects and additional statistical analysis involving covariate control are necessary to provide conclusive evidence about chemical effects on postural balance.

References

1. Baker, E. L.; Smith, T. J.; and Landrigan, P. J. 1850. The neurotoxicity of industrial solvents: a review of the literature. *Am. J. Ind. Med.* **8**: 207–217.
2. Knave, B.; Persson, H. E.; Goldberg, J. M.; and Westerholm, P. 1976. Long-term exposure to jet fuel. An investigation on occupationally exposed workers with special reference to the nervous system. *Scan. J. Work Environ. Health* **2**: 152–164.
3. Knave, B.; Anshelm-Olson, B.; Elofsson, S.; Gamberale, F.; Isaksson, A.; Mindus, P.; Persson, H. E.; Struwe, G.; Wennberg, A.; and Westerholm, P. 1978. Long-term exposure to jet fuel. II. A cross-sectional epidemiologic investigation on occupationally exposed industrial workers with special reference to the nervous system. *Scand. J. Work Environ. Health* **4**: 19–43.
4. Savolainen, K.; Riihimaki, V.; Seppalainen, A. M.; and Linnoila, M. 1980. Effects of short-term *m*-xylene exposure and physical exercise on the central nervous system. *Int. Arch. Occup. Environ. Health* **45**: 105–121.
5. Mikkelsen, S.; Gregersen, P.; Klausen, H.; Dossing, M.; and Nielsen, H. 1978. Presenile dementia as an occupational disease from industrial exposure to organic solvents. *Ugeskr. Laeg.* **140**: 1633–1637.
6. Gregersen, P.; Mikkelsen, S.; Klausen, H.; Dossing, M.; Nielsen, H.; and Thygesen, P. 1978. A chronic cerebral painter's syndrome. *Ugeskr. Laeg.* **140**: 1638–1644.
7. Allen, N.; Mendell, J. R.; Billmaier, D. J.; Fontaine, R. E.; and O'Neill, J. 1975. Toxic polyneuropathy due to methyl *n*-butyl ketone. *Arch. Neurol.* **32**: 209–218.
8. Cianchetti, C.; Abbritti, G.; Perticoni, G.; Siracusa, A.; and Curradi, A. 1976. Toxic polyneuropathy of shoe industry workers: a study of 122 cases. *J. Neurol. Neurosurg. Psychiat.* **39**: 1151–1161.
9. Seppalainen, A. M.; Husman, K.; and Martenson, C. 1978. Neurophysiological effects of long-term exposure to a mixture of organic solvents. *Scand. J. Work Environ. Health* **4**: 304–314.
10. Elofsson, S.; Gamberale, F.; Hindmarsh, T.; Iregren, A.; Isaksson, A.; Johnsson, I.; et al. 1980. Exposure to organic solvents. A cross-sectional epidemiologic investigation on occupationally exposed car and industrial spray painters with special reference to the nervous system. *Scand. J. Work Environ. Health* **6**: 239–273.
11. Arlien-Soborg, P.; Zilstorff, K.; Grandjean, B.; and Milling Pedersen, I. 1981. Vestibular dysfunction in occupational chronic solvent intoxication. *Clin. Otolaryngol.* **6**: 285–290.
12. Lindstrom, K. 1980. Changes in psychological performances of solvent-poisoned and solvent-exposed workers. *Am. J. Ind. Med.* **1**: 69–84.
13. Axelson, O.; Hane, M.; and Hogstedt, C. 1976. A case-referent study on neuropsychiatric disorders among workers exposed to solvents. *Scand. J. Work Environ. Health* **2**: 14–20.
14. Morgan, B. B., and Repko, J. D. 1974. Evaluation of behavioral functions in workers exposed to lead. In *Behavioral Toxicology. Early Detection of Occupational Hazards*, C. Xintaras, B. L. Johnson, and I. deGroot (eds.), pp. 248–266.
15. Lin-Fu., J. S. 1982. Evolution of childhood lead poisoning as a public health problem. In *Lead Absorption in Children*, J. J. Chisolm, Jr., and D. M. O'Hara, (eds.), Urban & Schwarzenberg, Baltimore, MD.
16. Lin-Fu, J. S. 1973. Vulnerability of children to lead exposure and toxicity. *N. Eng. J. Med.* **289**: 1229–1233, 1289–1293.
17. Sayre, J. W.; Charney, E.; and Vostal, J. 1974. House and hand dust as a potential source of childhood lead exposure. *Am. J. Dis. Child* **127**: 167–170.

18. Charney, E.; Sayre, J.; and Coulter, M. 1980. Increased lead absorption in inner city children: where does the lead come from? *Pediatrics* **65**: 226–231.
19. Bornschein, R. L.; Hammond, P. B.; Dietrich, K. N.; Succop, P.; Krafft, K.; Clark, S.; Berger, O.; Pearson, D.; and Que Hee, S. 1985. The Cincinnati prospective study of low-level lead exposure and its effects on child development: protocol and status report. *Environ. Res.* **38**: 4–18.
20. Landrigan, P. T.; Gehlbach, S. H.; and Rosenblum, B. F. 1975. Epidemic lead absorption near an ore smelter—the role of particulate lead. *N. Engl. J. Med.* **292**: 123–129.
21. Bornschein, R. L.; Grote, J.; Mitchell, T.; Succop, P.; Shukla, R.; and Dietrich, K. N. 1986. Effect of prenatal and postnatal lead exposure on fetal maturation and postnatal growth. Paper presented at the workshop on Lead Exposure and Neurobehavioral Effects of Children, Edinburgh, Scotland, Sept.
22. Dietrich, K. N.; Krafft, K. M.; Shukla, R.; Bornschein, R. L.; and Succop, P. A. 1986. The neurobehavioral effects of prenatal and early postnatal lead exposure. In *Toxic Substances and Mental Retardation: Neurobehavioral Toxicology and Teratology*, S. R. Schroeder (ed.), AAMD, Washington, DC.
23. Pentschew, A. 1965. Morphology and morphogenesis of lead encephalopathy. *Acta Neuropathol.* **5**: 133–160.
24. Pentschew, A., and Garro, F. 1965. Lead encephalomyelopathy of the suckling rat and its implications on the porphyrinopathic nervous disease. *Acta Neuropathol.* **6**: 266–278.
25. Thomas, J. A.; Dallenbach, F. D.; and Thomas, M. 1971. Considerations of the development of experimental lead encephalopathy. *Virchows Arch. Path. Anat.* **352**: 62–74.
26. Michaelson, I. A., and Sauerhoff, M. W. 1974. An improved model of lead-induced brain dysfunction in the suckling rat. *Toxicol. Appl. Pharmacol.* **28**: 88–96.
27. U.S. EPA. 1985. *Independent Peer Review of Selected Studies Concerning Neurobehavioral Effect of Lead Exposures in Nominally Asymptomatic Children: Official Report of Findings and Recommendations of an Interdisciplinary Expert Review Committee* (EPA-600/8-83-028A), Washington, DC.
28. Kober, T. E., and Cooper, G. P. 1976. Lead competitively inhibits calcium-dependent synaptic transmission in the bullfrog sympathetic ganglion. *Nature* **262** (London): 704–705.
29. Bull, R. J.; Lutkenhoff, S. D.; McCarty, G. E.; and Miller, R. G. 1979. Delays in the postnatal increase of cerebral cytochrome concentrations in lead-exposed rats. *Neuropharmacology* **18**: 83–92.
30. McCauley, P. T.; Bull, R. M.; Tonti, A. P.; Lutkenhoff, S. D.; Meister, M. V.; Doerger, J. V.; and Stober, J. A. 1982. The effect of prenatal and postnatal lead exposure on neonatal synaptogenesis in rat cerebral cortex. *J. Toxicol. Environ. Health* **10**: 639–651.
31. Krigman, M. R., and Hogan, E. L. 1974. Effect of lead intoxication on the postnatal growth of the rat nervous system. *Environ. Health Perspect.* **5**: 187–199.
32. Goyer, R. A. 1982. Lead toxicity. In *Absorption in Children*, J. J. Chisolm, Jr. and D. M. O'Hara (eds.), Urban & Schwarzenberg, Baltimore, MD.
33. Bellinger, D.; Leviton, A.; Waternaux, C.; Needleman, H.; and Rabinowitz, M. 1987. Longitudinal analysis of prenatal and post-natal lead exposure and early cognitive development. *New Engl. J. Med.* **316**: 1037–1043.
34. Needleman, H. L.; Gunnoe, C.; Leviton, A.; Reed, R.; Peresie, H.; Maher, C.; and Barrett, P. 1979. Deficits in psychologic and classroom performance of children with elevated dentine lead levels. *New Engl. J. Med.* **300**: 689–695.
35. Dietrich, K. N.; Krafft, K. M.; Bornschein, R. L.; Hammond, P. B.; Berger, O.

G.; Succop, P. A.; and Bier, M. 1987. Low-level fetal lead exposure effect on neurobehavioral development in early infancy. *Pediatrics* **80**: 721–730.
36. Hawk, B. A.; Schroeder, S. R.; Robinson, G.; Otto, D.; Mushak, P.; Kleinbaum, D.; and Dawson, G. 1986. Relationship of lead and social factors to IQ of low SES children: a partial replication. *Am. J. Ment. Defic.* **91**: 178–183.
37. Benetou-Marantidou, A.; Nakau, S.; and Micheloyannis, J. 1988. Neurobehavioral estimation of children with life long increased lead exposure. *Arch. Environ. Health* **43**: 392–395.
38. Roberts, T. M.; Hutchinson, T. C.; Paciga, J.; Chattopadhyay, A.; Jervis, R. E.; and Van Loon, J. 1979. Lead contamination around secondary smelters: estimation of dispersal and accumulation by humans. *Science* **186**: 1–20.
39. Bhattacharya, A.; Shukla, R.; Bornschein, R. L.; Dietrich, K. N.; and Kopke, J. 1988. Postural disequilibrium quantification in children with chronic lead exposure. *Neurotoxicology* **9**: 327–340.
40. Bhattacharya, A.; Shukla, R.; Bornschein, R.; Dietrich, K.; and Keith, R. 1990. Lead effects on postural balance of children. *Environ. Health Perspec.* **89**: 35–42.
41. Vander, A. J.; Sherman, J. H.; and Luciano, D. S. 1970. *Human Physiology: The Mechanisms of Body Functions*, McGraw-Hill, New York.
42. Nashner, L. M. 1985. Strategies for organization of human posture. In *Vestibular and Visual Control on Posture and Locomotor Equilibrium*, Igarashi and Black (eds.), 7th Int. Symp. Int. Soc. Posturography, Houston, TX; Karger, Basel, p. 108.
43. Sahlstrand, T.; Ortengren, R.; and Nachemson, A. 1978. Postural equilibrium in adolescent idiopathic scoliosis. *Acta Orthop. Scand.* **49**: 354–365.
44. Bhattacharya, A.; Morgan, R.; Shukla, R.; Ramakrishanan, H. K.; and Wang, L. 1987. Noninvasive estimation of afferent inputs for postural stability under low levels of alcohol. *Ann. Biomed. Eng.* **15**: 533–550.
45. Bhattacharya, A., and Linz, D. H. 1991. Postural sway analysis of a teenager with childhood lead intoxication—a case study. *Clin. Pediat.* **30**: 543–548.
46. Sack, D. M. 1988. Effects of chronic pesticide exposure on quantitative balance characteristics, M.S. thesis, Dept. Envir. Health, Univ. of Cincinnati Medical School.
47. Schuler, J., and Bhattacharya, A. 1989. Effect of solvent exposure on postural disequilibrium in painters. (Unpublished data.)
48. Dichigan, J.; Mauntz, K. H.; Allum, J. H.; and Brandt, T. 1976. Postural sway in normal and ataxic patients: analysis of the stabilizing and destabilizing effects of vision. *Agressologie* **17**:15–24.
49. DeWit, G. 1972. Analysis of the stabilographic curves. *Agressologie* **13**(c): 79–83.
50. Savolainen, K., and Riihimaki, V. 1981. An early sign of xylene effect on human equilibrium. *Acta Pharmacol. Toxicol.* **48**: 279–283.
51. Savolainen, K.; Riihimaki, V.; and Lane, A. 1982. Biphasic effects of inhaled solvents on human equilibrium. *Acta Pharmacol. Toxicol.* **51**: 237–242.
52. von Oettigen, W. F.; Neal, P. A.; and Donahue, D. D. 1942. The toxicity and potential dangers of toluene—preliminary report. *J. Am. Med. Assoc.* **118**: 579–584.
53. Matsushita, T.; Arimatsue, Y.; Veda A.; Saton, K.; and Nomura, S. 1975. Hematological and neuromuscular response of workers exposed to low concentrations of toluene vapor. *Ind. Health* **13**: 115–121.
54. Dick, R.; Bhattacharya, A.; and Shukla, R. 1990. Use of computerized postural sway measurement system for neurobehavioral toxicity. *Neurotoxicol. Teratol.* **12**: 1–6.
55. Horak, F. B.; Shumway-Cook, A.; Crowe, T. K.; and Black, F. O. 1988. Vestibular function and motor proficiency of children with impaired hearing, or

with learning disability and motor impairments. *Dev. Med. Child Neurol.* **30**: 64–79.

56. Lee, D. N., and Lishman, J. R. 1975. Visual proprioceptive control of stance. *J. Human Movement Stud.* **1**: 87–95.

21

Biological Exposure Indices

21.0 INTRODUCTION

The Biological Exposure Indices (BEI) Committee of the American Conference of Governmental Industrial Hygienists (ACGIH) first met in 1983 [1–3]. An earlier working group devoted to formulating Biological Limit Values (BLVs) was created in 1973, but no recommendations were approved by the ACGIH Threshold Limit Value (TLV) Committee. The TLV committee still recommends reference values of specific chemicals in air to help industrial hygienists evaluate the hazard to human health over a 5-day 8-h work period/16-h nonoccupational period, followed by two 24-h periods of nonoccupational exposure before the cycle is repeated.

BEIs represent [2] the concentrations of biological monitoring markers most likely to be observed in biological specimens collected from a healthy worker exposed to chemicals by inhalation at the appropriate workload physical activity and at the ACGIH-recommended Threshold Limit Value–Time Weighted Average (TLV-TWA).

The main kinds of information for specific chemicals considered by the BEI Committee include [2]: (1) the mechanism of absorption and elimination, including biotransformation in humans and animals; (2) all known adverse effects and the mechanism and pharmacodynamics of the most significant effect, observed usually at the lowest exposure level and including susceptible human populations; (3) field studies relating intensity of exposure (usually in air) or adverse effects to concentration of biological monitoring markers (dose-effect/dose-response); (4) controlled laboratory studies on volunteers providing pharmacokinetic data; and (5) simulation studies to extrapolate or match BEIs to TLVs. For the latter, simulation is done for a reference 70-kg male worker of height 170 cm doing light work with an energy expenditure of 50 W when exposed to a TLV-TWA. It is recommended that measurement of the biological monitoring marker be done at least twice, or compared with a group average of similarly exposed workers.

The BEI Committee compiles documentation to support its recommended reference value [4] in an analogous manner to the documentation for the TLVs [5]. As for TLVs, a recommendation is allowed public comment for one year, and a revised recommendation is published for public comment in the second year, with possible adoption at the beginning of the third year through the annual booklet *Threshold Limit Values for Chemical Substances and Physical Agents and Biological Exposure Indices* [6], which also contains the final action concentrations of other xenobiotics. As with the changes in TLVs themselves, the bases for the changes in recommendations are published throughout the year in the ACGIH journal *Applied Occupational and Environmental Hygiene*, and the official basis for the final recommendation is published in the ACGIH's *Documentation of the Threshold Limit Values and Biological Exposure Indices* after the two periods of public comment [5]. Thus changes in a TLV lead to changes in any appropriate BEI at a minimum of 2 years after the official change in the TLV. As new biological information becomes available relative to biological monitoring parameters, the BEI committee can initiate its own changes in recommendations.

The proceedings of a 1989 NSF symposium for U.S. and Japanese biological monitoring scientists showed the state of biological monitoring research, education, and concepts in Japan and the United States at that time [7]. Very few full courses in biological monitoring are taught in University courses although a special lecture on the topic often is encountered in a more general course.

21.1 BEIs AND THEIR ANALOGS IN OTHER COUNTRIES

The first recorded research to determine the critical toxic concentrations for air contaminants was done in Germany in 1883 [8] for carbon monoxide, where the nontoxic concentration for hens, rabbits, and the investigator himself was determined to be between 200 and 500 ppm. As early as 1926 in the United States, Cook used a combination of atmospheric and biological monitoring techniques to verify control of benzene exposures in a cable-insulating operation [9].

Since September 1989 Japan has had a compulsory annual/semiannual worker biological monitoring program superintended by physicians [10]. Usually, urine samples are collected during the last 2 h of a workshift except for the first workday of the week. Biological monitoring markers are reported in one of three ranges.

The European Economic Community organizes its biological monitoring activities through a Directorate General for Employment and Social Affairs with laboratory certification through a Community Bureau of Reference, and with dissemination of the rationale for biological monitoring through publication of monographs in a "Human Biological Monitoring of Industrial Chemicals Series" [11].

Germany first promulgated standards for worker health in 1886, and it now regulates the workplace through maximum concentrations (MAK-Werte), which factor in carcinogenicity, developmental effects, peak values, and skin absorption as proposed through the Commission for the Investigation of Health Hazards of Chemical Compounds in the Work Area [12]. The special working group of the German Commission called "Setting Limit Values in Biological Materials" began in 1979, and it has published Biological Tolerance Values for Work Materials (BAT-Werte) since 1981. MAK values aim at protecting groups of workers; BAT values apply for individuals. A BAT value is the maximum permissible quantity of a compound and/or its metabolites in biological specimens corresponding to the MAK-Werte as reference; it can also be defined as the maximum permissible deviation from the "reference range" of physiological parameters induced by the chemical at its MAK-Werte. The latter consideration allows BAT values to have more inherent scope than BEI values. The two concepts were compared by Fiserova-Bergerova [13].

Table 21.1 compares the BAT-Werte for those chemicals that have adopted BEIs with the corresponding MAKs, TLVs, and PELs [10–14]. The physical constants that are useful for pharmacokinetic modeling of these chemicals are provided in Table 3.1. Other countries such as Czechoslovakia, Finland, France, and Poland and the World Health Organization also have recommended biological monitoring biological exposure limits [15].

21.2 ACGIH PHARMACOKINETIC MODELS

Two simulation models are used, linear and nonlinear, to describe uptake, blood and tissue concentrations, and elimination of inhaled vapors and gases [16]. See Section 6.3.6 for a discussion of other models. Both models are five-compartment (the Japanese use seven-compartment models), where the tissues are pooled in compartments according to similarity in perfusion, solubility, and elimination/detoxification/excretion. The five compartments are: lung (lungs, alveolar air and arterial blood); liver; vessel-rich compartment (VRG), which comprises brain, gastrointestinal tract, glands, heart, kidney, pancreas, and spleen; muscle group (MG: muscles and skin); and the fat group FG: adipose tissue and white marrow), for males who are slim (65 kg), standard-weight (70 kg), and overweight (80 kg). Table 21.2 gives the reference physiological parameters for a standard 170-cm-tall man.

Usually the processes in the linear model are assumed to be first-order, with the metabolic rate constant derived from the intrinsic metabolic clearance. The mathematical solution proceeds by the Laplace transform [16]. The linear model usually applies at low absorbed doses. For the nonlinear model, metabolism is assumed to be a capacity-limited process where metabolic clearance depends on xenobiotic concentration at the metabolizing sites with the following metabolic rate, v_c:

$$v_c = c_a \times \sum_{i=1}^{i=n} [V_{max(i)}/(K_{m(i)} + c)] \tag{21.1}$$

where V_{max} and K_m are analogs to Michaelis–Menten equation parameters (Section 1.10), c_a is the concentration of inhaled xenobiotic at these sites, and i indicates the metabolic pathways. At saturation zero-order kinetics are obeyed.

TABLE 21.1. Comparison of TLV and PEL, MAK-Werte, biological markers, BEI, BAT-Werte, and Japanese reference values for chemicals having adopted BEIs.

Chemical[a]	TLV and PEL (mg/m³)	MAK (mg/m³)	Biological marker[b]	BEI[c]	BAT[c]
Aniline (s)	7.6	8	*p*-Aminophenol (eu)	50 mg/g	
	8		Methemoglobin (eb)	1.5% Hb	
			Aniline (eu)		1 mg/L
			Aniline Hb adduct (eb)		0.1 mg/L
Benzene	32	C	Total phenol (eu)	50 mg/g	C
	3.2		Benzene (pmea)	0.08 ppm	
			Benzene (peea)	0.12 ppm	
Cadmium	0.05	C	Cadmium (u)	0.010 mg/g	0.015 mg/g
	0.1		Cadmium (b)	0.010 mg/L	0.015 mg/L
Carbon disulfide	31	30	2-Thiothiazolidine-4-carboxylic acid (eu)	5 mg/g	8 mg/L
	12				
Carbon monoxide	57	33	Carboxyhemoglobin (eb)	<8% Hb	5% Hb
	40		Carbon monoxide (eea)	<40 ppm	
Chlorobenzene	46		Total 4-chlorocatechol (eu)	150 mg/g	
	350		Total 4-chlorophenol (eu)	25 mg/g	
Cholinesterase inhibitors			Acetylcholinesterase (b; red blood cells)	70% baseline	70% (eb) baseline
Chromium (VI)	0.05	C	Total Cr (eu)	0.010 mg/g	C
	0.01		Total Cr (weu)	0.030 mg/g	
	ceil				
N,N-Dimethyl-formamide	30		N-methylformamide (eu)	40 mg/g	
	30				
Ethylbenene	434		Mandelic acid (weu)	1.5 g/g	
	435		Ethylbenzene (eea)		
Fluorides	2.5	2.5	Fluoride (pu)	3 mg/g	4 mg/g
	2.5		Fluoride (eu)	10 mg/g	7 mg/g
Furfural	7.9	—	Total furoic acid (eu)	200 mg/g	
	8				
n-Hexane	176	180	2,5-Hexanedione (eu)	5 mg/g	9 mg/L
	180				
Lead	0.15	0.1	Lead (b)	0.5 mg/L	0.3, 0.7 mg/L (m, f)
	0.05				
			Lead (u)	0.15 mg/g	
			Zinc-protoporphyrin (b)	1 mg/L	
			δ-aminolevulinic acid (u)	2.5 mg/L red blood cells	6, 15 mg/L (m, f)
Methemoglobin inducers			Methemoglobin (eb)	1.5% of Hb	
Methyl alcohol (s)	262	260	Methanol (eu)	15 mg/L	30 mg/L
	260		Formic acid (wpu)	80 mg/g	
Methyl chloroform	1910	1080	Methyl chloroform (peea)	40 ppm	20 ppm
	1900		Trichloroacetic acid (weu)	10 mg/L	
			Trichloroethanol (weu)	30 mg/L	
			Trichloroethanol (web)	1 mg/L	
			Methyl chloroform (pu)		0.55 mg/L
Methyl ethyl ketone	590	590	Methyl ethyl ketone (eu)	2 mg/L	5 mg/L
	590				
Nitrobenzene (s)	5.0	5.0	*p*-Nitrophenol (weu)	5 mg/g	
	5		Methemoglobin (eb)	1.5% Hb	
			Aniline Hb adduct (eb)		0.1 mg/L

TABLE 21.1. *continued*

Chemical[a]	TLV and PEL (mg/m^3)	MAK	Biological marker[b]	BEI[c]	BAT[c]
Parathion (s)	0.1	0.1	*p*-Nitrophenol (eu)	0.5 mg/g	0.5 mg/L
	0.1		Acetylcholinesterase (red blood cells)	70% baseline	70% baseline
Pentachlorophenol (s)	0.5	0.5	Pentachlorophenol (wpu)	2 mg/g	0.3 mg/L
	0.5		Pentachlorophenol (ep)	5 mg/L	1 mg/L
Perchloroethylene	339	345	Perchloroethylene (wpeea)	10 ppm	9.5 ppm
	170		Perchloroethylene (wpb)	1 mg/L	1 mg/L
			Trichloroacetic acid (weu)	7 mg/L	
Phenol (s)	19	19	Phenol (eu)	250 mg/g	300 mg/g
	19				
Styrene (s)	213	85	Mandelic acid (eu)	800 mg/g	2 g/L
	215		Mandelic acid (pu)	300 mg/g	
			Phenylglyoxylic acid (eu)	240 mg/g	
			Phenylglyoxylic acid (pu)	100 mg/g	
			Styrene (eb)	0.55 mg/L	
			Styrene (pb)	0.02 mg/L	
			Mandelic + phenylglyoxylic acids (eu)		2.5 mg/L
Toluene	377	380	Hippuric acid (eu)	2.5 mg/g	
	375		Toluene (evb)	1 mg/L	1.7 mg/L
Trichloroethylene	269	270	Trichloroacetic acid (weu)	100 mg/g	100 mg/L
	270		Trichloroacetic acid + trichloroethanol (weu)	300 mg/g	
			Trichloroethanol (web)	4 mg/L	5 mg/L
			Trichloroethylene (eea)		
Xylenes	434	440	Methylhippuric acids (eu)	1.5 g/g	2 g/L
			Methylhippuric acids (last 4 h of shift u)	2 mg/min	
	435		Xylenes (eb)		1.5 mg/L

[a] (s) signifies skin absorption demonstrated; all TLV values are from reference 6; MAK-Werte are from reference 13; final rule OSHA PEL values are from reference 14. C, carcinogen.

[b] b, blood; peb, end of shift blood; eea, end-exhaled air postshift (all during-shift breath samples were eliminated in 1990); pmea, mixed exhaled air prior to next shift; peea, end exhaled air prior to next shift; wpeea, end exhaled air prior to last shift of workweek; ep, end of shift plasma; eu, end of shift urine; evb, end of shift venous blood; weu, end of shift urine at end of week; wpu, prior to last shift urine of workweek; f, female; m, male; pb, prior to the next shift blood; wbb, blood prior to the last shift of workweek; web, blood at end of shift at end of workweek; pu, prior to the next shift urine; u, urine.

The following samples are also taken at the end of the work week: aniline in urine; aniline–hemoglobin adduct in blood; acetylcholinesterase in blood BAT; methanol in urine BAT; formic acid in urine; methyl chloroform in end-exhaled air; trichloroacetic acid in urine; trichloroethanol in urine; trichloroacetic acid + trichloroethanol in urine; trichloroethanol in blood; methyl chloroform in blood; *p*-nitrophenol in urine for nitrobenzene; pentachlorophenol in urine for the BEI; all of the perchloroethylene markers; styrene in blood; trichloroethylene in end-exhaled air.

[c] Urine concentrations are in weight of marker/volume of urine or weight of marker/weight of creatinine.

Note: The BAT value for 2,5-hexanedione in urine includes 4,5-dihydroxy-2-hexane.

Japanese minimum and upper reference values [10]:

Urinary 2,5-hexanedione for *n*-Hexane: 2, 5 mg/L.
Blood lead: 0.2, 0.4 mg/L.
Red cell zinc protoporphyrin for lead: 1, 2.5 mg/L.
Urinary δ-aminolevulinic acid for lead: 5, 10 mg/L.
Urinary trichloroacetic acid for methyl chloroform: 3, 10 mg/L.
Urinary total trichloro compounds for methyl chloroform: 10, 40 mg/L.
Urinary mandelic acid for styrene: 0.3, 1 g/L.
Urinary trichloroacetic acid for tetrachloroethylene, 3, 10 mg/L.
Urinary total trichloro compounds for tetrachloroethylene, 3, 10 mg/L.
Urinary hippuric acid for toluene: 1.0, 2.5 g/L.
Urinary trichloroacetic acid for trichloroethylene: 30, 100 mg/L.
Urinary total trichloro compounds for trichloroethylene: 100, 300 mg/L.

TABLE 21.2. Physiological parameters for the ACGIH five compartment models for a 170-cm tall man [15].

	Perfusion (L/min)			
Compartment	Sleep	Sitting	50 W work	Volume (L)
Liver	1.5	1.6	1.6	2.6
Vessel-rich	2.9	3.0	3.2	3.8
Muscles/skin	1.05	1.75	5.0	34.4
Fat/white marrow				
Slim	0.08	0.17	0.23	5.2
Standard	0.15	0.34	0.45	10.2
Overweight	0.3	0.68	0.90	20.2
Lung	4.0	5.3	14.5	V_d

The lung compartment includes tissue and gas. The perfusions for the lung are for alveolar ventilation.
V_d = functional residual capacity + tidal volume/3 + arterial blood volume × partition coefficient for blood/gas + lung tissue volume × partition coefficient for lung/gas = 2.7 + 1.4 partition coefficient for blood/gas + 0.6 partition coefficient for lung/gas.
Note: The rest compartment volumes as % of lean body volume are: splanchnic 5.8; venous blood, 8.3; muscles/skin, 69; fat, body fat volume; lung, 8.3 comprised of tissue (0.9), air (5.5) and arterial blood (1.9); brain, 2–6; kidneys, 0.53; others, 1.0.

The perfusion rates in mL/min/mL at rest are: muscles and skin, 33; adipose tissues, 22; brain, 570; kidneys, 4520; splanchnic, 520; lung air, 0.8 × cardiac output in L/min; lung tissue, perfusion rate × compartment volume in L/min; others, 2830.

The solution of the nonlinear model is found by numerical integration using the Euler backward formula [17]. The non-linear model is most used at high absorbed doses. The solution of both models can be obtained on an Apple II Plus computer.

21.3 BEIs: SOME LIMITATIONS

The limitations of BEIs reflect those of the reference TLVs, the inherent limitations of biological monitoring/environmental data (Chapters 3–9), and specific limitations associated with each marker. This section addresses the first two items. The specific chemical limitations are discussed in Section 21.4.

21.3.1 Limitations of TLVs

The utility of BEI values depends on the toxicological basis of the TLV [6] because BEIs are set by utilizing TLVs as reference values. The TLV usually is recommended from a consideration of acute effects from exposure to the single specific chemical. TLVs for individual compounds during exposure to multi-component mixtures may or may not be protective.

The TLVs take only inhalation into account, with no other absorption routes accounted for. Just occupational inhalation exposures are assumed, for 8 h/day, 5 days/week. The toxicology for continuous 24-h exposures over a lifetime utilized for U.S. EPA risk assessment may be very different from this, especially for compounds of whole body half-times greater than 12 h; but there may be little difference for compounds of very short half-times such as <4 h, depending on the exposure concentration. Usually hygienic air concentrations are low relative to capacity-limiting processes, but not always. Immediately Dangerous to Life and Health (IDLH) concentrations are another matter.

Therefore, extrapolations back and forth are not valid. Thus ACGIH weekly exposures of 40-h compared with a U.S. EPA one of 168-h leaves a factor of 168/40 = 4.2. Similarly, a daily hour basis yields a factor of 24/8 = 3, and a monthly hour-basis a factor of 720/160 = 4.5. The division of TLV values by those factors to obtain U.S. EPA equivalent values is only valid when the time courses of both exposure toxicologies are the same.

The contributions of dermal and oral exposure (Chapter 3) to the absorbed dose of xenobiotic can be substantial, involving hygiene, work practices, existence and effectiveness of personal protective equipment (PPE), whether unit processes are open or enclosed, and whether ventilation is adequate relative to the source of emission and the worker.

The ACGIH, until recently, has not paid much attention to carcinogens, merely denoting confirmed (A1) and suspected (A2) human carcinogens. In 1992, the classifications were changed to: A1, confirmed human carcinogen based on epidemiologic or clinical evidence; A2, suspected human carcinogen because of conflicting epidemiologic data, or in animals at conditions relevant to worker exposure; A3, animal carcinogen under conditions not relevant to worker exposure; A4, not classifiable as a human carcinogen based on inadequate animal/human data; and A5, not suspected as a human carcinogen on the basis of epidemiologic studies.

When the OSHA permissible exposure limit (PEL) is lower than the corresponding TLV (Table 21.1), the BEI marker may be inadequate, practically speaking, because the PEL is the legal requirement in the United States, not the TLV. Under such circumstances the BEI value will not be protective enough. For example, the OSHA PEL for benzene is 1 ppm, and the TLV is 10 ppm; and the urinary phenol and blood benzene markers suitable for a 10 ppm TLV are inadequate at a 1 ppm PEL because they cannot be distinguished from background—that is, the sensitivity of the marker is insufficient [18]. The only viable classic biological monitoring marker at 1 ppm benzene is benzene in breath at the end of a shift [81, 19]. Examples of chemicals with lower PELs than TLVs for chemicals with BEIs include carbon disulfide, carbon monoxide, lead, and perchloroethylene The TLV for cadmium is lower than the PEL. Safe levels for carcinogens generally are not obtainable by the BEI approach because of problems with the sensitivity of analytical chemistry methods.

21.3.2 General Workplace/Nonworkplace Exposure Limitations

Nonwork exposures are not factored into the TLV values; and this is a problem for ubiquitous pollutants of relatively high concentration and/or high toxicity such as carbon monoxide and benzene, and oxidant gases such as ozone, nitrogen dioxide, and sulfur dioxide. If the TLV values approach recommended U.S. EPA air concentrations to within two orders of magnitude, that is cause to ascertain the extent of nonoccupational exposures. If the exposures are predominantly work-related, there is much greater confidence that the TLV value will be fully protective and thus the BEI as well. Therefore, environmental monitoring truly supplements biological monitoring and vice versa. Both are necessary to gauge the safety of workplaces as well as the ambient environment.

Nonwork carbon monoxide exposure, which can occur on highways, in the home, through smoking, at discos, and at recreational sites, is not factored into the TLV. In such situations personal baseline samples of biological materials must be taken to determine if the source of the marker is in the workplace, or if mixed exposure is occurring that requires baseline correction so that the workplace can be adjudged to be safe or not. Baseline correction also is necessary if there are endogenous sources of the marker, a situation often reflected by extreme interpersonal variability relative to concentrations of biological monitoring markers. Correction for a nonoccupational exposure still may result in extreme interpersonal variation, but now reflecting the type of work exposure rather than artifacts. It must be emphasized that biological monitoring integrates exposures over all exposure routes. If concentrations of biological monitoring markers exceed critical levels, baseline monitoring is the crucial next step to decide if the exposures are work-related or not. If exposures are work-related, work practices, PPE, ventilation, and unit processes become important to observe and adjudge.

It is the author's experience that group comparisons are inadequate when group data are not statistically homogeneous or if multimodal distributions are present. The BEI recommendations of group comparisons in the presence of large interpersonal variations thus may not be sufficiently protective of high exposure and susceptible individuals. A relative standard deviation of >30% in the time weighted average values of a group is cause for investigation of personal baselines, as well as further direct-reading instrument sleuthing or the design of an appropriate questionnaire to ascertain the incidence of nonoccupational exposures. Most often there are not enough data to assess whether multimodal exposures are occurring. In this case data acquired for the same worker over extended periods of time should be plotted (frequency versus time weighted average air concentrations or versus measured concentration of biological monitoring marker corrected as appropriate for baseline) to assess the exposure mode or the representative values and ranges.

Another aspect of exposure that has not received enough attention is the assessment of physical activity and its influence on body burden although the BEI Committee does factor it into its pharmacokinetic simulation models (Section 21.2). Comparison of results in different workplaces is difficult if the work forces do not have about the same physical activities, or if the data are not normalized to the same work activity. (This topic is discussed in Section 3.0.1.) Conclusions of epidemiology studies may be skewed by this factor. Sedentary or less active workers will inhale less and excrete less in the urine than very active workers exposed to the same ambient concentrations. Therefore, sedentary or inactive individuals are the most conservative human models in human volunteer studies, all other things being equal and in the absence of interactions.

BEIs (or any critical concentration for exposure to just one specific compound) are not to be used whenever known interactions exist, for example, for ingested/inhaled ethyl alcohol and inhaled trichloroethylene. The existence of interactions, marker specificity/selectivity, and occurrence of hypersensitivity are the intrinsic limiting factors of biological monitoring techniques when utilized to assess hazard through critical values. All these variables have been discussed. (Sections 5.2, 5.3, 6.0, 8.4 and 8.5).

The usual practice in BEI urine sampling is to take spot samples just after a shift, before the next shift, or before/after the shift at the end of a work week (Table 21.1). The discussion in Section 6.0.2 indicated that spot sampling can be a poor substitute for full-shift sampling or for cumulative sampling after the work day, depending on the half-time of the metabolite and the duration and the time of exposure. A compromise has to be reached relative to worker convenience, legalities, the politics of worker/owner relationships, and science, all of which will depend largely on the conditions in each plant and the personal cooperation of the workers.

The instructions for BEI sampling should be regarded as the minimum required, as for any NIOSH method for air sampling or EPA method for environmental sampling. They may be inadequate in some cases, especially in those that require strict timing. It is up to the professionals (industrial hygienists, occupational nurses, university academics, and occupational physicians) to recognize circumstances where rigid adherence to a protocol may not produce a representative sample that truly reflects a hazard. Additional environmental sampling and the use of direct-reading instruments may be necessary to determine the sources and times of exposure so that sampling durations of urines can be optimized to yield a representative sample. The time after the last exposure at which the sample was collected and any sampling durations must be documented for all samples for characterization of sample representativeness. Along with these factors, documentation of work practices, ventilation, PPE, hygiene, and type of unit process (closed or enclosed) is required. This means that computer and data-logging skills are also necessary.

Noninvasive sampling procedures are favored. Metabolites are adequate markers if they are sensitive/specific/selective (for example, urinary methylhippuric acids for xylenes), or if other sources of the metabolite are known not to be present (urinary aniline is specific for aniline if nitrobenzene or some other precursor is not also present). The best BEI markers often are those that involve the xenobiotic as long as the latter is not also produced by metabolism, as phenol, carboxyhemoglobin, and methanol can be. Thus, the most reliable urinary markers for specific chemicals are for fluorides, methyl ethyl ketone, pentachlorophenol, and methylhippuric acids for exposure to xylenes; the strongest breath markers similarly are for methyl chloroform and trichloroethylene. The nonspecific markers acetylcholinesterase, methemoglobin, formic acid, hippuric acid, and *p*-nitrophenol are most simply interpreted for exposures predominantly to one precursor xenobiotic. For the latter situation, a carefully designed questionnaire, knowledge of chemicals utilized and unit processes, and environmental monitoring data may be required.

Nonspecific markers are useful when mixtures of their precursors are exposing workers because the task of evaluating all specific markers produced from multicomponent chemical exposures is costly and time-consuming. However, the environmental exposure concentrations must be known or at least estimated to be able to interpret biological monitoring data from exposures to multicomponent mixtures. The industrial hygienist can weight the composition of the solvents provided in Hazardous Material Data Sheets for dermal exposures, and can utilize a TLV/PEL air concentration by assuming additivity as a first approximation in order to predict a critical BEI for inhalation exposure, to assess whether more air monitoring is required. The sampling time recommendations for the marker must be the same for the xenobiotics as those contained in the BEI documentation.

For example, we want to calculate the critical BEI for a methyl chloroform/perchloroethylene mixture at TLV concentrations. Both chemicals have a common urinary trichloroacetic acid marker under the same sampling time conditions of 10 mg/L and 7 mg/L, respectively, at the end of the work week, corresponding to TLVs of 350 ppm (1900 mg/m^3) and 50 ppm (335 mg/m^3), respectively. The combined BEI is the sum of the two BEI values, that is, 17 mg/L urine. If complete air concentrations are known for these two compounds, for example, 400 ppm of methyl chloroform and 30 ppm of perchloroethylene, the observed concentration/TLV ratios for the compounds are 1.14 and 0.6, respectively, with respective corresponding urine concentrations of $1.14 \times 10 = 11.4$ mg/L and $0.6 \times 7 = 4.2$ mg/L, or a total of 15.6 mg/L. In this case the BEI for methylchloroform is exceeded, but not that for perchloroethylene, and their sum does not exceed the expected BEI for both. The individual BEI data are the only important data for this case because individual air monitoring data are known. Any biological monitoring data above this value under these air concentration conditions may imply a dermal exposure component or another source of marker.

More usually all that the hygienist has is one air concentration and the concentration of a nonspecific biological monitoring marker. Let us assume that the air concentration for perchloroethylene is 30 ppm, but the biological monitoring data for trichloroacetic acid is 15.6 mg/L urine. If it is known that methyl chloroform and no other precursor to the trichloroacetic acid marker is also present, then the above calculation is easily reversed. Thus $(30/50 = 0.6) \times 7$ mg/L accounts for air perchloroethylene, or 4.3 mg/L. The unaccounted for trichloroacetic acid is thus $15.7 - 4.2 = 11.5$ mg/L. Because the methyl chloroform BEI of 10 mg/L corresponds to 350 ppm, the methyl chloroform exposure could be $11.5/10 = 1.15$ times above the BEI, and so could the air concentration relative to the TLV for methyl chloroform. However, the presence of dermal exposure to both solvents is still possible. Here the worker's work routine and personal protective equipment must be observed, before deciding to do further air or skin exposure monitoring.

If a complete air concentration data set is not available for all the components, the air concentrations can be based on solvent composition from the Hazard Material Data Sheets as a first approximation or, more correctly, these data weighted by the respective partial pressures of the components as a second approximation—the higher the vapor pressure, the greater the expected exposure.

To illustrate, let a solvent mixture consist of 50% heptane, 30% methyl chloroform, and 20% perchloroethylene, all percentages being on a weight/weight basis (density differences must be corrected for if percentages are on a v/v basis because masses, not volumes, are additive). Let us assume no interactions with heptane for the trichloroacetic acid biological monitoring marker, and no other trichloroacetic acid precursors. If the observed urinary trichloroacetic acid concentration under BEI Committee recommended conditions is 15.7 mg/L, and there are no other data, we proceed by one of two approaches: the equilibrium approach that utilizes Raoult's law to provide a maximum answer or the Henry's Law approach to account for solubility.

If we assume that Raoult's law applies, the partial pressure (p) at equilibrium reflects the mole fraction of solvent (x) modified by its vapor pressure (P), or:

$$p = XP \tag{21.2}$$

The Henry's law type of calculation replaces P in equation (21.2) with the appropriate Henry's law constant (k_H) to calculate the p (in equations 21.3 and 21.4). The p from Raoult's law is generally higher than the p calculated from equation (21.4).

$$k_H = \text{Equilibrium concentration in air/Equilibrium concentration in solution} \tag{21.3}$$

$$k_H = \text{Vapor pressure air concentration/Solubility in solution} \tag{21.4}$$

The chlorinated solvents are soluble in all proportions in heptane or one another, and therefore approach ideal solution behavior that obeys Raoult's law.

The P values from Table 3.1 are 19 and 14 mm Hg at 20°C for methyl chloroform and perchloroethylene, respectively. The respective molecular weights from Table 3.1 are 133.4 and 165.8. The mole fractions for methyl chloroform and perchloroethylene respectively are:

$$(30/133.4)/[(30/133.4) + (20/165.8) + \text{moles of heptane}]$$

and:

$$(20/133.4)/[(30/133.4) + (20/165.8) + \text{moles of heptane}]$$

The number of moles of heptane is 50/100.2 = 0.50; therefore the total number of moles, calculated for the common denominators just above, is 0.22 + 0.12 + 0.50 = 0.84.

Thus, utilizing equation (21.2), the respective p values for methyl chloroform and for perchloroethylene are 0.22/0.84 times 19 mm Hg and 0.12/0.84 times 14 mm Hg, that is, 5.0 and 2.0 mm Hg at 20°C.

These partial pressures can be converted into air concentrations in g/L using equation (3.2) at 20°C:

$$m/V = pM/RT = pM/(760 \times 0.08205 \times 293) = pM/18{,}271 \tag{21.5}$$

Thus the equilibrium air concentrations expected for these solvents, assuming Raoult's law at 20°C for methyl chloroform and perchloroethylene for this mixture, are 36.5 and 18 mg/L or 36,500 and 18,000 mg/m^3. This is the p just at the surface of the liquid. Both these equilibrium concentrations are well above the TLV-TWA concentrations. They are high because equilibrium is assumed.

The actual concentrations exposing the worker are not under equilibrium conditions but are a dilution of the maximum possible.

Generally for the effective air exposing concentration:

$$\text{Rate of accumulation} = \text{Rate of generation} - \text{Rate of removal}$$

$$VdC = Gdt - Q'Cdt \tag{21.6}$$

where:

C = concentration of the contaminant (mass/volume)
G = rate of generation (mass/time)
Q' = Q/K = effective rate of ventilation (volume/time) corrected for incomplete mixing, Q is the actual ventilation rate (volume/time), and K is the design distribution constant allowing for incomplete mixing and ranges from 1 to 10.
V = volume of the enclosure

At steady state, $dC = 0$, and equation (21.6) becomes:

$$Gdt = Q'Cdt \tag{21.7}$$

After integrating both sides of equation (21.7) with respect to t:

$$C = G/Q' \tag{21.8}$$

$$C = KG/Q \tag{21.9}$$

The open area of the container was $10\,\text{cm}^2$ and the linear velocity of vapor escape was measured to be 0.5 m/sec (ventilation at container top). Therefore the volume escaping in one second is $(10 \times 10^{-4}) \times 0.5 = 5 \times 10^{-4}\,\text{m}^3$; that is, $1\,\text{m}^3$ escapes in 2000 sec. Therefore G values for methyl chloroform and perchloroethylene are 18 and 9.0 mg/sec, respectively.

If $K = 5$ for both methyl chloroform and perchloroethylene, G is 18 and 9.0 mg/sec for methyl chloroform and perchloroethylene, respectively, and Q is $1000\,\text{ft}^3/\text{min} = 28.3\,\text{m}^3/\text{min} = 0.47\,\text{m}^3/\text{sec}$; and equation (21.9) becomes

$$C = 5G/0.47\,\text{mg/m}^3 \tag{21.10}$$

Values of C for methylchloroform and perchloroethylene are 191 and $96\,\text{mg/m}^3$. These concentrations are well below the TLV concentrations. If the velocity of vapor escape is unknown or below detection limit, the container can be treated like a diffusion tube, and a leak rate thus estimated from diffusion theory. Another approach is to estimate vapor loss rate by weighing the container and contents at least twice at known times.

The hygienist may be faced with a hot process so that correction of the vapor pressure using the Clausius–Clapeyron equation (equation 21.11) may be necessary:

$$\ln\,[p_1/p_2] = -(H/R)\,(1/T_1 - 1/T_2) \tag{21.11}$$

where p values can be partial or vapor pressures at two different temperatures, T_1 and T_2 in degrees Kelvin; H is the latent heat of vaporization for the liquid, obtainable from handbooks of physical constants; and R is the gas constant in the appropriate units, usually $1.98717\,\text{cal}\,\text{K}^{-1}\,\text{mol}^{-1}$ if H is in cal/mol. The logarithm term is to the base e. The extent of pyrolysis product formation must also be known if compounds like aldehydes, ketones, alcohols and carboxylic acids are being investigated.

The measured high urinary concentration may be from an analytical artifact (quality control and assurance problems), contamination (laboratory, worker, or hygienist), another trichloroacetic acid source (a second look at the Hazardous Materials Data Sheets is indicated, or environmental analysis of suspected sources), dermal exposure, oral exposure, or a nonworkplace exposure source (baseline samples need to be taken); or interactions may be present.

If the initial volume of solvent mixture can be measured and also the final volume, then a utilized mass can be used directly in equations (21.6) and (21.9); and because the solvent composition is known, an estimate for exposure to each chemical over the time of evaporation or usage can be calculated. If one assumes that all the solvent volume utilized is evaporated (or if all of it is), an estimate of the maximum air mass of each chemical can be calculated over the time sampled. To show the validity of this calculation, a gas chromatographic analysis of residual solvent must be done to assess whether enrichment of solvent has occurred, which would invalidate the assumed vapor composition. If enrichment does occur, a mass balance approach for the initial solvent and the residual solvent must be performed to obtain the maximum evaporated masses of specific chemicals for a given exposure time period. Such calculations are indispensable to interpret the environmental and monitoring data, and to assess whether more environmental measurements are required.

If the observed biological monitoring marker concentration is >50% of the BEI calculated from theoretical values, it is recommended that the air concentrations of the other xenobiotics contributing to the urinary marker be found explicitly, usually by the expensive charcoal tube/gas chromatography/mass spectrometry technique or at least maximum concentrations obtained from the less expensive charcoal tube/gas chromatography screening. This precalculation process, as outlined above, is not an infallible technique but is useful to justify monitoring to management and to convince workers that the workplace is safe.

Nonspecific markers can be excellent and inexpensive screening markers that may indicate the need for further investigation. The fact that biological monitoring integrates over all routes of exposure is especially important (note that the BEI only accounts for inhalation exposure) if extensive skin absorption occurs, and air concentrations thus may not be related to the measured concentrations of markers in biological fluids and to adverse effects.

The utility of biological monitoring in assessing the protectiveness of respirators, gloves, and other PPE is well known, the most famous instance being the use of blood lead to assess the effectiveness of PPE and workplace hygiene/work practices.

21.4 INDIVIDUAL BEI FACTORS

All the appropriate physical and BEI parameters for the chemicals with adopted BEIs are contained in Tables 21.1 and 3.1. The chlorinated organic solvents such as methylene chloride, methyl chloroform, perchloroethylene, and trichloroethylene, which have a maximum water solubility at 25°C of ~2% w/w (methylene chloride), form layers under a water layer beyond their saturation solubilities, unlike hydrocarbon organic solvents such as benzene, ethylbenzene, toluene, styrene, xylenes, and *n*-hexane, which float on top of water under similar circumstances. The vapors of the chlorinated solvents are also heavier than air so that volatilized vapors tend to sink. The chlorinated solvents also tend to bioaccumulate in fat: females having more fat may have lower metabolite concentrations in urine than males of the same weight exposed to the same concentration of xenobiotic. Chlorinated solvents are also absorbed dermally, and have long (>5 h) half-times of metabolism. In general the more water-soluble the chemical is at pH 7.4, the more likely it is to have a short whole-body half-time (<5 h) after inhalation, whether the excretion route is the breath, urine, or feces, or all of these. Aliphatic aldehyde, ketone, and alcohol solvents and their nitrogen and sulfur analogs tend to have high vapor pressures, water solubilities >2%, and high dermal penetration properties. As the vapor pressure increases in a series of chemically similar compounds, breath exhalation assumes greater importance although increasing water and tissue solubility are competing processes. Increased physical activity enhances uptake by inhalation but decreases lung retention because of increased exhalation rate. Inhalation also must be considered for nonvolatile chemicals (vapor pressures less than 10^{-4} mm Hg at 25°C) because particulates also are breathed in, the larger ones (>10–15 μm) in aerodynamic diameter) ultimately being ingested and the smaller ones being absorbed directly into the bloodstream or through the lymphatic system. These topics were treated in detail in earlier chapters (Chapters 3–6). Specific methods of analysis (that is, chromatography/detection) are meant to be utilized except for nitrobenzene, where only a colorimetric method is available, a situation that casts doubt on the interpretation of that assigned BEI.

Each documentation includes the following headings: Recommended BEI, Properties, Absorption, Possible Non-occupational Exposure, Elimination, Metabolic Pathways, TLV-TWA, and Summary; and the markers themselves are subdivided into sections such as: Methods, Sampling and Storage, Levels without Occupational Exposure, Kinetics, Factors Affecting Interpretation, Justification, Current Data Bases, and Recommendations.

The documentation publication includes an Introduction to the Biological Exposure Indices, Sources of Variability in Biological Monitoring (subdivided into Industrial Environment and the Human Body), Dermal Absorption, and Biological Specimens (Selection, Exhaled Air, Blood, and Urine), supplemented by special reviews and reports appearing in *Applied Occupational and Environmental Hygiene*.

We will concentrate on factors that are important to the interpretation of the biological monitoring data of the documentation chemicals [4].

21.4.1 Aniline

Aniline ($C_6H_5 \cdot NH_2$) is a clear liquid when pure (brown/yellow when diazo products are present), with a boiling point of 185°C. Aniline is present in many dyes, and is often used for their synthesis. Also it is in some medicinals, resins, varnishes, perfumes, shoe blacks, and vulcanized rubber. A TLV of 2 ppm (7.6 mg/m^3) (skin) is set to prevent methemoglobinemia, the first sign of toxic aniline exposure.

Aniline is readily absorbed through the skin from the vapor or the liquid form. Thus dermal and lung inhalation are known routes of exposure. About 90% is absorbed on inhalation. Aniline is a metabolite of: industrial chemicals such as singly substituted alkyl anilines, phenylhydroxylamine, *p*-nitroaniline, dimethylaniline, hydrazobenzene, *p*-toluidine, nitrobenzene, and acetanilide; the drugs phenacetin, *p*-phenetidin, and acetanilide; and phenazopyridine (disinfectant). It is a biodegradation product of the pesticides Propham, Carbetamide, Fenuron, and Siduron. About 13 to 40% of absorbed aniline is metabolized directly via ring hydroxylation and by acetylation to produce acetanilide ($C_6H_5 \cdot NHCO \cdot CH_3$) before ring hydroxylation to *p*-aminophenol [4-aminophenol ($HO \cdot C_6H_4 \cdot NH_2$)], partially conjugated as the *O*-glucuronide and the *O*-sulfate, with 89% of the total metabolite eliminated within 24-h postexposure and with less than 1% expelled unchanged in the expired breath and urine. The half-time is 3 to 5 h. *p*-Aminophenol is not produced endogenously, but interactions occur on ethanol ($CH_3 \cdot CH_2 \cdot OH$) ingestion (which increase the half-time) and after exposure to other xenobiotics producing hydroxylated intermediates. Hydroxylation of aniline also can occur at the nitrogen to form phenylhydroxylamine ($C_6H_5 \cdot NHOH$), responsible for methemoglobinemia, and it is further oxidized to nitrosobenzene ($C_6H_5 \cdot NO$). All these processes are reversible. The phenylhydroxylamine appears in the urine as its *N*-glucuronide and *N*-sulfate.

Equation (21.12) gives the aniline uptake (D) due to skin absorption and inhalation:

$$D = c_a t(X_i V + v) \tag{21.12}$$

where:

c_a = aniline concentration in ambient air
t = exposure duration
X_i = fraction of inhaled aniline absorbed
V = pulmonary ventilation
v = volume of air from which aniline is completely removed by dermal absorption

A standard worker has $c_a = 8\,\text{mg/m}^3$; $t = 8\,\text{h}$; $X_i = 0.9$; $V = 1.5\,\text{m}^3/\text{h}$; and $v = 0.47\,\text{m}^3/\text{h}$. Thus $D = 116\,\text{mg}$.

The daily urinary excretion of *p*-aminophenol (the BEI at end of shift is 50 mg/g creatinine) is about 30% of the absorbed dose, resulting in daily excretion of about 40 mg, equivalent to a urinary concentration at the end of a workshift of about 57 mg/L, assuming a half-time of 3 h and a mean urine volume of 1.2 L/day. There are considerable interpersonal variations; so a group test is recommended.

Methemoglobinemia is the basis of the TLV. Clinical cyanosis does not occur until the methemoglobin level reaches 10%, and levels >60% are life-threatening. The methemoglobin BEI for aniline is set at 1.5% of total hemoglobin.

21.4.2 Benzene

Benzene (C_6H_6) is a colorless liquid with a low boiling point of 80°C. It contains a resonating cyclic system of 3 Π C–C bonds on top of a cyclic framework of 6 σ C–C bonds (see Chapter 1). Six σ C–H bonds are attached also. Industrial uses of benzene (in synthesis of medicinals, dyes, artificial leather, linoleum, oil cloth, airplane dopes, varnishes, and lacquers, and as a solvent and paint remover) have been steadily decreasing since its leukemic properties were discovered. Traces (1.5%) of benzene occur in U.S. car gasoline and much more (up to 30%) in gasolines used in other countries. It is a trace contaminant of carbon disulfide and technical toluene. The TLV is set to avoid blood dyscrasias (but not to protect against leukemia (see Section 21.3.1)), the basis of the OSHA PEL value.

Both skin and inhalation absorption have been reported. About one-third of absorbed benzene is excreted as conjugated phenol ($C_6H_5 \cdot OH$) (as *O*-glucuronide and *O*-sulfate) and *o*- and *p*-cresols ($C_6H_4 \cdot (OH)_2$) and higher phenols. The urinary BEI is for total phenol, 50 mg/L, collected at the end of the shift. Approximately 12% of benzene is exhaled unchanged following 8 h of exposure at the TLV (triphasic half-times of 25 min, 2.5 h, and 30 h). It can act as a carbon source. Total phenol is also a metabolic product of proteins (background varies between 0 and 20 mg/L), in addition to being present in cough/throat medications, disinfectants, floor washes, germicidal paints, slimicides, mouthwashes, soaps, some drugs, the diet, and some atmospheric emissions from coal-fired power plants and certain hazardous waste dumps. The urinary BEI is based on human data for workers. The half-times of phenol for urine elimination are 5.7 and 28 h. A group test is recommended because of extreme individual variability.

The benzene in breath (0.12 ppm end-exhaled or 0.08 ppm mixed-exhaled) marker prior to the next shift also recommended is as a BEI, and is the only marker that can be used for a 1 ppm OSHA PEL standard (Section 21.3.1). It is greatly affected by physical activity, multiple exposures of benzene, and nonoccupational exposures to benzene before the sampling time. In recommending the breath BEI, the exposure duration has to be estimated, the equations utilized (equations 21.13 and 21.14) being invalid for single exposures.

For benzene in mixed-exhaled breath:

$$c_{16}[\text{mix}]/c_a = t/1000 \tag{21.13}$$

and for end-exhaled breath:

$$c_{16}[\text{end}]/c_a = 1.5t/1000 \tag{21.14}$$

where $c_{16}[\text{mix}]$, $c_{16}[\text{end}]$, and c_a are the benzene concentrations in mixed-exhaled air 16 h after exposure, in end-exhaled air 16 h after exposure, and during exposure, respectively; and t is the duration of exposure in hours.

21.4.3 Cadmium and Compounds

Cadmium and its compounds are mostly encountered in the workplace as oxide and metal fume produced during smelting, tapping, and pouring operations. It is present in many solders, easily fusible alloys, and photoelectric cells, and is used in electroplating processes, process engraving, amalgams, and nickel–

cadmium storage batteries. It is associated with zinc geologically. Tobacco smoke is an important source of cadmium exposure: the estimated absorption from nonsmoking areas is about 0.5 to 1.5 μg/day, whereas smoking 20 cigarettes/day adds about 0.5 to 2 μg/day. The TLV of 50 μg/m^3 for dusts, salts, and cadmium oxide production and the ceiling of 50 μg/m^3 for cadmium oxide fume are based on the prevention of urinary proteinuria after chronic exposure. Most workers exposed to 50 μg/m^3 are estimated to show proteinuria after 8 to 10 years of exposure; up to 20% are estimated to exhibit proteinuria after 10 years of exposure to 25 μg/m^3. In 1989 a recommendation was made to lower the TLV to 0.01 mg/m^3 for total dust, and 0.002 mg/m^3 for respirable dust, based on the potential for lung cancer and preclinical kidney dysfunction with urinary β_2-microglobulin excretion (considered to be a marker of proximal tubule defect) above 290 μg/L. Increased urinary excretion of *N*-acetyl-β-d-glucosaminidase represented functional enzymuria (isoenyme A) or damage to tubular cells (isoenzyme B). Enhanced excretion for both urinary markers of adverse effect occurred at >5 μg/g creatinine.

Inhalation of respirable particles is the major route of exposure. The average gastrointestinal absorption efficiency is usually about 3 to 7%, but it increases to up to 20% in nutritional deficiencies of iron, calcium, and protein. Between 40% and 80% of body cadmium is stored in the liver and kidneys, with one-third of that in the kidneys. Because cadmium has a long half-time of 10 to 30 years, the past history of exposure is important in interpreting biological monitoring data, the latter usually predicated on urinary cadmium, with some in the feces as well. Thus, timing is not critical in sampling time and duration. The background level for urinary cadmium is about 0.02 to 4.5 μg/L. The elimination is triphasic: the first phase reflects nonsaturation of binding sites in the kidney, the second phase results in an increase in urinary cadmium once all the binding sites are saturated, and the third phase is characterized by a steadily increasing excretion due to depletion of the kidney stores of cadmium because of renal dysfunction. The kidney thus stores cadmium until damage is such that it appears sharply increased in the urine, and thus is a marker of adverse chronic effect. Therefore, creatinine normalization of urinary concentrations is not adequate except during the first phase. The urinary BEI is 10 μg/g creatinine. There is an intent in 1992 to lower this concentration to 5 μg/g creatinine based on urinary excretion of markers of adverse effect and potential lung cancer effects.

Cadmium is transported by metallothionein. Red blood cells contain the most metallothionein of the blood cells; so blood cadmium is thought to reflect recent exposures. The BEI in whole blood of 10 μg/L is based on empirical information from several field studies. A recommendation has been made to lower the BEI to 5 μg/L based on adverse renal effects and potential lung cancer. OSHA in 1990 proposed annual monitoring of workers exposed to cadmium.

21.4.4 Carbon Disulfide

Carbon disulfide boils at 46.5°C, and is an inflammable liquid producing carbon dioxide and sulfur dioxide on burning. It is used in the manufacture of viscose rayon, carbon tetrachloride, xanthogenates, soil disinfectants, and electronic vacuum tubes. It is utilized in industrial hygiene chemistry for desorption of charcoal tubes. The TLV of 10 ppm is based on prevention of chronic neurological disturbances; the OSHA PEL is 4 ppm (Section 21.3.1).

The major route of entry is inhalation, but dermal absorption also is known. Absorbed carbon disulfide is concentrated in the red blood cells, in free and in acid-labile forms. Carbon disulfide is 10 to 30% exhaled after absorption, depending on physical activity, with a half-time less than 1 h. The initial short half-time is about 10 min. A longer half-time associated with the bound acid-labile form in blood has a half-time of about 2 to 3 days. Accumulation thus occurs in the tissues and blood. Less than 1% of the absorbed dose is excreted unchanged in the urine. The identified urinary metabolites include thiocarbamide ($NH_2 \cdot CS \cdot NH_2$), 2-thiothiazolidine-4-carboxylic acid ($C_3H_4NS_2 \cdot COOH$ or TTCA, the marker for the end-of-shift BEI of 5 mg/g creatinine), and 2-mercapto-2-thiazolin-5-one ($C_3H_3NOS_2$). TTCA is active in the sodium azide test traditionally utilized as a nonspecific biological monitoring test for carbon disulfide exposure concentrations greater than 16 ppm; it represents about 6% of the carbon disulfide absorbed. The urine is collected at the end of the shift, and results are normalized to creatinine. TTCA also is produced after exposure to Captan, Disulfiram (used in the management of alcoholism and in the rubber industry), and probably to other thiurams and dithiocarbamates often used as pesticides. Urinary sodium azide–sensitive metabolites produced by exposure to carbon disulfide have a half-time of about 1.4 h. TTCA in humans appears to show biphasic excretion half-times of 4 to 6 h and 2 to 3 days.

The BEI is set on human studies in viscose rayon plants based on end-of-shift values. The available studies disagree in their data, but two produce similar results. One of these studies correlated carbon disulfide in air in mg/m^3 (c_a) with TTCA concentration in mmol TTCA/mol creatinine in end-of-shift urines (c_u) of 19 workers with a correlation coefficient of 0.80:

$$c_a = 7.4\,c_u + 1.8 \tag{21.15}$$

21.4.5 Carbon Monoxide

Because carbon monoxide is a gas, the major route of absorption is through inhalation. Carbon monoxide is a ubiquitous product of combustion, and it is a component of natural gas, many deaths being caused through exposures to defective home heaters. Automobile exhaust may produce carbon monoxide concentrations of up to 100 ppm with carboxyhemoglobin of 5% or more. Other sources include tobacco smoke (carbon monoxide air concentrations may exceed 200 ppm; one pack of cigarettes per day produces blood carboxyhemoglobin levels of 5–6%, two to three packs produce 7 to 9% carboxyhemoglobin, and cigars can produce up to 20%) and internal combustion engines and motors. The TLV before 1992 was based on effects on cardiovascular performance under physical stress as a result of carbon monoxide binding 200 to 250 times more avidly to hemoglobin than oxygen to form carboxyhemoglobin. The TLV was lowered to 25 ppm in 1992, based on preventing neurobehavioral changes (decrease in vigilance and multitask performance), maintaining cardiovascular exercise capacity under strenuous conditions, and safeguarding susceptible groups such as pregnant workers (because of the greater affinity of fetal Hb for

CO than that of adult Hb after the placenta is crossed, and because mothers who smoke heavily give birth to babies of lower birthweight, increased infant mortality, and lower IQ than nonsmoking mothers) and those with cardiovascular (increased ventricular arrhythmias for patients with ischemic heart disease and arrhythmias conditions) and respiratory disease.

Carbon monoxide traditionally is detected in biological systems by blood carboxyhemoglobin. Carbon monoxide is formed endogenously (0.4–0.7% carboxyhemoglobin) as a metabolite of hemoglobin and other heme proteins (Section 2.11.5), and as a metabolite of methylene chloride (an industrial solvent often used for paint stripping that produces 3–5% carboxyhemoglobin after 8 h exposure at its TLV of 100 ppm). The half-time is about 5 h but is affected markedly by physical activity.

The relationship between percentage oxygen content in alveolar air ($\%O_2$) and carbon monoxide ambient air concentration (%CO) in terms of blood carboxyhemoglobin concentration (COHb) is given by the following equation:

$$\%\mathrm{CO} = (\%\mathrm{O_2}/a)\ [(\mathrm{COHb}/(100-\mathrm{COHb})] \tag{21.16}$$

where a is the ratio of affinities of CO and O_2 to hemoglobin (usually 200–250). The $\%O_2$ is about 14 to 15%, and COHb is measured at steady state.

Altitudes above 5000 feet cause lower $\%O_2$ and thus greater susceptibility to CO. The half-time for COHb ranges between 128 and 409 min. People with cardiovascular disease and those who are pregnant also may be more susceptible to CO. It is recommended that blood samples be collected at the end of a shift for the BEI of 8% of total hemoglobin. It was recommended in 1992 that this be lowered to 3.5% of hemoglobin.

Carbon monoxide (40 ppm) in end-exhaled breath sampled within 10 to 15 min of cessation of exposure is recommended as a BEI. It was recommended in 1992 that this value be lowered to 20 ppm. Endogenous CO concentration is <2 ppm. Values <30 ppm occur for patients with hemolytic anemia; 30 to 35 ppm for one pack/day smokers; 45 to 50 ppm for two to three packs/day smokers; up to 130 ppm for cigar smokers; >30 ppm in commuters exposed to automobile exhaust; and 15 to 30 ppm for workers exposed 8 h to methylene chloride at its TLV of 100 ppm. The half-time of CO in alveolar air following exposure ranges between 2 and 7 hours, depending on physical activity. Care must be taken to ensure that there is no infiltration of sampling equipment with workplace carbon monoxide.

21.4.6 Chromium[VI]

Chromium[VI] fume encountered in manual metal arc stainless steel welding operations contains about 60% water-soluble fume with 40% water-insoluble particulate. Water-soluble chromium[VI] mist is also produced during some electrochrome plating operations, but the BEI is not applicable to this situation. Chromium is an essential metal of at least 100 μg/day. Food, drinking water, ambient air, and tobacco smoke contain chromium. The TLV of 0.05 mg/m^3 is based on prevention of irritation of the respiratory tract and possible kidney and liver damage. The TLV does not protect against carcinogenic effects of Cr(VI).

Absorption of Cr[VI] increases with water solubility and decreases with increasing particle size. Dermal and gastrointestinal absorption also occur, with 10% of an oral dose being absorbed through the gastrointestinal tract. Background levels of urinary chromium are typically <1 ng/mL. The elimination of Cr[VI] is triphasic and is in the form of Cr[III] in the urine and the blood. The half-times are about 7 h, 15 to 30 days, and 3 to 5 years. The end-of-shift and end-of-work-week urinary BEI of 30 μg chromium/g creatinine (which requires a minimum bladder collection time of 2 h) and the during-shift BEI of 10 μg/g creatinine apply only to workers with a chronic history of chromium[VI] exposure because the chromium excretion rate increases with exposure duration. A baseline urine sample is also recommended to correct for accumulation. The BEIs are set on averaging the results of seven (end-of-shift) and four (during-shift) field studies on workers of at least 7 years' welding experience. Most of these studies did not correct for chromium[VI] baseline concentrations. Large interpersonal differences occur, but the average results agree "reasonably well." The BEI for new welding workers has been proposed as 7 μg/g creatinine end-of-shift. There is some evidence of urinary proteinuria at 5.3 ± 3.7 μg chromium[VI]/g creatinine (10% of 36 workers using special electrode welding on armored steel), but it was not associated with urinary chromium[VI].

21.4.7 Dimethylformamide

Dimethylformamide or *N,N*-dimethylformamide (DMF; $HCON(CH_3)_2$) is a liquid with a boiling point of 153°C. DMF is used as a solvent for Orlon and other polyacrylic synthetic fibers as well as in paint remover, printing ink, and shoe polish. The TLV of 10 ppm (30 mg/m^3) was set to prevent liver function and reproductive changes.

DMF is absorbed through the lung, skin, and gastrointestinal tract. The DMF concentration in blood declines rapidly with little excreted in the urine. DMF is oxidized to *N*-Methyl-*N*-hydroxymethylformamide ($HCONCH_3 \cdot CH_2OH$), *N*-methylformamide ($HCONH \cdot CH_3$), and formamide ($HCONH_2$) in that order, all being excreted in the urine. Other degradation products include formic acid (HCOOH), α-amino formic acid (NH_2COOH), formhydroxylamine (HCONHOH), and carbon dioxide (O=C=O). The urinary BEI is *N*-methylformamides (sum of *N*-methyl-*N*-hydroxymethylformamide and *N*-monomethylformamide) end-of-shift for the last 2 h at 40 mg/g creatinine. About 2 to 6% of absorbed inhaled DMF is excreted as *N*-methylmethylformamides, with preshift concentrations typically being about one-third end-of-shift concentrations. Half-time estimates vary, but average about 4 h in field and volunteer studies. Two different groups of investigators found the relationships (equations 21.17 and 21.18) between the daily urinary excretion rate of *N*-methylformamides in mg/day (r_u) and personal exposure air concentration of DMF in mg/m^3 (c_a) below 27 ppm to be:

$$r_u = 0.41\ c_a - 1.16 \qquad (r = 0.89) \tag{21.17}$$

$$r_u = 0.474\ c_{ah} + 0.894 \qquad (r = 0.90) \tag{21.18}$$

where c_{ah} is in units of ppm-h.

21.4.8 Ethylbenzene

Ethylbenzene is a colorless liquid with a boiling point of 136°C. It is a constituent of commercial xylenes often used as paint thinners, motor cleaners, or solvents. The TLV of 100 ppm (435 mg/m^3) is based on prevention of irritation and narcotic effects.

Inhalation exposure predominates, though ethylbenzene is absorbed through the skin and after ingestion. Ethylbenzene is metabolized to 1-phenylethanol ($C_6H_5 \cdot CHOH \cdot CH_3$, found in the urine as a glucuronide) and thence to mandelic acid ($C_6H_5 \cdot CHOH \cdot COOH$, 64% in the urine) and acetophenone ($C_6H_5 \cdot CO \cdot CH_3$) by competing paths, both finally forming phenylglyoxylic acid ($C_6H_5 \cdot CO \cdot COOH$, 25% in the urine), which is in equilibrium with mandelic acid. Traces of phenaceturic acid, hippuric acid, ethylphenols, and hydroxyacetophenones also are found in urine. Mandelic acid is the preferred urinary BEI marker at 2 g/L or 1.5 g/g creatinine, to be sampled at the end of the shift and the workweek. The urinary excretion of mandelic acid is characterized by a half-time of about 5 h for ethylbenzene, but its excretion after styrene exposure is biphasic with half-times of about 4 h and 25 h. The mandelic acid marker is not specific, as it can be produced from all long-chain singly substituted normal benzenes with an even number of carbons (through β-oxidation) as well as after exposure to 1-phenylethanol, 1-halo-phenylethyl compounds, ammonium mandelate, phenylglyoxylic acid, α-phenylaminoacetic acid, styrene, styrene glycol, and styrene oxide. The data on which the BEI is based are from laboratory studies, with urine collection recommended over the last 4 h of the last shift of a work week.

Ethylbenzene at 2 ppm in end-exhaled air collected before the last shift of the work week is recommended for the BEI breath marker. The marker is specific for ethylbenzene. The excretion is triphasic with half-times 3 min, 90 min, and 2 days. Ethylbenzene accumulates so that urinary mandelic acid levels and breath ethylbenzene concentrations increase steadily, even for the same ambient exposure. Both are affected by physical activity. The BEI was derived through a computer simulation.

21.4.9 Fluorides

The corresponding TLV of 2.5 mg/m^3 is for prevention of irritant effects and disabling bone changes after exposure to metallic fluorides (F^-), hydrogen fluoride (HF), and fluorine (F_2). Fluorides of alkali metals and of ammonium ion (monovalent) are more water-soluble than bivalent metal fluorides. Fluorides of higher valency generally hydrolyze in water except for the inert forms of cryolite (aluminum–potassium fluorides). Hydrofluoric acid is a weak acid that in concentrated solution attacks glass. Fluorine is a very reactive gas of high toxicity. Water supplies often are fluoridated, as are many toothpastes, mouthwashes, pills, and lozenges. Fluorides also are found in leaves, salt water fish, vegetables, and tea. The average daily input through the diet is 0.2 to 0.3 mg/day, and 1.0 mg/day (4 mg/L but with maximum concentrations of about 33 mg/L known) comes from drinking water. Environmental concentrations of fluorides may be high in water flowing over soils and geological strata rich in phosphate and cryolite and in regions near phosphate and aluminum plants. The release of fluorides by chlorofluorocarbons during metabolism is much less than the release of chloride ion or radicals. Some medications such as Fluoritab, Theraflur, Flurone ointment, fluorosteroids, fluorinated anesthetics, or Fluorvite decongestant contain fluoride. Exposure to household rust-removers or naval jelly may increase fluoride intake.

Toxicity from inhalation, dermal, and gastrointestinal absorption is known. About 90 to 97% of water-soluble fluoride is absorbed after oral ingestion. About 62% of calcium fluoride is absorbed. These data are not typical of pregnant women. Approximately half of the absorbed fluoride is excreted rapidly in urine, with a half-time of 4 to 7 h. The excretion rate is decreased by increased magnesium and calcium, and increased by increased iron intakes. Urinary pH also has been correlated with changes in fluoride excretion. About 5 to 30% of the fluoride ingested is excreted in the feces, with significant amounts also in the sweat and human milk. Fluoride elimination after intermittent exposure is triphasic, the soft tissues showing rapid excretion (on the order of weeks) with the skeletal component being biphasic (lasting for years). The urinary BEI requires sample collection preshift, preferably after 2 days without exposure (3 mg/L), and postexposure at the end of the shift (10 mg/L). Subtraction of the two gives the workplace contribution BEI for the fast excretion component of 7 mg/L. The BEI is not applicable to nonmetal fluorides or chlorofluorocarbons. Urine containers must be plastic. Showering is recommended before sampling.

The BEI was set on several field, environmental, and computer simulation studies, where effects such as hypertension and changes in bone structure (fluorosis) were considered in the presence of exposure data. For 24-h urines, the BEI was considered to be 5 mg/L which in end-of-shift specimens is equivalent to 9 mg/L and in preshift specimens 2 mg/L. A computer simulation model predicted preshift and end-of-shift urine concentrations of 2.1 and 16 mg/L, respectively, whereas all industrial field studies supported respective concentrations of 3.5 and 13 mg/L. The final respective BEIs were 3 and 10 mg/g creatinine.

Effects on the specific ion electrode used to measure fluoride militate against a blood BEI, the blood concentrations being one-tenth of those for urine and near the detection limit of the technique.

21.4.10 Furfural

Furfural ($C_4H_3O \cdot CHO$) is a colorless liquid when pure (technical furfural is brownish/yellowish), with a boiling point of 162°C, and is moderately soluble in water (about 8 g/100 mL). It is an aromatic system whose cyclic part (C_4H_3O) is flat, and which has continuous conjugation of the two ring C–C Π electron clouds with the Π electron clouds of the side-chain aldehyde group, as well as with the lone-pair electrons of the ring oxygen. Furfural is used as a herbicide and a fungicide, and traces are found in some cereal brans and essential oils. It is used in the manufacture of furfural–phenol plastics such as Durite and in varnishes, and is used as a solvent for the refining of petroleum oils, for nitrated cotton, for cellulose acetate, and for gums. It is used to accelerate rubber vulcanization. The TLV-TWA of 2 ppm (7.9 mg/m^3) is set to prevent lung and skin irritation. NIOSH reports that eye irritation, nasal stuffiness, and dryness of the mouth may be experienced above 5 ppm.

About 78% of inhaled furfural is absorbed, and 20 to 30% of the skin-applied chemical is absorbed at a rate of about 0.2 mg/cm^2/h. About 1% of absorbed furfural after 8 h of inhalation around the TLV-TWA is exhaled. Furfural is predominantly oxidized to furoic acid ($C_4H_3O \cdot COOH$), which then is conjugated with glycine to produce urinary furoylglycine ($C_4H_3O \cdot CONH \cdot CH_2COOH$). A very minor competing pathway (0.5–5% of the total absorbed dose) results in production of 2-furanacrylic acid ($C_4H_3O \cdot CH = CHCOOH$), which on glycine conjugation is excreted as urinary 2-furanacryluric acid ($C_4H_3O \cdot CH{=}CH \cdot CONH \cdot CH_2 \cdot COOH$). Free furoic acid may appear at high doses of furfural. The production of urinary furoylglycine is linear to a furfural concentration of 8 ppm. The urinary BEI is 200 mg/g creatinine at the end of a workshift or during the time of peak exposure if known, as analyzed after hydrolysis of urinary furoylglycine. The half-time is 2 h. Urine samples must be frozen on collection. The BEI was set on two volunteer studies using 2 and 8 ppm exposure concentrations and three field investigations. It includes the contribution of endogenous furoic acid.

Furoylglycine is naturally present in human urine at about 3 to 60 mg/g creatinine, depending on diet (especially in coffee drinkers), according to a circadian rhythm favoring greater day excretion. The average day level is about 15 mg/g creatinine. Furoylglycine also is excreted by people exposed to furfuryl alcohol, furfural diacetate, furfural hydrazone, furfuryl propionate, furylacrylic acid, and methylfuryl acrylate.

21.4.11 *n*-Hexane

n-Hexane (C_6H_{14}) is a colorless organic liquid with a boiling point of 69°C. Commercial hexane is a mixture of hexane isomers containing 20 to 80% *n*-hexane, and is widely used as industrial solvent. The other hexane isomers are much less toxic than *n*-hexane. *n*-Hexane is a ubiquitous component of lower-boiling fractions of petroleum ethers, and products such as glues and polishes contain it. Gasoline contains up to 1.5%. The TLV of 180 mg/m^3 or 50 ppm was set to prevent polyneuropathy.

n-Hexane is known to be absorbed by all routes of exposure. Because of its high vapor pressure, the major route in the occupational environment is inhalation, about 5 to 33% of inhaled *n*-hexane being absorbed. Thus exhalation is a major route of excretion; end-exhaled air concentrations during work for exposures of 45 to 400 ppm plateau at 85% of inhaled concentration, and 50 to 60% is exhaled after a 4-h exposure at the TLV. The exhalation process is biphasic with half-times of 14 min and 2.7 h.

About one-third of the absorbed amount is excreted in the urine, mostly as metabolites. The first step is oxidation to 2-hexanol ($CH_3 \cdot C(OH)H \cdot (CH_2)_3 \cdot CH_3$), which is further oxidized to either methyl-*n*-butyl ketone (2-hexanone, $CH_3 \cdot CO \cdot (CH_2)_3 \cdot CH_3$) or 2,5-hexanediol ($CH_3 \cdot C(OH)H \cdot (CH_2)_2 \cdot C(OH)H \cdot CH_3$), which both enventually produce 5-hydroxy-2-hexanone ($CH_3 \cdot CO \cdot (CH_2)_2 \cdot C(OH)H \cdot CH_3$). The latter can have three fates: (1) enolization, oxidation, and cyclization to 2,5-dimethylfuran ($C_4H_2O \cdot (CH_3)_2$); (2) oxidation to 2,5-hexanedione ($CH_3 \cdot CO \cdot (CH_2)_2 \cdot CO \cdot CH_3$); and (3) α-oxidation, decarboxylation, and further oxidation to 4-hydroxypentanoic acid ($CH_3 \cdot CO \cdot (CH_2)_2 \cdot C(OH)H \cdot CH_3$), which can cyclize further to a five-membered-ring compound, γ-valerolactone ($C_4H_5O_2 \cdot CH_3$). 2,5-Hexanedione causes the neurotoxic effect of both *n*-hexane and methyl-*n*-butyl ketone and is excreted in the urine (35% of the urinary metabolites of *n*-hexane). One BEI is thus end-of-shift 2,5-hexanedione in urine at 5 mg/L. Two field studies have shown that between 90 and 140 ppm of hexane the excretion of 2,5-hexanedione in end-of-shift samples is linear. Air concentrations of *n*-hexane lower than 1.5 ppm caused no excretion of 2,5-hexanedione. Higher-exposure air concentrations are thought to cause metabolism to be capacity-limited with eventual metabolic inhibition. Interactions with other solvents such as toluene have been observed. Toluene exposure inhibits *n*-hexane metabolism.

For end-of-shift samples collected after 8-h exposures, the regression equation between the urinary concentration of 2,5-hexanedione in mg/L (c_u) and the exposure air concentration of *n*-hexane in mg/m^3 (c_a) is:

$$c_u = 0.027\, c_a + 0.49 \tag{21.19}$$

where $r = 0.672$ and $n = 41$ for $p < 0.001$.

Because of the large experimental variation, it is recommended that the urinary BEI be a group test.

21.4.12 Lead

Lead metal vapor (Pb) is detectable at about 550 to 600°C, and it combines at the surface of the metal with the oxygen of the air to form lead oxides (PbO) ("fume") and, on deposition, dusts. Lead commonly is encountered in nonferrous (brass/bronze) foundries, where inhalation and gastrointestinal absorption both can be significant, especially in very dusty workplaces. Lead is a ubiquitous element in the environment. Formerly, a major U.S. source was leaded automobile exhaust. Leaded paint is little used by the general public, but it is still used for industrial and military installations. Leaded paint on buildings and that disseminated in the environment still may be major sources of adverse lead effects on young children. Lead also is found in solders, ceramic glazes, glass, the diet, drinking water, and air. Target shooting also may cause exposures to lead. Lead is more likely to be present in acidic soft drinking water than hard waters. The TLV-TWA is 0.15 mg/m^3 to prevent overt illness and long-term renal damage, but it does not protect for all blood effects. The OSHA PEL is 50 μg/m^3. Removal of the worker from the workplace occurs at 50 μg/dL of blood, or after 3 consecutuve months at >40 μg/dL. This is the only federally-mandated regulation based on biological monitoring.

About 35 to 50% of lead particles in the alveoli are absorbed. Workplace ingestion occurs with inhalation of large particles and the licking of dusty lips, or from contaminated food. Some lead compounds such as aqueous lead chloride also can be dermally absorbed, though oxides can not be to any great extent. The gastrointestinal absorption efficiency is higher in children than in adults. Lead is excreted in the urine and feces and eliminated in the hair and sweat. About 90% of ingested lead is excreted in the feces of adults. Approximately 76% of absorbed nonbone lead is excreted in the urine, 16% in gastrointestinal secretions, and less than 8% in hair, nails, and sweat. Human milk can have lead concentrations as high as 12 μg/L.

Lead inhibits the activities of key zinc-dependent enzymes in the heme synthetic pathway—δ-aminolevulinic acid dehydratase (ALAD) and δ-aminolevulinic acid synthase—as well as bone ferrochelatase. Urinary δ-aminolevulinic acid (ALA) and red cell and urinary coproporphyrinogen III and protoporphyrin IX increase.

Lead crosses the blood/brain and placental barriers. Lead concentrations in blood increase to a steady state after a month of occupational exposure. The relationship between steady-state blood lead and exposure concentration is not linear. Over 90% of the lead in blood is contained in the red blood cells. Blood lead is about 2% of the lead in the body and is an indicator of recent exposure, but it also reflects lead mobilization from the soft tissues. The timing of blood sample taking is not critical if the worker is in a steady state (after at least a month of exposure). The blood BEI is 50 μg/dL, as set from four studies. The OSHA critical value for blood is also 50 μg/dL. The elimination from blood is triphasic, with half-times of 35 to 40 days (soft tissues component), 6 months (bone/teeth), and 20 years (bone/teeth). The administration of chelating agents such as calcium disodium-EDTA and *d*-penicillamine upsets the blood/bone steady state for up to 6 weeks.

The other blood BEI is zinc protoporphyrin (ZPP), analyzed fluorimetrically or after extraction at 100 μg/dL blood or 250 μg/dL red blood cells after at least one month of exposure. Because ZPP is 95% of the free erythrocyte protoporphyrin (FEP), there is little difference between FEP and ZPP although both designations are used frequently. The endogenous adult background appears to average 20 μg/dL with a maximum of around 35 μg/dL, with increases with advancing age.

Increased ZPP occurs during erythropoietic protoporphyria, hemolytic anemia, and iron deficiency. Elevated carboxyhemoglobin may be correlated with low ZPP. ZPP persists in the red blood cells during their lifetime of about 120 days. The ZPP level thus reflects lead body burden and is a chronic marker of lead exposure. The half-time of ZPP in red cells is about 2 to 4 weeks. The relationship between ZPP concentration (ZPP) and lead concentration (Pb) in μg/dL is:

$$ZPP = 9.49 \exp(0.04Pb) \qquad r = 0.83 \tag{21.20}$$

Interindividual variability caused the BEI Committee to recommend that ZPP be utilized as a group test.

The urinary lead BEI from four studies is 150 μg/g creatinine. The sample can be taken at any time as long as the worker is in a steady state. Levels in the general population vary between 10 and 50 μg/L with 95% at <65 μg/L. Lead concentrations do not increase until about 10 days after exposure and reach a steady state after one month of exposure. Thereafter, the timing of sampling is not important as long as the worker has been exposed for at least one month. The BEI is not applicable after the administration of chelating agents. Because of interindividual variability, the BEI Committee recommends a group test.

21.4.13 Methemoglobin Inducers

Methemoglobinemia is the excess formation of methemoglobin, the oxidized form of hemoglobin in which the iron in the heme component is oxidized from the ferrous to the ferric state, thus impairing transport and release of oxygen to and from tissues. There is usually about 1% methemoglobin relative to total hemoglobin, mostly in the red blood cells. Methemoglobinemia is a nonspecific biological monitoring marker.

Methemoglobinemia is caused by many aromatic amines [aniline, dimethylaniline, *N*-methylaniline, 4,4-methylene*bis*(2-chloroaniline), *p*-nitroaniline, Paraquat, toluidines, and xylidines] and aromatic nitro-compounds (dinitrobenzenes, dinitrotoluenes, nitrobenzene, nitrotoluenes, and *p*-nitroaniline), as well as nitric oxide, nitrogen dioxide, nitrogen trifluoride, hydroxylamine, and some aliphatic nitrates (propylene glycol dinitrate, *n*-propylnitrate). The above-named compounds have methemoglobinemia as their principal toxic effect. Not all aromatic or aliphatic amines (anisidine, 2-naphthylamine, and cyclohexylamine) and nitro-compounds (2-nitropropane, tetranitromethane, and 2,4,6-trinitrotoluene (TNT)) have methemoglobinemia as their major toxicity end point. The presence of bacterial flora facilitates conversion of nitrates to nitrites, and probably to nitrosamines and to amines. The presence of the major reducing agents (vitamin C or ascorbic acid, glutathione, $NADH_2$, NADPH, and the inhibition/induction of methemoglobin reductase) also may be a factor. Thus diet and general health also are important. All compounds appear to take unique time courses for the development of methemoglobinemia. Baseline levels are crucial to determine if the observed methemoglobinemia is caused by work-related exposure. The BEI is set at 1.5% methemoglobin content of total hemoglobin in a sample taken during, or at the end of, a shift.

Exposure to many recreational drugs (amyl nitrate and butyl nitrite), medications (acetanilides, benzocaine, bismuth subnitrate, lidocaine, nitrites, nitroglycerine, phenacetin, prilocaine, silver nitrate, and sulfonamides), photographic developers (aminophenol), food preservatives (sodium nitrite), dyes (anilines, benzidine, and nitrobenzenes), commercial products (fuel additives, wax crayons, laundry markers, and waters with high bacterial content), fertilizers (nitrates), nitrogen dioxide–generating sources (such as silos, stack emissions, and ambient air), and the chloral salts used in matches and oxygen generators also may produce methemoglobinemia. Bacteria growing in burns and in topical nitrate agents applied to burns are sources also. People with congenital methemoglobinemia due to methemoglobin reductase deficiency may have 10 to 30% methemoglobin; acatalasemia, deficiency in NADH-reductase, and defective globin caused by congenital mutations also may produce elevated levels of methemoglobin. Storage may increase or decrease the levels, but analysis must be done within 1 h of taking the sample.

The half-time of methemoglobin (80–100%) varies between 6 and 24 h. Most kinetics are biphasic, signaling some component due to metabolic activation. There is much interindividual sensitivity. Cyanosis is usually intense at 10 to 15% methemoglobin; levels between 40% and 60% cause weakness, fatigue, breath shortness, rapid heart rate, dizziness, headaches, and disorientation;

and levels above 60% cause stupor, coma, and death. The mean ± standard deviation in the general population is (0.78 ± 0.37)% methemoglobin.

The TLV for aniline (Section 21.4.1) of 2 ppm was set to prevent methemoglobinemia, as was the TLV of 1 ppm for nitrobenzene (Section 21.4.17). Because many of the chemicals causing methemoglobinemia are efficiently absorbed through the skin, and because this nonspecific end point integrates absorbed doses over all exposure routes and for different chemicals, the marker is recommended as a screening marker for biological monitoring health effects and also is utilized as a medical monitoring marker.

21.4.14 Methyl Alcohol

Methyl alcohol or methanol ($CH_3 \cdot OH$) is a colorless liquid with a boiling point of 65°C that is miscible with water. Methanol is a component in many paint removers, methylated spirits, antifreeze, organic cleaners, fruit juices, foods, and alcoholic beverages. It is the active ingredient of gasohol (up to 15%). The TLV-TWA of 200 ppm or 262 mg/m^3 is set to prevent severe recurring headaches and sight impairment. The methanol in ingested methylated spirits is known to cause blindness and death. Ingestion of as little as 30 mL methanol can cause death.

Methanol distributes with water throughout the body. This means that the concentration of methanol in urine is independent of the urine volume, and thus creatinine corrections are not appropriate. About 58% of inhaled methanol vapor is absorbed independent of air concentration, duration of exposure, or physical activity. The dermal absorption rate is significant, with a predicted rate of 2.0 mg/cm^2/h and a measured rate on forearm skin of 11.5 mg/cm^2/h. Methanol is excreted in urine (BEI, 15 mg/L end-of-shift from four studies and two field exposure investigations) and exhaled breath, and part of it is oxidized by alcohol dehydrogenase to formaldehyde ($H_2 \cdot CO$) and then also to formic acid ($H \cdot COOH$) (BEI, 80 mg/g creatinine end-of-work-week-shift corrected for background, as set from one field study).

It is recommended that workers in plants not characterized for air methanol be sampled for urine during their 8-h shift after a baseline sample is taken. The BEI under 8-h collection conditions is 6.5 mg/L for workers at rest and 13 mg/L for workers with pulmonary ventilation of 21 L/min. The final BEI selected was an average of the end-of-shift and 8-h collection values. The samples for methanol in urine must be analyzed within 3 days even after refrigeration at 4°C. A steady state of methanol in blood takes longer than 8 h to attain.

Methanol is formed endogenously through the action of bacteria or as a common intermediate in C_1 metabolism. The range for methanol-unexposed subjects is 0.32 to 2.9 mg/L urine. Methyl esters ($R \cdot CO \cdot OCH_3$, where R is any alkyl or aryl group) are metabolized to the free acid and methanol. Methyl ethers ($R \cdot O \cdot CH_3$, where R is any alkyl or aryl group) such as ethylene glycol monomethyl ether (2-methoxyethanol, $HO \cdot CH_2 \cdot CH_2 \cdot OCH_3$) are less metabolized, to produce methanol and the other alcohol, $R \cdot OH$. Workers unexposed to methanol and alcoholic beverages have urinary methanol concentrations between <0.6 to 2.9 mg/L. Alcohol imbibers have up to 5 mg/L in their urines.

The metabolic oxidation of methanol to formic acid accounts for about 70 to

80% of the absorbed dose. The process is saturable with elimination half-times of about 1.5 to 2.0 h over the air concentration range 40 to 230 ppm. Long half-lives have been reported for poisoned patients. The accumulation of formic acid is responsible for the poisoning symptoms, metabolic acidosis, and optic neuropathy. The elimination of formic acid is pseudo first-order for exposures of 80 to 230 ppm at 8 h each. Formic acid concentrations in urine cannot be utilized at methanol air exposures below 150 ppm. Ethanol ($CH_3 \cdot CH_2 \cdot OH$) has more affinity than methanol for alcohol dehydrogenase, and methanol has to "wait in line" for metabolism, so that an antagonistic effect results with urine levels being much lower than expected and blood levels much higher. Formic acid also is formed endogenously in the range 4 to 47 mg/L in workers not exposed to methanol, the half-lives having variously been reported as 2.25 h below and at the TLV and >5 h, indicative of accumulation throughout the work week. Exposures to formaldehyde, ethylene oxide ($(CH_2)_2 \cdot O$), or propylene glycol increase urinary formic acid. Formic acid cannot be utilized as a valid marker for workers with renal failure.

21.4.15 Methyl Chloroform

Methyl chloroform ($CH_3 \cdot CCl_3$) or 1,1,1-trichloroethane is a heavier-than-water liquid with a boiling point of 74°C. It is much utilized in organic vapor degreasing of metallic machine parts and to clean plastic molds. Methyl chloroform is used as a solvent in many household products such as spot removers, adhesives, and aerosol spray cans. "Sniffing" has also been reported. It has been detected in ambient air (usually <1 ppb to a maximum of 100 ppb) and in drinking water (ppm concentrations). A TLV-TWA of 350 ppm or 1910 mg/m^3 was set to prevent anesthetic effects and odor perception.

Alveolar retention after exposure is about 40% after 30 min and 24% after 24 h. Dermal absorption also has been documented. Absorbed methyl chloroform is excreted unchanged (97%) in the breath with triphasic elimination kinetics of half-times 1, 5, and 32 h. After exposure, the concentration of methyl chloroform in end-exhaled air is 10 to 20% after 30 min relative to the exposing concentration (end-exhaled breath concentrations during exposure are commonly 60–80% of the exposure concentration). At 16 h after exposure the concentration detected relative to the exposure concentration is 2.4% after a single exposure and 4.1% after repeated exposures. The breath BEI from one field study is 40 ppm prior to the last shift and at the end of the work week (the end-exhaled air sample is collected in inert containers that have no rubber or plastic parts, 16 h after the end of exposure and after at least 2 consecutive days of exposure).

The small fraction that is metabolized is oxidized to 2,2,2-trichloroethanol ($CCl_3 \cdot CH_2OH$), which appears in the blood and the urine as a D-glucuronic acid conjugate as well as in the free form (also in the breath), the total of the two being 2 to 5% of the absorbed dose. The half-time for urine is 10 to 12 h, and the half-time for blood is 10 to 12 h for the fast-kinetics component. The BEI based on one field study for total trichloroethanol in blood at the end of a shift and at the end of a work week (after at least 2 consecutive workdays) is 1 mg/L blood. The BEI based on one field study and two independent computer simulation models for total trichloroethanol in urine collected at the end of a shift and at the end of the work week is 30 mg/L urine.

Trichloroethanol is a common intermediate of trichloroethylene (Section 21.4.25), chloral hydrate, perchloroethylene (Section 21.4.21), and tetrachloroethane and brominated trichloro-mixed halogenated analogs.

Further oxidation of trichloroethanol also occurs, to trichloroacetic acid ($CCl_3 \cdot COOH$), which constitutes 1 to 2% of the absorbed dose of methyl chloroform. The excretion kinetics are biphasic with the long half-time being about 3 days. The BEI based on one field study and a computer simulation model for urinary trichloroacetic acid collected at the end of the work week is 10 mg/L. The chemicals responsible for the positive interference effects of trichloroethanol exert the same effects for trichloroacetic acid.

The relationships between urinary total trichloroethanol, trichloracetic acid, and total trichlorocompounds are linear up to 500 ppm methylchloroform at least. Animal studies show that methyl chloroform must "wait in line" for metabolism when coexposed with perchloroethylene, resulting in higher blood and breath concentrations, and lower urinary metabolite concentrations than expected. Other chlorinated compounds also may affect the metabolic rate so that the breath BEI is the most reliable and specific. The urinary and blood BEIs are variable and constitute screening tests because the physical work rate is an extremely important variable in light of the small fraction metabolized. Trichloroethanol is a marker of recent absorbed dose, whereas trichloroacetic acid is more a subacute marker of absorbed dose.

21.4.16 Methyl Ethyl Ketone

Methyl ethyl ketone (MEK) or 2-butanone ($CH_3 \cdot CO \cdot CH_2CH_3$) is a colorless liquid with a boiling point of 80°C and with appreciable water solubility. It is utilized in glues, laminates, paints, cleaners, and many solvents. It also is used in the manufacture of smokeless powder and colorless synthetic resins. The TLV is 200 ppm (590 mg/m^3) to prevent injurious effects and to avoid respiratory irritation.

The pulmonary retention of inhaled MEK is about 50%, and it penetrates rapidly through skin, being found in the breath 2 to 3 min after forearm skin contact. The major fate is metabolism. MEK can be reduced to 2-butanol ($CH_3 \cdot C(OH)H \cdot CH_2CH_3$) or oxidized to 3-hydroxy-2-butanone ($CH_3 \cdot CO \cdot C(OH)H \cdot CH_3$), which is further reduced to 2,3-butandiol ($CH_3 \cdot C(OH)H \cdot C(OH)H \cdot CH_3$) in guinea pigs. Only methyl ethyl ketone and 3-hydroxy-2-butanone have been found in worker urine. The BEI based on two field studies is urinary MEK end-of-shift at 2 mg/L, usually analyzed by gas chromatographic headspace analysis. The BEI is relatively specific, though exposures to 2-butanol or 2-halobutanols could constitute positive interferences.

The linear regression equations connecting MEK by c_u, in µg/L urine, and c_a, the air exposure concentration in ppm, from two out of 4 reported field studies are as follows:

$$c_u = 9.4c_a + 196 \qquad n = 27 \qquad p < 0.001 \tag{21.21}$$

and

$$c_u = 9.4c_a + 320 \qquad n = 65 \qquad p < 0.01 \tag{21.22}$$

There is a neurotoxic interaction of MEK with *n*-hexane in animals.

21.4.17 Nitrobenzene

Nitrobenzene ($C_6H_5 \cdot NO_2$) is a colorless liquid when pure (technical grades are yellowish) with a boiling point of 211°C. It is used in the production of dyes, rubber formulations, shoe polishes, almond flavoring agents, perfumes, combustible propellants, and medicinals. The TLV of 1 ppm (5 mg/m^3) protects against methemoglobinemia (see Section 21.4.13).

Nitrobenzene is efficiently absorbed through the lungs (about 80%) and skin (for liquid, 0.2–0.3 mg/cm^2/h; for 1 ppm vapor, 1 mg/h). Increasing the relative humidity from 33% to 67% increases skin absorption rates by 40%. Trace amounts of unchanged nitrobenzene are detected in urine or expired air. The urinary excretions of *p*-nitrophenol ($HO \cdot C_6H_4 \cdot NO_2$; 6–37%) and *p*-aminophenol (<10%) account for only 20 to 30% of the nitrobenzene dose, the fate of the rest being unknown. The half-time for nitrobenzene is about 86 h. The half-time for *p*-nitrophenol is about 4 to 12 h, and that for *p*-aminophenol is about 4 h. The hydroxylation of nitrobenzene to nitrophenols (di- and monosubstituted) is mediated by a peroxidase in the presence of oxygen. Reduction also occurs to the hydroxy group for *ortho*-substituted amino phenol intermediates. Reduction of nitrobenzene by liver nitroreductases occurs also, to nitrosobenzene ($C_6H_5 \cdot NO$) and phenylhydroxylamine ($C_6H_5 \cdot NHOH$), the latter being a potent methemoglobinemic agent.

The urinary BEI based on one study with volunteers and a field study is 5 mg total *p*-nitrophenol/g creatinine end-of-shift at the end of the work week. The relationship between the amount of nitrobenzene absorbed m_a and exposure duration t in h, the pulmonary ventilation V, the pulmonary retention, P_r, and a, the coefficient of skin absorption, is provided in the following equation:

$$m_a = 5t(VP_r + a) \tag{21.23}$$

where P_r is 0.42 m^3/h at rest and 1.5 m^3/h at 50W, and a has been measured at 0.25 mg/h.

For an end-of-week urine sample, this equation can be utilized to obtain the excretion rate in μg/h:

$$\text{Excretion rate} = 10\,m_a \tag{21.24}$$

The urinary marker is also produced on exposure to parathion, to *p*-nitrophenol, or to *p*-nitrohalobenzenes. Baseline measurements are recommended to assess the contribution of nonworkplace exposures. Sulfates and glucuronides are the major phenolic conjugates in urine. Unfortunately, only data by a colorimetric method have been utilized, calling into question how specific the quantitation is, and how quantitative equations (21.23) and (21.24) are.

The blood BEI is methemoglobin, a very nonspecific marker, at 1.5% of hemoglobin (see Section 21.4.13).

21.4.18 Organophosphorus Cholinesterase Inhibitors

The marker is red cell cholinesterase activity, where a level 70% of baseline is the BEI. Organophosphate esters (RRXP′=O or=S where R and R′ are alkoxy and/or phenoxy and X is any functional group) often are used as pesticides [for example, the following have TLVs in mg/m^3: (0.2), demeton (0.11), diazinon (0.1), dichlorvos (0.9), dioxathion (0.2), EPN (0.5), ethion (0.4), fenamiphos (0.1), fensulfothion (0.1), fenthion (0.2), fonofos (0.1), malathion (10), methyl demeton (0.5), methyl parathion (0.2), mevinphos (0.092), naled (3), parathion (0.1), sulfotep (0.2), temephos (10), and TEPP (0.047)]. The TLVs usually are set on protection of the nervous system and all carry a '"skin" designation, except for femephos. The sulfur analogs are much less toxic than their oxygen analogs. Most of these compounds are applied as aerosols, sprays, or dusts, whereas other chemicals are often codispersed (see Chapter 22). Other compounds capable of producing cholinesterase inhibition are carbamate pesticides such as Sevin (TLV 5 mg/m^3), nerve gas components (tabun, sarin, soman, and VX), drugs such as echtothiophate, neostigmine, and physostigmine, and the anesthetic, succinyl choline. The carbamate pesticide inhibition is relatively brief (reversible inhibition) compared with that from organophosphates (irreversible inhibition), the red blood cell enzyme activity showing a recovery of about 1% per day. Factors causing enzyme increases include recovery from hemorrhages and successful treatments for pernicious anemia or megaloblastic anemia.

All routes of absorption are known, including the eyes. The dermal and ingestion absorption rates are dependent on the chemical structure, the more aromatic ones being efficiently ingested. Both temperature and humidity affect skin absorption. The oxon intermediates produced by the action of liver mixed-function oxidases generally are more cholinesterase-inhibiting than the original compounds. The esters eventually are hydrolyzed to the component alkyl phosphates and other water-soluble moieties (Chapter 22) in the liver and directly by plasma/tissue phosphoryl phosphatases. These hydrolysis products are excreted in the urine.

The BEI marker is inhibition of red blood cell acetyl cholinesterase (ChE) caused by binding of the inhibiting chemical/metabolite to the enzyme so that the excess acetylcholine cannot be hydrolyzed. This is an indirect marker of the nervous system enzyme where nervous signal transmission is disrupted between the synapse, the site of acetylcholine accumulation, and the adjacent nerve axon. Red cell ChE appears to have the same substrate affinity as nerve ending ChE unlike plasma ChE or "pseudocholinesterases," which are a family of isoenzymes produced in the liver whose activity is influenced by many other factors (early hepatitis, alcoholic cirrhosis, liver diseases, many drugs, and many chemical exposures). It is recommended that baseline levels of red blood cell ChE, at least 3 days prior to the exposure and at least 30 days after a known exposure, be measured by the same laboratory and analytical method because baselines vary greatly between individuals, and to assess whether exposure is acute or chronic. These two baseline values should differ by less than 20%. Laboratory values also often vary unpredictably, and laboratory reference ranges must be utilized for comparisons in the absence of personal baseline data—not compilations of general reference ranges. The laboratory doing the analysis should be consulted about which anticoagulant to use in the blood sampling tube. Blood samples should not be frozen, and should be analyzed as soon as possible because the enzyme loses activity over time.

There are several analytical methods, the Michel (Δ pH), the titrimetric (pH Stat), and the colorimetric (Ellman) being the most used. Many laboratories using the Δ pH method obtain reference values for the unexposed population between 0.58 and 0.95 Δ pH units; those using the pH Stat method obtain between 9 and 19 μmol acetyl choline/mL/min. The colorimetric test is much more nonspecific than the others but easier to automate. The reference range for the latter is extremely variable, but an average value is about 4.4 μmol acetyl choline/mL/min.

About 78% of red blood cell ChE activity compared with baseline is caused by circadian rhythms and normal daily variation. The appearance of toxic effects appears to be correlated to the rate of inhibition rather than the absolute value of the inhibition because acute exposures producing the same decrement as chronic exposures usually are accompanied by nervous symptoms. Ultimately there also is a critical value under chronic conditions because toxic symptoms can occur to chronically exposed people after a very small exposure that is insignificant by itself. The ChE activity has no relationship to the delayed neuropathy characteristic of the more potent organophosphates. The marker is a nonspecific one designed to be a screening marker for these chemicals where skin absorption is a major route and where air levels may not be representative of the major exposure route.

21.4.19 Parathion

Parathion [*O*,*O*-diethyl-*O*-(4-nitrophenyl) ester of phosphorothioic acid ($(C_2H_5O)_2 \cdot PS \cdot O \cdot C_6H_5 \cdot NO_2$)] is an organophosphorus insecticide that is a yellow liquid with a density of 1.26 g/mL at 25°C and a boiling point of 375°C. It is hydrolyzed in materials of higher pH than 7.5. The TLV of 0.1 mg/m^3 (skin) was set to prevent systemic toxicity. The moderate vapor pressure of 4.1×10^{-5} mm Hg at 20°C lessens high inhalation concentrations but the aerosol and dermal exposure routes become more important. Parathion home use products now are not marketed in the United States. Parathion has been detected in food at trace levels.

Parathion is absorbed by inhalation, skin, ingestion, the eyes, and mucous membranes. Dermal absorption is very variable among individuals. About 10% of the population absorbs twice the average amount, whereas 5% will absorb three times the average amount. Temperature and the pH of sweat also are important. Some investigators have measured slow dermal absorption rates of about 0.001 μg/min/cm^2 *in vitro*. After dermal administration of 4 μg/cm^2 of pure parathion through the skin of volunteers, most excretion was concluded by 48 h and constituted about 10% of the administered dose after 5 days.

The sulfur in parathion is exchanged for oxygen through the microsomal enzymes of the liver to form the paraoxon homolog, which inhibits the red blood cell acetylcholinesterase (see Section 21.4.18). The oxon derivative also can be produced in the environment after spraying through air and photochemical oxidation of residues on surfaces. Liver esterases cleave parathion to diethylphosphate ($(C_2H_5O)_2 \cdot P{=}O \cdot OH$) and 4-nitrophenol ($HO \cdot C_6H_4 \cdot NO_2$). Plasma/tissue esterases also produce diethylthiophosphate ($(C_2H_5O)_2 \cdot P{=}S \cdot OH$) and 4-nitrophenol. The phosphates and 4-nitrophenol are excreted in the urine within 48 h of exposure. The phenol is conjugated as sulfate and *O*-glucuronide, depending on the exposure dose.

The urinary BEI is total 4-nitrophenol in urine collected end-of-shift at 0.5 mg/g creatinine. Most analytical methods involve acidification (which hydrolyzes the conjugates), extraction, and GC/MS or GC analysis. The latter methods are preferable to the less specific colorimetric techniques. Background concentrations in unexposed populations range from 0.01 to 0.03 mg/L, mostly from exposures to other chemicals such as nitrobenzene (Section 21.4.17), methyl parathion, and the pesticide, EPN (*O*-ethyl-*O*-4-nitrophenyl-phenylphosphonothioate).

Urine concentrations of 4-nitrophenol do not correlate with red blood cell acetylcholinesterase activity inhibition <0.5 mg/L but do with serum parathion concentrations. The elimination half-time for 4-nitrophenol is about 3 h (ingestion) and 12 h (field studies). The excretion after ingestion is biphasic, 86% being excreted in 8 h. The BEI was calculated by assuming the 12 h half-time, no skin absorption, and a urinary output of 1 mL/min.

The red blood cell cholinesterase inhibition marker of 70% relative to baseline activity was discussed in Section 21.4.18.

21.4.20 Pentachlorophenol

Pentachlorophenol ($C_6Cl_5 \cdot OH$) is a white solid that melts at 190°C and boils at 310°C. Depending on the way it was manufactured, commercial pentachlorophenol may contain impurities such as chlorinated benzenes, phenols, phenoxyphenols, diphenyl ethers, hexachlorobenzene, chlorinated dibenzo-*p*-dioxins, chlorinated dibenzofurans, and chlorinated biphenylenes. Pentachlorophenol is widely used as a wood, leather, and paper preservative and as a fungicide. It is used in homes, log cabins, and telephone poles as a paint-on wood preservative. Significant exposures have been documented to occupants of log cabins, climbers of telephone poles, or dwellers of homes with interiors treated with pentachlorophenol. Pentachlorophenol has been detected in drinking water and foods; so most biological media will have some residues of it. The TLV of 0.5 mg/m^3 (skin) is supposed to prevent skin irritation and acute intoxication without consideration of the hazards of the impurities. In 1989, two technical grades of pentachlorophenol were found to be carcinogenic to mice down to 18 mg/kg/day ingested dose. The influence of the impurities was not determined. Pentachlorophenol is fetotoxic to rats. A No-Observed-Adverse-Effect Level of 3 mg/kg/day was determined by the U.S. EPA, and a reference dose of 0.03 mg/kg/day.

Pentachlorophenol is readily absorbed through the lungs, skin, and gastrointestinal tract, but no quantitative data are known. Death has occurred after skin absorption. Salt forms are known not to be so readily absorbed through the skin as the free phenol although any additional solvents will be important factors also. Pentachlorophenol is transported mostly (99%) in the blood plasma rather than the red blood cells. The elimination half-life of free pentachlorophenol in plasma is 30.2 ± 4.0 h, with a slower later component of half-time >30 days. Pentachlorophenol is found free in urine as well as in the form of an *O*-glucuronide. Very small amounts (<10% urinary pentachlorophenol concentration) of free tetrachlorohydroquinone (4-$C_6Cl_4(OH)_2$), tetrachloropyrocatechol (2-$C_6Cl_4(OH)_2$) and their glucuronides have been detected also. Exhalation of pentachlorophenol-derived material is negligible. The half-times for excreting urinary free pentachlorophenol were 33.1 ± 5.4 h, and for the glucuronide 12.7 ± 5.4 h. Peak excretion occurs 40 h after inhalation exposure. The excretion is probably triphasic, with the long half-time estimated variously between 4 and 72 days. Pentachlorophenol is also a metabolite of hexachlorobenzene, which also produces porphyria (Section 9.3.9).

The urinary BEI is 2 mg total pentachlorophenol/g creatinine on samples collected prior to the last shift of a workweek, with determination of baseline levels also recommended. Unexposed people usually have free pentachlorophenol urinary concentrations <0.007 mg/L corresponding to total pentachlorophenol <0.03 mg/L, as the free phenol is about 14% of the total pentachlorophenol. Pentachlorophenol appears to affect renal function, as measured by creatinine clearance at free pentachlorophenol between 0.59 and 0.95 mg/L, known to be no-effect concentrations. Urinary concentrations >29 mg/L have been reported in fatal poisoning incidents. The BEI is based on a pharmacokinetic model assuming a steady state, light work (50 W), an absorption of 3 mg of pentachlorophenol during 8 h of exposure at the TLV, an alveolar ventilation of 15 L/min, a urinary output of 1.2 L/day, no bio-accumulation, and no skin absorption. Total pentachlorophenol is independent of individual differences in conjugation abilities. The BEI is almost protective against fetotoxic effects, but would not be for carcinogenic effects.

The blood BEI is end-of-shift free pentachlorophenol in plasma at 5 mg/L (2.6 mg/L blood), with a baseline sample also recommended to ascertain chronic or nonoccupational exposure. Concentrations of free pentachlorophenol in blood for unexposed people are usually <0.3 mg/L. Fatal poisoning cases showed free pentachlorophenol blood levels between 16 and 170 mg/L. Plasma concentrations <2.6 mg/L cause no renal function changes; those <0.25 mg/L cause no hepatic function changes; and those <3.8 mg/L cause no eye irritation and inflammation. The BEI was set on a pharmacokinetic model of the following assumptions: renal clearance, 5 mL plasma/h; normal hematocrit; free pentachlorophenol accounting for 20% of total pentachlorophenol; daily urine output, 1.2 L; and excreting 0.6 mg of free pentachlorophenol.

21.4.21 Perchloroethylene

Perchloroethylene or tetrachloroethene ($Cl_2C{=}CCl_2$) is a colorless liquid with a boiling point of 121°C, which is used in dry cleaning and degreasing of metal parts. It is used therapeutically as an anthelmintic agent. Up to 10 ppb has been detected in ambient air and up to 2 ppb in drinking water. The TLV of 50 ppm and the Short Term Exposure Limit (STEL) of 200 ppm were set to prevent discomfort, as well as anesthetic and irritant effects. There is an intent to lower the TLV to 25 ppm in 1994.

Alveolar retention decreases during exposure, being 90% at exposure onset,

75% after 30 min of exposure, 60% at 4 h, and 47% after 8 h. Dermal absorption of the liquid is known, but that of the vapor is small (1% of exposure concentration). Most perchloroethylene is excreted in the breath with an estimated half-time of 3 days. Pharmacokinetic modeling resulted in triphasic half-times of 15 min, 4 h, and 4 days; half-times are directly proportional to body fat and inversely related to physical activity. Most perchloroethylene (97–99%) is exhaled unchanged, and only 1 to 3% is oxidized to urinary trichloroacetic acid (CCl_3COOH) via tetrachloroethylene epoxide (C_2Cl_4O) and trichloroacetyl chloride ($CCl_3 \cdot CO \cdot Cl$).

Three BEIs are recommended. Those based on gas chromatographic analysis of perchloroethylene are specific. All samplings must take into consideration the body content of fat and the physical activity during and following exposure.

The breath BEI of 10 ppm perchloroethylene in end-exhaled air should be collected prior to a shift and at the end of the work week (16 h after the previous day's exposure and prior to starting work on the last day of the work week, after at least 2 consecutive workdays). At the end of exposure, end-exhaled air has perchloroethylene concentrations that are 40 to 50% of exposure concentrations; 30 min after the exposure ends, these concentrations are 15 to 30% of the final exposure concentrations; after 16 h the concentration is 4–5% after a single exposure, and 8% after repeated 8-h exposures for 5 days. The half-times are 15 min, 4 h, and 4 days at the TLV at moderate work, and so bioaccumulation occurs. The BEI is set on a field study and a computer simulation assuming a moderate work load.

The blood BEI based on the field study and computer simulation is 1 mg perchloroethylene/L collected prior to the shift and at the end of a work week after at least 2 consecutive days of exposure at moderate work load. Baseline samples also are recommended because of perchloroethylene bioaccumulation. The arm used for blood collection must not be exposed dermally to perchloroethylene because higher levels would result. The blood elimination half-time is 3 to 4 days, with triphasic half-times of 15 min, 4 h, and 4 days. Since the recommended analytical method is by headspace analysis, the container should either be filled and stored refrigerated, or a headspace container utilized.

The urine BEI based on three field studies for end-of-work week trichloroacetic acid at 7 mg/L at moderate work load is a nonspecific marker, unlike the blood and breath BEIs, because exposure to chemicals such as methyl chloroform (Section 21.4.15), trichloroethylene (Section 21.4.25), and tetrachloroethane in the workplace or the home is a source of trichloroacetic acid after metabolism. The sedative, chloral hydrate, may also produce the acid. The half-time is not known experimentally, but blood trichloroacetic acid increases for 20 h after a single exposure to perchloroethylene and declines with a half-time of about 80 h. The marker is a subacute exposure screening indicator. Urine samples should be kept refrigerated.

21.4.22 Phenol

Phenol ($C_6H_5 \cdot OH$) is a white solid with a boiling point of 182°C and a melting point of 43°C. It is a common ingredient in disinfectants, cleaners, antiseptics, medicines, throat lozenges, calamine lotions, chemical dressings, and some antacids. The TLV of 5 ppm (19 mg/m^3) is based on acute irritant effects and systemic poisoning.

Phenol is absorbed rapidly on inhalation, skin contact of the vapor or solid/liquids, and ingestion. At the beginning of exposure to the TLV air concentration, lung retention is about 80%; at the end of 8 h, the retention is about 70%. Nearly all the absorbed phenol is eliminated within 16 h as unchanged phenol or sulfate/glucuronide conjugates in urine with <1% exhaled of the absorbed dose. Blood levels return to baseline about 24 h after dermal or TLV-TWA exposure. Traces of catechols (1,2-$C_6H_4(OH)_2$ and 1,2,3-$C_6H_3(OH)_3$) and hydroquinones (the keto forms of 1,4-dihydroxybenzenes) also are found in urine. The sulfate conjugate in urine dominates at low exposure doses, and glucuronides assume greater importance at higher phenol exposure concentrations. Below 5 ppm phenol, the sulfate/glucuronide ratio is 3.7 : 1. Phenol and conjugates also are produced after exposure to benzene (Section 21.4.2); so the marker is nonspecific. Individual concentrations of urinary phenol vary greatly so that the urinary BEI of 250 mg/g creatinine or 15 mg/h of total phenol collected at the end (last 2 h) of a shift should be applied as a group test. Thymol is recommended as a preservative. Phenol is stable in urine for 4 days at 25°C and at least 3 months when frozen. Accurate timing of voids is necessary. There is a NIOSH analytical method available.

Phenol is a product of protein metabolism relative to aromatic amino acids; the diet also may be important. Unexposed people have urinary phenol of <20 mg/L or 0.4 mg/h. The half-time is about 3.5 h whether absorption is by skin or the lungs. The use of noncolorimetric analytical methods is recommended. The rate of total phenol urinary excretion of volunteers correlates with the absorbed dose in the exposure range 5 to 25 mg/m^3, and also for workers in the field between exposure concentrations between 1.2 to 5.0 ppm, and can be simulated adequately with a computer one-compartment model.

21.4.23 Styrene

Styrene ($C_6H_5 \cdot CH_2{=}CH_2$) is a colorless liquid with a boiling point of 146°C that readily polymerizes in air and sunlight or at 200°C. Styrene is the starting compound for polystyrene polymers, and the monomer is used in some autobody patching agents. The TLV is 50 ppm (213 mg/m^3) based on preventing "styrene sickness" (drowsiness, headache, fatigue, and dizziness).

Pulmonary retention is about 60 to 70%, and decreases in chronically exposed workers. Styrene concentration in mixed-exhaled air is about 35% of the exposure concentration. Skin absorption is significant and is between 0.03 to 12 mg/cm^2/h. Fat solubility also is high; so body fat content must be known to interpret biological monitoring data. Metabolic clearance is the major fate (95%) of absorbed styrene, with trace quantities (<1%) of styrene found in both urine and exhaled air after absorption. The breath elimination half-times are 13 to 52 min, 4 to 20 h, and 3 days (fat mobilization). The latter half-time reflects adipose tissue clearance. Venous blood half-times for styrene are 35 min, 13 h, and 3 days, the latter reflecting adipose tissue clearance. The first metabolic oxidation step is epoxidation to form styrene oxide ($C_6H_5 \cdot CH_2CH_2O$), which is further degraded to styrene glycol ($C_6H_5 \cdot HCOH \cdot CH_2OH$), which, on continued oxidation at the ring β carbon, forms mandelic acid ($C_6H_5 \cdot CHOH \cdot COOH$), which is 85% of the excreted urinary products. About 10% of the last compound is further oxidized to phenylglyoxylic acid ($C_6H_5 \cdot CO \cdot COOH$), which also is found in the urine. Less than 4% is excreted as benzyl alcohol ($C_6H_5 \cdot CH_2OH$) and benzoic acid ($C_6H_5 \cdot COOH$), the latter being conjugated with glycine to form hippuric acid ($C_6H_5 \cdot CO \cdot NH \cdot CH_2COOH$) (Section 21.4.24). The metabolism is capacity-limited, being pseudo first-order up to exposure concentrations of 80 ppm, with saturation occurring beyond an exposure concentration of 200 ppm. The correlation with exposure concentration is linear up to 150 ppm. Exposure to concentrations >200 ppm results in smaller amounts of phenylglyoxylic and mandelic acids excreted in the urine than at 200 ppm, with exhalation of styrene the overflow pathway. This may indicate the threshold of an adverse effect. Interactions with other xenobiotics, notably ethyl alcohol or other alcohols, are known, leading to underestimation of air exposure levels from urinary markers but especially mandelic acid and overestimation of exposure from breath styrene concentrations. The alcohol interference can be assessed by measurements of blood mandelic acid and styrene glycol. If the ratio drops below 1:30, the urine measurements for styrene are invalid. Trichloroethylene, xylenes, toluene and acetone competitively inhibit styrene metabolism also. Styrene also induces liver enzymes so that repeated exposures to styrene result in lower blood concentrations and higher urinary metabolite concentrations than expected.

There are two urinary BEIs: end-of-shift mandelic acid at 1 g/L or 800 mg/g creatinine set from three field studies, or 300 mg/g creatinine prior to the next shift; and end-of-shift phenylglyoxylic acid at 250 mg/L or 240 mg/g creatinine set from two field studies, or 100 mg/g creatinine prior to the next shift. Neither marker is specific because both are produced after exposures to ethylbenzene (Section 21.4.8), styrene glycol, acetophenone, styrene oxide, phenaceturic acid, phenylglycol, and α-phenylaminoacetic acids. The half-times for urinary mandelic acid after styrene inhalation are 3 to 4 and, 25 to 40 h. The half-time for urinary phenylglyoxylic acid is about 7 to 10 h. All of these half-times vary in the presence of other solvents whose metabolisms are mediated by the cytochrome P-450 enzyme system.

The regression equations linking styrene air concentrations in ppm (c_a) and urinary mandelic acid in g/L (c_u) are as follows for c_a <150 ppm and samples collected at the end of an 8-h exposure in the absence of interferences.

$$c_a = 54.3c_u - 8.1 \tag{21.25}$$

for urines of unknown specific gravity.

$$c_a = 80c_u - 14.5 \tag{21.26}$$

for urines of specific gravity 1.016.

$$c_a = 65c_u - 3.6 \tag{21.27}$$

for c_u in g/g creatinine.

The regression equations linking styrene air exposure in ppm (c_a) and urinary phenylglyoxylic acid concentrations in mg/L (c_u) collected at the end of an 8-h exposure for <150 ppm TWA are as follows:

$$c_a = 0.37c_u - 29 \tag{21.28}$$

for urines of unknown specific gravity.

$$c_a = 0.25c_u - 20 \tag{21.29}$$

for urines of specific gravity 1.016.

$$c_a = 0.25c_u - 9.5 \tag{21.30}$$

for c_u in mg/g creatinine.

A field study and a pharmacokinetic model support 300 mg mandelic acid/g creatinine, and 100 mg phenylglyoxylic acid/g creatinine in urines taken prior to the next shift of the next day.

The venous blood BEIs based on one volunteer study after a single 8-h exposure at the TLV-TWA are 0.55 mg/L collected end-of-shift and 0.02 mg/L collected 16 h after the last exposure and prior to the next shift, both at the end of a work week for workers at rest, and utilizing EDTA anticoagulant in the Vacutainers. After 8 h exposure to 50 ppm styrene, the styrene concentration in blood (c_{bt}) in mg/L at time t in h after the end of exposure and sampling is:

$$c_{bt} = 0.5e^{-1.21t} + 0.044e^{-0.0534t} \tag{21.31}$$

This equation does not reflect induction of liver enzymes after repeated exposures; so the BEI probably is overprotective. The blood BEI is specific, but is recommended only as confirmatory unless all interferences are known quantitatively.

21.4.24 Toluene

Toluene ($C_6H_5 \cdot CH_3$; methylbenzene) is a colorless liquid with a boiling point of 111°C utilized in the manufacture of benzoic acid (food preservative sodium benzoate), dyes, benzaldehyde, and some explosives. It is often found in paints, paint removers, varnishes, lacquers, gums, glues, household cleaners, adhesives, and resins as a solvent, and is a component of automobile exhaust. The TLV changed to 50 ppm (188 mg/m^3) from 100 ppm in 1992/93 to prevent central nervous system effects.

The lung retention at 100 ppm toluene is about 50%. Skin absorption is known for the liquid but not the vapor. More toluene is absorbed by fat people than thin. Physical activity markedly affects absorption and retention. About 15 to 20% of the absorbed dose is excreted unchanged in the breath following a 5-h inhalation exposure at 100 ppm toluene with complete clearance after 24 h. Toluene is bound by blood lipoproteins, especially in the chylomicra (Section 2.8.2). Urinary levels of toluene are negligible. The remaining 80 to 85% is mostly metabolized successively to benzyl alcohol ($C_6H_5 \cdot CH_2OH$), benzaldehyde ($C_6H_5 \cdot CHO$), and benzoic acid ($C_6H_5 \cdot COOH$). The latter is then 80% conjugated with glycine (NH_2CH_2COOH) to form urinary hippuric acid ($C_6H_5 \cdot CONH \cdot CH_2COOH$), and <20% conjugated with D-glucuronic acid to form benzoylglucuronide at around the TLV. Glucuronidation is the overflow pathway at higher toluene exposure concentrations. Toluene is also 1% metabolized through a 2,3-epoxide to form urinary 2-, 3-, 4-cresols ($HO \cdot C_6H_4 \cdot CH_3$) as sulfate and glucuronide conjugates. The half-time for hippuric acid urinary excretion is about 1 to 2 h, and it is completely eliminated after exposure ends within 24 h. Toluene does accumulate in fatty tissues following repeated exposures but is eliminated quickly after exposure.

The urinary BEI in 1992/1993 based on a 100 ppm TLV-TWA is end-of-shift hippuric acid at 2.5 g/g creatinine based on many studies, or 3 mg/min for the last 4 h of a shift equivalent at moderate work activity based on five studies. Because hippuric acid is produced endogenously as a product of aromatic amino acid metabolism and nitrogen excretion, background reference values (0.5–1.5 mg/g creatinine or 0.15–1.2 mg/min) vary from individual to individual, resulting in the recommendation of the BEI as a group test. Baseline samples also are recommended to assess the effects of diet and exogenous sources. The data from collections in the last 4 h correlate better with toluene exposure concentrations than do spot sample data. Lowering of the TLV to 50 ppm renders the hippuric acid BEI untenable because the 1.25 mg/g creatinine BEI is within the reference range for background values.

Exposure to styrene (Section 21.4.23), ethyl benzene (21.4.8), benzoic acid, and sodium benzoate food preservative increases urinary hippuric acid concentrations. Such acidic foods as fruits, berries, plums, cranberries, and prunes contain high concentrations of hippuric acid. Hippuric acid appears not to bind to blood proteins. Thymol or nitric acid is recommended as a urine preservative. Frozen samples are stable for at least one month.

End-of-shift venous blood toluene is recommended as a BEI for 100 ppm toluene at 1 mg/L based on extrapolation of the biological tolerance value (BAT) data of the West German Commission for Investigation of Health Hazards of Chemical Compounds in the Work Area, and on six other studies, mostly on volunteers. These studies report blood toluene concentrations between 0.3 and 1.3 mg/L after 8-h exposure to 100 ppm toluene. Blood concentrations are related to average exposure conditions rather than instantaneous exposure concentrations. The blood marker for toluene exposure concentrations of less than 50 ppm has advantages, as it is specific and has a lower detection limit relative to background concentrations, especially if specific headspace or gas chromatographic methods are used for analysis. Coexposure to ethanol increases venous blood toluene concentrations relative to toluene exposure alone. Heparin is recommended as the anticoagulant for blood samples stored at 2 to 5°C, which are stable for 5 to 7 days. Ethanol intake must be avoided for 24 h prior to sampling. Blood toluene in "unexposed" humans is generally <0.015 mg/L. After 8-h exposure to 100 ppm the blood concentration (c_b) in μg/L declines at time t in minutes after exposure according to the following equation:

$$c_b = 355e^{-0.335t} + 352e^{-0.0197t} + 129e^{-0.00339t} \tag{21.32}$$

The half-times are 2 min, 33 min, and 3.4 h.

The 1992/93 Documentation indicates that timing of blood sampling is so critical that the blood BEIs are confirmatory and not quantitative. A new urinary BEI of *o*-cresol at 1 mg/g creatinine sampled end-of-shift was recommended in 1991 but is not adopted for 1992/93. This marker is also nonspecific, as 2-cresol, 2-halotoluene (halo being chloro-, bromo-, and iodo-) and other molecules producing 2-cresol *in situ* are positive interferences. This marker is more sensitive than the hippuric acid marker in spite of a lower metabolic production because there are fewer endogenous sources of the marker.

21.4.25 Trichloroethylene

Trichloroethylene ($CCl_2{=}CHCl$), a denser liquid than water, has a boiling point of 87°C. It is used as a solvent for fats, cleaners, spot removers, adhesives, waxes, resins, oils, rubbers, paints, and varnishes, and is a degreasing and dry-cleaning agent. Trichloroethylene is an animal carcinogen, and its industrial use in the United States has been restricted. It has been detected in ambient air and drinking water. People have been known to sniff it for highs. The TLV-TWA is 50 ppm (270 mg/m^3), based on prevention of central nervous system effects and of adverse reactions when coexposure to alcohol occurs.

About 60% of inhaled trichloroethylene is absorbed under steady-state conditions at the TLV. About 9% of the absorbed mass is exhaled. The half-times of exhalation are 20 min, 3 h, and 30 h. Liquid trichloroethylene penetrates the skin (0.27 mg/cm^2/h) and crosses the placental barrier. Significant absorption after ingestion occurs.

Oxidative metabolism produces successively the following intermediates: 1,1,2-trichloroethylene oxide (CCl_2CHClO), 1,1,1-trichloroacetaldehyde (CCl_3CHO), and chloralhydrate ($CCl_3CH(OH)_2$). The latter can be reduced (33% of pulmonary absorbed dose) to 2,2,2-trichloroethanol (CCl_3CH_2OH), which is excreted in urine as a glucuronide; or the hydrate can be further oxidized (about 18% of the pulmonary absorbed dose) to trichloroacetic acid, which also is excreted in the urine. No chloral hydrate has been detected in the urine but has been in the blood. There is also a reversible oxidative pathway from 2,2,2-trichloroethanol to the trichloroacetic acid. Blood 2,2,2-trichloroethanol has a half-time of about 12 h with about 50% in the glucuronide form. Traces of urinary monochloroacetic acid ($ClCH_2COOH$) and exhaled chloroform (Cl_3CH) also are detected. About 8% of absorbed trichloroethylene is excreted as conjugates in the feces and sweat. The rest of the absorbed dose, especially at >50 ppm usually is stored in the fat tissues or bound to blood proteins as trichloroethylene, or accumulates in the blood as 2,2,2-trichloroethanol. The half-time for urinary trichloroacetic acid is 50 to 100 h, and that for urinary 2,2,2-trichloroethanol is 12 to 26 h. Total trichlorometabolites decline to one-third in urine 2 days after the end of 5 days of exposure to the TLV concentration. Glucose absorption or insulin administration decrease these half-times. Therefore, the diet is a major factor for these excretion rates. The extent of metabolism may vary more for Chinese who have high incidences of deficiencies in aldehyde and alcohol dehydrogenases.

There are two urinary BEIs. The one for trichloroacetic acid of 100 mg/g creatinine sampled at the end of the work week is based on a linear relation between trichloroethylene air concentrations and urinary trichloroacetic acid concentrations at <50 ppm trichloroethylene. This BEI does not protect susceptible groups. Negative interference occurs for urinary concentrations on coexposure/prior exposure to ethanol and Disulfiram/thiram pesticides, but blood concentrations are higher than expected. There is much interindividual variation; so a group test is recommended.

The second BEI is for total trichloro- metabolites (trichloroacetic acid/2,2,2-trichloroethanol, free and conjugated) at 300 mg/g creatinine in terms of trichloroacetic acid equivalents sampled at the end of the shift and end of the work week or after 3 consecutive days of exposure. Urinary 2,2,2-trichloroethanol has a half-time of about 12 to 26 h; so the ratio of the alcohol to acid markers varies, depending on the time after exposure but usually is between 1 and 2 on a molar basis for workers after five consecutive exposures at the TLV. This should be compared with a ratio of 10 at the end of the first day of exposure. The ratio was about 1 for urines sampled on the morning prior to the fifth day of daily exposure. Most of the trichloroethanol conjugates are in the glucuronide form.

The urinary concentration (c_u) of trichloro metabolites in mg/L collected from Japanese workers t days after the last 8-h exposure at trichloroethylene air concentration (c_a) in ppm was described by the following equation:

$$c_a = (1/6)c_u 10^{kt} \tag{21.33}$$

where k is the elimination rate constant (males = 0.23 day; females = 0.20 day).

This relationship was also obeyed by European volunteers exposed 8 h/day, 5 days/week to the same TLV concentrations, less or greater than 50 ppm trichloroethylene. However, the relationship does not hold for Chinese workers who excrete 5.5-fold less metabolites. Creatinine normalization appears to improve correlations.

Both urinary markers are nonspecific. Exposures to 1,1,1,2-tetrachloroethane ($CCl_3 \cdot CH_2Cl$), 1,1,2,2-tetrachloroethane ($CCl_2 \cdot CCl_2$), perchloroethylene (Section 21.4.21), methyl chloroform (Section 21.4.15), trichloroacetaldehyde ($Cl_3C \cdot CHO$), and chloral hydrate produce positive interferences. Exposures to alcohol and thiurams cause negative interferences. Large interindividual differences occur; so a group test is recommended. The metabolism to trichloroacetic acid is saturable above 50 ppm trichloroethylene vapor inhaled at TWA conditions, and above 1000 ppm for the trichloroethanol marker.

Another relationship also has been derived for Japanese workers:

$$\mathrm{c_u} = 8.37\mathrm{c_a} + 17.2 \tag{21.34}$$

where $\mathrm{c_u}$ and $\mathrm{c_a}$ are the same as in equation (21.33).

The blood free 2,2,2-trichloroethanol BEI based on many studies on volunteers is 4 mg/L at the end of a shift at the end of a work week, or after at least 3 consecutive days of exposure, using a specific gas chromatographic method for the headspace at 60°C or hexane extraction techniques. The anticoagulant should be heparin. The same influences that affect urinary trichloroacetic acid and total trichloro- compounds influence this marker. The neurological symptoms associated with trichloroethylene exposure are better correlated with blood trichloroethanol than trichloroethylene air exposure concentrations. Interindividual and intraindividual variation are much less with this marker than with the urinary ones. The marker is an indicator of same-day exposure. About 50% of the total 2,2,2-trichloroethanol (free alcohol plus glucuronide) is free <100 ppm trichloroethylene.

The breath BEI in end-exhaled air is trichloroethylene at 0.4 ppm collected prior to the last shift of the work week or 16 h after the fourth consecutive day of exposure. The steady-state mixed-exhaled air concentration is 40% of the inhaled concentration. For a single 8-h exposure to 50 ppm trichloroethylene, the concentration in alveolar air c_{ba} in ppm at t hours after the end of exposure is:

$$c_{ba} = 2.6e^{-2.3t} + 1.6e^{-0.23t} + 0.25e^{-0.023t} \qquad (21.35)$$

Sixteen hours after one 8-h exposure to 50 ppm trichloroethylene c_{ba} is 0.21 ppm. After sampling of breath from volunteers under the BEI conditions, c_{ba} is 0.44 ppm, which is also confirmed by a computer simulation. The marker is specific, unlike those using trichloro- compounds. This breath test should be utilized only for confirmatory or screening purposes because quantitation is so dependent on physical activity, preexposure history, and sampling time.

In 1991 and in 1992, a trichloroethylene in blood index was similarly recommended as a screening or confirmatory test when the headspace gas chromatography/electron capture technique was used. The sampling time is critical, and sampling for a venous sample from the cubital vein must be performed. The concentration in blood in mg/L (c_{bl}) after a 6-h exposure to 100 ppm of trichloroethylene declines at time t for resting volunteers according to the following equation:

$$c_{bl} = 0.89e^{-0.65t} + 0.11e^{-0.031t} \qquad (21.36)$$

The half-times were about 1 h and 22 h. There is significant accumulation during a work week. Computer simulation studies showed that equation (21.36) did describe a single TLV exposure under resting conditions.

Similarly for 8 h/day, 5 days/week exposures with modeling after the last exposure on the fifth day, equation (21.37) was derived for conditions simulating resting volunteers:

$$c_{bl} = 0.96e^{-0.83t} + 0.085e^{-0.023t} \qquad (21.37)$$

The calculated half-times were 50 min and 40 h. Computer modelling confirmed that the blood concentration is very dependent on work load, sampling time, and preexposure history, thus relegating it to the status of a screening/confirmatory test. Samples should be taken at least 3 h after the last exposure.

21.4.26 Xylenes

Commercial xylenes (1,2-, 1,3-, and 1,4-dimethylbenzenes; $C_6H_4(CH_3)_2$) consist of a mixture of these isomers plus ethylbenzene (Section 21.4.8), the mixture boiling at 137–140°C. The predominant isomer is 1,3-dimethylbenzene. The mixture is used in the syntheses of benzoic acid, isophthalic and terephthalic acids and esters, leather dyes, and phthalic anhydride, as well as in sterilizing catgut, oil immersion microscopy, scintillation fluids, varnishes, thinners, adhesives, and paints, and as a solvent. The TLV based on irritant and central nervous system effects is 100 ppm (435 mg/m^3).

The average retention of inhaled xylene over an 8-h period is 60 to 65%. About 3 to 6% of absorbed xylenes is exhaled after 8-h exposure with half-times of 1 h and 20 h. Skin absorption through the hands has been documented at 0.15 $mg/cm^2/h$. Rapid absorption after ingestion has been measured.

Most (about 95%) of the absorbed xylene isomers are metabolized to urinary methylhippuric acids ($C_6H_4CH_3 \cdot CONH \cdot CH_2COOH$) via 1-, 2-, and 3-methylbenzoic acids ($C_6H_4CH_3 \cdot COOH$), the latter being conjugated with glycine in a manner analogous to benzoic acid (Section 21.4.24). A small fraction (<1%) of xylenes undergo ring hydroxylation to form urinary xylenols ($C_6H_3 \cdot CH_3 \cdot (OH)_2$). The xylenes also are stored in fatty tissues and accumulate in blood bound to proteins after repetitive exposures. Urinary excretion of unchanged xylenes is negligible. The half-times for urinary methylhippuric acids are about 3.6 h and 30 h (reflecting adipose tissue release) with almost complete elimination after 3 days.

The urinary BEI based on many studies is end-of-shift "spot/composite sample" total methylhippuric acids at 1.5 g/g creatinine or 2 mg/min in a composite sample over the last 4 h of a shift for moderate physical activity. The concentrations are decreased (50% inhibition) by alcohol intake, which also elevates blood concentrations of xylenes. Since ethylbenzene inhibits xylene isomer metabolism, the BEI applies only for technical grades not pure xylene isomers. Aspirin also inhibits. Thymol and acid are the recommended urine preservatives, with frozen samples being stable for over 4 weeks. There are large interindividual differences.

21.4.27 Other Topics

While compounds are considered in alphabetical order, the short entries do not have Documentation issued for public comment as of November 1992.

There is a 1992 intent to establish a BEI for acetone ($CH_3 \cdot CO \cdot CH_3$) in urine at 100 mg/L, sampling at the end of the shift, to account for acetone TLV-TWA exposure of 1780 mg/m^3. C_1 and C_2 compounds, and diabetes patients give rise to acetone in urine and breath (Section 6.3.5), as well as endogenous processes (Section 2.6).

Arsenic (and its water-soluble inorganic compounds) and arsine have TLVs of 0.2 mg/m^3 and 0.16 mg/m^3 (0.05 ppm), respectively. The TLV for water-soluble arsenicals is based on widely varying acute local effects on the skin and mucous membranes. The TLV for arsine is set on the same considerations as above, but arsine causes hemolysis and renal damage >0.5 ppm. OSHA regulates arsenic as a carcinogen with a PEL of 10 $\mu g/m^3$ and there is a 1992 intent to change the TLV to the OSHA value. Pulmonary deposition of arsenic in cigarette fumes ranges from 25% to 40%; and absorption depends on solubility, which also depends on particle size. Smelter studies suggest triphasic kinetics with half-times of 4 days, 10 days, and unspecified years. About 60%

of the water-soluble inorganic arsenic absorbed is excreted in the urine, mostly as dimethylarsinic acid ($HO\cdot(As{=}O)\cdot(CH_3)$)) and lesser amounts of methylarsonic acid ($(HO)_2(As{=}O)CH_3$). The concentrations of both of these metabolites are related to biologically effective trivalent arsenic at <500 μg oral intake, the methylation being saturable above this intake. The half-times of urinary elimination after exposure are 2, 3.5, and 8 days in volunteers. Arsenic has been detected in hair, fingernails, and blood. Accumulation occurs during the work week. Trivalent arsenic is reversibly oxidized to pentavalent arsenic, the latter also appearing in urine. In contrast the organoarsenicals in seafood (mostly in the forms of arsenobetaine and arsenocholine), the major food source, are minimally metabolized.

The estimated daily intake of arsenic in food aside from seafood is 0.04 mg, but it is 20.19 mg with seafood. Other estimated daily intakes are <15 μg from drinking water, <0.2 μg from breathing ambient air, and 12 to 42 μg/cigarette. Endogenous urinary concentrations range from 0.013 to 0.25 μg/L, and baseline sampling is essential, particularly if total arsenic is being measured. The BEI for inorganic As metabolites in the urine from samples at the end of the work week is 50 μg/g creatinine. Hydride generation atomic absorption spectrophotometry is the recommended analytical chemistry method after separation of the inorganic arsenic from organic arsenic.

A new (1992/93) BEI is for chlorobenzene ($C_6H_5\cdot Cl$), whose TLV is 10 ppm (46 mg/m^3) based on liver effects in rats. The OSHA PEL is 75 ppm. The BEIs are end-of-shift urinary total 4-chlorocatechol ($(HO)_2\cdot C_6H_3\cdot Cl$) at 150 mg/g creatinine and end-of-shift urinary total 4-chlorophenol ($HO\cdot C_6H_4\cdot Cl$) at 25 mg/g creatinine, both nonspecific markers.

There is a 1992 intent to establish a BEI for TLV-TWA exposure to 2-ethoxyethanol ($CH_3CH_2\cdot O\cdot CH_2\cdot CH_2\cdot OH$) (18 mg/m^3) and 2-ethoxyacetate (27 mg/m^3) using a BEI of end of shift at the end of the work week 2-ethoxyacetic acid ($CH_3CH_2\cdot O\cdot CH_2\cdot COOH$) at 100 mg/g creatinine.

There is an intent to establish a BEI for methyl isobutyl ketone or MIBK ($CH_3\cdot(C{=}O)\cdot CH_2\cdot CH\ (CH_3)_2$). It has a boiling point of 115.8°C with the following partition coefficients: blood/gas, 90; oil/gas, 926; water/gas, 79; and urine/gas, 73. The TLV is 50 ppm (205 mg/m^3), based on protection from irritative and nephrotoxic effects. MIBK is used extensively as an industrial and household product (paint thinner) solvent. The pulmonary absorption is 60% of the exposure dose, and skin/gastrointestinal absorption is significant. The excretion of the parent compound is small in the urine but sufficient to be the basis for a BEI of 2 mg/L sampled end-of-shift. The elimination is biphasic, with half-times of about 40 min and 6.9 h. Following a single, 6-h exposure to 50 ppm MIBK, the urinary concentration of MIBK (c_u) t hours after the end of exposure is found by:

$$c_u = 2.90e^{-1.04t} + 0.95e^{-0.10t} \tag{21.40}$$

where e is the base of natural logarithms.

The timing of sampling is crucial, as is prevention of contamination of the sample. Individual variation and physical work-load effects are large. Because MIBK is very soluble in water, it distributes with body water. The major human metabolite appears to be 4-methyl-2-pentanol ($CH_3\cdot C(OH)H\cdot CH_2\cdot CH(CH_3)_2$). Presumably further oxidation can occur.

Another intended BEI is for total inorganic mercury (Hg), whose TLV is 0.05 mg/m^3 (elemental mercury vapor) and 0.1 mg/m^3 (aryl and inorganic mercury compounds), based on brain accumulation and attendant central nervous system effects characterized by tremor and neuropsychiatric disturbances. The ratio of total urinary mercury, in units of mg/L adjusted to specific gravity of 1.024, to personal TWA mercury in the breathing zone, in mg/m^3, varied from 1.1 to 4.7, with clustering between 2.3 and 3.0. The highest ratios were shown after mercuric oxide exposures, with the lowest after exposure to alkyl mercurials, indicative of a speciation difference. The urinary BEI recommended is preshift total inorganic mercury at 35 μg/g creatinine. The blood BEI is end-of-shift total inorganic mercury at the end of the work week at 15 μg/L. The highly variable endogeneous backgrounds make baseline sampling desirable also.

Compounds whose BEIs are being reexamined or investigated include: acrylonitrile, antimony, benzene, 2-butoxyethanol, cobalt, dichlorobenzene, N,N-dimethylacetamide, formaldehyde, lead, 2-methoxyethanol, 2-methoxyethanol acetate, 4,4′-methylene*bis*(2-chloroaniline), methylene chloride, nickel, perchloroethylene, synthetic pyrethrins, toluene, and vanadium. Other issues being considered include: quality control, effect of medication and illness, effect of exposures to mixtures, biological monitoring strategies, and control charts.

Further Reading

American Conference of Governmental Industrial Hygienists. 1988. *Industrial Ventilation: a Manual of Recommended Practice*, ACGIH, Cincinnati, OH.

American Conference of Governmental Industrial Hygienists. 1991. *Documentation of the Biological Exposure Indices*, 6th ed., ACGIH, Cincinnati, OH.

American Conference of Governmental Industrial Hygienists. 1991. *Documentation of the Threshold Limit Values and Biological Exposure Indices*, 6th ed., ACGIH, Cincinnati, OH.

American Conference of Governmental Industrial Hygienists. 1991. Biological Exposure Indices Committee. *Appl. Occup. Environ. Hyg*. **6**: 798–799.

American Conference of Governmental Industrial Hygienists. 1991. Notice of intended change for:
Arsenic. *Appl. Occup. Environ. Hyg*. **6**: 1049–1056.
Cadmium. *Appl. Occup. Environ. Hyg*. **6**: 703–711.
Carbon monoxide. *Appl. Occup. Environ. Hyg*. **6**: 896–902.
Methyl isobutyl ketone. *Appl. Occup. Environ. Hyg*. **6**: 712–714.
Trichloroethylene. *Appl. Occup. Environ. Hyg*. **6**: 715–727.

References

1. Thomas, V. 1988. Five years of the biological exposure indices committee. *Appl. Ind. Hyg*. **3**: F-26–F-28.
2. Fiserova-Bergerova (Thomas), V. 1987. Development of biological exposure indices (BEIs) and their implementation. *Appl. Ind. Hyg*. **2**: 87–92.
3. Fiserova-Bergerova (Thomas), V. 1990. History and concept of biological exposure indices. In *Biological Monitoring of Exposure to Industrial Chemicals*, V. Fiserova-Bergerova (Thomas) and M. Ogata (eds.), ACGIH, Cincinnati, OH, pp. 19–23.
4. American Conference of Governmental Industrial Hygienists. 1991. *Documentation of the Biological Exposure Indices*, 6th ed., ACGIH, Cincinnati, OH.

5. American Conference of Governmental Industrial Hygienists. 1986. *Documentation of the Threshold Limit Values and Biological Exposure Indices*, 5th ed., ACGIH, Cincinnati, OH.
6. American Conference of Governmental Industrial Hygienists. 1990. *1990–1991 Threshold Limit Values for Chemical Substances and Physical Agents and Biological Exposure Indices*, ACGIH, Cincinnati, OH.
7. Fiserova-Bergerova, V.; and Ogata, M. (eds.). 1990. *Biological Monitoring of Exposure to Industrial Chemicals*, ACGIH, Cincinnati, OH.
8. Gruber, M. 1883. Uber den Nachweis und die Wichtigkeit des Kohlenoxyds and sein Vorkommen in Wohnraumen. *Arch. Hyg.* **1**: 145–168.
9. Cook, W. 1990. Introduction: supplemental values of atmospheric and biologic monitoring. In *Biological Monitoring of Exposure to Industrial Chemicals*, V. Fiserova-Bergerova and M. Ogata (eds.), ACGIH, Cincinnati, OH, pp. xi–xxii.
10. Ogata, M. 1990. Goals and activities of the biological monitoring group in Japan. In *Biological Monitoring of Exposure to Industrial Chemicals*, V. Fiserova-Bergerova and M. Ogata (eds.), ACGIH, Cincinnati, OH, pp. 3–7.
11. Alessio, L. 1990. History and concept of biological monitoring in the European Communities. In *Biological Monitoring of Exposure to Industrial Chemicals*, V. Fiserova-Bergerova and M. Ogata (eds.), ACGIH, Cincinnati, OH, pp. 15–18.
12. Henschler, D. 1990. Biological monitoring and exposure limits as perceived in Germany. In *Biological Monitoring of Exposure to Industrial Chemicals*, V. Fiserova-Bergerova and M. Ogata (eds.), ACGIH, Cincinnati, OH, pp. 25–30.
13. Fiserova-Bergerova (Thomas), V. 1990. Comparison of biological exposure indices (BEIs) and biological tolerance values (BATs). In *Biological Monitoring of Exposure to Industrial Chemicals*, V. Fiserova-Bergerova and M. Ogata (eds.), ACGIH, Cincinnati, OH, pp. 31–33.
14. OSHA. 1989. OSHA–Final rule air contaminants–permissible exposure limits (Title 29 CFR Part 1910.1000). *Am. Ind. Hyg. Assoc. J.* **50**: A-257–A-293.
15. Bardodej, Z.; Urban, J.; and Malonova, H. 1987. Important considerations in the development of biological monitoring methods of determine occupational exposure to organic chemicals. In *Biological Monitoring of Exposure to Chemicals: Organic Compounds*, M. H. Ho and H. K. Dillon (eds.), Wiley-Interscience, New York, pp. 17–28.
16. Fiserova-Bergerova, V. 1987. Simulation model as a tool for adjustment of biological exposure indices to exposure conditions. In *Biological Monitoring of Exposure to Chemicals: Organic Compounds*, M. H. Ho and H. K. Dillon (eds.), Wiley-Interscience, New York, pp. 29–57.
17. Vlach, J. 1983. Simulation. In *Modeling of Inhalation Exposure to Vapors: Uptake, Distribution, and Elimination*, Vol I, V. Fiserova-Bergerova (ed.), CRC Press, Boca Raton, FL, pp. 133–153.
18. Drummond, L.; Luck, R.; Afacan, A. S.; and Wilson, H. K. 1988. Biological monitoring of workers exposed to benzene in the coke oven industry. *Br. J. Ind. Med.* **45**: 256–261.
19. Perbellini, L.; Faccini, G. B.; Pasini, F.; Cazzoli F.; Pistoia, S.; Rosellini, R.; Valsecchi, M.; and Brugnone, F. 1988. Environmental and occupational exposure to benzene by analysis of breath and blood. *Br. J. Ind. Med.* **45**: 345–352.

22

Biological Monitoring and Pesticides

22.0 INTRODUCTION

Pesticides are agents (chemical or physical) designed to rid humans of anything they deem a "pest." This usually is done by killing the pest, repelling it, or stopping it from reproducing. Legislatively, such agents, when they are chemicals, are collectively termed "economic poisons."

Their major advantages are to tilt the cost/benefit ratio to lower values to enhance human activities, prevent disease, enhance economic productivity, and extend human control over large land areas. Thus, increasing crop production, reducing insect-borne disease (for example, DDT is used to kill the larvae of the *Anopheles* mosquito, which causes malaria), controlling rodents, fungi, weeds, insects, and invertebrates that might lessen crop/animal productivity, and disinfecting water supplies to safeguard human health are some examples of desirable traits of pesticides when they are used properly.

When used in large doses, pesticides may kill humans or cause illness; perturb, affect, or kill nontarget species; and cause environmental contamination. If pesticides bioaccumulate, they may affect food chains and ultimately humans, as, for example, DDT and DDE in fish and shellfish used for human consumption. Because they often are designed to be selective to the target species, pesticides may be more toxic to that species than to any other, but this is not necessarily so for all pesticides. Quite often toxic impurities, as, for example, 2,3,7,8-substituted polychlorinated dibenzo-*p*-dioxins (PCDDs) and dibenzofurans (PCDFs) in chlorinated phenolic fungicides and phenoxyacetic herbicides may be of more importance to human health than the pesticidal ingredient ("active ingredient") itself. Another problem may occur if an environmental degradation product accumulates, such as photodieldrin from dieldrin, that is more toxic than the original pesticide. Furthermore, the oxon forms produced after metabolism of thionoorganophosphate pesticides are more toxic to mammals than the original pesticide (Sections 21.4.18 and 21.4.19).

The major types of pesticides can be named in several ways. In terms of target species, there are acaricides, avicides, bactericides, fungicides, herbicides, ichycides, insecticides, molluscides, nematocides, and rodenticides. In terms of type of action, there are attractants, biocides, biological control agents, contact pesticides, disinfectants, fumigants, larvicides, miticides, nerve agents, ovicides, recombinant DNA organisms, repellants, slow-release or controlled-release agents, systemic pesticides, and wood preservatives. As preapplication storage/transport forms, pesticides can be found as dusts, emulsion concentrates, granules, soluble powders, and wettable powders. They may be applied to the target species as aerosols, dusts, water- or diesel oil–diluted emulsions, granules, soluble powders, slow-release forms, and wettable powders. During application the concentration of the pesticidal active ingredient must be optimal for selectivity against the target species.

If aerosols are involved in the applications, the droplet or particle diameter must be controlled to enable adequate coverage, whether from a boom-sprayer rig, a spraying vehicle, a spray can, or aircraft. Drift ("non-target deposition") also must be minimized. To enhance water solubility in aqueous sprayings of herbicides, surfactants must be added if the pesticide is organic and water-insoluble. To control droplet diameters for application of diluted emulsion concentrates, a fraction of diesel, paraffinic, or petroleum ethers (the "inert components") often is added to lower the surface tension of the solution, with final adjustment through specific "adjuvants." Even in spray can applications, a propellant is required—still mostly chlorofluorocarbons so that aerosol exposure occurs around the home also.

Thus pesticide application often is accompanied by exposure to many other nonpesticidal chemicals constituting multicomponent chemical exposures. Such exposures may enhance or inhibit entry of the pesticide into the human body relative to the pure active ingredient alone, especially via the skin. This is especially important in recommending reentry intervals for workers after spraying and the type of protective equipment to be worn. In pesticide-formulating areas, many pesticides and many solvents, surfactants, inert ingredients, and adjuvants may be handled simultaneously, often in confined spaces that also result in high-level, multicomponent exposures to several pesticides and many other nonpesticidal chemicals. In manufacture of the active ingredient itself, often there is little exposure because many of the processes are enclosed. However during maintenance, cleaning, and sampling of reactor contents, high exposures may occur in the confined space of the enclosed reactors.

To complicate the issue further, just about every chemical ever manufactured has been used for a pesticidal purpose. Thus, sulfuric acid was the major herbicide utilized in the United States in the first 30 years of the twentieth century, and the use of inorganic and organic acids and bases as contact pesticides is still prevalent in many countries. Some common inorganic and organic chemicals used or formerly used as pesticides are listed in Table 22.1 [1–5]. This enormous list of specific chemicals is continually growing. It is no wonder that very few biological monitoring methods have been developed for these chemicals. The chief chemical groupings are: the organophosphate

TABLE 22.1. Common inorganic and organic chemicals used as pesticides. Synonyms are not provided. [1–5].

Pesticide type	Chemicals
Acaricides	azocycloten; benzomate; bromophos; bromophos-ethyl; cyolane; cytrolane; danitol; dazomet; DDVP; delnav; demeton; diazinon; dibrom; dichloropropene; dimethoate; dinobuton; disulfoton; endosulfan; EPN; ethion; ethyl guthion; FAC; fenthion; folimat; formothion; guthion; hostathion; imidan; malathion; menazon; mercarbam; metaldehyde; metasystox-R; methamidophos; methyl parathion; morestan; morocide; omite; parathion; pentac; phenthoate; phosalone; phosdrin; phosphamidon; plictran; supracide; temik; thimet; thiometon; torak; trithion; vamidothion; vendex.
Algicide	quinonamid.
Animal repellents	ammonium soaps of fatty acids (Hinder); big game repellent; bone tar oil; hot sauce animal repellent.
Attractants	juvenille hormones (insects).
Avicides	3-chloro-*p*-toluidine hydrochloride (starlicide); dieldrin; endrin (bird perch); ornitrol; queletox.
Bactericides	*m*-cresol; formalin; hexachlorophene; gallex; methyl isocyanide; phenol; streptomycin; terramycin; thiurams; 2,4-xylenol.
Biocides	biological agents: bacteria (anthrax, brucellosis, cholera, glanders, plague, *Salmonella*, tularemia, typhoid fever); biotoxins (aflatoxins, botulinus, ricin, tricothenes); fungi (anti-plant fungi used in World War II, coccidiodmycosis); rickettsia (Q fever, Rocky Mountain spotted fever, other spotted fevers, typhus or nonspotted fevers (Brill-Zinsser disease, epidemic typhus, murine typhus, rickettsial pox, scrub typhus)); viruses (dengue fever, encephalitis, immune deficiency viruses, influenza, meningitis, psittacosis, rift valley fever, smallpox, yellow fever).
	chemical blister agents (arsenicals: ED, L, MD, PD; mixes: HL, HT; mustards: HD; nitrogen mustards: HM-1, HN-2, HN-3; oximes: CX; others: Q, T).
	chemical blood agents (AC, CK, SA).
	chemical choking agents [chlorine, DP (diphosgene), CG (phosgene)].
	chemical herbicides (Agents BLUE, bromacil, 2,4-D, orange, 2,4,5-T).
	chemical incapacitating agents: central nervous system stimulants (amphetamine, cocaine, dexamphetamine, methamphetamine); central nervous system depressants (BZ); psychedelic drugs (lysergic acid, mescaline, morphine, opiates, phenylcyclidine, psilocybin); moderate incapacitating agents (cannabis, methaqualone, nitrazepam); agents mimicking noradrenaline and serotonin.
	chemical nerve gases [bicyclophosphinates, GA (Tabun), GB (Sarin), GD (Soman), GF, peptides, VE].
	chemical riot control agents: vomitants (DA, DC, and DM (adamsite); tear agents (CA, CN, CNB, CNC, CNS, CS).
Biological agents	*Bacillus thuringienses* (spores inducing disease in certain larvae); cactoblastis (cacti-eating larvae); chlorophenols (animal repellers secreted by many plants); Collego (spores used as a herbicide); DeVine (plant disease used as herbicide); elcar (ovicide viral agent); mycar (miticide); myxomotosis (rabbit virus); noloc (grasshoppers); padan; pyrethrums; rotenones.
Bird repellents	4-aminopyridine (avitrol); 9,10-anthraquinone.
Disinfectants	chlorine; chlorine dioxide; ozone; peroxozone; phenol; 2-phenylphenol (Dowcide 1); 2-phenylphenolates (Dowcide A); Triton X detergents.
Fungicides	cadmium chloride; calcium polysulfide; basic copper carbonate; basic copper chloride; copper hydroxide; basic copper sulfate (Bordeaux mixture); basic zinc sulfate; copper ammonium carbonate; copper sulfate; cuprous oxide; sulfur.
	acti-dione; alicylanilide; aluminum tris-*O*-ethylphosphonate (aliette); 2-aminobutane (deccotane); baycor; bayleton; baytan; benodanail; biphenyl; blasticidin; 2-bromo-2-nitropropan-1-diol (bronopol); bupirimate; busan-72; cadmium succinate (cadminate); calixin; captan; carbamates (benlate, previcur-

TABLE 22.1. *Continued*

Pesticide type	Chemicals
	N, rovral); chloranil; copper complexes with cyclopentanecarboxylates and quinolinolates; copper salts of fatty and rosin acids (citcop); curzate; cyprofuram; daconil 2787; DFX-H 6573; dichloro-2,5-dimethoxybenzene (demosan); 2,3-dichloro-1,4-naphthoquinone (dichlone); 2,6-dichloro-4-nitroaniline (dicloran); difolatin; dithiocarbamates (anthracol, basfungin; denmert; dikar, dimethirimol; dithane M-45, dithianon; dodemorphacetate; dodine; drazoxolon; Ferbam, Maneb, nabam, polyram, Zineb, Ziram); dwell; dyrene; EL-228; EL-291; ethirimol; euparen; fenarimol; fenfuran; fenpropimorph; ferric methanoarsonate (neoasozin); folpet; fongarid; formalin; fuji-one; furavax; furfural; furmecyclox; galben; glyodin; guazatine; hexachlorophene; imadazoles (bavistin; fuberidazole, imazalil, prochloraz, thiabendazole); impact; karathane; kasumin; kayabest; kumulan; lesan; mepronil; metalaxyl; mildiomycin; monceron; moncut; morestan; morocide; organomercurials; organophosphates (afugan, hinosan, kitazin, plondrel, rizolex); oturanic; pentachloronitrobenzene; pentachlorophenol; phenzain; phenol; phenyl mercuric acetate (pma); 2-phenylphenolates (Dowcide A); 2-phenylphenol (Dowcide 1); piomy; pipron; plantvax; polyoxins; potassium sorbate/sodium lauryl sulfate (MP-11); probenazole; rabcide; salclomide; sandofan; serinal; spartcide; sumilex; tachigaren; techlofthalan; terrazole; thiophanate; thiophanate methyl; thiurams (Thiram; triforine); tilt; triphenyltin acetate (brestan); triphenyltin hydroxide (du-ter); vigil; vinclozolin; vitavax.
Growth regulators (plants)	silicon dioxide. AC 94377; accel; 3-acetyl-thiazolidine-4-carboxylic acid (ergostim); acti-aid; ancymidol; atrinal; captan; CGA-15281; 2-chloroethylphosphonic acid (ethrel); 2-chloroethyl-trimethylammonium chloride (Cycocel); 2-chloroethyl-tris-(2′-methoxyethoxy)-silane (alsol); cytex; *n*-decanol (off-shoot-t); dinoseb; diphenylamine; embark; ethandial dioxime (PIK-OFF); ethoxyquin; ethylene; figaron; gibberelic acid; harvade; hybrex; indolebutyric acid; isopropyl-*m*-chlorocarbanilate (chlorpropham, CIPC); maleic hydrazide; methyl esters of fatty acids (off-shoot-o); morphactin; naphthaleneacetamide; 1-naphthylacetic acid; 1-naphthyl methylcarbamate (Sevin, Carbaryl); NC-9634; phenoxy acids, esters and amines [fruitone CPA-528; 4-chlorophenoxyacetic acid; 2,4-D; silvex (fruitone-T)], PIX; polado; polaris; PP 333; prime+; promaline; 3-propyl-3-t-butylphenoxyacetate; release; SN-49537; sodium dinitro-*o*-cresylate (DNOC); stemtrol; tamex; terpal; 2,3,5,6-tetrachloronitrobenzene (Fusarex); tomaset; tributyl phosphorotrithoate (DEF); tributyl phosphorotrithioite (folex).
Herbicides	ammonium sulfamate; calcium hydroxide; copper sulfate; mercuric chloride; mercurous chloride; sodium arsenate; sodium borate; sodium chlorate; sulfuric acid. AC-222,293; AC-252,925; acetanilides (acetochlor; alachlor, antor, butachlor, dual, L-flamprop isopropyl, metazachlor, potablan, propachlor, propanil, URIBEST, vistar); acrolein; alloxydim-sodium; allyl alcohol; aromatic nitro compounds (balan, basalin, dinoseb, dinoseb acetate, ethalfluralin, paarlan, prowl, surflan, trifluralin, vertac); aromatic oils; avenge; basagran; bensulide; benzamizole; benzoic acid esters and amine salts [alanap; 3-amino-2,5-dichlorobenzoic acid (amiben), benazolin, bromoxynil, butam, dicamba, dyanap, endothall, 2,3,6-trichlorophenylacetic acid (fenac)]; bromacil; buthidazole; cacodylic acid; carbamates and thiocarbamates [asulam, barban, betanal, betanex, carbetamide, CIPC, diallate (avadex), drepamon, eptam, eradicane, IPC, karbutilate, krenite, Ro-Neet, Sutan, SWEP, thiobencarb, Tillam, triallate (FARGO), verdinal, Vernam]; chinch; dacthal; dalapon; devrinol; 2,6-dichlorobenzonitrile (Casoron); 2,6-dichlorothiobenzamide (Prefix); dimethachlor; dinoseb; diphenamid; diquat; disodium methanearsonate (DSMA); Dowco 356; erbotan; faneron; fenoxaprop-ethyl; fenthiapropethyl;

TABLE 22.1. *Continued*

Pesticide type	Chemicals
	fluazifop; fluridone; glufosinate; glyphosate; halogenated diphenyl ethers (blazer, CGA-82725, diclofop, Dowco 453, fomesafen, goal, lactofen, MO, nitrofen, TOK, X-52); ioxynil; kayametone; kerb; lenacil; maleic hydrazide; mataven; merpelan-AZ; methanearsonate (AMA); modown; mogeton; norflurazon; nortron; ordram; organophosphates (anilofos, cremart, krenite); oust; paraquat; petroleum oils; phenoxyalkanoic salts and esters [2,4-D; 2,4-DB; 2,4-DP; Dow 233; herbit; MCPA; MCPB; MCPP (mecoprop); Sesone; silvex; 2,4,5-T]; picolinic acids (Dowco 233, Dowco 290, picloram); piperophos; poast; pyridate; pyrazon; ronstar; scepter; sinbar; sodium dinitro-*o*-cresylate (DNOC); sodium methanearsonate (MSMA); sodium-2,2,3,3-tetrafluoropropionate (Frenock); suffix; tar oils; triazines (ametryn, amitrole, atrazine, aziprotryn, BAY-SSH-0860, bladex, dimethametryn, glean, goltix, igran, prometone, prometryn, propazine, sancap, semeron, sencor, simazine, sumitol, terbumeton, terbuthylazine, velpar); trichloroacetic acid; undecylenic acid; urea compounds (benathiazuron, chlorbromuron, chloroxuron, dicuran, difenoxuron, diuron, dymron, fluometuron, isoproturon, isuon, lorox, methyldymron, metoxuron, monolinuron, monuron, neburon, patoran, tebuthiuron, tribunil, tupersan, UROX, ustilan); URIBEST.
Ichyicide	fintrol
Insect fumigants	aluminum phosphide; carbon dioxide; carbon disulfide; hydrogen cyanide; magnesium phosphide; sodium cyanide; sulfur dioxide; sulfuryl fluoride.
	acrylonitrile; basamid (dazomet); carbon tetrachloride; chloropicrin (trichloronitromethane); dichlorobenzenes; 1,2-dibromo-3-chloropropane; 1,2-dichloropropane; 1,3-dichloropropane; 1,3-dichloropropene; dimethyl carbamate; dimethylphthalate; dioxane; ethyl formate; ethylene dibromide; ethylene dichloride; ethylene oxide; formaldehyde; indalone; methyl bromide; methyl chloride; methylene chloride; methylisothiocyanate; naphthalene; paraformaldehyde; perchloroethylene; propylene dichloride; sodium *N*-methyldithiocarbamate (Vapam); telone; trichloroethylene; validamycin.
Insect growth regulator	BAY SIR 8514; CGA-72662; ENSTAR.
Insecticides	arsenic oxides; arsenites; arsenates; barium fluorosilicate; basic lead arsenate; borax; boric acid; cryolite; lead arsenate; mercuric chloride; silica aerogel; sodium arsenite; sodium fluoride; white phosphorus.
	altosid; amdro; amitraz; applaud; bollex; carbamates (BAS-263, baycarb, baygon, butocarboxime, butoxicarboxim, carbamult, carbofuran, carbosulfan, croneton, dioxacarb, etrofolan, ficam, formetanate, lannate, larvin, macbal, matacil, meobal, mesurol, MTMC, nem-a-tak, oxamyl, padan, pirimor, sevin, temik, terbam, UC-21865, UC-56295); chlorinated aromatic compounds [ACORAL, baygon-meb, chlorodimeform, chlorobenzilate, dichlorobenzenes, DDT, dicofol (kelthane), diflubenzuron, methoxychlor, pydrin, qikron, sappiran, tedion]; *o*-chlorophenol; cyclodienes (aldrin, chlordane, dieldrin, endosulfan, endrin, heptachlor, kepone, mirex); evisect; lethane 384; lindane; metaldehyde; morestan; naled; naphthalene; nifluridide; omite; organophosphates (abate, agritox, alfracron, aphidan, aspon, azodrin, baythion-C, bidrin, BOLSTAR, bomyl, bromophos, CELATHION; chlorfenvinphos, chlormephos, ciodrin, co-ral, counter, curacron, cyanox, cyolane, cytrolane, dasanit, DDVP, delnav, demeton, diazinon, dibrom, dimethoate, disulfoton, dowco 214, dursban, dyfonate, dylox, EPN, ethion, ethyl guthion, etrimfos, FAC, famphur, fenitrothion, fenthion, folimat, formothion, guthion, hodson, hostaquick, hostathion, imidan, iodofenphos, karphos, malathion, menazon, mercarbam; methamidophos, metasystox-R, methacrifos, methyl parathion, MIRAL, mocap, nemacur, nem-a-tak, ofnak, oftanol, orthene, parathion, phenthoate, phosalone, phosdrin, phosphamidon, phoxim, pirimiphos, pirimiphos-ethyl, propetamphos, quinalphos, rabon, RH-0994, ronnel, salithion, S-seven, supracide, surecide,

TABLE 22.1. *Continued*

Pesticide type	Chemicals
	thimet, thiometon, tokuthion, torak, trithion, vamidothion); pentac; pentachlorophenol; petroleum oils; plictran; pyrethrum; rotenone; SN-72129; synthetic pyrethroids (baythroid, cypermethrin, danitol, decamethrin, Dowco 417, mavrik, pay-off, permethrin, phenothrin, pydrin, pyrethrin, resmethrin, tetramethrin); tetrachlorophenols; toxaphene.
Insect repellents	dibutylsuccinate; 2-ethyl-1,3-hexandiol; 2-hydroxy-n-octyl sulfide; MGK 326.
Miticides	DPX-3792; RH-0994; UBI-T930.
Molluscicides	cupric sulfate; frescon; mesuron; metaldehyde.
Nematocides	carbofuran; dasanit; dazomet; dibromochloropropane; dichloropropene; formetanate; lannate; MIRAL; mocap; nemacur; nem-a-tak; oxamyl; temik; UC-21865.
Ovicides	chlordimeform; elcar; trithion.
Rodenticides	arsenic phosphides; barium carbonate; thallium sulfate; zinc phosphide. alphakil; antu; calciferol; castrix; α-chlorohydrin; chlorophacinone; diphacin; diphenylsulfone; endrin; fluoroacetate; fluoroacetamide; fumarin; maki; pival; racumin; ratak; scilliroside; strychnine; talon; tomorin; valone; warfarin.
Virucide	Terramycin.

Reference 5 was utilized for the biocide data; references 1–4 were utilized for the rest of the data. The reader should consult these references to obtain the exact chemical nature of the pesticides.

insecticides/acaricides/fungicides; the carbamate/thiocarbamate insecticides/herbicides/fungicides; the chlorophenoxy herbicides; the chlorophenolic fungicides; and acid/base contact chemicals, inorganic and organic. The organic pesticides have the advantage that many may act systemically and therefore require much smaller amounts to be applied to achieve their pesticidal effect than contact pesticides require. However, because most organic pesticides are relatively insoluble in water, they often need other chemicals in the formulation to allow cheap spraying and adequate coverage.

The pesticides considered in Chapter 21 include: cadmium and its compounds as fungicides (Section 21.4.3); carbon disulfide fumigant (Section 21.4.4); furfural fungicide (Section 21.4.10); organophosphorus cholinesterase inhibitors used as insecticides, acaricides, fumigants, and nematocides (Section 21.4.18); parathion insecticide and acaricide (Section 21.4.19); pentachlorophenol fungicide (Section 21.4.20); perchloroethylene fumigant (Section 21.4.21); phenol disinfectant/bactericide (Section 21.4.22); and trichloroethylene fumigant (Section 21.4.25). We will not consider the specific biological monitoring of these compounds here.

Certain biological monitoring markers considered in Chapter 21 also suffer positive interference from the chemicals listed in Table 22.1. Thus formalin fungicide, formaldehyde fumigant, paraformaldehyde fumigant, and the degradation of the organophosphates dicrotophos (Bidrin) and monocrotophos (Azodrin) will enhance the urinary formic acid marker for methanol (Section 21.4.14). Lead arsenates and basic lead arsenates used as insecticides will increase blood lead, urinary lead, and blood zinc protoporphyrin concentrations (Section 21.4.12). Sodium fluoride, barium fluorosilicate, and cryolite insecticides and sulfuryl fluoride insect fumigant affect the measurement of urinary fluoride (Section 21.4.9), whereas the organic fluoride organophosphates [for example, the nerve gases GB (sarin), GD (soman), and GF] and herbicides (for example, trifluralin) also must be considered. Phenol disinfectant/bactericide exposure also will increase the apparent benzene exposure (Section 21.4.2). The urinary *p*-nitrophenol marker of nitrobenzene (Section 21.4.17) is enhanced by exposure to parathion. The urinary *p*-aminophenol marker for aniline (Section 21.4.1) is increased by applications of Carbetamide, Fenuron, Propham, and Siduron because aniline is generated as a metabolite from these pesticides; thus the nonspecific methemoglobinemia marker (Section 21.4.13) also may be affected by high exposures to these four pesticides. If in addition the inert components of emulsion sprays contain toluene (Section 21.4.24), benzene (Section 21.4.2), ethylbenzene (Section 21.4.8), xylenes (Section 21.4.26), and *n*-hexane (Section 21.4.11), exposure to pesticide spray drift, to the spray itself, to the vapor drift, and to residues/vapors at reentry may cause increases in the biological markers for these solvents.

Interactions also may occur. Thus the effects of the chlorinated aliphatic solvent fumigants and fungicidal thiurams on methanol metabolism are well known (Section 21.4.14), and vice versa. The same effect has been also noted for ethanol. This is an area of much-needed research because interactions are the weakest area of biological monitoring interpretation.

Like other chemicals, the concentrations of pesticide residues in the diet are important, especially for the less volatile compounds [6]. Health and safety considerations of workers exposed to pesticides have been widely reported [7–12], and medical surveillance (Chapters 7–9) is crucial. Hypersusceptibility (Section 13.3) of people to pesticides and to other chemicals even at low concentrations also has been noted, due to genetic factors, chemical interactions, or predisposing life-style or dietary factors [13]. Such hypersusceptibility is one of the chief drawbacks to the use of exposure and biological monitoring as surrogates for the health of individuals relative to typical susceptibilities. The interrelationship of biological monitoring data with health effects also may be confounded by the presence of toxic impurities in the formulations used and by any simultaneous exposure to several pesticides and solvents.

Biological monitoring for pesticides containing metals has traditionally been in terms of total metal, in the body tissue or fluid. Classical analyses by atomic absorption, emission, inductively coupled plasma, neutron activation, X-ray fluorescence and other techniques for metals have been discussed in Section 6.0.6 and 2.13.4. We will limit further discussion to the organic pesticides and biological monitoring markers not already discussed elsewhere, utilizing various books and symposia published on the topic [7, 11–18]. Therefore, attention will be focused on the organophosphate, carbamate, and organochlorine pesticides.

22.1 ORGANOPHOSPHATES

There are several basic sources for the following summary [19–21], in addition to the relevant sections in Chapter 21.

22.1.1 Activation and Detoxification

The general formula for organophosphates is: $(R_1R_2){\cdot}P{=}O(S){\cdot}X$, where X can be almost any other functional group, and R_1 and R_2 can be any substituted alkyl, aryl, alkoxy, aryloxy group, thioxy, phenoxythio, or amide groups. If X is F [GB (Sarin), GD (Soman), and GF] or cyano (GA) and R_1 is $-NR_3R_4$ [for example, in GA (Tabun)] or $-S-R_5$ (VE, VX) where R_3, R_4, and R_5 are alkyl, alkoxy, aryl, aryloxy, and acyl, very acutely potent agents result with respect to central nervous system effects and inhibition of cholinesterase (Section 21.4.18). Activation to more potent intermediates occurs via five mechanisms: oxidative desulfurization of the thiophosphoryl compounds; oxidation of a sulfur to sulfoxides or sulfones; oxidation of amides (methylphosphoramides form *N*-oxides or *N*-methylols, and *N*-alkylcarboxyamides form the dealkylated analogs); hydroxylation of alkyl groups to produce eventually cyclic phosphate esters or ketones; and nonoxidative and nonenzymic processes such as the rearrangement of α-hydroxy-β-haloalkylphosphonates to vinyl phosphates, dehalogenation by reaction with such molecules as glutathione (Section 2.11.4), thiono–thiolo rearrangements, and dehalogenation–hydroxylation. The oxidative reactions predominate in the mixed-function oxidase enzymes of the endoplasmic reticulum of the liver and require molecular oxygen, NADPH, cytochrome P-450, and other components (Section 2.9). Oxidation–reduction processes often occur on the same enzyme complex (Sections 2.12 and 2.13.1).

The major deactivation processes usually are classified in terms of those that attack at the phosphorus atom, and those that do not. Such attacking species include phosphatases, phosphoramidases, carboxyesterases, amidases, alkaline and acid phosphatases (Section 9.0.5), and Phase II processes that may occur before or after these other processes (Sections 2.13.2 and Section 5.1). The phosphatases attack only triesters and anhydrides of orthophosphoric acid, whereas the alkaline and acid phosphatases hydrolyze partial esters of orthophosphoric acid. Thus for oxidative hydrolysis of organophosphorothionates [$(RO)_2\cdot(P{=}S)\cdot O-R_1$; for example, parathion, methyl parathion, fenitrothion, P-S-demeton, and diazinon] and organophosphorothiolothionates [$(RO)_2\cdot(P{=}S)\cdot S-R_1$; for example, disulfoton, phorate, metidathion, dimethoate, and malathion], the net deactivation reaction is through oxidative dealkylation, esterase hydrolysis, and the participation of glutathione-*S*-alkyl transferase:

$$\begin{aligned}&\tfrac{1}{2}\,O_2 + (RO)_2\cdot(P{=}S)\cdot S(\text{or } O)-R_1 + H_2O \rightarrow\\&(RO)_2\cdot(P{=}S)\cdot OH + HS(\text{or } HO)\cdot R_1\end{aligned} \tag{22.1}$$

where R_1 is a substituted aryl (for example, parathion, methyl parathion, and fenitrothion) or alkyl group, and the R groups are alkyl (usually methyl or ethyl groups).

This process competes with oxidative desulfurization activation to produce the potent oxon analog:

$$\begin{aligned}&\tfrac{1}{2}\,O_2 + (RO)_2\cdot(P{=}S)\cdot S(\text{or } O)-R_1 + H_2O \rightarrow\\&\underset{\text{oxon}}{(RO)_2\cdot(P{=}O)\cdot S(\text{or } O)-R_1} + -SH^- + OH^-\end{aligned} \tag{22.2a}$$

When R is methyl for organophosphorothionates (for example, in methyl parathion, fenitrothion, methidathion, dimethoate, and malathion), activation predominates over deactivation but not at longer chain lengths. This oxidative desulfurization activation in organophosphorothiolothionates also occurs with nonaromatic leaving R_1 groups such as the maleate moiety in malathion.

The enzymic cleavage of the anhydride bond of phosphate esters occurs through the A-esterases of the serum and the liver. They do not hydrolyze organophosphorothionates, but do hydrolyze organophosphorothiolates ($(RO)_2{\cdot}(P{=}O){\cdot}S{-}R_1$; for example, P–O–demeton, and diazinon) as well as organophosphoates (for example, dichlorvos, dicrotophos, monocrotophos):

$$H_2O + (RO)_2{\cdot}(P{=}O){\cdot}O(\text{or } S){-}R_1 + H_2O \rightarrow (RO)_2{\cdot}(P{=}O){\cdot}OH + HO(\text{or } S)R_1 \tag{22.2b}$$

Most of the A-esterases in humans are calcium-activated (unlike those in insects, which cannot deactivate the compound efficiently thus leading to its insecticidal action; insect and microbiol A-esterases generally have a manganese activator and mammals also have some of these enzymes, the ratio between the manganese and calcium forms being related in some people to hypersusceptibility to these insecticides). $S{-}R_1$ cleavage is believed to occur in phosphorothiolates but is minor.

The third major mechanism by which the anhydride bond can be cleaved involves nonenzymic and enzymic conjugation with glutathione (Section 2.11.4):

$$(RO)_2{\cdot}(P{=}O(\text{or } S)){\cdot}O{-}R_1 + GSH \rightarrow (RO)_2{\cdot}(P{=}O(\text{or } S)){\cdot}OH + GSR_1 \tag{22.3}$$

where GSH is the tripeptide glutathione.

Alkyl ester bond cleavage does occur but is not as important as anhydride bond cleavage. Oxidative dealkylation, hydrolysis, and glutathione conjugation also occur:

$$0.5O_2 + (RCH_2O)_2{\cdot}(P{=}O){\cdot}X \rightarrow (R{\cdot}HCOH{\cdot}O)\ (RCH_2O){\cdot}(P{=}O){\cdot}X \rightarrow RCHO + (HO)(RCH_2O){\cdot}(P{=}O){\cdot}X \tag{22.4}$$

where R is an alkyl group and X a leaving group (for example, trichlorfon and the organophosphoates). Ethyl esters produce the most alkyl ester bond cleavage. The aldehyde product can undergo further oxidation to the corresponding carboxylic acids, reduction to the corresponding alcohols, and transamination. Oxidative dealkylation is more important for phosphate triesters than for phosphorothionates.

A liver hydrolase also catalyzes hydrolysis of the alkyl ester bond of phosphate esters:

$$(RCH_2O)_2{\cdot}(P{=}O){\cdot}X + H_2O \rightarrow RCH_2OH + (HO)(RCH_2O){\cdot}(P{=}O){\cdot}X \tag{22.5}$$

Methyl phosphate and phosphorothionate esters are primarily demethylated in the liver by reaction with GSH:

$$(CH_3O)_2 \cdot (P{=}O(\text{or } S)) \cdot X \rightarrow (HO)(CH_3O) \cdot (P{=}O(S)) \cdot X + GS{-}CH_3 \quad (22.6)$$

The liver GSH-*S*-transferase enzymes are inactive toward phosphonates and the monomethylated by-products of equation (22.6). Cleavage of P–N bonds in phosphoramides also may occur.

Metabolic reactions to not only occur at the phosphate moiety. For those organophosphate compounds containing a carboxyester or carboxythiolo linkage (for example, malathion), enzymic hydrolysis is mediated by the B-esterases found in almost all human tissues except serum. Insects have low activities of these enzymes. Although this is a major pathway for malathion, it is not for mevinphos, where degradation by phosphatases is predominant. For malaoxon, the diethyl carboxyester of the maleic acid leaving group is hydrolyzed to the free diacid (dominates) and a monacid. The carboxyamide group in organophosphorus pesticides (for example, in methidathion, dicrotophos, dimethoate, and some nerve gas peptides) is hydrolyzed by amidases in the liver endoplasmic reticulum:

$$-(C{=}O) \cdot N \cdot R_1R_2 + H_2O \rightarrow -(C{=}O) \cdot OH + H \cdot NR_1R_2 \quad (22.7)$$

Both *N*-mono- and *N,N*-dialkyl amides can be cleaved, though binding may depend on the chain length and the parent acid. Dimethoate, a phosphorothiolothionate that contains the *N*-methyl amide of ethanoic acid, readily undergoes amide cleavage to yield the corresponding dimethoate acid. The oxygen analog is not cleaved. Amide cleavage occurs also in dicrotophos, which has the *N,N*-dimethylamide of the methylpropenoic acid moiety. No amide cleavage has been observed for phosphamidon, which is a phosphate ester containing the *N,N*-diethylamide of methylchloropropenoic acid. Liver phosphatases compete with carboxyamidases.

The reduction of aromatic nitro groups to amino groups is important for organophosphates such as parathion, methyl parathion, and fenitrothion. The conjugation of the cleaved moieties of degraded organophosphate esters promotes detoxification. Urine excretion occurs for those cleavage products below the biliary excretion molecular weight cutoff (MW 410–435 in humans) and for those high molecular weight compounds that undergo enterohepatic circulation (Section 3.1) after microbial action in the gastrointestinal tract. Glucuronides (Section 5.1.1) are produced competitively on in situ production of hydroxy, carboxyl, phenolic, amino, and thio functional groups (for example, for the dichlorovinyl alcohol from dichlorvos and trichlorfon; for the trichloroethanol from trichlorfon). Sulfation (Section 5.1.1) also occurs for alcohols, phenols, and aromatic amines. Methylation (Section 5.1.3) of thiols to methyl sulfides, thence to sulfoxides and sulfones, also occurs (for example, for P-S-demeton, P-O-demeton, disulfoton, phorate, and the methyl sulfide from the thiadiazole leaving group of methidathion).

22.1.2 Biological Monitoring Markers

If a number of dimethoxyorganophosphates are being sprayed (e.g., methyl parathion, fenitrothion, trichlorfon, dichlorvos, methidathion, dicrotophos, monocrotophos, dimethoate, and malathion), then after the X group leaves and any –P=S bond is converted to –P=O (methyl parathion, fenitrothion, methidathion, dimethoate, and malathion), *O*,*O*-dimethylphosphate is a nonspecific urinary and blood biological monitoring marker. Other alkyl phosphates found in urine and blood include: *O*,*O*-dimethyl phosphorothionate (from, e.g., methyl parathion, fenitrothion, methidathion, dimethoate, and malathion); *O*,*O*-dimethyl phosphorothiolate (from, e.g., P-O-demeton directly and indirectly from disulfoton, phorate, methidathion, dimethoate, and malathion); *O*,*O*-dimethylphosphorodithioate (from, e.g., disulfoton, phorate, methidathion, dimethoate, and malathion); *O*,*O*-diethylphosphate (from, e.g., parathion, P-S-demeton, P-O-demeton, disulfoton, phorate, and diazinon); and the other diethyl analogs of the dimethyl derivatives. Monoalkyl phosphates also are found in the urine and blood.

About 30% of acutely ingested ethyl parathion is excreted in humans as urinary *O*,*O*-diethyl phosphate (within 72 h) and as the lesser metabolite, *O*,*O*-diethylphosphorothionate (within 4 h) as a dose-effect. The dimethyl analogs also show a dose-effect in 24 h on acute ingestion of methyl parathion. Other studies have shown a high correlation between urinary alkyl phosphates excreted in 2 days and guthion sprayed. Urinary alkyl phosphates correlate with red blood cell cholinesterase activities for phorate, but not for guthion or some other organophosphates, especially at low doses. Urinary dimethylthiophosphate concentrations after methyl-azinphos exposure are suggestive of excretion of 1 μg in 48 h for every 10 μg of pesticide applied dermally [16].

The necessity of taking 24- or 48-h urine samples has made the urinary dialkyl phosphates an inconvenient choice as biological monitoring markers. The analytical techniques are difficult also. The use of disposable extraction cartridges has facilitated collection and cleanup [22]. However, alkyl phosphates do exhibit a dose-effect at exposure levels far below those necessary to elicit lowering of blood cholinesterase. The patterns of alkyl phosphates may help identify the type of exposing organophosphate if this is unknown (e.g., the presence of both *O*,*O*-dimethyl phosphate and *p*-nitrophenol implies methyl parathion exposure; the presence of *O*,*O*-diethyl phosphate, *O*,*O*-diethyl phosphorothionate, and *p*-nitrophenol implies ethyl parathion).

Biological monitoring of the original organophosphate in blood is not done because of fast metabolism and the fact that the storage of blood samples causes organophosphates to decrease rapidly, unlike the organochlorine pesticides. This does not mean that the organophosphates cannot be detected in fat, liver, or brain after autopsy. The major problem lies in the interpretation of the data. Massive amounts of pesticide naturally require little interpretation.

Medical monitoring apart from serum cholinesterase has shown that organophosphates may induce pancytopenia [23] (the reduction of all formed elements of the blood) and hemoglobin decreases [24]. Immune system effects have been reported [24]; for example, host defense mechanisms have been impaired by carbophenothion, crufomate, DEP, diazinon, dichlorvos, dimethoate, leptophos, malathion, methylmercaptophos, ronnel, trichlorofon, and triisopropylphosphate. Serum paraoxonase and lymphocyte/platelet neuropathy target esterase (for agents causing delayed neuropathy) activities have also been recommended as markers [25].

The connection of biological monitoring data with health effects is influenced not only by interindividual human variations but also by the presence of toxic impurities, which may or may not have been present in the manufacturer's organophosphorus formulation. Thus for example, the fenitrothion *S*-methyl isomer often is present between 0.5% and 1.5%, and increases with storage, ultraviolet irradiation, and increasing temperature [26]. This isomer is two to three orders of magnitude more effective at inhibiting cholinesterase than fenitrothion in human serum, and even at 1% the isomer accounts for 35% of the inhibition versus 12% for the major organophosphate [26]. Malathion also contains isomalathion, depending on the temperature, packing material, humidity, and manufacturing process. Isomalathion concentrations >1.8% (w/w) in malathion formulations will produce unexpected toxicity [26]. Sulfotepp (acute rat oral LD_{50} of 5 mg/kg) in diazinon (0.01–0.53% in fresh formulations [27, 28]), demeton (3.1–3.6%), coumaphos (0.04–0.06%), and parathion (0.07%) may make these pesticides more toxic than expected from biological monitoring data on the major active ingredients [27]. The LD_{50} for pure diazinon is 300 to 850 mg/kg [28]. Chlorpyrifos, fensulfothion, phosalone, disulfoton, and terbufos generally have <0.03% sulfotepp in freshly received formulations [27].

The occurrence of delayed neurotoxicity has been observed for mipatox, DFP, dimefox and its ethyl derivative, BFP, tri-*o*-cresylphosphate (TOCP), trichloronate, methamidophos, leptophos, chlorpyrifos, and trichlorofon, the roles of impurities in these effects being unclear [29–31].

Although red blood cell cholinesterase activity is the major biological monitoring marker for organophosphates because it measures the net effect of exposure to many organophosphates by any exposure route, urinary dialkyl and alkyl phosphate determination is a useful adjunct. Other newer markers include vagal tone (obtained by measurement of the decrease in heart period with inspiration and the increase with expiration) and salivary and plasma cholinesterase [32]. Another nonspecific medical monitoring index that is much used in a screening manner is urinary mutagenicity. The following organophosphates are known to be mutagenic in bacterial reversion-assay systems with five strains of *Salmonella typhimurium* (TA98, TA100, TA1535, TA1537, and TA1538) and strain WP2 *her* of *Escherichia coli* [33]: acephate (orthene), chlorfenvinphos (birlane), dichlorvos (DDVP), dimethoate, disulfoton (disyston), ESP (estox), fenitrothion (sumithion), formothion (anthio), monocrotophos (azodrin), phosmet (PMP), pirimiphosmethyl (actellic), salithion, thiometon (ekatin M), trichlorfon (dipterex), and vamidothion (kilval). Those known not to be mutagenic include: bensulide, chlorpyrifos, chlorpyrifosmethyl, cyanopyrifosmethyl, diazinon, dichlofenthion, dimethylvinphos, edinphos, EPBP, EPN, ethephon, ethion, etrimfos, glyphosate, IBP, isofenfos, isoxathion, malathion, mecarbam, naled, phenthoate, phoxim, piperophos, propaphos, phosdifen, prothiophos, pyrazophos, pyridaphenthion, and tetrachlorvinphos. Amiprofosmethyl and krenite tested negative with TA98 and TA100 [33].

22.2 CARBAMATES

Carbamates ($R_1 \cdot O \cdot (C{=}O) \cdot N \cdot (R_2R_3)$) by agreement also include thiocarbamates ($R_1 \cdot O \cdot (C{=}S) \cdot N \cdot (R_2R_3)$) and dithiocarbamates ($[R_2R_3N \cdot (C{=}S) \cdot S \cdot]_nX$), where R_1, R_2, and R_3 can be alkyl or aryl groups with $n = 1$, and

X can be a metal group for $n > 1$ [for example, DDC (sodium; $n = 1$), Ferbam (iron; $n = 3$), TTCA (arsenic; $n = 3$), and Ziram (zinc; $n = 2$)], or $(\text{–S}\cdot(\text{C=S})\cdot \text{NR}_2\text{R}_3)$ as for thiram and EMSC. The $(\text{–CH}_2\text{N}\cdot(\text{C=S})\cdot\text{S}\cdot)_n\text{X}$ configuration also is common, as in maneb (X = Mn; $n = 2$); zineb (X = Zn; $n = 2$); polyram (X = Zn; $n = 1$ or 2); dithane M-45 (mixture of maneb and zineb); and nabam (X = Na; $n = 2$). The dithiocarbamates very quickly have their weak disulfide bonds cleaved to form thiocarbamates in blood, and the sulfur in these carbamates often is replaced by oxygen in a process very similar to the replacement of S by O for organophosphates (Section 22.1.1) through oxidative carbamylation. Commonly R_2 and R_3 and methyl groups, as for chloropropham, DDC, EMSC, ferbam, formetanate, pirimor, polycarbamate, propamocarb, propham, thiram, TTCA, and ziram. The substitution $R_2 = H$ and R_3 = methyl is even more common [for example, for BAS-263, BASSA, baygon (propoxur), butocarboxime, butoxicarboxim, carbamult, carbaryl (sevin), carbofuran, carbosulfan, croneton, DIOXACARB, etrofolan, ficam, knockbal, lannate, macbal, matacil, MEOBAL, mesurol, MTMC, oxamyl, temik, and UC-21865]. R_2 and R_3 are ethyl for benthiocarb and Vegedex, and R_1 is aromatic for BAS-263, BASSA, baygon, betanal, carbamult, carbaryl, carbetamide, carbofuran, carbosulfan, CARBYNE, chloropropham, croneton, DIOXACARB, etrofolan, ficam, formetanate, knockbal, macbal, matacil, MEOBAL, mesurol, MTMC, pirimor, propham, and SWEP. R_1 also can be an oxime [for example, TEMIK (aldicarb)], or an alicyclic group.

The mode of action of carbamates involves competition for the acetyl choline receptor sites on cholinesterase, unlike organophosphates, which act by phosphorylating the acetyl cholinesterase enzyme, thereby leading to accumulation of acetylcholine. Because the carbamylation of the enzyme is less favored than decarbamylation (unlike the situation for phosphorylation) the cholinesterase inhibition can be reversed far more easily (reversible inhibition, compared with irreversible inhibition for organophosphates). Although hydrolysis of carbamylated cholinesterase is 50% complete in about 30 min, the same quantity for the phosphorylated enzyme takes 80 to 480 min. The severe symptoms of carbamate poisonings are the same as for organophosphate poisoning: constriction of the pupils of the eyes, muscular weakness or spasms, respiratory failure, lowered blood pressure, and cardiac arrest. Convulsions can be tonic leading to rigid limbs, or clonic leading to rapid uncontrolled movements. At sublethal doses, headaches, vomiting, blurred vision, and diarrhea are common. Mild poisoning affects behavioral patterns, reduces mental capacity, and reduces concentration ability. Atropine is the antidote rather than the methioidide of pyridine-2-aldoxime (PAM) used for organophosphate poisonings.

22.2.1 Activation and Detoxification

The metabolism of carbamates, thiocarbamates, and thiolcarbamates has been reviewed [34].

Like the organophosphorothionates and organophosphorothiolates, the S atoms in thiocarbamates and thiolcarbamates can be replaced with O atoms through oxidative desulfurization (Section 22.1.1). Similarly, esterases attack the bond to the oxygen side of the –C=O or –C=S bond, especially for R_1

substituents that are aromatic or heterocyclic. Amidases also attack the carboxamide group to cleave the C–N bond of the amide link. This is more important for aliphatic R_1 groups, and if the R_2 and R_3 groups are aromatic. The aromatic rings and heterocyclic rings are hydroxylated via monoxygenases. Such hydroxylated derivatives then can be glucuronidated, glutathionated, or sulfated, or undergo further oxidation. Aromatic ring hydroxylation also may lead to loss of aromaticity of one ring for biannulated aromatic systems and above. *N*-Methyl hydroxylation leading to dealkylation or direct alkylation also may occur. 5-Hydroxycarbaryl is twice as potent an inhibitor of cholinesterase as carbaryl itself so that hydroxylation is not necessarily deactivating.

The three most important carbamates probably are aldicarb, methomyl, and oxamyl. All three have R_1 oxime substituents ending with a methyl thioether linkage. In between these two functional groups, the major functional groups are the propionaldehyde, ethylidineamino, and dimethylacetamide moieties, respectively. All three are toxic. Aldicarb ($CH_3{\cdot}S{\cdot}C(CH_3)_2{\cdot}CH{=}N{\cdot}O{\cdot}CONH{\cdot}CH_3$) can cross the placental barrier. The S in the thioether link is oxidized mostly to the sulfoxide (–(S=O)–) with a small amount of sulfone ($-SO_2-$) also produced. The N–O bond α to the carbonyl group of the amide then is cleaved, with the oxime, the sulfoxide, and the sulfone as products. A small amount of reduction of the amide group of the sulfoxide to the sulfoxide nitrile also has been reported. The oxime sulfoxides and sulfones then are oxidized to the parent aldehydes, which are oxidized further to carboxylic acids, which then are conjugated for excretion in the urine.

Methomyl ($CH_3{\cdot}S{\cdot}(CH_3)C{=}N{\cdot}O{\cdot}CONH{\cdot}CH_3$), in contrast to aldicarb, does not produce sulfoxides or sulfones because the S is not easily oxidizable. Instead an oxime ($CH_3{\cdot}S{\cdot}(CH_3)\ C{=}N{\cdot}OH$) is produced that first is oxidized to its ketone ($CH_3{\cdot}S{\cdot}CO{\cdot}(CH_3)$), which eventually is oxidized further to carbon dioxide. Methyl cyanide also is produced in small amounts.

The metabolism of oxamyl ($CH_3{\cdot}S{\cdot}[(CH_3)_2{\cdot}N{\cdot}CO]C{=}N{\cdot}O{\cdot}CONH{\cdot}CH_3$) has not been much studied in humans. Oxime production would be expected to occur again ($CH_3{\cdot}S{\cdot}[(CH_3)_2{\cdot}N{\cdot}CO]C{=}N{\cdot}OH$), with subsequent ketone formation as for methomyl. The dimethylacetyl group may hydrolyze to form *N*,*N*-dimethylformamide, excreted as *N*-methylformamide and formamide in urine (Section 21.4.7) or *N*,*N*-dimethyl carbamic acid.

The metabolism of the soil-acting herbicidal phenyl carbamates or carbanilates to substituted anilines, *N*-acetylated derivatives, and the 4-hydroxy unhydrolyzed herbicide (for chlorpropham and chlorbufam) and its *N*-acetylated hydrolysis products in the form of sulfate and glucuronides is commonly found. Thus chlorpropham [$(CH_3)_2HC{\cdot}O{\cdot}CONH{\cdot}R_2$, where R_2 is the 3-chlorophenyl group] produces 3-chloroaniline and thence 3-chloroacetanilide as well as 4-hydroxychlorpropham, after which are produced 3-chloro-4-hydroxyaniline and then 3-chloro-4-hydroxyacetanilide. The isopropoxy group also is hydroxylated at one of the terminal methyl groups, and is oxidized to an aldehyde and then a carboxylic acid. The latter pathway appears to be be minor, however.

Thiolcarbamates ($R_2R_3N{\cdot}CO{\cdot}S{\cdot}R_1$; for example, benthiocarb, butylate, cycloate, diallate, EPTC, molinate, pebulate, triallate, and vernolate) have a very exchangeable S with subsequent liberation of carbon dioxide and a dialkylamine. The latter is excreted in the breath for the lighter R_2 and R_3 groups (di-*n*-propyl for EPTC and vernolate; diisobutyl for butylate; and diisopropyl in diallate and triallate), but in the urine for the heavier groups such as found for the (ethyl, cyclohexyl) group in cycloate. Light R_1 groups such as ethyl (butylate, cycloate, and EPTC), *n*-propyl (vernolate), and 2,3-dichloroprop-2,3-enyl (diallate) and 2,3,3-trichloroprop-2,3-enyl (triallate) may lead to exhalation of volatile products. However, all these C_2 and C_3 hydrocarbon fragments also may be incorporated in the carbon pools (Chapter 2). There is some evidence for sulfoxide and sulfone formation for cycloate.

22.2.2 Biological Monitoring Markers

All three of the oxime carbamates, aldicarb, methomyl, and oxamyl, will produce the *N*-methylformamide ($H \cdot CONH \cdot CH_3$) and *N*-methylamino formic acid ($HOOC \cdot NH \cdot CH_3$) as a result of R_1 cleavage. The former is a urinary biological monitoring marker for *N,N*-dimethylformamide (Section 21.4.7). Demethylation will also occur to provide urinary formamide ($H \cdot CO \cdot NH_2$) and carbamic acid ($HOOC \cdot NH_2$), respectively. All of these urinary biological monitoring markers thus will be nonspecific, and the *N*-methylformamide and formamide markers will have dimethylformamide as a positive interference. Thus the *N*-methylamino formic acid and carbamic acid markers probably are more indicative of carbamate exposure. The type of R_1 group in these carbamate oximes also may be retained in urinary metabolites, as discussed in the introduction to Section 22.2. Metabolism is fast ($t_{0.5} < 4\,h$) for most carbamates.

A common fate of the thiocarbamates is cyclization to substituted dithiazolidines and dithiazolidones, which often are excreted in the urine as carboxylate derivatives after β oxidation of a hydrocarbon side chain. The metabolism of thiram to dimethyl dithiocarbamic acid and cyclization to thiazolidones is very similar to the metabolic route for the antialcoholic drug Antabuse. The breath also contains carbon disulfide and methylamine, the characteristic products of bacterial metabolism. Thus after ziram exposure, thiram and dimethyl dithiocarbamic acid were found in the urine, and carbon disulfide and methylamine in the breath.

The most used biological monitoring test for carbamates is cholinesterase inhibition, as discussed in the introduction to Section 22.2. Whole blood and plasma cholinesterase inhibition usually are measured, with the plasma marker being the more sensitive of the two.

Bendiocarb or Ficam (2,2-dimethyl-1,3-benzodioxol-4-yl-methylcarbamate) is completely metabolized within 4 h, and its metabolites are eliminated within 16 h. The major urinary metabolite is the 2,2-dimethyl-1,3-benzodiox-4-ol (NC 7312) with about a 20% equivalent of the applied dermal dose excreted within 28 h, the rate of excretion depending on the ambient temperature [35].

Propoxur ($R_1 \cdot O \cdot CONH \cdot CH_3$, where R_1 is the 2-isopropoxyphenyl moiety) has a biological half-time of $<1\,h$ [36]. The preferred urinary metabolite for biological monitoring is 2-isopropoxyphenol, which is excreted as sulfate and glucuronide conjugates released after action of esterases [36]. This metabolite is excreted completely during 24 h. Hemoglobin adducts of propoxur also have been utilized (Chapter 12). The cholinesterase inhibition correlates better with the hemoglobin adduct concentration than does the urinary excretion [36].

The biological half-time for carbaryl excretion (1-naphthyl methylcarbamate) has been estimated at 1670 h with 90% excretion complete in 5548 h [32]. An ELISA technique (Section 11.1.2) for aldicarb is available, and it has been utilized on urine and saliva at a detection limit of 300 ppb [37].

Because many dithiocarbamate fungicides are metabolized to dialkylcarbamic acids in the urine and to carbon disulfide and dialkylamines in the breath [38], these compounds could constitute nonspecific biological monitoring markers. In addition the urinary iodine-azide test for reducing compounds (dithiocarbamates, dithiazolines, and dithiazolidones) used commonly for carbon disulfide exposure may be useful as a nonspecific test [39].

One mutagenic pesticidal carbamate in five strains of *Salmonella* and one strain of *E. coli* is carbofuran [33], whereas others known not to be mutagenic include asulam, benomyl, BPMC, butoxycarboxim, carbaryl, chloropropham, cycloate, EPTC, isoprocarb, methomyl, MPMC, MTMC, orthobencarb, oxamyl, phenmedipham, pirimicarb, propoxur, SWEP, and XMC. Most of the dithiocarbamates studied are not mutagenic [33], including amobam, mancozeb, maneb, metamammonium, milneb, and zineb; whereas mutagenic dithiocarbamates include DDC, EMSC, ferbam, polycarbamate, thiram, TTCA, and ziram. Some carbamates known to alter host immune defense mechanisms include: carbaryl, carbofuran, and dicresyl; some thiocarbamates known to do the same are: maneb, thiram, zineb, and ziram [24].

22.3 ORGANOCHLORINE PESTICIDES

Organochlorine pesticides include a vast array of compounds ranging from chlorinated fumigants such as the dichloropropanes to aromatic polychlorinated fungicides such as pentachlorophenol (Section 21.4.20). The major organochlorine insecticides can be divided into compounds related to DDT (*p,p′*-dichlorophenyl-1,1,1-trichloroethane; $R_1 \cdot CHCCl_3 \cdot R_1$, where R_1 is *p*-chlorophenyl), lindane or γ-BHC (hexachlorocyclohexane; CH_6Cl_6), and the chlorinated cyclodiene family (alicyclic biannulated cyclohexene rings, with each ring also having a bridgehead carbon connecting with the ring carbons adjacent to the two dicyclohexenyl bridgehead carbon atoms). The chlorines facilitate entry into the target pest, but this same property means that entry of these chemicals into humans by skin, inhalation, or oral ingestion also will be fast. The bioaccumulation of such materials in the fat is well documented, as is the similar bioaccumulation of such other chlorinated compounds as PCDDs and PCDFs (Section 6.7.1).

The organochlorines are all potentially neurotoxic at high-enough concentrations, the DDT-like family (for example, DDT, methoxychlor, dicofol, and chlorbenzilate) affecting the peripheral nervous system; whereas the lindane family (α-, β- and γ-1,2,3,4,5,6-hexachlorocyclohexane) and the chlorinated cyclodienes [for example, aldrin, chlordane, dieldrin, endosulfan, endrin (used also as a bird perch agent and rodenticide), heptachlor, isodrin, kepone, mirex, and thiodan] attack the central nervous system. The phenoxyacetic acid herbicides (2,4-D; 2,4-DB; 2,4,5-T; silvex; MCPA; sesone; MCPP; MCPB) are so quickly excreted that there is little time to develop nervous symptoms except at massive doses. This is not so for the chlorinated diphenyl ether herbicides such as bifenox, CFNP, MO, nitrofen, RH-2512, RH-2915, and X-52.

22.3.1 Activation and Detoxification

The major fate of chlorines bonded to aliphatic carbons is dehalogenative hydroxylation or reduction. Hydroxylation without dehalogenation, as for trichloroethylene (Section 21.4.25) and methyl chloroform (Section 21.4.15), occurs when a hydroxylatable site is available, as in a chlorinated isolated double bond. In chlorinated benzene groups (for example, *o,p′*-DDT, 2,4-D, 2,4,5-T, and silvex) dehalogenative hydroxylation and reduction are favored for chlorines *ortho* to *ortho/para*-directing functional groups and for chlorines *meta* to *meta*-directing groups. Chlorines *para* to *ortho/para*-directing groups in benzene rings (for example, in *p,p′*-DDT, 2,4-D, 2,4,5-T, and silvex) tend to be stable and to direct hydroxyl attack (*ortho/para*) to the ring. Where both *o*- and *p*-substituted chlorines occur (for example, in 2,4-D, 2,4,5-T, and silvex), the *o*-dehalogenative hydroxylation and reduction process occurs first in metabolism, then the ring hydroxylation.

We now consider the DDT family. *p,p′*-DDT dechlorinates reductively at the trichlorinated carbon atom in the ethane group to form *p,p′*-DDD (rhothane or TDE). Dehydrohalogenation results in the loss of HCl by the agency of a DDT dehydrochlorinase (GSH-dependent) to produce a double bond in the ethane moiety to form *p,p′*-DDE. The latter is known to be carcinogenic and is the chief form of DDT in fat. "DDT" is usually the sum of DDT, DDE, and DDD. Ultimately, the $-CCl_3$ portion is replaced with a $-COOH$ to form DDA. This is excreted in the feces in free or conjugated form. Methoxychlor is identical to *p,p′*-DDT except that the two ring chlorines have been replaced by methoxy groups. As expected, it does not bioaccumulate as much as *p,p′*-DDT. DDE and DDD analogs are produced as metabolites. One or both methyls are removed by microsomal *O*-demethylases to form phenols, which can be sulfated and glucuronidated. Dicofol, also a minor metabolite of DDT, is identical to *p,p′*-DDT except that the hydrogen on the ethane group is replaced by a hydroxy group. A DDD analog is produced as a metabolite, as well as an epoxide after dehydrohalogenation. Chlorobenzilate is identical to Dicofol except that the trichloromethyl group is replaced with an ethylformate group. The ester group is hydrolyzed to the free acid, which is the same acid produced by replacement of the trichloromethyl group of Dicofol with a carboxyl group.

Lindane exists as several isomers, but only the γ isomer (HCH or BHC) is a potent insecticide. It is in the chair conformation with alternating axial chlorines at the 1, 2, and 3 positions and alternating equatorial chlorines at the 4, 5, and 6 positions. Dehydrohalogenation produces 1,2,4-trichlorobenzene, which eventually is hydroxylated to produce chlorophenols, which are sulfated and glucuronidated. 2,4,6-Trichlorophenol also has been detected. Mercapturic acid derivatives in urine also indicate participation of GSH in the detoxification.

The numerous chlorinated cyclodienes synthesized by Diels-Alder condensation of hexachlorocyclopentadiene with suitable cyclic hydrocarbons containing five to seven carbon atoms have complex stereochemistries. Aldrin (which has one *exo* and one *endo* bridge) is oxidized rapidly to its epoxide (carbon atoms 6 and 7), dieldrin, by a NADPH-dependent monooxygenase. Similarly, isodrin (which has two *endo* bridges) is oxidized to endrin. Chlordane

(8 chlorines) and Mirex (12 chlorines) and dimers of chlorinated cyclopentadienes. Both are saturated and hence less reactive than the cyclodienes.

Dehydrohalogenation produces olefines (analogs of aldrin), which then can epoxidize to give oxychlordane. Because Mirex is very stable, this process is not favored. The epoxides can be hydroxylated at unsubstituted double bonds by the action of monooxygenases (as for dieldrin), or the epoxide link is unhooked by hydrolases to form *trans* diols. These hydroxyl groups can be oxidized further to keto groups (for example, as for 2-ketodieldrin, the most important urinary metabolite of dieldrin).

The chlorinated nitrobenzenes that are contact fungicides, quintozene (PCNB or 2,3,4,5,6-pentachloronitrobenzene), Tecnazene (TCNB or 2,3,4,6-tetrachloronitrobenzene) and dicloran (2,6-dichloro-4-nitroaniline) have their nitro group quickly reduced to an amino group, which eventually is oxidized to a hydroxy group via the hydroxylamine to produce a phenol that can be sulfated and glucuronidated and excreted in the urine; one of the *ortho*-chlorine positions is glutathionated, and any hydrogen-substituted carbons in the benzene ring can be hydroxylated. Other organochlorine compounds that are contact fungicides, chlorothalonil (2,4,5,6-tetrachloro-1,3-dinitrilobenzene) and dichlone (2,3-dichloro-1,4-naphthoquinone), are detoxified by reaction of glutathione; the nitrile group(s) in chlorothalonil is (are) oxidized to a carboxyl group, which then is excreted in the urine as glycine or alanine conjugates. Other chlorinated systemic fungicides include fenarimol ((2-chlorophenyl)-(4-chlorophenyl)-(pyrimidin-5-yl)methanol), triadimefon (4-chlorophenoxy-*t*-butylcarbonyl-(1,2,4-triazol-1-yl)methane), and chloroneb (1,4-dichloro-3,6-dimethoxybenzene); their human metabolism has not been investigated. Glutathione detoxification is expected to be important for these compounds.

The chlorinated herbicides are another enormous class of compounds. Chlorines substituted on a benzene ring (for example, alanap, amiben, anilofos, barban, benazolin, blazer, casoron, chlorbromuron, chloroxuron, chlortoluron, CIPC, 2,4-D, dacthal, dicamba, diuron, Dowco 356, 2,4-DP, 3,6-DPA, dynanap, fenac, fenoxaprop-ethyl, fenthiaprop-ethyl, L-flamprop-isopropyl, fomesafen, glean, GOAL, herbit, hoelon, kerb, linuron, mataven, MCPA, MCPB, MCPP, metoxuron, MO, Modown, monolinuron, monuron, neburon, nitrofen, NORFLURAZON, pentachlorophenol, potablan, prefix, propanil, PYRAZON, quinonamid, Ronstar, silvex, sesone, suffix, swep, 2,4,5-T, thiobencarb, tordon, triclopyr, and X-52) may suffer (as already discussed above for ring substituted compounds) hydroxylative or reductive dechlorination, glutathionation with subsequent excretion as thioethers in the urine, or direct hydroxylation of the ring with subsequent excretion in the urine as glucuronides and sulfates. The major detoxicative processes in green plants appear to involve hydroxylation at the ring, but this usually is minor in humans. However, whether these events are major or minor depends on the side chains on the benzene ring. Thus because pentachlorophenol (Section 21.4.20) has no side chains, it must undergo these transformations; much faster processes than these occur if there are functional groups such as carboxyl groups that facilitate elimination.

Thus the chlorinated phenoxyalkanoic foliar herbicides (for example, 2,4-D, 2,4-DB, DEP, 2,4-DP, erbon, herbit, MCPA, MCPB, MCPP, sesone, silvex, and 2,4,5-T, whether sprayed as esters or as amine/alkanolamine salts [40]) are converted to the free acid, which then is excreted free and as glycine and alanine conjugates in the urine. Phenoxy side-chain hydrolysis to the appropriate chlorinated phenol (2,4-dichlorophenol for 2,4-D, 2,4-DB, DEP, 2,4-DP, and sesone; 2,4,5-trichlorophenol for erbon, silvex, and 2,4,5-T; 2-methyl-4-chlorophenol for herbit, MCPA, MCPB, and MCPP) usually is minor for humans. Animals are known to lose the ability to regulate body temperature at very high doses of the phenoxyalkanoic herbicides. Peripheral neuropathy induced by 2,4-D also has been demonstrated in animals [41] and in humans [42]. The embryotoxic, teratogenic, and carcinogenic properties of the impurities (2,3,7,8-substituted PCDDs and PCDFs) in the herbicides synthesized from 2,4,5-trichlorophenol (erbon, silvex, and 2,4,5-T) are well known [40, 42]. The PCDDs and PCDFs derived from 2,4-dichlorophenol and 2-methyl-4-chlorophenol are not so toxic as the preceding substances.

The chlorinated benzoic acid herbicides (for example, alanap, amiben, benazolin, dacthal, dicamba, dynanap, fenac, and 2,3,6-TBA) are more effective soil herbicides than the phenoxyalkanoic acids. The two most important members are dicamba (3,6-dichloro-2-methoxybenzoic acid) and 2,3,6-TBA (2,3,6-trichlorobenzoic acid) formulated as esters or amine/alkanolamine salts. They have the same kind of metabolic fate as the phenoxyalkanoic herbicides.

Other chlorinated benzenoid herbicides include the anilide analogs of the phenoxys (for example, anilofos, CARBYNE, CIPC, L-flamprop isopropyl, metoxuron, pentanochlor, potablan, propanil, suffix, and SWEP). Most of these produce the corresponding aniline through amidase cleavage (3,4-dichloroaniline from propanil, suffix, and SWEP; 3-chloro-4-methylaniline from pentanochlor; 3-chloro-4-methoxyaniline from metoxuron; 3-chloroaniline from CIPC and CARBYNE; 4-chloroaniline from anilofos and potablan; and 3-chloro-4-fluoroaniline from L-flamprop isopropyl). The chlorines may be replaced by hydroxy groups, or hydroxylative attack on the ring may occur on the ring to produce phenols, which are excreted in the urine as sulfates and glucuronides. The chlorinated benzenoid ureas are analogs of the anilides considered above. Some of these compounds are: chlorbromuron, chloroxuron, dicuran, diuron, linuron, lorox, metoxuron, monolinuron, neburon, and UROX. The ureides usually are utilized as soil herbicides, and their metabolism in humans has scarcely been investigated. It might be expected that chloroanilines would be produced and that ring hydroxylation (at C_6) would occur, similar to that in the acetanilides. Demethylation and demethoxylation at the urea terminal N may occur to produce the dehydro terminal N derivative as for carbamates (Section 22.2.1). Other chlorinated benzenoid herbicides include: casoron, chlorthiamid, dichlobenil, Dowco 356, fenoxaprop-ethyl, fenthiaprop-ethyl, kerb, prefix, ronstar, thiobencarb, and the chlorinated diphenyl ethers (for example, blazer, fomesafen, GOAL, hoelon, MO, modown, nitrofen, and X-52).

Some other chlorinated benzenoid insecticides include: agritox, BAY SIR 8514, benzomate, bromophos, bromophos-ethyl, CELATHION, chlorfenvinphos, chlorodimeform, curacron, iodofenphos, mavrik, MEB-6046, pydrin, qikron, rabon, ronnel, sappiran, S-Seven, tedion, tokuthion, trithion, and UBI-T930. Chlorinated aromatic rodenticides include: castrix, chlorophacinone, and tomorin.

Other nonbenzene chlorinated aromatic herbicides include: the triazines (atrazine, bladex, cyprazine, propazine, simazine, terbuthylazine, and trietazine with a chlorine on C_2), the picolinic acid derivatives (3,6-DPA, tordon, and triclopyr), other heterocyclics (PYRAZON and pyridate), and the quinones (Mogeton and quinonamid). For the triazines, hydroxylative dechlorination at C_2, and GSH conjugation at the chlorine have been observed; the secondary amines at the 4- and 6-carbon atoms may be dealkylated. Nonbenzene chlorinated aromatic insecticides include: DOWCO 214, dursban, pentac, and phosalone.

The major aliphatic organochlorine pesticides include: carboxylic acid herbicides [dalapon (2,2-dichloropropionic acid), TCA (sodium trichloroacetic acid salt)]; herbicides and insecticides with double bonds that are partially or fully chlorinated (herbicides: Avadex, FAR-GO; insecticides: BAY-FCR 1272; chlorfenvinphos, CO-RAL, cypermethrin, DDVP, DOWCO 417, permethrin, phosphamidon, and rabon); and pesticides in which the chlorine(s) is (are) substituted on a terminal saturated carbon (herbicides: acetochlor, alachlor, CARBYNE, dimethachlor, dual, machete, metazachlor, propachlor, quinonamid, and randox; insecticides: aphidan, BAS-263, DDT, dibrom, dylox, kelthane, MEB-6046, methoxychlor, and torak; rodenticides: alphakil and epibloc). See Table 22.1 for the many fumigants that have chlorinated terminal carbons and chlorinated double bonds.

Most of these pesticides have not been investigated in humans.

22.3.2 Biological Monitoring Markers

Only selected chlorinated pesticides will be considered here.

Endrin has been the object of intensive biological monitoring research because of its high toxicity (poisoning has been detected in humans at doses as low as 0.2 mg/kg body weight), and because it causes convulsions above a blood concentration above 50 ng endrin/mL blood [43]. It also has been implicated in several poisoning incidents, via bread contamination in Wales in 1956, in Qatar and Hofuf in Saudi Arabia in 1967, and in Egypt in 1967. Endrin has been detected in tissues including blood and urine after acute poisoning incidents. The half-time in blood is estimated to be 1 to 2 days. *Anti*-12-hydroxyendrin has been detected in the feces of factory workers exposed to endrin. Its urinary β-glucuronide, which varied between 0.010 and 0.14 μg/mL was detected in a dose-effect manner with endrin exposure [44]. The toxic metabolite 12-ketoendrin was variably present in the urine, from undetectable to 0.13 μg/mL, but 3-hydroxyendrin or the 4,5-*trans*-dihydroisodrindiol were not detected. A urinary *anti*-12-hydroxyendrin concentration of 0.13 mg/g creatinine was considered to be the threshold level below which enzyme induction, as shown by urinary D-glucaric acid excretion (Section 9.3.8), did not occur [45]. The D-glucaric acid concentration did not return to baseline until 6 weeks after exposure. This was confirmed in another investigation [46]. *Anti*-12-hydroxyendrin also was detected in the urine of workers in another workplace [47].

Lindane used in malaria control in India in 1975–77 caused no skin and coordination problems in 464 sprayers, nor did it cause higher SGPT and serum alkaline phosphatase activities or serum whole cell counts relative to 201 controls [48]. The serum protein concentration was affected, as was serum glucose [48]. Serum lindane ($\beta > \alpha > \gamma$) was higher in all exposed sprayers. For a similar study in Argentina [49] with 48 sprayers, the serum residues in 1978 found in greatest concentrations were β-HCH, γ-HCH, DDT, DDE, dieldrin, and α-HCH relative to five controls. No significant differences were observed for serum GOT, GPT, alkaline phosphatase, cholinesterase, lactate dehydrogenase, and creatine phosphokinase; and no differences were noted for serum α-fetoprotein. Another Indian investigator [50] reported higher DDT and lindane serum concentrations in males, with toxic signs and symptoms in the HCH formulators. In the latter study on 19 formulators and 26 manufacturing process personnel (14 controls), lactate dehydrogenase, γ-glutamyl transpeptidase, leucine aminopeptidase, and immunoglobulin M were significantly higher in the formulators than in the other groups. The formulators also had the highest serum β, α, γ, and δ-HCH isomer concentrations. Electrocardiogram monitoring 1 h after the end of exposure showed evidence of cardiac effects in 15% of the workers [50].

The phenoxyalkanoic herbicides with more than one chlorine are metabolized to their corresponding acids, which then are excreted within one day in the urine. 2,4-D/2,4-5-T butoxyethyl esters (4 Swedish applicators) and MCPA/2,4-DP salts (8 applicators and 13 farmers) sprayed as 2% aqueous emulsions from a tractor were absorbed [51] from both inhalation and dermal routes and detected in the serum (sampled at 0, 12, 24, and 36 h after end of exposure and at the end of the work week) and the urine (baseline, end-of-workday, and 12-h samples). 2,4-D/2,4,5-T ester air concentrations were 0.1 to 0.2 mg/m^3. MCPA air concentrations ranged up to 26 ng/m^3, and 2,4-DP was detected up to 36 ng/m^3. Sprayers had much higher levels in their urine than farmers. MCPA and 2,4-DP eliminations took longer than 24 h. A Canadian study [52] showed that urinary acid equivalent 2,4-D (24-h samples) was correlated with the dermal exposure of four farmers (eight controls) to its amine salts expressed as acid equivalents. The urine samples also were collected for 4 to 7 days after the end of spraying. All baseline samples showed a 2,4-D presence. The half-time was estimated to be 10 to 28 h. The kinetics for single exposures are different from those for multiple exposures, the maximum concentration being reached 3 days after exposure for a single exposure. Also baseline levels were reached only for a single exposure after 8 days. Much interindividual variation was noted.

The extreme interindividual variability has been commented upon by Lavy and Mattice [53], who considered data only in terms of each individual monitored rather than group data. Aerial application of 2,4-D was shown to be maximal 2 to 3 days after exposure in five aircraft crew members, and avoidance of exposure for at least one week was recommended to allow interpretation of the biological monitoring data. Over 95% of 2,4-D absorbed was excreted within 5 days. A picloram/2,4-D exposure (Tordon 101-R) showed that picloram did not perturb the kinetics of 2,4-D excretion, with picloram being >96% excreted within 24 h in 60 applicators. Dermal studies have shown that 0.18% of picloram dermally applied is excreted in urine, and 6% of the dermally applied 2,4-D. The presence of 2,4-DP does not affect 2,4-D excretion kinetics.

In another review paper, Lavy and Mattice [54] emphasized that spot sampling of urines is insufficient for chemicals of long half-times. They also reported that pydrin is 62% excreted in the urine [54]. The half-time of 2,4,5-T in urine after oral administration to men has been found [32] to be about 23 h, identical to the plasma half-time. The respective data for 2,4-D were 18 and 12 h; and for silvex, biphasic plasma half-times of 4.0 and 17 h and urine half-times of 5 and 26 h [32]. MCPA provided orally had a half-time of >24 h [32], whereas when it was applied dermally to the thigh, the maximum concentration in urine appeared after 2 days and maximum plasma concentration in 12 h, with urine excretion over 5 days. 2,4-D also has been detected in sweat [32]. 2,4-D glucuronide also has been detected [55] in human urine at varying ratios relative to "free acid" (ratios of 0 to 37%).

A review of occupational exposure to the chlorophenoxyalkanoic herbicides is provided by IARC [56]. Data from production workers showed that 2,4-D could be detected in the urine (0.06–9.5 mg/L), and PCDDs and PCDFs could be detected in the fat; ground spraying operators in Australia, Canada, Finland, New Zealand, Sweden, and the United States had urine concentrations up to 33 mg/L; tractor spraying workers had urine concentrations of up to 20 mg/L; and aerial spraying personnel had urine concentrations up to 1.1 mg/L. Epidemiology studies concerning the chlorophenoxys are reviewed also by IARC [56]. In summary, exposure to these herbicides has not been found to cause teratogenicity after male or female exposure, chromosomal aberrations, or sister chromatid exchanges, and there has been no overall increase in cancer incidence. There were increases in soft-tissue sarcoma rates and lung cancer, but these were confounded by multicomponent exposures for exposures to MCPA, MCPP, 2,4-D, and 2,4-DP. The soft-tissue sarcoma effect has been reproduced in studies in Denmark, Sweden (four investigations), and Italy but not in other studies in Finland and New Zealand. Malignant lymphoma excess was observed in studies in Sweden but not in studies in Denmark and New Zealand. IARC adjudged that there is limited evidence that chlorophenoxy herbicides are carcinogenic to humans.

Quintozene (pentachloronitrobenzene), applied as a powder and as an aqueous emulsion, has been detected [57] in Finnish pine nursery sprayers through pentachloroaniline concentrations in 24-h urines. The highest breathing zone air concentrations caused the highest urinary concentrations of metabolite. No hexachlorobenzene impurity was monitored.

Chlordimeform exposure to workers in a packaging plant caused urinary tract irritation leading to bloody urine, dysuria, hesitancy, and abdominal pain [58]. This was associated with a urinary concentration of chlordimeform and metabolites of >1 mg/L [58]. Investigation of aerial applicators exposed for 4 years showed that adequate protective measures were implemented, as urinary levels of chlordimeform were only about 90 μg/L, 8 to 18 h after the start of an 8-h exposure [59]. Chlordimeform was detected in urine 4 h after the start of exposure. Another investigation [60] involving 2489 workers in the years 1978 through 1984 showed that fewer than 2% of the workers had total 4-chloro-2-toluidine containing urinary metabolites [61] >5 μg/mL, with 75% of the results <0.3 μg/mL. The kinetics of plasma elimination after a single dermal application in water for 9 h is triphasic, with half-times of 8, 22, and 40 h. The urinary metabolites were mostly chlordimeform conjugates that were labile in basic solution. Total 4-chloro-2-toluidine–containing metabolites accounted for

40% of the applied dose excreted for 48 h. The half-time varied between 5.9 and 12 h.

Diuron is metabolized in the liver to 3,4-dichloroaniline, is acetylated, and then is excreted in the urine as 3,4-dichloroacetanilide [36]. This occurs with only 60% of diuron-exposed persons (urinary concentrations of total aniline and acetanilide varied between 40 and 510 μg/g creatinine). In 40% of people (slow acetylators), the urine contains mostly free 3,4-dichloroaniline, and hemoglobin adduct concentrations are higher than in fast acetylators. No cyanosis is observed at these low blood levels [36]. The reference upper value is 10 μg/g creatinine.

The chlorinated carbamate triademefon is metabolized to 4-chlorophenol, which can be detected in the blood and urine [36], the latter as a sulfate and glucuronide conjugate. Urinary concentrations varied between 250 and 810 μg/g creatinine. Much interindividual variation was seen for hemoglobin adducts of the original compound [36].

Lavy and Mattice [54] report that chlorpyrifos is 70% excreted in urine in humans as 3,5,6-trichloro-2-pyridinol, presumably as sulfate and glucuronide conjugates.

The fumigant 1,3-dichloropropene has been monitored [62] in three male workers by urinary analysis of the metabolite (*N*-acetyl-*S*-*cis*-3-chloroprop-2-enyl)cysteine, a specific mercapturic acid. Peak urine concentrations after exposure were variable (0–16 h), but there appeared to be a dose relationship of 24-h urine concentrations with air concentrations. Baseline samples were adjudged to be essential for interpretation of biological monitoring data.

Absorbed alachlor applied [63] as emulsifiable concentrate, microencapsulated, or water-dispersible granules was >87% excreted in the urine of 36 applicators within 5 days, mostly as diethylaniline (80%) and 2-(1-hydroxyethyl)ethylaniline (20%) at 24-h urine total concentrations of up to 14 ng/mL. Monsanto submitted three biological monitoring studies to the U.S. EPA as part of its effort in the continuing registration of this herbicide [64].

IARC also has reviewed the biological monitoring data associated with occupational exposures to chlorophenols [65]. Five chlorophenols are important: 2,4-dichloro-, 2,4,5-trichloro-, 2,4,6-trichloro-, 2,3,4,6-tetrachloro-, and pentachlorophenol. Biological monitoring for these phenols and their glucuronide and sulfate conjugates in urine show highly variable data. Urinary pentachlorophenol (Section 21.4.20) ranges up to 3.4 mg/L for production plant workers, to 5.6 mg/L in wood treatment personnel, to 10 mg/mL in sawmill personnel, to 9.7 mg/L during dipping and spraying and during loading of freshly treated timber, and to 36 mg/L during pest control operations. Chlorophenol exposure during textile impregnation and fabric sewing has been detected up to 0.8 mg/L, and at tanneries up to 11 mg/L. Blood concentrations also have been reported with averages of 4.7 μg/mL common and up to 0.92 μg/mL in serum. Blood PCDD and PCDF concentrations also have been given, with hepta and octa congeners predominating. The only other known metabolite of pentachlorophenol is tetrachlorohydroquinone. The half-time becomes longer with increasing exposure. Oral pentachlorophenol is excreted with a half-time of 33 h, with the glucuronide having a half-time of 13 h. More than 40% of urinary pentachlorophenol exists as the glucuronide.

The urinary half-times for 2,4,6-tri-, 2,3,4,6-tetra-, and pentachlorophenols are 0.75, 2 to 5.1, and 16 days, respectively. 2,4,6,-Tri- and 2,3,4,6-tetrachlorophenols are mostly present in urine as conjugates, 2,4-Di-, 2,4,6-tri, and pentachlorophenols bind reversibly to human serum albumin.

There appears to be no association between chlorophenol exposure and adverse pregnancy outcomes. The literature is contradictory on whether the chlorophenols are genotoxic. Soft-tissue sarcoma associations were shown in two Swedish studies but not in a New Zealand investigation. The incidence of malignant lymphoma with exposure to chlorophenols was noted in a Swedish study and marginally in a New Zealand investigation. A Swedish study observed a correlation between nose and nasopharyngeal cancer and exposure to chlorophenols. IARC concluded that there was limited evidence for human carcinogenicity [65].

Captan (*N*-(trichloromethylthio)-4-cyclohexene-1,2-dicarboximide) fungicide exposure of California strawberry pickers in 1987 [66] was monitored by tetrahydrophthalimide concentrations in 24-h urines. This metabolite constitutes about 15% of the urinary metabolites, which comprise 85% of the absorbed dose.

Because so many chlorinated pesticides are detoxified through glutathionation with subsequent urinary excretion of thioethers, the urinary thioether test (Section 9.3.7) assumes special importance here for its integrative function. Specific thioether species may enable identification of the exposing pesticide as for 1,3-dichloropropene. Pancytopenia results from the exposure of DDT, lindane, and chlordane [23].

Chlorinated pesticides known to alter host immunologic defense mechanisms are [24]: barban, chlordane, chlorobenzilate, *p,p'*-DDT, dichlorvos, dieldrin, endrin, heptachlor, hexachlorobenzene, lindane, linuron, mirex, monuron, toxaphene, and trichlorofon. The immunologic effects of 2,4,5-T, pentachlorophenols, tetrachlorophenols, and hexachlorobenzene have been attributed to the presence of the 2,3,7,8-substituted polychlorinated dibenzofurans and dibenzo-*p*-dioxins. The dibenzofuran derivatives also have been postulated to be responsible for the eye and immunologic effects of commercial PCBs.

The following chlorinated pesticides are known to be mutagenic in at least five bacterial strains [33]: butachlor, captafol, captan, chlomethoxynil, chlorfenvinphos, chloropicrin, DBCP, D-D, dichlofluanid, 1,2-dichloroethane, dichlorvos, dienochlor, echlomezol, folpet, and nitrofen. Some chlorinated pesticides known not to be mutagenic in five bacterial strains are [33]: ACN, alachlor, aldrin, α-BMC, anilazine, benzomate, bifenox, butachlor, chlorfenethol, chlorfenson, chlorobenzilate, chloroneb, 4-chloro-(2-hydroxymethyl) phenoxyacetic acid, 4-chlorophenoxyacetic acid, chloropropham, chloropropylate, chlorothalonil, chlorpyrifos, chlorpyrifosmethyl, chlorthiamid, CNP, cyanazine, 2,4-D, dacthal, dalapon, DCIP, *p,p'*-DDD, *p,p'*-DDE, *p,p'*-DDT, dicamba, dichlofenthion, dicofol, dieldrin, diflubenzuron, dimethylvinphos, dinoseb acetate, diuron, endosulfan, endrin, EPBP, ethephon, fthalide, heptachlor, heptachlor epoxide, informe, linuron, MCPA, MCPB, MCPP, naled, pentachloronitrobenzene, pentachlorophenol, permethrin, phenothiol, phosdifen, propanil, propyzamide, prothiophos, ronstar, swep, terbacil, tetrachlorvinphos, tetradifon, thiochlormethyl, trichlorfon, trichloroacetic acid, and triclopyr.

22.4 MISCELLANEOUS PESTICIDES

Exposure to pyrethrins has been monitored [67] by biological monitoring of an acid metabolite in 24-h urines, by 14 blood biochemistry parameters, and by peripheral nerve velocities. Because 78% of the maximum amount of *trans* metabolite and 32% of the *cis* were excreted in 24 h, the *trans* metabolite was chosen as the index marker. An investigation [68] that involved measurement of cypermethrin, permethrin, fenvalerate, and deltamethrin in spot urine and serum samples after the work shift for a greenhouse spraying crew of 11 revealed an immunotoxicological effect resulting in a decrease of T-cells related to cypermethrin exposure. Metabolite excretion was observed for one sprayer only. Sprayers exposed to permethrin and fenvalerate have complained of itching, burning sensations, paresthesia, nasal secretion, coughing, and eye irritation [69].

Fluazifop-butyl (the butyl ester of fluazifop) exposure to backpack and vehicle sprayers was mostly accounted for by skin absorption [70]. Monitoring of the major metabolite, the free acid fluazifop, (4-(5-trifluoromethyl)-2-pyridyloxy) phenoxypropionate, in the 24-h urines of three volunteers after a 5 mg oral exposure showed that 80 to 93% of the administered dose was excreted free in the urine with undetectable amounts in the feces. About 10% in the urine was conjugated. The half-time was 9 to 21 h, or an average of 14 h. Excretion was complete after 4 days. Two groups of three sprayers also excreted fluazifop with an estimated half-time of 27 to 36 h, or an average of 30 h, with complete excretion 7 days after exposure. Patch sampling showed that the exposure was mostly through the dermal route. Absorption efficiency varied greatly (0.2–56%), depending on the area of the body exposed and the exposing amount; the pharmacokinetic models that assumed uniform absorption percentage always underestimated the exposure dose. The assumption of a constant absorption rate of 0.04 to 0.05 $\mu g/cm^2/h$ (range, 0.003–0.12) yielded better results.

The herbicide amitrole (3-amino-1,2,4-triazole) produces changes in the thyroid gland at high exposure levels [36]. Urinary amitrole correlates with air concentrations. Hemoglobin adducts also reflect a dose-effect, thyroid disturbances being evident at concentrations >100 μg/L in whole blood. Because the hemoglobin adduct has a long half-time, the sampling time is no longer a crucial variable, unlike whole blood or spot urine sampling for metabolites. Another triazole fungicide, bitertanol [β-((1,1′-biphenyl)-4-yloxy)α-(1,1-dimethylethyl)-1H-1,2,4-triazole-1-ethanol] can be detected by urinary excretion of 4-phenylphenol (mostly as glucuronide), which also forms hemoglobin adducts [36]. Interindividual variation in the hemoglobin adducts limits the utility of this technique for this fungicide. The advantage of the technique is that although urinary metabolites reflect detoxification, the hemoglobin adducts are more closely related than urinary metabolites to the effects on target tissues, that is, they are better markers of the biologically effective dose.

Fumigants such as ethylene oxide, trichloroethylene (Section 21.4.25),

1,2-dichloroethane, methyl chloroform (Section 21.4.15), toluene (Section 21.4.24), perchloroethylene (Section 21.4.21), and xylene (Section 21.4.26) have been detected in the breath of humans [71]. Such other fumigants as chloropicrin, methylisocyanate, HCN, sulfuryl fluoride, vapam, dichloropropane, dichloropropylene, naphthalene, *p*-dichlorobenzene, methyl bromide, diesel fuel, kerosene, methanol, and petroleum distillates also may be amenable to such monitoring.

Diquat and paraquat have been monitored by quantitation of the parent compound in the urine [32]. Diquat after an intravenous dose to humans has been estimated to have a half-time of 204 h [32]. Thus urine sampling after dermal exposure is not very practical with respect to sensitivity.

Health surveillance has been attempted for genotoxic pesticides. Chromatid aberrations, and the micronucleus incidence have been measured for urothelial cells in 21 orchardists exposed to a variety of pesticides [72]. The micronucleus data were inconclusive, but chromatid aberrations were observed only during the spraying season. However, urines were sampled only for 8 h after the work day, and this may be too short a urine collection time.

The application of ELISA techniques (Section 11.1.2) to pesticide analysis in biological fluids has been reported for paraquat, but assay results are better for the simpler matrices of environmental samples, particularly waters [73].

References

1. Thomson, W. T. 1982. *Agricultural Chemicals*, Book I: *Insecticides*, 1982–83, Thomson Publications, Fresno, CA.
2. Thomson, W. T. 1983. *Agricultural Chemicals*, Book II: *Herbicides*, 1983–84, Thomson Publications, Fresno, CA.
3. Thomson, W. T. 1983. *Agricultural Chemicals*, Book III: *Fumigants, Growth Regulators, Repellants, and Rodenticides*, 1983, Thomson Publications, Fresno, CA.
4. Thomson, W. T. 1984. *Agricultural Chemicals*, Book IV: *Fungicides*, Thomson Publications, Fresno, CA.
5. Compton, J. A. F. 1987. *Military Chemical and Biological Agents: Chemical and Toxicological Properties*, Telford Press, Caldwell, NJ.
6. World Health Organization. 1990. Principles for the toxicological assessment of pesticide residues in food. *Environ. Health Criteria* **104**, WHO, Geneva, Switzerland.
7. International Labour Office. 1979. *Guide to Health and Hygiene in Agricultural Work*, ILO, Geneva, Switzerland.
8. International Labour Office. 1985. *Safe Use of Pesticides*, ILO, Geneva, Switzerland.
9. U.S. Department of Health, Education and Welfare. 1977. *NIOSH Health and Safety Guide for Pesticide Formulators*, U.S. Government Printing Office, Washington, D.C.
10. van Heemstra, E. A. H., and Tordoir, W. F. (eds.). 1982. *Studies in Environmental Science 18: Education and Safe Handling in Pesticide Application*, Elsevier Scientific Publishing, New York.
11. U.S. Department of Health, Education and Welfare. 1978. *NIOSH Criteria for a Recommended Standard: Occupational Exposure during the Manufacture and Formulation of Pesticides*, U.S. Government Printing Office, Washington, DC.
12. Tordoir, W. F., and van Heemstra-Lequin, E. A. H. 1980. *Studies in Environmental Science 7: Field Worker Exposure during Pesticide Application*, Elsevier Scientific Publishing, New York.

13. Ashford, N. A., and Miller, C. S. 1991. *Chemical Exposures: Low Levels and High Stakes*, Van Nostrand Reinhold, New York.
14. Baselt, R. C. 1988. *Biological Monitoring Methods for Industrial Chemicals*, 2nd ed., PSG Publishing, Littleton, MA.
15. Ho, M. H., and Dillon, H. K. (eds.). 1987. *Biological Monitoring of Exposure to Chemicals: Organic Compounds*, Wiley-Interscience, New York.
16. van Heemstra-Lequin, E. A. H., and van Sittert, N. J. 1986. Biological Monitoring of Workers Manufacturing, Formulating and Applying Pesticides. *Toxicol. Lett.* **33**.
17. Wang, R. G. M.; Franklin, C. A.; Honeycutt, R. C.; and Reinert, J. C. 1989. *Biological Monitoring for Pesticide Exposure: Measurement, Estimation, and Risk Reduction*, Am. Chem. Soc. Symp. Ser. **382**.
18. Fiserova-Bergerova, V., and Ogata, M. 1990. *Biological Monitoring of Exposure to Industrial Chemicals*, ACGIH, Cincinnati, OH.
19. Eto, M. 1977. *Organophosphorus Pesticides: Organic and Biological Chemistry*, CRC Press, Boca Raton, FL.
20. Dillon, H. K., and Ho, M. H. 1987. Biological monitoring of exposure to organophosphorus pesticides. In reference 15, pp. 227–287.
21. Derache, R. (ed.). 1977. *Organophosphate Pesticides*, Pergamon Press, Oxford, Great Britain.
22. Weisskopf, C. P., and Seiber, J. N. 1989. New approaches to analysis of organophosphate metabolites in the urine of field workers. In reference 17 pp. 206–214.
23. David, A., and Fairchild, E. J. 1980. Occupational pesticide hazards in the activities of WHO's office of occupational health: hematological criteria for health assessment. In reference 12, pp. 3–15.
24. Sharma, R. P., and Reddy, R. V. 1987. Toxic effects of chemicals on the immune system. In *Handbook of Toxicoloty*, T. J. Haley and W. O. Berndt, (eds.), Hemis phere pp. 555–591.
25. Maroni, M.; Jarvisalo, J.; and La Ferla, F. 1986. The WHO–UNDP epidemiological study on the health effects of exposure to organophosphorus pesticides. In reference 16, pp. 115–123.
26. Rosival, L., and Batora, V. 1980. Consequences for field exposure of impurities in pesticide formulations. In reference 12, pp. 163–172.
27. Turle, R., and Levac, B. 1987. Sulfotepp in diazinon and other organophosphorus pesticides. *Bull. Environ. Contam. Toxicol.* **38**: 793–797.
28. Karr, J. J. 1985. Analysis of diazinon for impurities and degradation materials. *J. Assoc. Off. Chem.* **68**: 929–934.
29. Baron, R. L. (ed.). 1976. *Pesticide-Induced Delayed Neurotoxicity: Proceedings of a Conference*, EPA-600/1-76-025.
30. Lotti, M. 1986. Biological monitoring for organophosphate-induced delayed polyneuropathy. In reference 16, pp. 167–172.
31. Lotti, M. 1989. Neuropathy target esterase in blood lymphocytes. In reference 17, pp. 117–123.
32. Nigg, H. N., and Stamper, J. H. 1989. Biological monitoring for pesticide dose determination. In reference 17, pp. 6–27.
33. Moriya, M.; Ohta, T.; Watanabe, K.; Miyazawa, T.; Kato, K.; and Shirasu, Y. 1983. Further mutagenicity studies on pesticides in bacterial reversion assay systems. *Mutat. Res.* **116**: 185–216.
34. Hassall, K. A. 1982. *The Chemistry of Pesticides: Their Metabolism, Mode of Action and Uses in Crop Protection*, Verlag Chemie, Deerfield Beach, FL, pp. 97–119.
35. Bonsall, J. L., and Goose, J. 1986. The safety evaluation of bendiocarb, a residual insecticide for vector control. In reference 16, pp. 45–59.

36. Lewalter, J., and Korallus, U. 1986. Erythrocyte protein conjugates as a principle of biological monitoring for pesticides. In reference 16, pp. 153–165.
37. Brady, J. F.; Fleeker, J. R.; Wilson, R. A.; and Mumma, R. O. 1989. Enzyme immunoassay for aldicarb. In reference 17, pp. 262–284.
38. Hassall, K. A. 1982. Reference 34, pp. 197–205.
39. NIOSH. 1977. *Criteria for a Recommended Standard: Occupational Exposure to Carbon Disulfide*, U.S. DHEW No 77–156, U.S. Government Printing Office, Washington, DC, pp. 123–125, 169–173.
40. Que Hee, S. S., and Sutherland, R. G. 1981. *The Phenoxyalkanoic Herbicides*, Vol. I, *Chemistry, Analysis and Environmental Pollution*, CRC Press, Boca Raton, FL.
41. Heene, R. 1975. *Experimental Myopathies and Muscular Dystrophy: Studies in the Formal Pathogenesis of the Myopathy of 2,4-Dichlorophenoxyacetate*, Springer-Verlag, New York.
42. Hassall, K. A. 1982. Reference 34, pp. 266–270.
43. U.S. EPA. 1984. *Research and Development Drinking Water Criteria Document for Endrin*, ECAO-CIN-423, ECAO, Cincinnati, OH.
44. Baldwin, M. K., and Hutson, D. H. 1980. Analysis of human urine for a metabolite of endrin by chemical oxidation and gas liquid chromatography as an indicator of exposure to endrin. *Analyst* **105**: 60–65.
45. Ottevanger, C. F., and van Sittert, N. J. 1979. Relation between *anti*-12-hydroxyendrin excretion and enzyme induction in workers involved in the manufacture of endrin. In *Chemical Porphyria in Man*, J. J. T. W. A. Strik and J. H. Koeman (eds.) Elsevier/North-Holland Biomedical Press, New York, pp. 123–129.
46. Vrij-Standhardt, W. G.; Strik, J. J. T. W. A.; Ottevanger, C. F.; and van Sittert, N. J. 1979. Urinary D-glucaric acid and urinary total porphyrin excretion in workers exposed to endrin. In *Chemical Porphyria in Man*, J. J. T. W. A. Strik and J. H. Koeman (eds.) Elsevier/North-Holland Biomedical Press, New York, pp. 113–121.
47. Kummer, R., and van Sittert, N. J. 1986. Field studies on health effects from the application of two organophosphorus insecticide formulations by hand-held ULV to cotton. In reference 16, pp. 7–24.
48. Kashyap, S. K.; Gupta, S. K.; Karnik, A. B.; Parikh, J. R.; and Chatterjee, S. K. 1980. Scope and need of toxicological evaluation of pesticides under field conditions—medical surveillance of malaria spraymen exposed to HCH (hexachlorocyclohexane) in India. In reference 12, pp. 53–61.
49. Astolfi, E.; Maccagno, A.; Gotelli, C.; and Higa de Landoni, J. 1980. Study of public health secretariat pesticide applicators during the anti-malaria campaign 1978. In reference 12, pp. 67–71.
50. Kashyap, S. K. 1986. Health surveillance and biological monitoring of pesticide formulators in India. In reference 16, pp. 107–114.
51. Kolmodin-Hedman, B.; Erne, K.; and Akerblom, M. 1980. Field application of phenoxy acid herbicides. In reference 12, pp. 73–77.
52. Grover, R.; Franklin, C. A.; Muir, N. I.; Cessna, A. J.; and Riedel, D. 1986. Dermal exposure and urinary metabolite excretion in farmers repeatedly exposed to 2,4-D amine. In reference 16, pp. 73–83.
53. Lavy, T. L., and Mattice, J. D. 1986. Progress in pesticide exposure studies and future concerns. In reference 16, pp. 61–71.
54. Lavy, T. L., and Mattice, J. D. 1989. Biological monitoring techniques for humans exposed to pesticides. In reference 17, pp. 192–205.
55. Ritter, L., and Franklin, C. A. 1989. Use of biological monitoring in the regulatory process. In reference 17, pp. 354–367.
56. IARC. 1986. *Some Halogenated Hydrocarbons and Pesticide Exposures*, Lyon, France. **41**: 357–406.

57. Kangas, J.; Koskinen, A.; and Husman, K. 1980. Exposure of Finnish forestry nursery workers to quintozene and maneb. In reference 12, pp. 79–84.
58. Folland, D. S.; Kimbrough, R. D.; Cline, R. E.; Swiggart, R. C.; and Schaffner, W. 1978. Acute hemorrhagic cystitis: industrial exposure to the pesticide chlordimeform. *J. Am. Med. Assoc.* 1052–1055.
59. Maddy, K. T.; Knaak, J. B.; and Gibbons, D. B. 1986. Monitoring the urine of pesticide applicators in California for residues of chlordimeform and its metabolites 1982–1985. In reference 16, pp. 37–44.
60. Balu, K. 1989. Evaluation of field worker exposure to chlordimeform by using urine monitoring. In reference 17, pp. 47–55.
61. Cheung, M. W.; Kahrs, R. A.; Nixon, W. B.; Ross, J. A.; and Tweedy, B. G. 1989. Determination of chlordimeform residues as 4-chloro-*o*-toluidine in human urine using high-performance liquid chromatography. In reference 17, pp. 231–239.
62. Osterloh, J. D.; Wang, R.; O'Connell, L.; Jacob, P., III; and Maddy, K. T. 1989. Pilot study for biological monitoring of 1,3-dichloropropene. In reference 17, pp. 215–230.
63. Dubelman, S., and Cowell, J. E. 1989. Biological monitoring technology for measurement of applicator exposure. In reference 17, pp. 240–250.
64. Lunchick, C.; Burin, G.; Reinert, J. C.; and Warkentien, K. E. 1989. The Environmental Protection Agency's use of biological monitoring data for the special review of alachlor. In reference 17, pp. 327–337.
65. IARC. 1986. *Some Halogenated Hydrocarbons and Pesticide Exposures*, Lyon, France. **41**: 319–356.
66. Maddy, K. T.; Krieger, R. I.; O'Connell, L.; Bisbiglia, M.; and Margetich, S. 1989. Use of biological monitoring data from pesticide users in making pesticide regulatory decisions in California. In reference 17, pp. 338–353.
67. Prinsen, G. H., and van Sittert, N. J. 1980. Exposure and medical monitoring study of a new synthetic pyrethroid after one season of spraying on cotton in Ivory Coast. In reference 12, pp. 105–120.
68. Desi, I.; Palota, M.; Vetro, G.; Csolle, I.; Nehez, M.; Zimanyi, M.; Ferke, A.; Huszta, E.; and Nagymajtenyi, L. 1986. Biological monitoring and health surveillance of a group of greenhouse pesticide sprayers. In reference 16, pp. 91–105.
69. Kolmodin-Hedman, B.; Swensson, A.; and Akerblom, M. 1982. Occupational exposure to some synthetic pyrethroids (Permethrin and Fenvalerate). *Arch. Toxicol.* **50**: 27–33.
70. Chester, G., and Hart, T. B. 1986. Biological monitoring of a herbicide applied through backpack and vehicle sprayers. In reference 16, pp. 137–149.
71. Morgan, M. S.; Phillips, G. S.; and Kirkpatrick, E. M. 1989. Convenient field sampling method for monitoring volatile compounds in exhaled breath. In reference 17, pp. 56–69.
72. San, R. H. C.; Rosin, M. P.; See, R. H.; Dunn, B. P.; and Stich, H. F. 1989. Use of urine for monitoring human exposure to genotoxic agents. In reference 17, pp. 98–116.
73. Van Emon, J. M., and Lopez-Avila, V. 1992. Immunochemical methods for environmental analysis. *Anal. Chem.* **64**: 79A–88A.

23

Biological Monitoring, Hazardous Wastes, and Environmental Pollution in the United States

23.0 THE TOTAL EXPOSURE CONCEPT

23.0.1 The TEAM Study

The Total Exposure Assessment Methodology (TEAM) approach planned by the U.S. EPA since 1979 utilizes breath biological monitoring as a critical tool to assess whether humans have been exposed [1–8]. Volatile organics were investigated in 1980–87 [2–8], carbon monoxide in 1982–83, pesticides in 1986–89, and particulates from 1987 to 1990. The goals of the studies were to develop estimates of the exposures and body burdens of urban populations exposed to toxic and carcinogenic organic chemicals in several U.S. cities (Chapel Hill and Greensboro, NC; Bayonne–Elizabeth, NJ; Devil's Lake, ND; Los Angeles, Antioch, and Pittsburg, CA) on group and individual bases.

Data are needed from various sources. Pollution cannot be identified if historical baseline data do not exist in time as well as space. Also, the impact of hazardous waste dumps on the environment cannot be assessed without such data. It is important too to know what natural cycling patterns exist in addition to the anthropogenic contributions. Because homes, offices, and schools often are sealed hermetically and employ recirculation ventilation systems, they constitute confined spaces just as much as underground storage tanks, enclosed reactors, and underground sewers do in the workplace. Frequent deaths from carbon monoxide poisoning from gas-fired heaters in homes or from leaking exhausts in traveling or stationary cars with their engines on support this assertion. Finally, realistic risk assessment requires accurate and representative exposure data because the U.S. EPA has as part of its risk assessment procedure a section to estimate lifetime exposure from all routes and at all times, not just from workplace air on a 8 h/day for 5 days/week routine as done by the American Conference of Governmental Industrial Hygienists, NIOSH, and OSHA.

Most of the environmental data base is for given points in time instead of being continuous or cross-sectional; so it is extremely difficult to know whether pollution for most compounds is increasing or not. Good examples are carbon dioxide or ozone concentrations in the atmosphere relative to ignorance on long-term trends.

Ten of the 11 volatile chemicals (benzene; carbon tetrachloride; chloroform; *m*- and *p*-dichlorobenzene; ethylbenzene; methylchloroform; perchloroethylene; styrene; trichloroethylene; *m*- and *p*-xylene; *o*-xylene) measured in the breath correlated with indoor air concentrations of New Jersey residences, which, in general, were higher than outdoor concentrations. Thus for perchloroethylene, breath concentrations were 90% of indoor concentrations, which were twice outdoor concentrations. Benzene breath concentrations were 75 to 80% of indoor concentrations from gasoline. The rest of the compounds showed breath concentrations that were 30 to 40% of those of indoor air. Each subject wore a personal air sampler of Tenax GC solid sorbent in the breathing zone for 24 h and provided a breath sample at the end of the day. The variation of concentrations was two orders of magnitude or more. Over 400 people from three states participated in this first study [2–18]. The total number in the TEAM study eventually was 591 [1]. Drinking water in the New Jersey study did not contain any chemicals in high concentrations apart from chloroform (up to 170 ppb), bromodichloromethane (up to 54 ppb), dibromochloromethane (up to 8.4 ppb), trichloroethylene (up to 8.3 ppb), methyl chloroform (up to 5.3 ppb), perchloroethylene (up to 9.3 ppb), toluene (up to 2.7 ppb), vinylidene chloride (up to 2.4 ppb), and benzene (up to 4.8 ppb). Chlorobenzene and bromoform were not detected. The one chemical for which breath and indoor air concentrations did not correlate was chloroform. Here breath concentrations correlated to concentrations in drinking water. The frequent air inversions in California increased [1, 8] outdoor air concentrations of volatile chemicals relative to those in New Jersey, but even in California indoor concentrations generally exceeded outdoor air concentrations. *n*-Decane, dodecane, 1,4-dioxane, α-pinene, undecane, *n*-octane, 1,2-dichloroethane, and 1,1,2,2-tetrachloroethane were added to the list of chemicals investigated for the California study. The California study also resulted in better correlations between indoor air concentrations and breath concentrations than those for outdoor air situations. Breath perchloroethylene increased when subjects visited dry cleaners. Smoking or exposure to tobacco smoke enhanced breath benzene, *p*-xylene, ethylbenzene, and styrene concentrations. Breath benzene increased after visits to gasoline stations. Breath aromatics also were increased by exposure to wet paint, chemical plants, plastics manufacturing products, printing works, and furniture refinishing.

Although the authors of the study claim that breath concentrations reflected absorbed dose, it is unclear that the indoor exposures ceased long enough before breath sampling for only the absorbed dose to be reflected (Sections 6.3 and 21.1). Efforts to address this point were foiled by experimental difficulties [9]. Physical activity also is known to be an important factor in interpreting breath results (Sections 3.0 and 6.3), and this factor was not accounted for in most of the early work. Instrumentation to record personal activity by a data logger is now available [10]. However, there is no doubt that people were exposed, and that they breathed in the test chemicals. Over 200 chemicals were identified in the air in the New Jersey study. The TEAM project also resulted in the development of an alveolar air sampling method [11].

The same relationship of indoor air with higher concentrations than outside air was noted for the pesticides chlordane, chlorpyrifos, diazinon, dichlorvos, heptachlor, *o*-phenylenediamine, and propoxur [12].

The Elizabeth–Bayonne area of New Jersey was revisited in 1987, but Tenax GC solid sorbent area sampling was used for the indoor/outdoor comparison [13]. Although higher concentrations were observed for aromatics in inside air at Elizabeth because of smokers, the outside air was important at Bayonne. Methyl chloroform concentrations were similar indoors and outdoors at Elizabeth; Bayonne homes had much higher trichloroethylene indoor concentrations than Elizabeth homes because more were newly painted in Bayonne, and because of large amounts of adhesives that had been applied. Indoor perchloroethylene concentrations were much higher than those outside because of dry-cleaned clothes. Correlations between personal air samples and breath were noted for the volatiles emitted continuously from specific indoor sources. Air stagnation and inversion conditions increased the influence of outdoor air, and the micrometeorology had to be well-characterized so that results could be interpreted. Thus, aromatics from automobile emissions were clearly increased indoors and outdoors during stagnation and inversion periods.

The TEAM approach has generated related studies on chemicals not studied by TEAM: pentachlorophenol studies related to urine concentrations [14] (Sections 21.4.20 and 22.3); prediction of 2,3,7,8-tetrachlorodibenzo-*p*-dioxin and chloroform in milk and fat, modeled from the major sources [15] (Section 6.7); radionuclides such as ^{210}Po in urine [16]; carboxyhemoglobin and carbon monoxide [17] (Section 21.4.5); pulmonary function parameters and exposures to nitrogen dioxide, sulfur dioxide, and total suspended particulates [17]; lead and cadmium in breathing zone air as correlated with blood and fecal concentrations [18]; urinary cotinine and nicotine from exposure to environmental tobacco smoke [19] (Sections 5.3.2 and 8.4.10); blood, urine, and hair analyses for up to 13 metals in German citizens [20] (Chapter 6); the inadequacy of blood lead to represent tissue concentrations of lead [21]; and the TCDD equivalency method to measure exposure to toxic PCDDs and PCDFs to provide a relationship to health effects [22] (Section 6.7.2). For the latter, some International Toxicity Factors for specific PCDDs and PCDFs are: 2,3,7,8-TCDD, 1.00; 1,2,3,7,8-PeCDD/PeCDF and 2,3,4,7,8-PeCDF, 0.5; 1,2,3,4,7,8-HxCDD/HxCDF, 1,2,3,7,8,9-HxCDD/HxCDF, 1,2,3,6,7,8-HxCDD/HxCDF, and 2,3,4,6,7,8-HxCDF, 0.1; 1,2,3,4,6,7,8-HpCDD/HpCDF and 1,2,3,4,7,8,9-HpCDF, 0.01; and OCDD and OCDF, 0.001.

23.0.2 Modeling Total Exposure from Multiple Pathways

How to predict exposure from multiple pathways of exposure was dealt with descriptively in Chapter 3. Nevertheless, we provide a generalized scheme below [15].

Population risk R in disease incidence per year resulting from a contaminant rclcased at a source S (in kg/year) is assumed to be comprised of several factors:

$$R = N \cdot f\{S, E(S),\ D(E), a\} \tag{23.1}$$

where N is the population size; E is the exposure duration that is equivalent to lifetime equivalent contact; D is the dose that is absorbed, depending on whither the body or a target organ is being considered; and a is the risk per unit dose rate or potency

Estimation of exposure and risk includes temporal and/or spatial relations and a knowledge of the interdependencies among the source, exposure, dose, time, and incidence of the health effects. Thus the function E is divided into a series of terms that relate route and mode of exposure:

$$E = \text{sum}_i\ \text{sum}_j\ c_i(S)F_{ij} \tag{23.2}$$

where $c_i(S)$ is the concentration of the chemical in the environmental compartment (air, soil, water) (denoted by subscript i) associated with source S, and F_{ij} is the pathway exposure factor that relates the compartment concentration to the mode of exposure (inhalation, ingestion, dermal absorption, eye absorption) (denoted by subscript j) in units of mg chemical/kg body weight/day. F_{ij} incorporates information on anatomy, physiology, detoxification, activation, diet, physical activity, and environmental partitioning. Thus concentrations in mg/L water, mg/m^3 air, and mg/kg soil are translated into a daily exposure. The major compartments are generally thought to be: air (gas phase), air (particulate phase), soil, drinking water, and surface water. The major modes of exposure are: inhalation, ingestion (water, fruits and vegetables, grains, meat, fish, milk, and soil), and dermal (chloroform in water) absorption. Though drinking water contains negligible particulate matter, the latter may become important for surface waters.

Estimates involve assumptions and errors also. A child aged 1 to 15 years consumes approximately 1.4 ± 0.6 L fluid/day, breathes $14.3 \pm 4\,\text{m}^3$ air/day, drinks 0.39 ± 0.26 L milk/day, and weighs 27 ± 14 kg; an adult aged 15 to 70 years consumes 1.7 ± 0.7 L fluid/day, drinks 0.22 ± 0.44 L milk/day, breathes $22.3 \pm 6\,\text{m}^3$ air/day, and weighs 66 ± 14 kg. The standard deviation is one standard deviation. The log transforms between water intake and body weight and between inhalation volume and body weight are assumed to have correlations of about 0.7. If the distributions of these parameters are assumed to be lognormal and each medium is assumed isotropic (equal concentration), F_{ij} values can be calculated, but with a great error.

Often deposition factors (wet and dry) relating air concentration in mg/m^3 to vegetation deposition V_{dp} in mg/m^2/day must be estimated as follows:

$$V_{dp} = v_g + bRW_p \tag{23.3}$$

where v_g is the dry deposition velocity onto vegetation in m/day (usually 0.9 to 155,000 m/day), b is the fraction of material retained on vegetation from wet deposition (usually 0.1–0.3), R is the annual average rainfall rate in m/day, and W_p is the washout factor for particles (unitless; usually 10^5–10^6).

The factor v_g depends on total deposition velocity v_t:

$$v_g = v_t\,[1 - \exp(-dM_v)] \tag{23.4}$$

where d is the foliar interception constant in m^2/dry kg (usually about 2.8), and M_v is the dry mass inventory of vegetation per unit area in kg/m^2 (usually about $0.6\,kg/m^2$).

Thus v_g is about $0.8v_t$ for pasture crops. The uncertainty in V_{dp} is about 0.1% for particles of <5 mm aerodynamic diameter.

The biotransfer factor B_k between animals and their milk often is required in risk assessment to estimate food chain concentration probabilities. The regression equation is utilized:

$$\log B_k = \log K_{ow} - 8.1, \text{ with } n = 28 \text{ and } r = 0.74 \tag{23.5}$$

where K_{ow} is the octanol/water partition coefficient (Section 3.2).

23.1 BIOLOGICAL MONITORING AND HAZARDOUS WASTE SITES

The purpose of this section is to provide a general introduction to the topic rather than a literature survey of current knowledge.

23.1.1 General Considerations

After chemical spills or at hazardous waste sites, exposure to many chemicals may occur through all routes of absorption [23–26]. One of the major functions of biological monitoring is to ensure that the cumulative and multiroute exposures (Section 23.0.2) cause no adverse health effects. As discussed quantitatively in Section 21.3.1, biological monitoring is extremely important in defining whether unsuspected sources and routes of absorption are present, especially if air concentrations are too low to account for the observed effects.

The tasks of analyzing single xenobiotics, metabolities, or adducts in biological media are potentially infinite after/during exposure to a complex mixture of chemicals. Even if such analysis is possible, interpretation of the results may be confounded by a lack of knowledge of interactions, the ubiquitous interindividual variability, and hypersensitivity. Specific markers can be used, as detailed in the previous chapters, if the identities of specific exposing chemicals are known. Use of the BEI recommendations for 24-h exposures, as discussed in Section 21.3, are not appropriate except for personnel working on-site 8 h/day, 5 days/week, or a similar regimen where work-site exposure is the only exposure to the chemical of concern, and where the other conditions for applications of the specific BEIs are appropriate. However, the identities of the exposing chemicals generally are not known.

Health effects and medical monitoring therefore are the chief means of detecting an overall adverse effect, on an individual and a population basis, after hazardous wastes exposures. Hence the ideal medical surveillance program should be one generally similar to that described in Section 7.1 for workers at hazardous waste sites. Such oversight for the general population is not enforceable, and it is expensive. At least annual medical examinations are recommended, however. It is much more important to determine the health status of an individual than to ascertain whether exposure occurred (a fact often deducible from acute symptomology). Thus it is important to measure markers capable of integrating exposure to multiple chemicals when the exposing chemicals are unknown. The most important of these markers are discussed in Chapter 9.

The Agency for Toxic Substances and Disease Registry (ATSDR), created by the Superfund (CERCLA) statute is the U.S. government agency whose mission is to prevent/mitigate adverse human health effects or the diminished quality of life resulting from exposure to hazardous substances in the environment [27]. The U.S. EPA is the regulatory agency. ATSDR undertakes health assessments of hazardous waste sites and facilities; health consultations provided to citizens, community groups, private groups, and government agencies; exposure registries exposed to substances prioritized by the U.S. EPA and ATSDR; pilot assessment studies; research to elucidate mechanisms of toxicity including that of biomarkers; accumulation of reference data; prospective and retrospective epidemiological studies; clinical referrals; issuances of health advisories; recommendations to other federal, state, county, and local government agencies; health education; development and distribution of toxicological profiles to set forth the important data in a way understandable to the public; and development of specialty information to facilitate reduction of exposure. Of high priority is the assessment of risk to pesticidal wastes and to their precursor/formulation chemicals. (The biological monitoring markers for organic pesticides are discussed in Chapter 22.)

23.1.2 Some Examples of Useful Markers

Urinary thioethers were measured [28] by the present author for workers at the North Wastewater Treatment Plant in Memphis, Tennessee after a spill from a pesticide manufacturer occurred for chemicals used in the synthesis of the chlorinated cyclodiene pesticides (Section 22.3). End-of-shift spot urines also were analyzed for the pesticidal precursors (hexachlorocyclopentadiene and hexachlorobicycloheptadiene) and β-glucuronidase. Of the ten workers sampled, only two had total thioethers >5.9 mmol SH/mol creatinine, considered the upper reference limit (Section 9.3.7). There was an inverse relationship of urinary thioethers to urinary hexachlorobicycloheptadiene concentrations. This decreased thioether excretion might signify damage to the liver, which lessens the capacity of the liver to produce the thioethers. Such an observation is not classic because dose-effect relationships usually are interpreted to mean greater response with increased exposing concentration. An equally valid explanation is that the presence of interactions due to exposure to a multicomponent mixture might cause a "wait-in-line" phenomenon for endogenous compounds that are thioether precursors. Another interpretation could be saturation of a particular metabolic pathway with shunting of the alternative metabolites through another excretory route like the breath or feces. Another study on a group of Hardeman County residents exposed to the same type of waste reported lower urinary cholylglycine concentrations [26].

A book written about health effects of hazardous waste sites [29] collected a large amount of the pertinent data for U.S. hazardous wastes sites up to 1984. The U.S. EPA lists certain industrial wastes as hazardous, and so categorizes unlisted wastes that have any of the four characteristics of ignitability, corrosivity, reactivity, and environmental toxicity (above critical concentrations after leaching of the waste, simulating groundwater contamination, through the EP and TCLP leaching protocols). The major health effects are [30]: symptoms such as rashes and eye irritation; signs such as rashes, paralysis, tremor, convulsions, and so forth; diseases or disorders [apparent disorders: atypical reproductive outcomes, growth and developmental disorders, behavioral or psychological disorders, cancer, mortality, other disorders (such as autoimmune diseases, blood dyscrasias, coronary artery diseases, and so on); nonobvious biochemical abnormalities (cholinesterase, erythrocyte protoporphyrin, liver function tests); immunologic abnormalities (lymphocyte tests); chromosomal abnormalities; nerve conduction abnormalities; and other test abnormalities (for example, pulmonary function)]. The "not apparent" disorders category contains most of the medical markers discussed in Chapter 9.

Analytic indices of reproductive dysfunction include [30, 31]: sexual dysfunction (decreased libido, impotence); sperm abnormalities (decreased number, decreased motility, abnormal morphology); subfecundity (abnormal genitalia, ducts, gonads; abnormal pubertal development; infertility; amenorrhea; anovulatory cycles); illness during pregnancy and parturition (toxemia, hemorrhage); early fetal loss to 28 weeks; perinatal death (late fetal loss after 28 weeks and stillbirth, intrapartum death, death in first week); decreased birth weight; gestational age at delivery (prematurity, postmaturity); altered chromosomal sex ratio; multiple births; birth defects (major, minor); chromosomal abnormalities (early fetuses, through amniocentesis, in perinatal deaths, in livebirths); infant mortality; childhood morbidity; childhood malignancies; and age at menopause. A comprehensive review is available on biological markers of reproductive toxicology [31]. See also Section 6.7.5 for semen markers and Section 6.8.5 for menses markers, as well as Section 8.5.7 on gender markers, Section 8.5.12 on menstrual cycle variations, and Section 9.3 on chromosomal, cancer, and urinary health surveillance markers.

Markers used to assess the integrity of the fetus include [31]: lecithin/sphingomyelin ratio and phosphoglycerol in amniotic fluid as related to fetal lung maturity; genetic screening of amniotic cells; concentration of estriol in maternal urine and serum; and direct measures of growth including femur length and biparietal diameters. Serum maternal α-fetoprotein increases above reference ranges when fetuses have open neural tube defects. The presence of low amniotic fluid α-fetoprotein as well as normal anatomy as deduced from sonography suggests that a pregnancy is at high risk for preterm labor, low birth weight, and fetal wastage. Birth defects can be genetic, but also can be due to maternal diseases such as rubella (discovered in the early 1940s) and to chemicals such as thalidomide (in the 1960s). Adverse effects on the neonate have been documented for the following drugs: azathiopine (decreased immunologic competence), cannabis or marijuana (neuorobehavioral effects), chloramphenicol (Gray syndrome), cocaine (neonate withdrawal and cerebral infarction), diazepam (floppy baby syndrome), ethanol (heart malformations and mental retardation), heroin and other narcotics (growth retardation, neonate withdrawal, and microcephaly), lithium (heart malformations), oxytocin (hyperbilirubinemia), phenobarbital (neonatal bleeding), propranolol (hypoglycemia and bradycardia), reserpine (nasal congestion), salicylates (platelet dysfunction), thiazides (thrombocytopenia and electrolyte imbalance), tobacco (intrauterine growth retardation), and warfarin (bleeding). Ultrasonography allows direct visualization of the fetus during organogenesis to birth, and morphological, physiological, and surface abnormalities can be detected. Microcephaly is not detectable, however. Doppler blood flow measurements of uterine blood flow, umbilical blood flow, and fetal heart rate also are much used.

Neurodevelopmental markers also are important, these usually being detected by behavioral studies [31]. Lead is the best-known neurodevelopmental toxicant, children and the fetus being far more susceptible than adults. Biological monitoring markers of neurobehavioral effect of lead include: urinary homovanillic acid, a metabolite of dopamine that is correlated to blood lead concentration above 2.5 micromolar in young children exposed to lead paint, with a reference range between 3 and 8 mg/m^3/day of homovanillic acid below this blood lead threshold; and cerebrospinal fluid γ-butyric acid and enkephalins in animal models. Some blood lead thresholds include [31]: heme pathway effects (10 μg/dL for 5′-Pyri, and decreased δ-aminolevulinic acid dehydratase activity; 15 μg/dL for increased free erythrocyte protoporphyrin; 40 μg/dL for decreased heme production; 50 μg/dL for basophilic stippling; and 60 μg/dL for frank anemia); central nervous system effects (35 μg/dL for quantitative electroencephalogram abnormalities; 10 μg/dL for evoked potential abnormalities); psychologic effects (15 μg/dL for decreased IQ; 10 μg/dL for decreased attention deficits; 35 μg/dL for appearance of speech and language deficits); and other effects (12 μg/dL for alteration of 1,25-vitamin D hydroxylase activity; 20 μg/dL for alteration of Na–K ATPase activity).

Ionizing radiation is a well known physical factor that induces hyperactivity in males (like lead) but hypoactivity in females [31]. (See also Sections 8.5.3 and 8.5.4.) Animal experiments have shown that eye defects and forebrain defects occurred after irradiation during early embryo development, but cerebellar malformations occurred during fetal and neonatal life. Learning acquisition and visual/tactile discrimination were impaired also by X-ray irradiation of the hippocampus of newly born rats. Whether this models human effects is still uncertain. Brain damage caused by *N*-methyl-4-phenyltetrahydropyridine, a contaminant in some designer drugs or meperidine derivatives with opiate-like characteristics, resembles idiopathic Parkinson's disease by damaging the same target nigrostriatal dopaminergic pathways [31].

The neurotoxicants most investigated include lead, mercury, cadmium, PCBs, phenytoin, ethanol, and methadone. Drugs such as clonidine, diazepam, imipramine-like agents, and reserpine also are often utilized as reference compounds; all produce hyperactivity.

Some general central spinal fluid markers of development and cell injury include [31]: markers of the status of central nervous system neurons such as protein I, neural tube D2, and B50; P5D 95 for the status of the postsynaptic receptors; myelin basic protein for the status of the oligodendroglia and myelin sheath; myelin-associated glycoprotein to reflect the status of the oligodendroglia; and GFAP to relect the astrocytes of the glioma.

Brain tissue markers include protein III and synapsin I to reflect cell loss at the nerve terminals [31]. These markers, apart from the behavioral and urinary end points, are necessarily invasive and thus difficult to use in epidemiological studies. Newer techniques such as computed axial tomography, positron emission tomography (used to diagnose *N*-methyl-4-phenyltetrahydropyridine brain damage), and magnetic resonance imaging (which might be useful for lead exposures because energy transfer from phosphate groups is visualized, and lead affects Na–K ATPase activities) are noninvasive and allow visualization of physiologic/biochemical processes of the brain in living people. These techniques are very expensive; they also are not portable.

Some behavioral end points often studied include [31]: nerve conduction time (in children exposed to lead); sensory psychophysical functions and scotopic vision (where visual acuity in the dark is diminished by lead exposure); evoked potentials (where auditory evoked potentials responding to pure tones or clicks are diminished by exposure to lead, carbon monoxide, and trichloroethylene; visual evoked potentials are diminished by exposure to xylene, dimethyl mercury and *n*-hexane; and somatosensory evoked potentials are diminished by exposure to lead but not by *n*-hexane); auditory discrimination (in children exposed to lead); vibration sense (for exposure to pharmaceuticals such as isoniazid, phenytoin, vincristine, amd glutethimide, and to chemicals such as acrylamide, arsenic, *n*-hexane, lead, mercury and methyl butyl ketone; see also Chapter 20); motor function (in children exposed to lead); attention (in children exposed to lead); visual–motor integration; speech and language function; psychometric intelligence (for lead, polybrominated biphenyls, and fetal-alcohol exposures using the Bayley Scales of Infant Development for children 6 months to 3 years of age, using the McCarthy Scales for children 3 to 5 years old, and using the revised Wechsler Intelligence Scales for children older than 5 years); and social behavior (lead-exposed children being more dependent, nonadaptive, and hyperactive than those not exposed).

A book on the markers used in pulmonary toxicology has been published [32]. Most of these markers are discussed in Sections 3.0, 6.3, 6.6, and 8.2.4.

Biological monitoring plays an important role in proving asbestos exposure. Plasma malondialdehyde, a nonspecific marker of lipid peroxidation, was elevated (11.5 ± 2.8 nmol/mL) in 59 male workers exposed to asbestos dust for 15.6 ± 4.5 years relative to 31 male workers exposed to silica dust (10.5 ± 1.7 nmol/L) for 21.3 ± 8.3 years and also to 52 age-matched healthy male controls (9.46 ± 2.2 nmol/L) [33]. The effects of silica exposure also were significantly different from controls [33]. Smoking appeared not to be a confounding factor. Both diseases were postulated to evoke malondialdehyde through the susceptibility of alveolar macrophages to release fibrogenic factors. Because the plasma concentrations of the marker were no different whether lung fibrosis could be detected or not, the malondialdehyde marker is a predictive marker of adverse effect at least 10% above the plasma concentration of controls. Another predictive marker of early fibrosis due to asbestos exposure in 36 male workers (exposed 2 to 27 years) was serum type III procollagen peptide cleaved from procollagen by peptidases during secretion of newly formed collagen from the collagen-producing cells [34]. The reference range in control workers was 7.0 to 12 ng/mL, with the asbestos workers showing values from 7 to 20 ng/mL, the data not being distributed normally. Alcohol ingestion and smoking were not confounding factors. As for the plasma malondialdehyde marker, the concentrations of the peptide were significantly different, independent of whether fibrosis was detectable or not.

The conventional noninvasive bronchoalveolar lavage by bronchofiberscopy also revealed asbestos bodies, long (>5 μm) asbestos fibers coated with ferroprotein by macrophages, in 563 workers in an exposure-duration–related manner [35]. Workers with asbestosis showed positive asbestos bodies in 98.3% relative to controls, as did 95% of those with benign pleural disease and 75% of those with malignant mesothelioma. Thus this marker is a biological monitoring marker of exposure to asbestos. Asbestos fibers also have been detected in urines (only 10 workers from an asbestos cement factory were examined), and there appeared to be no correlation with extent of asbestos exposure [35]. Chrysotile and crocidolite asbestos, all <2.5 μm in length, were detected in the urines of asbestos workers and "control" foundry workers. The chrysotile was of workplace origin, but not the crocidolite. Thus some long thin asbestos fibers can pass through the bronchiolar epithelium and gastrointestinal tract and be transported to distant parts of the body. Other markers utilized to detect asbestos exposure include [36]: asbestos bodies in sputum, asbestos fibers in feces, measurement of cell-mediated immunity, white cell modified nucleoside, and urinary pseudouridine (Section 10.1.1). This is a good example of the possible applications of biological monitoring methods to characterize exposure and to predict or monitor health effects of a xenobiotic not thought to be suitable for biological monitoring. The application to asbestos exposures in hazardous waste situations also is obvious.

23.1.3 Some Epidemiological Considerations

Epidemiological investigations around waste sites generally are limited by lack of statistical power, at least 100 people being required to have an accuracy of 99% at 95% confidence limits [30]. Usually, the number of people showing adverse health effects after exposure to hazardous wastes is much smaller than this. Problems related to representative controls (selection bias) and highly variable control population responses often limit the successful detection of subtle effects. Dose-effects and responses are merely correlations, not necessarily cause and effect. Actual population exposures usually are poorly defined and nonuniform. Life-style and genetic factors are hard to allow for in statistical analyses. Latent periods often exist that go unrecognized. Questionnaires often are inappropriate and can be misunderstood, and many contain leading questions. Also many questions may be poorly designed. The answers to questionnaires often are incomplete and selective. Suspicion, paranoia, selectivity, and nonrepresentativeness of the population may bias results. Confounders may exert bias if they are not thought of by the questionnaire designer.

The variation in the characteristics of the populations and the variation in the quality of the data must be separable if correct interpretation of group data is to be achieved. The hardest error to correct for generally is the systematic one leading to misclassification (information bias). Such errors include: instrumental errors, where it is not known whether the instruments are in calibration; recall bias, related to answering questionnaires; interview procedure and questionnaire bias; the use of environmental data without error estimation; the use of a parameter that is not related to the variable being studied; and positive or negative bias from making an assumption about an event that may lead to a set of questions that are compatible with other causes, and not just the one being studied.

The question of interactions, as in the case of multicomponent exposures, may be extremely complicated, and may upset any dose-effect/response relationship expected for single chemicals. Because exposure or biological monitoring data in general often are not measured for the majority of studies, all means of correcting for interactions are arbitrary and may involve much error. Incomplete data present another problem.

For cross-sectional studies involving a comparison between two matched groups, if a background illness occurred at the rate of 0.1%, a comparison study with 25,500 exposed and 25,500 control people would be necessary to detect a frequency of 0.2% in the exposed group at a two-tailed 5% significance level with a statistical power of 80%. Detection of a similar 1% incidence in the exposed cohort would require about 1000 people in each group. The relationship to group size and statistical power varies with the square root of the group number. For unmatched case-control studies, the power to discriminate effects is maximized when the proportion of exposed controls is around 0.25 to 0.5. Power can be increased by individual matching (personal baseline determinations) and/or by using multiple controls for each case. Some background frequencies commonly quoted include [30]: (a) for reproductive effects using 1981 data—azospermia, 10^{-2}; live-birth birth weight <2500 g, 7×10^{-2}; spontaneous abortion after 8 to 28 weeks of gestation, 0.1 to 0.2; chromosomal anomaly among fetuses aborted spontaneously, 0.3 to 0.4; birth defects in live births, 0.02 to 0.03; and neural tube defects in live- and stillbirths, 10^{-4} to 10^{-2}; (b) for cancer incidence for individuals using age-adjusted 1970 incidence rates and data from 1973 through 1976 at all SEER sites—all sites, 3.2×10^{-3}; 9.8×10^{-5}; colon, 3.3×10^{-4}; lung and bronchus, 4.5×10^{-4}; bladder, 1.5×10^{-4}; kidney, 6.4×10^{-5}; lymphomas, 1.2×10^{-4}; and leukemias, 9.5×10^{-5}; and (c) for 1970 U.S. mortality rates—all causes, 9.5×10^{-3}; all cancer sites, 1.6×10^{-3}; liver cirrhosis, 1.4×10^{-4}; and congenital anomalies, 8.4×10^{-5}.

Most studies of an exposed population involve an initial ecological and environmental assessment to identify contamination and any hot spots; the next phase is a pilot study on the most exposed individuals to the test chemical or physical agent; the third step is a community survey to identify matched controls and those who are exposed; and the fourth step is a cohort study that is prospective (that is, with health effects monitored in time), retrospective (for a past exposure with the data at hand), or ambispective (a combination of both approaches). The prospective design is too expensive for effects having a long lag time such as cancer but is excellent for acute effects or for studies on children soon after their birth, as, for example, to assess the effect of environmental lead exposure on children. The retrospective design is better for chronic effects such as asbestosis and cancer. Ambispective design is excellent when an exposed population that shows health effects from a retrospective analysis must be followed in the future. Unfortunately, the retrospective design may have incomplete data and information, whereas a prospective design will be much more flexible than the retrospective type. An ambispective design combines the best of the two extreme approaches. Space/time cluster studies also may be desirable, depending on the exposure source, geography, meteorology, and population movement.

In all of studies on populations, the frequency of response/effect versus class response/effect interval histograms must be utilized to decide the applicable distribution curves—that is, normal, lognormal, bimodal, trimodal, and so on. Then one can decide how the most representative value and the variance of each population are to be calculated. Often nonparametric statistics must be utilized when two different distributions are to be compared.

It is well known that most exposure data gathered occupationally are lognormally distributed for frequency of response/effect versus class response/effect interval plots. However, the assignment of population distribution still must be performed for each individual study, as is the case for environmental exposure investigations. Biological monitoring data characteristically have much scatter, with low and high control group reference values over a span of two to three orders of magnitude not uncommon (Section 8.3).

23.2 SYNOPSIS OF PUBLISHED AND UNPUBLISHED STUDIES OR STUDY PROTOCOLS RELATED TO HEALTH EFFECTS EVALUATIONS AT HAZARDOUS WASTE SITES IN THE UNITED STATES TO 1984

The following case control studies are reproduced from Appendix C of reference 29 [37]. Though not up to date, the list illustrates the general approaches, critical factors to evaluate the quality of each study, and major study variables that must be considered.

I. Reference: CDC. Polychlorinated Biphenyls (PCBs) Exposure at Superfund Waste Sites (draft), August 23, 1983 Study Protocol

II. Facility:
   A. Location: Superfund sites with PCB exposures to humans
   B. Physical condition:
   C. Hazardous materials: PCBs and possibly other chemicals
   D. Principal routes of exposures: Various

III. Study:
   A. Motivation of study: There are three reasons given for studying PCBs:
      1. They are the most prevalent chemicals found in Superfund sites.
      2. They can be reliably measured in serum.
      3. Serum levels reflect body burdens over many years due to equilibration between fat PCB stores and serum levels.
   B. Population studied: It is proposed to study people exposed to PCBs from Superfund sites.
   C. Health measurements: Not stated at present.
   D. Exposure measurements: Serum collected from people; questionnaire regarding possible contamination.
   E. Study design:
      Stage 1: Assess the presence of PCBs at waste sites and possible PCB

contamination to humans. The presence of other toxic chemicals will also be assessed.

Stage 2: A pilot study will be conducted of the potentially "most exposed" people at the high priority sites chosen in Stage 1.

Stage 3: Community surveys will be conducted at sites found important in Stages 1 and 2.

Stage 4: Registries of PCB-exposed cohorts will be designed and implemented for cohorts detected by Stage 3.

I. Reference: Halperin, W., Landrigan, P. J., Altman, R., Iaci, A. W., Morse, D. L., and Needham, L. L. Chemical fire at toxic waste disposal plant: Epidemiologic study of exposure to smoke and fire. *J. of Med. Soc. of N.J.* Vol. 78, No. 9, pp. 591–594, August, 1981.

II. Facility:

A. Location: Southern New Jersey

B. Physical condition: Waste-chemical disposal plant consisting of storage tanks, high-temperature incinerators, ancillary buildings

C. Hazardous materials: Diverse chemicals including PCB, benzene, methylene chloride, aniline

D. Principal routes of exposures: Air, direct contact

III. Study:

A. Motivation of study: Exposed people developed symptoms. Also there was a possibility that TCDD or TCDF may have been produced in the combustion of PCB.

B. Population studied: All people present at the fire.

C. Health measurements: Questionnaires measured previous medical history, complaints of respiratory problems, headache, eye and throat irritation, nausea, etc.

D. Exposure measurements: Soil samples throughout fire zone and wipe samples of fire equipment measured for TCDD and TCDF. Closeness of people to fire site and duration of exposure were noted.

E. Study design: Names of people at the fire were obtained by contacting fire companies, police, rescue squads, civil defense groups and other groups that participated, as well as general media appeal. 440 of the 459 people known to have been present at the fire were surveyed. Followup questionnaires were administered to people who reported respiratory symptoms on the first questionnaire.

F. Limitations of study: No control group of unexposed people, or people exposed to a "non-toxic" fire. There was no measurement of fumes.

G. Results: A positive association of symptoms with duration of exposure. No evidence of TCDD or TCDF in any environmental sample.

I. Reference: Kreiss, K., Zack, M. M., Kimbrough, R. D., Needham, L. L., Smrek, A. L., and Jones, B. T. Cross-sectional study of a community with exceptional exposure to DDT. *JAMA* 245, #19, (1926–1930), 1981.

II. Facility:

A. Location: Triana, Alabama

B. Physical condition: Between 1947 and 1971, DDT was manufactured 10 km from Triana. Industrial waste was dumped into a rural stream.

C. Hazardous materials: DDT and related compounds

D. Principal routes of exposures: Food chain (fish)

III. Study:

A. Motivation of study: Publicity concerning high DDT residues in fish caught near Triana.

B. Population studied: All residents of Triana and its rural environs were asked to participate; not all did. 518 people were registered for the study; 499 gave blood.

C. Health measurements: Demographic, diet, sources of insecticide exposure, medical history, blood analysis, blood pressure, urinalysis.

D. Exposure measurements: Serum DDT residues.

E. Study design: Cross-sectional survey of a population likely to be exposed to DDT through food.

F. Limitations of study: No control group. Complete ascertainment of population at risk was not addressed.

G. Results: Serum triglyceride was positively correlated with DDT. There was no association with other measured health effects such as history of heart disease, hypertension, diabetes.

I. Reference: Rothenberg, R. Morbidity study at a chemical dump—New York. *MMWR*, Vol. 30, No. 24, pp. 293–294, June 26, 1981.

II. Facility:

A. Location: Hyde Park landfill, north of Niagara Falls, New York.

B. Physical condition: It was used from 1953 to 1975 as disposal site for approximately 80,200 tons of chemical waste. A compacted clay cover was installed in 1978 and a drainage system around the perimeter in 1979.

C. Hazardous materials: Diverse chemicals, including many chlorinated hydrocarbons

D. Principal routes of exposures: Air

III. Study:

A. Motivation of study: Not stated

B. Population studied: People who worked or lived near Hyde Park landfill. There was a 59% participation rate.

C. Health measurements: Questionnaire (from HANES) and a limited physical examination, urine and blood tests. Compared to matched controls from HANES study.

D. Exposure measurements: Exposures to people were checked through urine and blood tests. NIOSH had found lindane, mirex and dioxins in dust samples of rafters of nearby companies.

E. Study design: Cross-sectional study.

F. Limitations of study: Low participation rate. Lack of sufficient interval for exposures to produce outcomes such as cancer.

G. Results: Of 180 evaluated variables, 9 were statistically significant; hiatal hernia survey was highest, O.R. = 7.6.

I. Reference: Oudbier, A. J., Eyster, J. T., and Lock, J.M. Berlin-Farro respiratory study, Michigan Department of Public Health, December, 1981.

II. Facility:

A. Location: Genesee County, Michigan

B. Physical condition: Berlin-Farro Liquid Incinerator Company operated from about 1970 to 1974. It was shut down because of resident complaints of fumes and health problems. In 1981 the contaminated sludge was hauled away.
C. Hazardous materials: Diverse chemicals
D. Principal routes of exposures: Air

III. Study:
A. Motivation of study: Resident complaints.
B. Population studied: All residents, 16 years and older, within a 2-square mile around the site.
C. Health measurements: Self-reported respiratory complaints.
D. Exposure measurements: Soil sampling. The exposure measurement of people was self-reported exposure to fumes and length of residence.
E. Study design: Questionnaire survey.
F. Limitations of study: Self-selection and self-reporting bias.
G. Results: Among males, there was an association between respiratory complaints and self-reported exposure, accounting for age and cigarette smoking. Among females there was no association.

I. Reference: New Jersey State Dept. Health. A Health Census of a Community with Groundwater Contamination—Jackson Township, 1980.

II. Facility:
A. Location: Jackson Township landfill, Ocean County, New Jersey
B. Physical condition: Landfill operating from 1972 to 1980. Not insulated from underlying groundwater.
C. Hazardous materials: Chemicals include various halogenated organic compounds.
D. Principal routes of exposures: Groundwater, air.

III. Study:
A. Motivation of study: Demonstrated contaminated well water. A previous health survey showed some complaints. Health department was concerned about long-term effects.
B. Population studied: Affected residents and controls. Total of 560 people from 150 households.
C. Health measurements: Health questionnaire.
D. Exposure measurements: Household water sample. Home air sample. Information on water supply.
E. Study design: Cross-sectional study of exposed and nonexposed controls.
F. Limitations of study: Possibility of recall bias. Residents were aware of problems. There had been previous surveys, and there was a class-action suit in 1980.
G. Results: Increased risk of skin complaints. Among users of shallow wells there was increased kidney illness, but a causal relationship is not biologically plausible.

I. Reference: New Jersey State Dept. of Health. A Health Survey of the Population Living Near Gloucester Environmental Management Services (GEMS) Landfill. April, 1982.

II. Facility:
A. Location: Camden County, New Jersey

B. Physical condition: Landfill was opened in 1960 as sanitary landfill. It is believed that chemical dumping took place in 1970s. It is now covered, but erosion is evident with leachate flowing into an adjacent creek.
C. Hazardous materials: Diverse chemicals
D. Principal routes of exposures: Groundwater, air

III. Study:
A. Motivation of study: Resident complaints of odors and health problems
B. Population studied: Residents living near GEMS landfill and controls living 5 miles away.
C. Health measurements: Questionnaire covering problems like eye and throat irritation, coughing, medical problems. Lung function test.
D. Exposure measurements: Air sampling for volatile organics inside and outside of homes of residents and controls.
E. Study design: Cross-sectional survey of residents and controls.
F. Limitations of study: The initial lung function testing was wrong, so people had to return. Volunteering twice could possibly be source of selection bias. Also, they invited only some subgroups and not everyone.
G. Results: Increased respiratory complaints in residents, but no medical problems. Pulmonary results were not consistent with questionnaire survey.

I. Reference: New Jersey State Dept. Health. A Health Survey of the Population Living Near the Price Landfill. July, 1983.

II. Facility:
A. Location: Price Landfill, Atlantic County, New Jersey
B. Physical condition: 26-acre site. Sanitary Landfill 1972 to 1980. Closed, inactive, covered, with erosion with leachate on western edge of site.
C. Hazardous materials: Diverse chemicals including cadmium, lead, chloroform, vinyl chloride, benzene
D. Principal routes of exposures: Groundwater

III. Study:
A. Motivation of study: Contamination of private and public wells had already been established by EPA, DEP, and Atlantic County Health Department.
B. Population studied: Households thought to be affected by contaminated groundwater and suitable controls.
C. Health measurements: Health questionnaire on exposure to toxic substances, presence of symptoms and reported medical problems.
D. Exposure measurements: Well water samples showed that Water Quality Criteria was exceeded for many chemicals including cadmium, lead, chloroform, vinyl chloride.
E. Study design: Cross-sectional survey of exposed residents and non-exposed controls.
F. Limitations of study: Bias due to resident knowledge and concern of water problems is unknown.
G. Results: Female exposed residents reported excess of several symp-

toms compared to controls. There was no difference in reported medical problems.

I. Reference: Janerich, D. T., Burnett, W. S., Feck, G., Hoff, M., Nasca, P., Polednak, A. P., Greenwald, P., and Vianna, N. Cancer incidence in the Love Canal Area, *Science* 212, 1404–1407, 1981.
II. Facility:
   A. Location: Love Canal, New York.
   B. Physical condition: Waste burial 1920 through 1953, population grew rapidly afterwards, though it was affected in 1978 when concern started regarding health hazards. Inactive landfill in residential area.
   C. Hazardous materials: Over 80 chemicals identified (though not all toxic), including benzene and halogenated hydrocarbons. Largely residues from pesticide production.
   D. Principal routes of exposures: Direct, air, water.
III. Study:
   A. Motivation of study: This was one of later studies of a recognized problem area.
   B. Population studied: Exposed: Exposed people taken from census tract surrounding Love Canal (LC). Unexposed: Unexposed people taken from Niagara Falls census tracts and New York state rates. Estimated from 1960, 1967, and 1970 censuses.
   C. Health measurements: All sites cancer incidence as reported to the New York Cancer Registry.
   D. Exposure measurements: None in this study.
   E. Study design: Ecologic design. Age/sex-specific cancer rates of LC area were first compared to 25 Niagara Falls census tracts, then New York state incidence rates. All sites compared for 1966 to 1977 (better data). Liver, lymphoma, leukemia compared for 1955 to 1965 as well.
   F. Limitations of study: Population at risk ill-defined. Completeness and accuracy of registry data not known; it could be a factor since there were only a few deaths per census tract per age/sex category in several cancers.
   G. Results: There was high rate of respiratory cancer, but it seemed to be related to entire city of Niagara Falls. Standardized incidence ratios based on New York state rates found the 2 female 1955 to the 1965 liver cancers significant. Another look at age-specific rates comparing LC to Niagara Falls census tract found LC to be high. But the authors discounted all positive findings because of the small number of cases.

I. Reference: Indian et al. Health Survey of a Population in the Proximity of a Chemical Waste Disposal Site, Lorain County, Ohio Department of Health. December, 1980.
II. Facility:
   A. Location: Lorain County, Ohio
   B. Physical condition: Chemical disposal site, begun in 1950s. Began with open burning of chemical wastes but has since used a series of improved incinerators. Clay lined landfills and lagoons are utilized.
   C. Hazardous materials: Diverse chemicals.

D. Principal routes of exposures: Air.

III. Study:

A. Motivation of study: Request by EPA to investigate resident complaints.

B. Population studied: Northern Eaton township residents were target population.

C. Health measurements: Cancer mortality and interview survey on health complaints.

D. Exposure measurements: None, but there was an interview survey of nuisance complaints.

E. Study design: Ecologic design. In the part of the study discussed here, death certificates were obtained from the Ohio Department of Health. Observed cancer mortality for study area was compared to expected based on mortality from control populations. Also, house-to-house survey done on health complaints.

F. Limitations of study: The rural control populations differed by socioeconomic factors in the mortality study. Lifestyle factors were not considered. Small populations meant small statistical power to detect differences. Survey results were not compared to any controls.

G. Results: No significant increase of mortality. Residents complained of odors from waste site.

I. Reference: Lyon et al. Cancer clustering around Point Sources of Pollution: Assessment by a Case-Control Methodology. *Env. Res.* 25, 29–34, 1981.

II. Facility:

A. Location: Utah

B. Physical condition: Uranium tailing dump

C. Hazardous materials: Radon gas

D. Principal routes of exposures: Air

III. Study:

A. Motivation of study:

B. Population studied: People living in the two counties containing dump site between 1966 and 1975.

C. Health measurements: None—just what was reported to cancer registry.

D. Exposure measurements: Environmental measurements were taken around dump, but not for individuals.

E. Study design: Ambidirectional design. Cases and controls were drawn from Utah Cancer Regstry, their addresses determined. Distance from site was used as substitute exposure measurement.

F. Limitations of study: Distance from site may not be a good exposure measurement. It does not account for wind direction. Assumption that migration and ascertainment for cases and controls be equal may not be valid. An excess of lung cancer in males might be due to men living close to where they work.

G. Results: No significant differences between cases and controls for radiogenic malignancies (acute leukemia, multiple myeloma, osteogenic sarcoma).

I. Reference: Clark et al. An Environmental Health Survey of Drinking Water Contamination by Leachate from a Pesticide Waste Dump in Hardeman County, Tennessee. *Arch. Environ. Health* Vol. 37, 9–18, 1982.
Meyer, C. R. Liver Dysfunction in Residents Exposed to Leachate from a Toxic Waste Dump. *Environ. Health Pers.* 48, 9–13, 1983.

II. Facility:
  A. Location: Hardeman County, Tennessee
  B. Physical condition: Land dump operated from 1964 to 1972 by local pesticide manufacturer. 200 acres. 3,000,000–500,000 55-gallon barrels of liquid and solid waste in shallow trenches. Closed in 1972 because of contaminated water in test wells.
  C. Hazardous materials: Diverse, including chlorinated organic compounds.
  D. Principal routes of exposures: Ground water, air.

III. Study:
  A. Motivation of study: In-progress study of Memphis wastewater treatment plant workers who treated contaminated water plus complaints of local citizens of skin and eye irritation, muscle weakness, shortness of breath, nausea, vomiting, diarrhea, abdominal pain.
  B. Population studied: Hardeman County resident wells were tested. People were divided into exposed, intermediate, control. It is not clear who was eligible for study, how many were tested, etc.
  C. Health measurements: Medical Questionnaire (alcohol/drug consumption, history of liver problems), blood (liver profile), bile acid survey, urine analysis.
  D. Exposure measurements: Air and water samples from some homes.
  E. Study design: In November 1978 a survey of 36 exposed individuals was conducted. In January 1979 another survey was done; people were categorized by exposure: 49 were exposed, 33 were intermediate-exposed, 57 were nonexposed. 31 people participated in both studies. It was a hasty study because by end of 1978 people were not using wells (being closed).
  F. Limitations of study: Population at risk and controls ill-defined. Study initiated by complaints of residents (bias).
  G. Results: Apparently, the November 1978 exposed were compared to the January 1979 nonexposed to find significant differences in liver enzyme profiles (alkaline phosphatase, SGOT). However, there was a decrease of liver enzyme values in the 31 people measured in November 1978 and January 1979. So, January 1979 study found nothing significant. Result: a subclinical transitory liver insult. No differences in skin or eye abnormalities.

I. Reference: Parker, G. S., and Rosen, S. L. Woburn: Cancer Incidence and Environmental Health Hazards, 1969–1978. Massachusetts Department of Public Health. January 23, 1981.

II. Facility:
  A. Location: Woburn, Massachusetts
  B. Physical conditions: In 1979 industrial wastes were discovered in a

section of Woburn called Industri-plex. Two drinking water wells were closed.

C. Hazardous materials: Chemicals include lead, arsenic, organic contaminants.

D. Principal routes of exposure: Groundwater.

III. Study:

A. Motivation of study: Detection of wastes and suspected high incidence of cancer.

B. Population studies: Residents of Woburn

C. Health measurements: Vital statistics on childhood leukemia, renal, liver and bladder cancer.

D. Exposure measurements: Possible exposure to known carcinogens were obtained through interviews. Several wells were tested for arsenic, chromium, and lead.

E. Study design: Ambidirectional design. Cases of Cancer of residents were ascertained for the years 1969 to 1978. Two matched controls were chosen for each case. Cases and controls (or their nearest relatives) were interviewed.

F. Limitations of study: There were small numbers: twelve cases of childhood leukemia, thirty cases of renal cancer.

G. Results: Although the leukemia and renal cancer rates were higher than expected by comparison to data from the Third National Cancer Survey, the case-control interviews revealed no association with environmental exposure.

I. Reference: Pennsylvania Department of Health. Health Surveillance Protocol: Planned Health Activities Related to the Drake Chemical Superfund Site, Lock Haven, Clinton County, Pennsylvania. November 15, 1983.

II. Facility:

A. Location: Clinton County, Pennsylvania

B. Physical condition: Kilsdonk Chemical Corporation operated from 1948 to 1962. Drake Chemical Company continued operations until 1981, when it went bankrupt. There is concern about chemical storage problems at the site.

C. Hazardous materials: Diverse chemicals, including β-naphthylamine, DCB, TCPAA.

D. Principal routes of exposure: Air, direct contact

III. Study:

A. Motivation of study: Previous health studies revealed adverse health effects related to the site. Request for Pennsylvania Department of Health involvement came from EPA, DER, and local citizens.

B. Population studied: There will be different populations associated with the different substudies.

1. Clinton County residents will be studied in the mortality survey.
2. Residential population at risk (retrospective) will be studied in morbidity study.
3. Occupational study will cover employees at Drake who worked at least 3 months from 1940 to 1981.

C. Health measurements:
   1. Cancer mortality
   2. Mortality and morbidity ascertained through survey questionnaires and followup of hospital/medical records
   3. Medical surveillance includes urinalysis
D. Exposure measurements: Unspecified determination of environmental and occupational exposure.
E. Study design:
   1. Ecologic examination of cancer mortality rates 1950 to present
   2. Cross-sectional survey of residents
   3. Medical surveillance of former workers

I. Reference: Talbott, E., Radford, T., Schmeltz, R., Murphy, P., Kuller, L., Portocarrero, C., and Doll, R. Distribution of thyroid abnormalities in a community exposed to low levels of gamma radiation. Submitted to *Amer. J. Epidemiol.*, 1983.
II. Facility:
   A. Location: Strabane/Canonsburg, Pennsylvania
   B. Physical condition: A refinery processing uranium began its operation in 1910. Radioactive waste continued to be dumped around the plant until 1958. A survey in 1977 showed that onsite levels of gamma radiation were high (500 R/hr). Liquid wastes were discharged into an open drain which emptied into a swamp.
   C. Hazardous materials: Radioactive waste.
   D. Principal routes of exposures: Air, direct contact.
III. Study:
   A. Motivation of study: A DOE report of onsite and offsite gamma radiation levels became public. Graduate School of Public Health, University of Pittsburgh initiated a study.
   B. Population studied: Exposed: current full-time resident, at least 21 years of age who lives within 1/3 miles of site and has been a resident in the area for at least 15 years. 514 people were eligible for the study. Unexposed: residents of a nearby community, Muse, Pennsylvania, who are at least 21 years of age and have lived in the vicinity for at least 15 years.
   C. Health measurements: Thyroid evaluations, medical history, demo.
   D. Exposure measurements: None. Length of residence was the indirect measure of exposure.
   E. Study design: Cross-sectional study of prevalence of thyroid disease in an exposed population and unexposed population matched for several demographic variables.
   F. Limitations of study: Definition of outcome: defining which thyroid diseases are rad-related is difficult. There may be a self-selection bias in the decision to participate; thyroid disease may be more frequent among participants than nonparticipants.
   G. Results: Rate of radiation-related thyroid diseases in exposed population was marginally higher than in the nonexposed population.

I. Reference: Paigen and Goldman. Lessons from Love Canal. The Role of the Public and the Use of Birthweight, Growth and Indigenous Wildlife to Evaluate Health Risk. 4th Annual Symposium on Environmental Epidemiology.

II. Facility:
   A. Location: Love Canal, New York
   B. Physical condition: Residential area over and near capped toxic waste dump
   C. Hazardous materials: Diverse chemicals, residues from pesticide production.
   D. Principal routes of exposures: Direct, air, water

III. Study:
   A. Motivation of study: Concern of local residents. Residents received grant money and initiated a study not involving New York state or Feds.
   B. Population studied: 523 children, 18 months to 16 years living in Love Canal area; 440 controls.
   C. Health measurements: Birth weight, birth height
   D. Exposure measurements: None. The only exposure-related measurement was distance from dump site.
   E. Study design: Ambidirectional design. Comparison of birth weights and birth heights of exposed and unexposed residents and controls.
   F. Limitations of study: The possibilities of selection or misclassification biases are discussed in the chapter. Regarding misclassification bias, there is no certainty whether those classified as exposed really had exposure, or whether those classified as unexposed really were unexposed.
   G. Results: Odds ratio for low birth weight children among Love Canal homeowners was 3.0. Children living in Love Canal were also shorter than the controls.

References

1. Air and Waste Management Association. 1990. *Total Exposure Assessment Methodology*, Air and Waste Management Association, Pittsburgh, PA.
2. Wallace, L. A. 1987. *The Total Exposure Assessment Methodology (TEAM) Study*. EPA/600/S6-87/002.
3. Wallace, L. A.; Pellizzari, E.; Hartwell, T.; Rosenzweig, M.; Erickson, M.; Sparacino, C.; and Zelon, H. 1984. Personal exposure to volatile organic compounds. I. Direct measurements in breathing-zone air, drinking water, food, and exhaled breath. *Environ. Res.* **35**: 293–319.
4. Wallace, L.; Pellizzari, E.; Hartwell, T.; Zelon, H.; Sparacino, C.; Perritt, R.; and Whitmore, R. 1986. Concentrations of 20 volatile organic compounds in the air the drinking water of 350 residents of New Jersey compared with concentrations in their exhaled breath. *J. Occup. Med.* **28**: 603–608.
5. Wallace, L. A.; Hartwell, T. D.; Sparacino, C.; Whitmore, R.; Sheldon, L.; Zelon, H.; and Perritt, R. 1987. The TEAM study: personal exposures to toxic substances in air, drinking water, and breath of 400 residents of New Jersey, North Carolina, and North Dakota. *Environ. Res.* **43**: 290–307.
6. Wallace, L. A.; Pellizzari, E.; Leaderer, B.; Zelon, H.; and Sheldon, L. 1987. Emissions of volatile organic compounds from building materials and consumer products. *Atmos. Environ.* **21**: 385–393.
7. Colome, S.; Daisey, J.; Dellarco, M.; Pellizzari, E.; and Quackenboss, J. 1991.

Total Exposure and Assessment Methodology, Princeton Scientific Publishing, Princeton, NJ.

8. Wallace, L. A.; Pellizzari, E.; Hartwell, T. D.; Whitmore, R.; Zelon, H.; Perritt, R.; and Sheldon, L. 1988. The California TEAM study: breath concentrations and personal exposures to 26 volatile compounds in air and drinking water of 188 residents of Los Angeles, Antioch and Pittsburg, CA. *Atmos. Environ.* **22**: 2141–2163.
9. Gordon, S. M.; Wallace, L. A.; Pellizzari, E. D.; and Moschandreas, D. J. 1990. Residence times of volatile organic compounds in human breath following exposures to air pollutants at near-normal environmental concentrations. In reference 1, pp. 247–256.
10. McMaster, L. R., and Hinton, D. O. 1990. Wearable personal activity logger (PAL). In reference 1, pp. 335–344.
11. Pellizzari, E. D.; Raymer, J.; Thomas, K.; and Cooper, S. D. 1990. Development of an alveolar air sampling method. In reference 1, pp. 368–381.
12. Immerman, F., and Schaum, J. 1990. *Final Report of the Nonoccupational Pesticide Exposure Study*, U.S. EPA, Research Triangle Park, NC.
13. Lioy, P. J.; Wallace, L.; and Pellizzari, E. 1990. Indoor/outdoor and personal monitor relationships for selected volatile organic compounds measured at three homes during New Jersey TEAM-1987. In reference 1, pp. 17–37.
14. Levin, H. 1990. General population exposure to pentachlorophenol. In reference 1, pp. 86–97.
15. McKone, T. E., and Daniels, J. I. 1990. Predicting human exposure from multiple pathways: integrated approach. In reference 1, pp. 154–165.
16. Cohen, N., and Fellman, A. 1990. A new look at old data: consideration for reassessment of internal radiation doses. In reference 1, pp. 277–288.
17. Silverman, F.; Urch, R. B.; Corey, P.; and Shephard, R. J. 1990. Dose response for selected air pollutants: symptoms and pulmonary function changes. In reference 1, pp. 289–299.
18. Berglund, M.; Lind, B.; and Vahter, M. 1990. UNEP/WHO human exposure assessment location (HEAL) pilot project on lead and cadmium. In reference 1, pp. 323–334.
19. Winiwarter, W.; Gunther, K.; Belnap, D.; Tang, H.; Crawford, J.; Hansen, L. D.; Eatough, D. J.; Lewis, E. A.; Schwartz, S. L.; and Balter, N. J. 1990. Elimination of nicotine and cotinine by nonsmokers exposed to sidestream tobacco smoke under controlled conditions. In reference 1, pp. 526–540.
20. Seifert, B.; Chutsch, M.; Henke, M.; Huber, M.; Kliem, C.; Krause, C.; Schulz, C.; and Schwarz, E. 1990. Trace elements in the blood, urine, and hair of a representative population of the Federal Republic of Germany. In reference 1, pp. 541–552.
21. Blancato, J. N. 1990. Physiologic pharmacokinetic modeling and biomarkers of exposure. In reference 1, pp. 577–587.
22. Kutz, F. W.; Barnes, D. G.; Bottimore, D. P.; and Bretthauer, E. W. 1990. The toxicity equivalency factor (TEF) method for estimating risks associated with exposures to complex mixtures. In reference 1, pp. 619–629.
23. Lurker, P. A.; Clark, C. S.; Elia, V. J.; Gartside, P. S.; and Kinman, R. N. 1983. Worker exposure to chlorinated organic compounds from the activated sludge wastewater treatment process. *Am. Ind. Hyg. Assoc. J.* **44**: 109–112.
24. Lurker, P. A.; Clark, C. S.; and Elia, V. J. 1982. Atmospheric release of chlorinated organic compounds from the activated sludge process. *J. Water Pollut. Control. Fed.* **54**: 1566–1573.
25. Clark, C. S.; Meyer, C. R.; Gartside, P. S.; Majeti, V. A.; Specker, B.; Balistreri, W. F.; and Elia, V. J. 1982. An enviromental health survey of drinking water

contamination by leachate from a pesticide waste dump in Hardeman County, Tennessee. *Arch. Environ. Health* **37**: 9–18.
26. Elia, V. J.; Clark, C. S.; Majeti, V. A.; Gartside, P. S.; Macdonald, T.; Richdale, N.; Meyer, C. R.; Van Meer, G. L.; and Hunninen, K. 1983. Hazardous chemical exposure at a municipal wastewater treatment plant. *Environ. Res.* **32**: 360–371.
27. Johnson, B. L.; Straight, J. M.; Grissom, R. E.; Gift, J. S.; and Holler, J. S. 1990. Monitoring human exposures that involve hazardous waste. In *Biological Monitoring of Exposure to Industrial Chemicals*, V. Fiserova-Bergerova and M. Ogata (eds.), ACGIH, Cincinnati, OH, pp. 83–88.
28. Que Hee, S. S.; Igwe, O. J.; and Clark, C. S. 1987. Thioether excretion of workers in a wastewater facility receiving pesticide wastes. In *Biological Monitoring of Exposure to Chemicals*, M. H. Ho and H. K. Dillon (eds.), John Wiley and Sons, New York, pp. 219–225.
29. Andelman, J. B., and Underhill, D. W. (eds.). 1987. *Health Effects from Hazardous Waste Sites*, Lewis Publishers, Chelsea, MI.
30. March G. M., and Caplan, R. J. 1987. Evaluating health effects of exposure at hazardous waste sites: a review of the state-of-the-art, with recommendations for future research. In reference 29, pp. 3–80.
31. National Research Council. 1989. *Biologic Markers in Reproductive Toxicology*, National Academy Press, Washington, DC.
32. National Research Council. 1989. *Biologic Markers in Pulmonary Toxicology*, National Academy Press, Washington, DC.
33. Kamal, A. M.; Gomaa, A.; El Khafif, M.; and Hammad, A. S. 1989. Plasma lipid peroxides among workers exposed to silica or asbestos dusts. *Environ. Res.* **49**: 173–180.
34. Cavalleri, A.; Gobba, F.; Bacchella, L.; Luberto, F.; and Ziccardi, A. 1988. Serum type III procollagen peptide in asbestos workers: an early indicator of pulmonary fibrosis. *Br. J. Ind. Med.* **45**: 818–823.
35. De Vuyst, P.; Dumortier, P.; Moulin, E.; Yourassowsky, N.; and Yernault, J. C. 1987. Diagnostic value of asbestos bodies in bronchoalveolar lavage fluid. *Am. Rev. Respir. Dis.* **136**: 1219–1224.
36. Guillemin, M. P.; Litzistorf, G.; and Buffat, P. A. 1989. Urinary fibres in occupational exposure to asbestos. *Ann. Occup. Hyg.* **33**: 219–233.
37. Reference 29, pp. 267–281.

APPENDIXES

APPENDIX A

Reference Ranges

Reference ranges are valuable guidelines for the clinician, but they should not be regarded as absolute indicators of health and disease. Reference ranges should be used with caution since values for "healthy" individuals often overlap significantly with values for persons afflicted with disease. In addition, laboratory values may vary significantly due to methodological differences and mode of standardization. This is especially true for immunological tests, which utilize antibodies that may have different characteristics. As a result, laboratory values in individual institutions may differ from those listed in this appendix. Reference ranges given in other chapters of this book reflect the authors' experience and are specific for the methods discussed. Thus, these values may also differ from those listed here.

The values in this chapter are for adults in the fasting state unless otherwise stated. Values for other age groups, when included, are clearly identified. Most of this material was extracted from *Clinical Guide to Laboratory Tests*, N. W. Tietz, Ed.; Philadelphia, W. B. Saunders Company, 1983. Other sources are listed at the end of Appendix B.

All laboratory values are given in conventional and international units. In general, the international units given conform to the SI system (Système International d'Unités). However, in some cases the recommendations of the International Union of Pure and Applied Chemistry (IUPAC) and the Commission on World Standards of the World Association of Societies of Pathology (COWS of WASP) are used, since it is felt that these have found wider acceptance in clinical laboratories and offer advantages over the units recommended in the SI system. If the exact molecular weight of a compound has not been established, e.g., for some proteins, values in the conventional unit are converted to values expressed in mass/L.

Throughout this appendix, we have used the prefixes for units as approved by the CGPM (Conférence Générale des Poids et Mésures), 1964, and the International Union of Pure and Applied Chemistry (IUPAC) and International Federation of Clinical Chemistry (IFCC), Clinica Chimica Acta, 96:157F–183F, 1979.

For convenience and to preserve space, we have used standard abbreviations commonly used in laboratory medicine. Less common abbreviations and some non-standard abbreviations are given below.

Abbreviations

AAS	atomic absorption spectrophotometry	Ox	oxalate
ACD	acid-citrate-dextrose	P	plasma
Amf	amniotic fluid	Pericf	pericardial fluid
Ascf	ascitic fluid	Placent	placental
Br	breath	Plf	pleural fluid
Cit	citrate	Plt	platelets
CSF	cerebrospinal fluid	post-stim	post-stimulation
EDTA	ethylenediaminetetraacetate, acetic acid	pp	postprandial
F	feces	RBC	red blood cells
F−	fluoride	RIA	Radioimmunoassay
F−/Ox	fluoride and oxalate	S	serum
Gast Cont	gastric contents	Sal	saliva
Gastf	gastric fluid	SD	standard deviation
Gast Res	gastric residue	SE	standard error
GLC	gas liquid chromatography	Semf	seminal fluid
H	hair	Serf	serous fluid
Hep	heparin	Swt	sweat
IU	international units	Synf	synovial fluid
NAA	neutron activation analysis	T	tissue
Occup. exp.	occupational exposure	U	urine
		WB	whole blood

Prefix Abbreviations

G	10^9	n	10^{-9}
M	10^6	p	10^{-12}
k	10^3	f	10^{-15}
d	10^{-1}	a	10^{-18}
m	10^{-3}		
μ	10^{-6}		

CLINICAL CHEMISTRY AND TOXICOLOGY.

Test	Specimen	Reference Range	Conversion Factor	Reference Range (International Units)
Acetaldehyde	WB (F^-/Ox)	*mg/L*		μmol/L
		<0.2	× 22.7	<4.5
		Occup. exp.: <0.5		<11.4
		Toxic: 1–2		22.7–45.4
Acetoacetate				
Semiquant.	S or P	Negative (< 3 mg/dL)	× 0.098	Negative (<0.3 mmol/L)
	(F^-/Ox) U	Negative (< 50 mg/dL)		Negative (<4.9 mmol/L)
Acetone				
Semiquant.	S or P (F^- or Ox)	Negative (<3 mg/dL)	× 0.172	Negative (<0.52 mmol/L)
		mg/dL		*mmol/L*
Quant.		0.3–2.0	× 0.172	0.05–0.34
		Ketoacidosis: 10–70		1.72–12.04
		Occup. exp.: <10		<1.72
		Toxic: >20		>3.44
Semiquant.	U	Negative		Negative
Quant.		0.3	× 0.172	0.05
		Occup. exp.: >27		>4.64
		mg/L		*μmol/L*
	Br	0.003	× 17.2	0.52
		Occup. exp.: <0.006		<1.03
Acetonitrile	WB (F^-/Ox)	*mg/L*		*μmol/L*
		CN^-: <0.04	× 38.4	<1.5
		SCN^-: <12	× 17.2	<206
		Occup. exp., CN^-: <0.1	× 38.4	<3.8
		Toxic,		
		CN^-: 3–11	× 38.4	115–422
		SCN^-: 160–230	× 17.2	2752–3956
	U	SCN^-: <17		<292
		Occup. exp., SCN^-: <20		<344

Clinical chemistry and toxicology (*Continued*).

Test	Specimen	Reference Range	Conversion Factor	Reference Range (International Units)
Acetylcholinesterase in Erythrocytes	WB (ACD, EDTA, or Hep)	Adult:		
		36.9 ± 3.83 U/g Hb (SD)	× 0.0645	2.38 ± 0.23 MU/mol Hb
		1070 ± 111 U/10^{12} RBC	× 10^{-3}	1.07 ± 0.11 nU/RBC
		12.5 ± 1.30 U/mL RBC	× 1	12.5 ± 1.30 kU/L RBC
		Lower in newborns		
α_1-Acid-Glycoprotein (Orosomucoid)	S	Adult: 55–140 mg/dL	× 10	550–1400 mg/L
	U	0.29–0.68 mg/d		0.29–0.68 mg/d
	CSF	0.41 ± 0.13 mg/dL (SE)	× 10	4.1 ± 1.3 mg/L (SE)
Acrylonitrile	WB (F^-/Ox)	*mg/L*		*µmol/L*
		CN^-: 0.04	× 38.4	1.5
		SCN^-: 0.12	× 17.2	2.1
		Toxic (SCN^-),		
		Nonsmokers: >20		>344
		Smokers: >30		>516
		Toxic (CN^-): >0.1	× 38.4	>3.8
		Toxic (SCN^-): >20	× 17.2	>344
	U			
Adrenocorticotropic Hormone (ACTH)	P (EDTA)	*pg/mL*		*ng/L*
		Cord: 143 ± 7.0 (SD)		143 ± 7.0 (SD)
		1–7 d: 120 ± 8.3	× 1	120 ± 8.3
		Adult,		
		0800 h: 25–100	× 1	25–100
		1800 h: <50		<50
	Amf			
		10–18 wk: 209 (mean)		209 (mean)
		26–30 wk: 430		430
		35 – 36 wk: 162 and maintained thereafter		162 and maintained thereafter

Test	Specimen		Reference range (conventional)	Factor	Reference range (SI)
Adrenocorticotropic Hormone-Insulin Stimulation Test	S: fasting, 15, 30, and 60 min post-stim	Cortisol:	>20 µg/dL, and 10 µg/dL rise ½ h after max. fall in blood glucose	× 0.028	>0.56 µmol/L and 0.28 µmol/L rise ½ h after max. fall in blood glucose
Dose: 0.05–0.15 U insulin/kg. IV. after overnight fast		Glucose:	50% below base or signs of hypoglycemia	× 0.01	0.50 (concentration fraction) below base or signs of hypoglycemia
Adrenocorticotropic Hormone Stimulation Test (Prolonged Infusion)	U, 24 h	17-KGS:	2–4-fold rise		Same
		17-KS:	2-fold rise		
		17-OHCS:	2–5-fold rise		
Dose: 500 µg *Cortrosyn/d × 3*	S	Cortisol:	25–50 µg/dL	× 0.028	Cortisol: 0.7–1.4 µmol/L
Adrenocorticotropic Hormone Stimulation Test (Rapid Test)	S: baseline, 30 and 60 min post-stim	Cortisol,		× 0.028	
		Baseline:	>5.0 µg/dL		Baseline: >0.14 µmol/L
Dose: 250 µg Cortrosyn, *IM*		After Cortrosyn:	2 × baseline		Same
Alanine			*mg/dL*		*µmol/L*
	S	Premature, 1 d:	3.34 ± 0.45 (SD)	× 112.2	375 ± 50 (SD)
		Newborn, 1 d:	2.10–3.65		236–410
		1–3 mo:	2.45 ± 0.63 (SD)		275 ± 71 (SD)
		2–6 mo:	1.58–3.68		177–413
		9 mo-2 y:	0.88–2.79		99–313
		3–10 y:	1.22–2.71		137–305
		6–18 y:	1.72–4.85		193–545
		Adult:	1.87–5.88		210–661

Clinical Chemistry and Toxicology (*Continued*).

Test	Specimen	Reference Range		Conversion Factor	Reference Range (International Units)
			mg/d		*μmol/d*
	U, 24 h	10 d-7 wk:	4–10	× 11.2	45–112
		3–12 y:	9–39		101–437
		Adult:	8–48		90–538
Alanine Aminotransferase (ALT, GPT)	S				
Henry, optimized, 30°C			*U/L*		
		Newborn/Infant:	5–28		Same
		Adult:	8–20		
		>60 y, M:	7–24		
		F:	7–16		
IFCC, with P-5′-P. 30°C			<30		
Albumin					
Nephelometric, colorimetric	S	Adult:	3.5–5.0 g/dL	× 10	35–50 g/L
		>60 y:	3.4–4.8 g/dL		34–48 g/L
		Avg. ~0.3 g/dL higher in upright individuals			Avg. ~3 g/L higher in upright individuals
Nephelometric, rate	CSF	10–30 mg/dL		× 10	100–300 mg/L
	U	At rest:	<80 mg/d		Same
		Ambulatory:	50–80 mg/d		
Alcohol Dehydrogenase (ADH) *340 nm, 30°C*	S	⩽2.8 U/L			⩽2.8 U/L
Aldolase	S	1.0–7.5 U/L (30°C)			Same
		0.3–3.0 U/L at bed rest			
		1.5–12.0 U/L (37°C)			

Test	Specimen		Conventional	Factor	SI
Aldosterone	S or P (Hep, EDTA)		*ng/dL*		*nmol/L*
		Newborn:	5–60	× 0.0277	0.14–1.66
		1 wk–1 y:	1–160		0.03–4.43
		1–3 y:	5–60		0.14–1.66
		3–5 y:	<5–80		<0.138–2.22
		5–7 y:	<5–50		<0.138–1.39
		7–11 y:	5–70		0.138–1.94
		11–15 y:	<5–50		<0.138–1.39
		Adult, *average sodium diet*			
		Supine:	3–10		0.083–0.28
		Upright, F:	5–30		0.138–0.83
		M:	6–22		0.166–0.609
		2–3 × higher during pregnancy			
		Adrenal vein:	200–800		5.54–22.16
		Low sodium diet:			
		Increases	2–5-fold		
		Florinef suppression:	<4 ng/dL		<0.11
		ACTH or angiotensin stimulation, 1 h: 2–5-fold increase			

U. 24 h

Total Urinary Na mEq/d	*Plasma Renin Activity (ng AI*/h)/mL*	*Urinary Aldosterone µg/d*	Factor	*Urinary Aldosterone nmol/d*
<20	5–24	35–80	× 0.277	97–222
50	2–7	13–33		36–91.4
100	1–5	5–24		13.8–66.5
150	0.5–4	3–19		8.3–52.6
200		1–16		2.7–44.3
250		1–13		2.7–36

(assuming normal serum Na, K, and extracellular vol)

*Angiotensin I

Clinical chemistry and toxicology (*Continued*).

Test	Specimen	Reference Range	Conversion Factor	Reference Range (International Units)
Aluminum (Al)		*μg/dL*		*μmol/L*
	S	0.4	× 0.371	0.15
	P	0.6–0.7		0.22–0.26
		Patients on Al medication: <3.0 μg/dL		<1.11
	U, random	None detected		None detected
α-Amino Acid Nitrogen (AAN)				
Ninhydrin	P (EDTA)	3.2–5.5 mg/dL	× 0.714	2.28–3.93 mmol/L
Naphthoquinone and FDNB	U, 24 h	50–200 mg/d	× 0.0714	3.57–14.28 mmol/L
δ-Aminolevulinate Dehydratase *Colorimetric, 38°C*	RBC (Hep)	139–211 U/mL erythrocytes	× 1	139–211 kU/L
δ-Aminolevulinic Acid (δ-ALA)	S	15–23 μg/dL; lower in children	× 0.076	1.14–1.75 μmol/L
	U	1.3–7.0 mg/d	× 7.626	9.9–53.4 μmol/d
Ammonia Nitrogen				
Resin or enzymatic	S or P (NaHep)	*μg N/dL*		*μmol N/L*
		Newborn: 90–150	× 0.714	64–107
		0–2-wk: 79–129		56–92
		>1 mo: 29–70		21–50
		Adult: 15–45		11–32
Conway diffusion		40–110		29–79
		(values for arterial plasma are lower than for venous plasma)		
	U, 24 h	140–1500 mg/d	× 0.0714	10–107 mmol/d
Ammonium Chloride Loading Test *Dose: 0.1 g ammonium chloride/kg orally at 0800 h after complete midnight fast*	*U, hourly* between 1000–1600 h	pH should fall to ≤5.2 between 2 and 8 h after the dose		H^+ concentration should increase to >6 μmol/L between 2 and 8 h after the dose

Test	Specimen	Reference Range	Factor	SI Reference Range
Amniotic Fluid Analysis ΔA_{450nm} L/S Ratio, see Lecithin/ sphingomyelin ratio	Amf	28 wk: 0–0.048Δ*A* 40 wk: 0–0.02Δ*A*		Same
Amylase *UV-method,* *Beckman; BMD*	S	Adult: 25–125 U/L >70 y: 25–60 U/L		Same
	U, timed	1–17 U/h		1–17 U/h
Amylase/Creatinine Clearance Ratio	S and U, random	1–4%	× 0.01	Clearance fraction: 0.01–0.04
Amyloid-Associated Protein (Amyloid A Protein, AA Protein)	S	0–50 y: <20 mg/dL (Conc. increases after 50 y of age)	× 10	<200 mg/L
Androstenedione	S	*ng/dL* (mean ± *SE*) *M* / *F*		*nmol/L* (*mean* ± *SE*) *M* / *F*
		Cord: 85 ± 27 / 93 ± 28	× 0.0349	2.97 ± 0.94 / 3.25 ± 0.98
		1–3 mo: 34 ± 11 / 19 ± 4		1.19 ± 0.38 / 0.66 ± 0.14
		3–5 mo: 24 ± 15 / 14 ± 5		0.84 ± 0.52 / 0.49 ± 0.17
		Adult: 107 ± 25 / 151 ± 38		3.73 ± 0.87 / 5.27 ± 1.33
	Amf	Midpregnancy, *ng/mL* Male fetus: 1.0 Female fetus: 0.7 Term: 0.7–3.5	× 3.49	*nmol/L* 3.49 2.44 2.44–12.22
Angiotensin I	P (K EDTA), periph-vein	11–88 pg/mL	× 1	11–88 ng/L
Angiotensin II	P (K EDTA)	Arterial: 2.4 ± 1.2 ng/dL (SD) Venous: 50–75% of arterial conc	× 10 × 0.01	24 ± 12 ng/L (SD) Fraction of arterial conc.: 0.50–0.75
Anion Gap $[Na - (Cl^- + HCO_3^-)]$	P (Hep)	7-16 mEq/L	× 1	7-16 mmol/L
α_1-Antichymotrypsin(α_1AC)	S	Newborn: ~1 mg/dL Adult: 30–60 mg/dL	× 10	~10 mg/L 300–600 mg/L

Clinical Chemistry and Toxicology (*Continued*).

Test	Specimen	Reference Range		Conversion Factor	Reference Range (International Units)
Antidiuretic Hormone	P (EDTA)	*Plasma*	*Plasma ADH*		*Plasma ADH*
(hADH, Vasopressin)		*mOsmol/kg*	*pg/mL*		*ng/L*
		270–280:	<1.5	× 1	<1.5
		280–285:	<2.5		<2.5
		285–290:	1–5		1–5
		290–295:	2–7		2–7
		295–300:	4–12		4–12
Antimony		0.052 ± 0.019 µg/dL (SD)		× 82.1	4.27 ± 1.56 nmol/L (SD)
NAA. AAS	P (Hep)	<10 µg/L		× 8.21	<82.1 nmol/L
	U	Toxic:	>1 mg/L	× 8.21	>8.21 µmol/L
α_1-Antitrypsin	S	Newborn:	145–270 mg/dL	× 0.1	1.45–2.70 g/L
Nephelometric		Adult:	78–200 mg/dL		0.78–2.00 g/L
Arsenic	WB (Hep)		*µg/dL*		*µmol/L*
			0.2–6.2	× 0.133	0.03–0.83
		Chronic poisoning:	10–50		1.33–6.65
		Acute poisoning:	60–930		7.98–124
	U, 24 h	5–50 µg/d		× 0.0133	0.07–0.67 µmol/d
Ascorbic Acid, *see Vitamin C*					
Aspartate	S		*U/L*		
Aminotransferase		Newborn/Infant:	25–75		Same
(AST, SGOT),		Adults:	8–20		
(30°C)		>60 y, M:	11–26		
		F:	10–20		
		With P-5′-P:	12–29		
Base Excess	WB (Hep)		*mmol/L*		Same
		Newborn:	(−10)–(−2)		
		Infant:	(−7)–(−1)		
		Child:	(−4)–(+2)		
		Adult:	(−2)–(+3)		

Test	Specimen	Conventional			Factor	SI	
Benzene	S	Negative				Negative	
			mg/L			*μmol/L*	
		Toxic:	>1.0		× 12.8	>13	
	U	As phenol:	<10.0		× 10.6	<106	
		Toxic, as phenol:	>75.0			>795	
Beryllium *Fluorometric, AAS*	U, 24 h	None detected				None detected	
		Toxic:	>20 μg/L		× 0.111	>2.22 μmol/L	
Bicarbonate (HCO_3^-)	S	Art.:	21–28 mmol/L			Same	
		Ven.:	22–29 mmol/L				
			mEq/L			*mmol/L*	
	WB, arterial (Hep; anaerobic)	Newborn:	17.2–23.6		× 1	17.2–23.6	
		Infant:	19.0–23.9			19.0–23.9	
		2 mo-2 y:	16.3–23.9			16.3–23.9	
		Adult:	18–23			18–23	
Bile Acid Breath Test *Dose: 300 mL test meal containing 10 μ Ci of* [14] *C-glycocholic acid and cholyl-2, 4-*[3]*H taurine to fasting subjects at 0800 h*	Br	Radioactivity expressed as a % of the original dose; only minute quantities (0.11% ± 0.15%, SD) of radiation are detected at 2 h (0.52 ± 0.09%, SD, cumulative excretion at 4 h)			× 0.001	Fraction of radiation detected at 2 h: 0.0011 ± 0.0015 (SD) Cumulative fraction excreted at 4 h: 0.0052 ± 0.0009 (SD)	
Bile Acids, Total *GLC*	S	0.3–2.3 μg/mL			× 2.45	0.74–5.64 μmol/L	
	S, 1 h pp	1.8–3.2 μg/mL				4.41–7.84 μmol/L	
	F	120–225 mg/d				294–551 μmol/d (Conv. factor based on cholic acid, M. W. 408.6)	
Bilirubin *Total*	S		*Premature* *mg/dL*	*Full Term* *mg/dL*		*Premature* *μmol/L*	*Full Term* *μmol/L*
		Cord:	<2.0	<2.0	× 17.1	<34.2	<34.2
		0–1 d:	<8.0	<6.0		<137	<103
		1–2 d:	<12.0	<8.0		<205	<137
		3–5 d:	<16.0	<12.0		<274	<205
		>5 d:	<2.0	0.2–1.0		<34.2	3.4–17.1

Clinical chemistry and toxicology (*Continued*).

Test	Specimen	Reference Range		Conversion Factor	Reference Range (International Units)
	U	Negative			Negative
	Amf	28 wk:	0.075 mg/dL	× 17.1	1.28 μmol/L
			(or ΔA_{450} <0.048)		
		40 wk:	0.025 mg/dL		0.43 μmol/L
			(or ΔA_{450} < 0.02)		
Conjugated (direct)	S	0–0.2 mg/dL		× 17.1	0–3.4 μmol/L
Bismuth	P (Hep)	<1.0 μg/dL		× 47.85	<47.9 nmol/L
	U, 24 h	<20 μg/L		× 4.785	<95.7 nmol/L
Blood Volume	WB (Hep)	M:	52–83 mL/kg	× 0.001	0.052–0.083 L/kg
		F:	50–75 mL/kg		0.050–0.075 L/kg
Borate	S		*mg/L*		*μmol/L*
		Child:	<7	× 17.0	<119
		Adult, M:	<2		<34
		Toxic:	>20		>340
Bromosulfophthalein (BSP) Test (5 mg/kg)	S	<6% retention at 45 min		× 0.01	Fraction dye retained: <0.06
C-Peptide	S		*ng/mL*		*μg/L*
		Adult:	≤4.0	× 1	≤4.0
		>60 y, M:	1.5–5.0		1.5–5.0
		F:	1.4–5.5		1.4–5.5
C-Reactive Protein	S	Cord blood:	1–35 μg/dL	× 10	10–350 μg/L
		Adult:	6.8–820 μg/dL		68–8200 μg/L
Cadmium	WB (Hep)	0.1–0.5 μg/dL		× 8.897	0.89–4.45 nmol/L
		Toxic:	10–300 μg/dL	× 0.089	0.89–26.70 μmol/L
	U, 24h	<15 μg/d		× 0.0089	<0.13 μmol/d
Calcitonin (hCT)	S or P (Hep or EDTA)		*pg/mL*		*ng/L*
		Newborn,			
		Term, cord:	30–240	× 1	30–240
		48 h:	91–580		91–580
		7 d:	77–293		77–293

		Premature, cord:	30–265		30–265
		48 h:	108–670		108–670
		7 d:	79–570		79–570
		Adult, M:	<100		<100
		F:	4 times lower (increases in preg)		
		Concentrations decrease with age			
Calcitonin-Calcium Infusion Stimulation Test *Dose: 15 mg Ca (as gluconate)/kg. IV infusion/4h*	S or P (Hep or EDTA): baseline, 3 and 4 h	Peak hCT level,			
		M:	<265 pg/mL	× 1	M: <265 ng/L
		F:	<120 pg/mL		F: <120 ng/L
Calcium, Ionized (Ca_I)	S, P, or WB (Hep)		*mg/dL*		*mmol/L*
		Cord, venous:	5.5 ± 0.3 (SD)	× 0.25	1.38 ± 0.08 (SD)
		Newborn,			
		3–14 h:	4.3–5.1		1.08–1.28
		24–48 h:	4.0–4.7		1.00–1.18
		Adult:	4.48–4.92		1.12–1.23
		or	2.24–2.46 mEq/L	× 0.5	1.12–1.23
		>60 y:	2.25–2.60 mEq/L		1.13–1.30
Calcium, Total	S		*mg/dL*		*mmol/L*
		Cord:	9.0–11.5	× 0.25	2.25–2.88
		Newborn,			
		3–24 h:	9.0–10.6		2.25–2.65
		24–48 h:	7.0–12.0		1.75–3.0
		4–7 d:	9.0–10.9		2.25–2.73
		Child:	8.8–10.8		2.20–2.70
		Adult:	8.4–10.2		2.10–2.55
		M, >60 y:	8.4–10.0		2.10–2.50
	CSF	2.1–2.7 mEq/L or		× 0.50	1.05–1.35 mmol/L
		4.2–5.4 mg/dL		× 0.25	1.05–1.35 mmol/L
	U, 24 h	*Ca in diet*	*mg/d*		*mmol/d*
		Ca-free:	5–40	× 0.025	0.13–1.00
		Low to average:	50–150		1.25–3.75
		Average (800 mg/d):	100–300		(20 mmol/d): 2.50–7.50
		Average:	<0.64 g/d	× 25	16 mmol/d

Clinical chemistry and toxicology (*Continued*).

Test	Specimen	Reference Range		Conversion Factor	Reference Range (International Units)
Cannabinoids	P (Hep or EDTA)	Negative: THC after smoking 10 mg: 0.09–0.026 mg/L		× 3.18	0.060–0.083 μmol/L
	U	Negative			Negative
Carbon Dioxide, Partial Pressure (pCO_2)	WB, arterial (Hep)		*mm Hg*		*kPa*
		Newborn:	27–40	× 0.133	3.59–5.32
		Infant:	27–41		3.59–5.45
		Adult, M:	35–48		4.66–6.38
		F:	32–45		4.26–5.99
Carbon Dioxide, Total (tCO_2)	S or P (Hep)		*mmol/L*		Same
		Cord:	14–22		
		Newborn:	13–22		
		Premature, 1 wk:	14–27		
		Infant:	20–28		
		Child:	20–28		
		Adult:	22–29		
		>60 y:	23–31		
Carbon Disulfide *GLC, color (metabolites)*	WB (F^-/Ox)	Negative			Negative
		Occup. exp.:	<0.3 mg/L	× 13.1	<3.9 μmol/L
	U	Toxic:	>0.5 mg/L		>6.6 μmol/L
		Exposure index:	6–10		6–10
Carbon Monoxide	WB (EDTA)		*% HbCO*		*HbCO Fraction*
		Nonsmokers:	0.5–1.5	× 0.01	0.005–0.015
		Smokers,			
		1–2 pack/d:	4–5		0.04–0.05
		>2 packs/d:	8–9		0.08–0.09
		Toxic:	>20		>0.20
		Lethal:	>50		>0.5
Carboxyhemoglobin, *see Carbon Monoxide*					
Carcinoembryonic Antigen (CEA)	S	Nonsmokers:	0–3.0 ng/mL	× 1	0–3.0 μg/L
		Smokers:	0–5.0 ng/mL		0–5.0 μg/L

Test	Specimen	Conventional		Factor	SI
β-Carotene *Petroleum ether extraction*	S		*µg/dL*		*µmol/L*
		Infant:	20–70	× 0.0186	0.37–1.30
		Child:	40–130		0.74–2.42
		Adult:	60–200		1.12–3.72
β-Carotene Absorption Test *Dose: 15,000 U carotene orally, 3 × daily with meals for 3 d*	S	Increase by ≥35 µg/dL after loading		× 0.0186	Increase by ≥0.65 µmol/L after loading
Catecholamines	U, 24 h				
HPLC		<110 µg/d		× 5.91	<650 nmol/d
Fluorometric		<280 µg/d			<1655 nmol/d (Conv. factor based on norepinephrine, M. W. 169.18)
Catecholamines, Fractionated	U, 24 h	Norepinephrine,	µg/d		*nmol/d*
		1–4 y:	0–29	× 5.91	0–171
		4–10 y:	8–65		47–384
		10–15 y:	15–80		89–473
		Adult:	0–100		0–591
		Epinephrine,	µg/d		*nmol/d*
		1–4 y:	0–6.0	× 5.46	0–32.8
		4–10 y:	0–10.0		0–54.6
		10–15 y:	0.5–20		2.7–109
		Adult:	0–15		0–81.9
		Dopamine,	*µg/d*		*nmol/d*
		1–4 y:	40–260	× 6.53	261–1698
		>4 y:	65–400		425–2610
Catecholamines, Free	P (EDTA and Na metabisulfite)		*pg/mL*		*pmol/L*
		Epinephrine, random:	<88	× 5.46	<480
		Norepinephrine, random:	104–548	× 5.91	615–3239
		Dopamine, random:	<136	× 6.53	<888
		Lower values with patient supine			
Cerebrospinal Fluid Volume	CSF	Child:	60–100 mL	× 0.001	0.06–0.10 L
		Adult:	100–160 mL		0.10–0.16 L

Clinical chemistry and toxicology (*Continued*).

Test	Specimen	Reference Range		Conversion Factor	Reference Range (International Units)
Ceruloplasmin	S		*mg/dL*	× 10	*μmol/L*
RID		Newborn:	1–30		10–300
		6 mo-1 y:	15–50		150–500
		1–12 y:	30–65		300–650
		Thereafter:	15–60		150–600
Chenodeoxycholic Acid, Total	S	0.31 ± 0.32 μg/mL		× 2.55	0.79 ± 0.82 μmol/L
Chenodeoxycholyl-glycine, Conjugated	S	0.09 ± 0.01 μg/mL		× 2.22	0.2 ± 0.03 μmol/L
Chloride	S or P (Hep)		*mmol/L*		Same
		Cord:	96–104		
		Newborn:	96–110		
		Thereafter:	98–106		
	CSF	Infant:	111–130		
		Adult:	118–132		
	U, 24 h		*mmol/d*		Same
		Infant:	2–10		
		Child:	15–40		
		Thereafter:	110–250		
		(vary greatly with Cl intake)			
	Swt		*mmol/L*		Same
		Normal:	0–30		
		Cystic fibrosis:	60–200		
	RBC, lysed		49–54		
	Sal		*mmol/L*		Same
		Without stimulation:	5–20		
		After stimulation:	44		
	WB		77–87		

Cholesterol, Total	S or P (EDTA)		*mg/dL*		*mmol/L*
		Cord:	45–100	× 0.0259	1.17–2.59
		Newborn:	53–135		1.37–3.50
		Infant:	70–175		1.81–4.53
		Child:	120–200		3.11–5.18
		Adolescent:	120–210		3.11–5.44
		Adult:	140–310		3.63–8.03
		Recommended (desirable) range for adults:	140–220		3.63–5.70
Cholic Acid, Total	S	0.20 ± 0.17 μg/mL		× 2.45	0.49 ± 0.42 μmol/L
Cholinesterase II (S-Pseudocholinesterase)					
RID	S	0.5–1.5 mg/dL		× 10	5–15 mg/L
DuPont aca		8–18 U/mL			8–18 kU/L
Dibucaine:		83.6 ± 1.3% (SD) inhibition		× 0.01	Fraction of activity inhibited: 0.84 ± 0.013 (SD)
Fluoride:		79.7 ± 1.2% (SD) inhibition			0.80 ± 0.012 (SD)
Cholylglycine, Conjugated	S	0.13 ± 0.01 μg/mL		× 2.15	0.27 ± 0.03 μmol/L
Chorionic Gonadotropin, β- Subunit (β-hCG)	S or P (EDTA)		*mIU/ml*		*IU/L*
		M and nonpregnant F:	<3.0	× 1	<3.0
		F, post-conception,			
		7–10 d:	>3.0		>3.0
		30 d:	100–5000		100,5000
		40 d:	>2000		>2000
		10 wk:	50,000–140,000		50,000–140,000
		14 wk:	10,000–50,000		10,000–50,000
		Trophoblastic disease:	>100,000		>100,000
	U, 24 h	Pregnancy (wk),	*IU/d (mean)*		Same
		6th:	13,000		
		8th:	30,000		
		12–14th:	105,000		
		16th:	46,000		
		Thereafter	5000–20,000		

Clinical chemistry and toxicology (*Continued*).

Test	Specimen	Reference Range	Conversion Factor	Reference Range (International Units)
Chromium	WB (Hep)	70 ng/dL (Includes Cr^{6+} bound to RBC)	× 0.192	13.4 nmol/L
	S	14 ng/dL	× 0.192	2.7 nmol/L
	U, 24 h	0.8 μg/d	× 19.23	15.4 nmol/d
	H	0.21 ± 0.14 μg/g (mean ± SD)	× 19.23	4.0 ± 2.7 nmol/g (mean ± SD)
Chymotrypsin	S or P EDTA and polybrene	~10 μg/L		~10 μg/g
	F	120–1265 μg/g stool (mean: 290)	× 1	120–1265 mg/kg stool (mean: 290)
Citrulline	S	*μg/dL*		*μmol/L*
		Newborn, 1 d: 158–508	× 0.057	9–29
		1–3 mo: 368 ± 193 (SD)		21 ± 11 (SD)
		2–6 mo: 543–876		31–50
		9 mo–10 y: 210–526		12–30
		6–18 y: 333–911		19–52
		Adult: 210–964		12–55
	U, 24 h	Adult: 0.4–8 mg/d	× 5.71	2–46 μmol/d
		or 2 ± 1 mg/g creatinine (SD)	× 0.65	or 1.3 ± 0.7 mmol/mol creatinine (SD)
Cobalt	WB (no anti-coagulant)	0.20–0.28 μg/dL	× 169.7	33.9–47.5 nmol/L
	U	1–7 μg/L	× 16.97	17.0–118.8 nmol/L
Complement Components				
Total hemolytic complement activity	P (EDTA)	75–160 U/mL or	× 1	75–160 kU/mL
		>33% of plasma CH50	× 0.01	Fraction of CH50: >0.33
Total complement	P (EDTA)	~10–20%		Fraction decay rate:

decay rate (functional)		Deficiency: >50%		~0.10–0.20 >0.50
Classic pathway components		*mg/dL*		*mg/L*
C1q	S	6.5 ± 0.7 (SD)	× 10	65 ± 7 (SD)
C1r	S	2.5–3.8		25–38
C1s (Cl esterase)	S	2.5–3.8		25–38
C2	S	2.8 ± 0.6 (SD)		28 ± 6 (SD)
C3 (β₁ C-globulin)	S	80–155		800–1550
C4 (β₁ E-globulin)	S	13–37		130–370
C5 (β₁ F-globulin)	S	6.4 ± 1.3 (SD)		64 ± 13 (SD)
C6	S	5.6 ± 0.80 (SD)		56 ± 8.0 (SD)
C7	S	4.9–7.0		49–70
C8	S	4.3–6.3		43–63
C9	S	4.7–6.9		47–69
Alternative pathway components				
C4 binding protein (reliable assay not presently available)	S	18–32	× 10	180–320
Factor B (C3 proactivator)	S	20–45	× 10	200–450
Properdin	S	2.8 ± 0.4 (SD)	× 10	28 ± 4 (SD)
Regulatory proteins				
β_1 H-globulin (C3b inactivator accelerator)	S	56.1 ± 7.8 (SD)	× 10	561 ± 78 (SD)
C1 inhibitor (Esterase inhibitor)	P (EDTA)	17.4–24.0	× 10	174–240
C1 inhibitor by complement decay rate (functional)	P (EDTA)	~10–20% Deficiency: >50%	× 0.01	Fraction decay rate: ~0.10–0.20 >0.50
C3b inactivator (KAF)	S	4.0 ± 0.7 (SD) mg/dL	× 10	40 ± 7 (SD) mg/L
S protein	S	41.8 – 60.0 mg/dL		418–600 mg/L

Clinical chemistry and toxicology (*Continued*).

Test	Specimen	Reference Range		Conversion Factor	Reference Range (International Units)
Copper	S	Copper	*μg/dL*		*μmol/L*
		Birth-6 mo:	20–70	× 0.157	3.14–10.99
		6 y:	90–190		14.13–29.83
		12 y:	80–160		12.56–25.12
		Adult, M:	70–140		10.99–21.98
		F:	80–155		12.56–24.34
		Pregnancy at term:	118–302		18.53–47.41
		Values for blacks ~8–12% higher			Blacks ~8–12% higher
	RBC (Hep)	90–150 μg/dL		× 0.157	14.13–23.55 μmol/L
	U, 24 h	15–30 μg/d		× 0.0157	0.24–0.47 μmol/d
Coproporphyrin	U, 24 h	34–234 μg/d		× 1.5	51–351 nmol/d
	F, 24 h	<30 μg/g dry wt		× 1.5	<45 nmol/g dry wt
		400–1200 μg/d			600–1800 nmol/d
Corticobinding Globulin (CBG), *see Transcortin*					
Corticosterone	S or P (Hep, EDTA, or Ox)	0.13–2.3 μg/dL		× 28.9	3.8–66.5 nmol/L
Cortisol	S or P (Hep)	0800 h:	5–23 μg/dL	× 27.6	138–635 nmol/L
		1600 h:	3–15 μg/dL		83–414 nmol/L
		2000 h:	≤50% of 0800 h	×0.01	Fraction of 0800 h: ≤0.50
Cortisol, Free	U, 24 h		*μg/d*		*nmol/d*
		Child:	2–27	× 2.76	5.5–74.5
		Adolescent:	5–55		13.8–152
		Adult:	10–100		27.6–276

Test	Specimen		Conventional units	Factor		SI units
Creatine	S or P	M:	0.17–0.70 mg/dL	× 76.3	M:	13–53 µmol/L
		F:	0.35–0.93 mg/dL		F:	27–71 µmol/L
	U, 24 h	M:	0–40 mg/d	× 7.63	M:	0–305 µmol/d
		F:	0–80 mg/d		F:	0–609 µmol/d
Creatine Kinase (CK)	S					
Total, 30°C			*U/L*	Same		
		Newborn:	10–200			
		Adult, M:	12–80			
		F:	10–55			
		>60 y, M:	20–110			
		F:	16–80			
		>70 y, M:	22–90			
		F:	16–80			
		Ambulatory,				
		M:	25–90			
		F:	10–70			
		Higher after exercise				
Total, CK-NAC, 30°C		Newborn:	68–580			
		Adult, M:	25–130			
		F:	10–115			
Isoenzymes		Fraction 2 (MB):	<4–6% of total (method dependent)	× 0.01		Fraction of total: <0.04–0.06
Creatinine	S or P		*mg/dL*			*µmol/L*
Jaffe, kinetic or enzymatic		Cord:	0.6–1.2	× 88.4		53–106
		Newborn, 1–4 d:	0.3–1.0			27–88
		Infant:	0.2–0.4			18–35
		Child:	0.3–0.7			27–62
		Adolescent:	0.5–1.0			44–88
		Adult, M:	0.6–1.2			53–106
		F:	0.5–1.1			44–97

Clinical chemistry and toxicology (*Continued*).

Test	Specimen	Reference Range		Conversion Factor	Reference Range (International Units)
Jaffe, manual	S or P	0.8–1.5 mg/dL		×88.4	71–133 μmol/L
	Amf	After 37 wk gestation: >2.0 mg/dL		×88.4	After 37 wk gestation: >177 μmol/L
	U, 24 h		*(mg/d)/kg*		*μmol·d^{-1}·kg^{-1}*
		Infant:	8–20	×8.84	71–180
		Child:	8–22		71–195
		Adolescent:	8–30		71–265
		Adult, M:	14–26		124–230
		F:	11–20		97–177
		Declines with age to (10 mg/kg)/d at age 90 or			
		M: 800–1800 mg/d		×0.00884	7.1–15.9 nmol/d
		F: 600–1600 mg/d			5.2–14.1 nmol/d
Creatinine Clearance (Endogenous)	S or P, and U	<40 y, M: (97–137 mL/min)/1.73 m^2 skin area		×0.00963	(0.93–1.32 mL/s)/m^2 skin area
		F: (88–128 mL/min)/1.73 m^2 skin area			(0.85–1.23 mL/s)/m^2 skin area
		Decreases (~6.5 mL/min)/1.73 m^2 skin area per decade			Decreases (~0.06 mL/s)/m^2 skin area per decade
Cyanide	S		*mg/L*		*μmol/L*
		Nonsmokers:	0.004	×38.4	0.15
		Smokers:	0.006		0.23
		Nitroprusside therapy:	0.01–0.06		0.38–2.30
		Toxic:	>0.1		>3.84
	WB (Ox)	Nonsmokers:	0.016		0.61
		Smokers:	0.041		1.57
		Nitroprusside therapy:	0.05–0.5		1.92–19.20
		Toxic:	>1		>38.40
Cyclic AMP	P (EDTA)	M: 5.6–10.9 ng/mL		×3.04	M: 17–33 nmol/L
		F: 3.6–8.9 ng/mL			F: 11–27 nmol/L
	U, 24 h	<3.3 mg/d		×344	<10 μmol/d

Test	Specimen	Conventional		Factor	SI
Cystine and Cysteine					
Qual.	U, random	Negative			Negative
Quant.	U, 24 h	10–100 mg/d		×8.254	83–830 μmol/d Conversion based on cysteine (M.W. 121.16)
Dehydroepiandros terone (DHEA)					
Total	S		*ng/mL*		*nmol/L*
		Cord:	5.6–20.0	×3.47	19–69
		Child:	1.0–3.0		3–10
		Adult, M:	1.7–4.2		6–15
		F:	2.0–5.2		7–18
		Pregnancy:	0.5–12.5		2–43
Unconjugated	U, 24 h		*mg/d*		*μmol/d*
		Child,		×3.47	<0.3
		0–5 y:	<0.1		<0.7
		6–9 y:	<0.2		<1.4
		10–15 y:	<0.4		0–8.0
		Adult, M:	0–2.3		0–4.2
		F:	0–1.2		
Dehydroepiandros-terone Sulfate (DHEA-SO_4)	S or P (Hep or EDTA)	*μg/mL*			*μmol/L*
		Newborn:	<300	×2.6	<780
		1–4 d:	<20		<52
		5–7 d:	<45		<117
		Child:	0.60–2.54		1.6–6.6
		Adult, M:	1.99–3.34		5.2–8.7
		F, Premenopausal:	0.82–3.38		2.1–8.8
		Postmenopausal:	0.11–0.61		0.3–1.6
		Pregnancy, term:	0.23–1.17		0.6–3.0
	Amf	10–50 ng/mL		×2.6	26–130 nmol/L

Clinical chemistry and toxicology (*Continued*).

Test	Specimen	Reference Range	Conversion Factor	Reference Range (International Units)
Deoxycholic Acid, Total	S	0.22 ± 0.13 μg/mL (SD)	× 2.55	0.56 ± 0.33 μmol/L (SD)
11-Deoxycorticosterone (DOC)	S or P (Hep, EDTA, or Ox)	Ad lib diet, 0800 h: 4.3–12.3 ng/dL	× 0.0303	0.13–0.37 nmol/L
11-Deoxycortisol (Compound S)	P (Hep, EDTA, or Ox)	*μg/dL* <1 without metyrapone >7 after metyranpone	× 0.029	*μmol/L* <0.029 >0.203
Dexamethasone Single Dose Overnight Suppression Test *Dose: 1 mg orally at 2300 or 2400 h*	S, 0800 h	Cortisol: Suppression to 5–10 μg/dL or to <50% of baseline	× 27.59	Cortisol: Suppression to 138–276 nmol/L or fraction of baseline: <0.50
Dexamethasone Suppression Test (Standard) *Low dose, adult: 0.5 mg q 6 h × 8*	S, 0800 h Control, day 2 and 3	Cortisol: Suppression on day 3 to <50% of baseline or to <5 μg/dL	× 0.01 × 27.59	Cortisol: Suppression on day 3; fraction of baseline: <0.50 or <138 nmol/L
	U, 24 h Control, day 1, 2, and 3	17-KGS: Suppression on day 2 to <7.5 mg/d	× 3.467	17-KGS: Suppression on day 2 to <26 μmol/d
		17-OHCS: Suppression on day 2 to <4.5 mg/d	× 2.76	17-OHCS: Suppression on day 2 to <12.4 μmol/L
		Free cortisol: <50% of baseline	× 0.01	Free cortisol: Fraction of baseline: <0.50

Test	Specimen	Conventional Units	Factor	SI Units
High dose, adult *2.0 mg q 6 h × 8*		Cortisol, 17-KGS, 17-OHCS: Suppression on day 3 to <50% of baseline	× 0.01	Cortisol, 17-KGS, 17-OHCS: Suppression on day 3; fraction of baseline: <0.50
Dihydrotestosterone (DHT)	S	*ng/dL*		*nmol/L*
		Pubertal *M* *F*		*M* *F*
		stage I: <10 <10	× 0.0344	<0.34 <0.34
		II: <20 <15		<0.69 <0.52
		III: <35 <25		<1.20 <0.86
		IV–V: <75 <25		<2.58 <0.86
		Adult: 60–300 10–40		2–10.3 0.34–1.4
Disaccharide Absorption Test	S	*mg/dL*		*mmol/L*
		Change in glucose from fasting value: >30	× 0.055	Change in glucose from fasting value: >1.67
		Inconclusive: 20–30		1.11–1.67
		Abnormal: <20		<1.11
Estradiol, (E_2), Total	S or P (Hep or EDTA)	*pg/mL*		*pmol/L*
		M, Pubertal stage I: 2–8	× 3.67	7–29
		II: 11		40
		III: >20		>73
		Adult, M: 8–36		29–132
		F, Pubertal stage I: 0–23		0–84
		II: 0–66		0–242
		III: 0–105		0–385
		IV: 20–300		73–1100
		Follicular: 10–90		37–330
		Midcycle: 100–500		367–1835
		Luteal: 50–240		184–881
		(Lower on oral contraceptives)		
		Pregnancy,		
		6–8 wk: 7.6–11.4		28–42
		25–28 wk: 41.8–158		153–580
		Term: 127–281		466–1031
		Postmenopausal: 10–30		37–110

Clinical chemistry and toxicology (*Continued*).

Test	Specimen	Reference Range		Conversion Factor	Reference Range (International Units)
Estradiol, (E_2), Total (*continued*)					
	U, 24 h		*μg/d*		*nmol/d*
		Adult, M:	0–6	× 3.67	0–22
		F, Follicular:	0–3		0–11
		Ovulatory peak:	4–14		15–51
		Luteal:	4–10		15–37
		Postmenopausal:	0–4		0–15
Estriol (E_3), Free	S	Pregnancy (wk),	*μg/L*		*nmol/L*
		25–28:	3.5–12.5	× 3.47	12.1–43.4
		30–32:	4.5–16.0		15.6–55.5
		34:	5.5–18.5		19.1–64.2
		36:	7.0–25.0		24.3–86.8
		37:	8.0–28.0		27.8–97.2
		38:	9.0–32.0		31.2–111.0
		39:	10.0–34.0		34.7–118.0
		40–41:	10.5–25.0		36.4–86.8
	Amf		*ng/mL*		*nmol/L*
		Pregnancy (wk),	*(95% range)*		*(95% range)*
		16–20:	1.0–3.2	× 3.47	3.5–11.1
		20–24:	2.1–7.8		7.3–27.1
		24–28:	2.1–7.8		7.3–27.1
		28–32:	4.0–13.6		13.9–47.2
		32–36:	3.6–15.5		12.5–53.8
		36–38:	4.6–18.0		16.0–62.5
		38–40:	5.4–19.8		18.7–68.7
Estriol (E_3), Total	S	Pregnancy (wk),	*ng/mL*		*nmol/L*
		24–28:	30–170	× 3.47	104–590
		28–32:	40–220		139–763
		32–36:	60–280		208–972
		36–40:	80–350		278–1215
		Adult, M and nonprep F:	<2		<7
	U, 24 h	Pregnancy (wk),	*mg/d*		*μmol/d*
		30:	6–18	× 3.47	21–62

Test	Specimen	Reference Range		Factor	SI Reference Range
		35:	9–28		31–97
		40:	13–42		45–146
		Decrease of >40% of previous value suggests fetus at risk			Fraction of previous value of <0.60 suggests fetus at risk
	Amf	Pregnancy (wk), *ng/mL*		× 3.47	*nmol/L*
		<20	1–7		3.5–24.3
		21–32:	5–50		17–174
		33–35:	9–240		31–833
		36–41:	150–213		521–739
Estrogen Receptor Assay (ERA)	T		*fmol/mg protein*		*nmol/kg Protein*
		Negative:	<3.0	× 1	<3.0
		Borderline positive:	3–20		3–20
		Positive:	>20.0		>20.0
Estrogens, Total	S		*pg/mL*		*ng/L*
		Child:	<30	× 1	<30
		Adult, M:	40–115		40–115
		F, cycle-days,			
		1–10 d:	61–394		61–394
		11–20 d:	122–437		122–437
		21–30 d:	156–350		156–350
		Pregnancy (wk),			
		0–12:	700–8700		700–8700
		36–42:	8000–31,000		8000–31,000
		Prepubertal and postmenopausal:	≤40		≤40
	U, 24 h		*μg/d*		Same
		Child:	1.0 (mean)		
		M, pubertal stage I:	2.5 (mean)		
		II:	5.9 (mean)		
		III:	6.2 (mean)		
		Adult, M:	5–25		
		F, Preovulation:	5–25		
		Ovulation:	28–100		
		Luteal peak:	22–80		
		Pregnancy:	<45,000		
		Postmenopause:	<10		

Clinical chemistry and toxicology (*Continued*).

Test	Specimen	Reference Range		Conversion Factor	Reference Range (International Units)
Estrone (E_1)					
Unconjugated	S		*pg/mL*		*pmol/L*
		M, Pubertal stage I:	11	× 3.70	41
		II:	16		59
		III:	21		78
		Adult:	30–170		111–629
		F, Pubertal stage I:	0–29		0–107
		II:	10–35		37–130
		III:	15–45		56–167
		IV:	20–80		74–296
		Follicular:	20–150		74–555
	U, 24 h		*µg/d*		*nmol/d*
		Adult, M:	3–8	× 3.70	11–30
		F, Ovulatory peak:	11–31		41–115
		Luteal:	10–23		37–85
		Postmenopausal:	1–7		4–26
Conjugated	Amf	38–40 wk:	8.0 ng/mL (mean)	× 2.24	18 nmol/L (mean)
Unconjugated	Amf	Term:	2.5–5.6 ng/mL	× 3.70	9–21 nmol/L
Ethanol	WB (Ox) or S		*mg/dL*		*mmol/L*
		Toxic:	50–100	× 0.217	11–22
		Depression of CNS:	>100		>21.7
		Fatalities reported:	>400		>86.8
Ethylene Glycol	P (EDTA)	0 mg/L		× 16.1	0 µmol/L
	U	0 mg/L		× 16.1	0 µmol/L
Fat, Fecal	F, 72 h		*g/d*		Same
		Infant, breast-fed:	<1		
		0–6 y:	<2		
		Adult:	<7		
		Adult (fat-free diet):	<4		

Fatty Acid Profile	S or P (Hep)		*% of Total Nonesterified Fatty Acids*		*Fraction of Total Nonesterified Fatty Acids*
		Oleic:	26–45	× 0.01	0.26–0.45
		Palmitic:	23–25		0.23–0.25
		Stearic:	10–14		0.10–0.14
		Linoleic:	8–16		0.08–0.16
Fatty Acids, Nonesterified (Free)	S or P (Hep)		*mg/dL*		*mmol/L*
		Adult:	8–25	× 0.0354	0.30–0.90
		Child and obese adults:	<31		<1.10 (Conv. factor based on oleic acid, M.W. 282.47)
Fatty Acids, Total	S	190–420 mg/dL		× 0.0352	7–15 mmol/L
Ferric Chloride Test	U, random	Negative			Negative
Ferritin	S		*ng/mL*		*μg/L*
		Newborn:	25–200	× 1	25–200
		1 mo:	200–600		200–600
		2–5 mo:	5–200		50–200
		6 mo–15 y:	7–140		7–140
		Adult, M:	15–200		15–200
		F:	12–150		12–150
α_1-Fetoprotein (AFP)	S	Adult:	<30 ng/mL	× 1	<30 μg/L
		Fetal:	Peak of 200–400 mg/dL in first trimester, falls to 1% of peak (<5 mg/dL) in cord blood	× 0.01	Peak of 2–4 g/L in first trimester, falls to 1% of peak (<0.05 g/L) in cord blood
		1 y:	<30 ng/mL	× 1	<30 μg/L

Clinical chemistry and toxicology (*Continued*).

Test	Specimen	Reference Range			Conversion Factor	Reference Range (International Units)	
α_1-Fetoprotein (AFP) (*continued*)							
	S, maternal		*µg/dL 10th–90th*			*µg/L 10th–90th*	
		Pregnancy (wk)	*Percentile*	*Median*		*Percentile*	*Median*
		6–9	<1.0–1.5	<1.0	× 10	<10–15	<10
		10–12	<1.0–2.5	<1.0		<10–25	<10
		13–15	<1.0–4.4	1.9		<10–44	19
		16–18	<1.0–7.1	3.6		<10–71	36
		19–21	2.1–9.6	5.9		21–96	59
		22–24	5.1–15.0	7.6		51–150	76
		25–27	5.6–17.0	9.9		56–170	99
		28–30	7.9–19.8	14.0		79–198	140
		31–33	8.4–34.4	14.9		84–344	149
		34–36	6.0–33.5	12.3		60–335	123
		37–40	6.3–16.5	13.5		63–165	135
	Amf		*mg/dL*			*mg/L*	
		Pregnancy (wk)	*Median*	*±2 log SD*		*Median*	*±2 log SD*
		11–12	2.4	1.0–5.0	× 10	24	10–50
		13–14	2.3	1.3–4.1		23	13–41
		15–16	1.8	0.9–3.5		18	9–35
		17–18	1.5	0.6–3.3		15	6–33
		19–20	1.0	0.5–2.5		10	5–25
		21–25	0.7	0.4–1.4		7	4–14
		26–30	0.6	0.3–1.0		6	3–10
		31–35	0.2	0.05–0.7		2	0.5–7
		36–40	0.1	0.02–0.3		1	0.2–3
Fibrinogen	P (NaCit)	200–400 mg/dL			× 0.01	2.00–4.00 g/L	
FIGLU *Dose: 5 g histidine q 4 h × 3*	U, 24 h, after initial dose	<35 mg/d			× 5.74	<201 µmol/d	

Test	Specimen	Conventional units	Factor	SI units
Fluoride		*μg/mL*		*μmol/L*
	P (Hep)	0.01–0.2	× 52.6	0.5–10.5
	U	0.2–1.1		10.5–57.9
		Occup. exp.: 4–5		210–263
Folate	S	1.8–9 ng/mL	× 2.265	4.1–20.4 nmol/L
		>60 y: 2–12 ng/mL		4.5–27.2 nmol/L
	RBC (EDTA)	150–450 ng/mL packed cells		340–1020 nmol/L packed cells
		>60 y: 95–500 ng/mL packed cells		215–1132 nmol/L packed cells
Folate Absorption Test	U, 24 h	45 ± 7% of dose	× 0.01	Fraction of dose: 0.45 ± 0.07
Follicle Stimulating Hormone (hFSH)	S or P (Hep)	*mIU/mL (IRP-2-hMG)**		*IU/L*
		Birth 1 y, M: <1–12	× 1	<1–12
		F: <1–20		<1–20
		1–8 y, M: <1–6		<1–6
		F: <1–4		<1–4
		9–10 y, M: <1–10		<1–10
		F: 2–8		2–8
		11–12 y, M: 2–12		2–12
		F: 3–11		3–11
		13–14 y, M: 3–15		3–15
		F: 3–15		3–15
		Adult, M: 4–25		4–25
		F:		
		Premenopause: 4–30		4–30
		Midcycle peak: 10–90		10–90
		Pregnancy: Low to undetectable		Low to undetectable
		Postmenopause: 40–250		40–250

* 2nd International Reference Preparation of Human Menopausal Gonadotropin

Clinical chemistry and toxicology (*Continued*).

Test	Specimen	Reference Range		Conversion Factor	Reference Range (International Units)
Follicle Stimulating Hormone (hFSH) (*continued*)					
	U, 24 h	*IU/d (IRP-2-hMG)**			Same
		Birth-1 y, F:	<0.5–1.4		
		1–8 y, M:	<0.5–4.5		
		F:	<0.5–4.0		
		9–10 y, M:	1–5		
		F:	1–4		
		11–12 y, M:	1.5–5		
		F:	1–8		
		13–14 y, M:	2–12		
		F:	1–10		
		Adult, M:	4–18		
		F:	3–12		
		Higher in males >60 y			
		* 2nd International Reference Preparation of Human Menopausal Gonadotropin			
Formaldehyde	WB (F^-/Ox)	Occup. exp.:	0.6–4.0 mg/L	× 33.3	20–133 µmol/L
	U	Formic acid:	<17 mg/L	× 21.7	<369 µmol/L
Free Thyroxine Index (FT_4I) *with normalized* T_3RU	S		*FT_4 Index*		Same
			1.2–5.0		
		1–3 d:	9.3–26.6		
		1–4 wk:	7.6–20.8		
		1–4 mo:	7.4–17.9		
		4–12 mo:	6.1–14.5		
		1–6 y:	5.7–13.3		
		>6 y:	5.5–10.0		
		Borderline low:	4.8		
		Borderline high:	14.0		

Free Triiodothyronine, *see Triiodothyronine, Free*					
Free Triiodothyronine Index (FT_3I)	S	1–5 y:	165		Same
		5–10 y:	150		
		10–15 y:	130		
Fructose	S	1–6 mg/dL		× 55.5	55.5–333 µmol/L
	U	<60 mg/d		× 5.55	<333 µmol/d
	Semf	>150 mg/dL		× 0.0555	>8.33 mmol/L
Fructose Loading Test	S	Peak:	15–25 mg/dL	× 0.0555	0.83–1.39 mmol/L
	U	1–2% of administered dose		× 0.01	Fraction of administered dose: 0.01–0.02
Galactose	S	Newborn:	0–20 mg/dL	× 0.0555	0–1.11 mmol/L
		Thereafter:	<5 mg/dL		<0.28 mmol/L
	U	Newborn:	≤60 mg/dL	× 0.0555	≤3.33 mmol/L
		Thereafter:	<14 mg/d	× 0.00555	<0.08 mmol/d
Galactose Tolerance Test *Dose: 40 g in 250 ml H_2O, orally*	WB (Hep with NaF)	60 min:	40–60 mg/dL	× 0.0555	2.22–3.33 mmol/L
		Sum of 30, 60, 90, 120 min specimens:	<110 mg/dL		<6.11 mmol/L
	U, 5 h	≤3 g/5 h		× 5.55	<16.7 mmol/5 h
Gastric Acid	Gast Res		*Without Stimulation mmol/L*		Same
		Free:	0–40		
		Combined:	10–20		
		Total:	10–50		
Gastric Content	Gast Res	Volume:	20–100 mL	× 0.001	0.02–0.1 L
		pH:	1.5–3.5		H^+ concentration: 32–316 µmol/L
Gastric Secretion Rate	Gast Cont, total; six 15-min spec.	BAO:	0–5 mmol/h		Same
		PAO:	5–20 mmol/h (post Pentagastrin)		
		BAO/PAO:	0.20		

Clinical chemistry and toxicology (*Continued*).

Test	Specimen	Reference Range		Conversion Factor	Reference Range (International Units)
Gastrin	S		*pg/mL*		*ng/L*
		Cord, venous:	64 ± 12.5 (SEM)	× 1	64 ± 12.5 (SEM)
		4d:	151 ± 15.8		151 ± 15.8
		<3 y:	32.7 ± 22.3		32.7 ± 22.3
		>3 y:	14.8 ± 14.3		14.8 ± 14.3
		<60 y:	<100		<100
		>60 y:	<100 (15% have values of 100–800 pg/mL)		<100 (15% have values of 100–800 pg/mL)
Gastrin-Calcium Infusion Stimulation Test	S	Gastrin:	Slight or no increase		Same
		Z.E. syndrome:	>450 pg/mL	× 1	Z.E. syndrome: >450 ng/L
Gastrin-Secretin Stimulation Test *IV dose: 5 U secretin/kg*	S: baseline and 15-min intervals for 1 h	Gastrin: No response or slight suppression			Same
		Z.E. syndrome: Increase > 110 pg/mL if baseline is 80–500 pg/mL; increase >1400 pg/mL if baseline is high			Z.E. syndrome: Increase >110 ng/L if baseline is 80–500 ng/L; increase > 1400 ng/mL if baseline is high
Glomerular Selectivity Test (IgG/Albumin Ratio)	U	<0.16 indicates high selectivity			Same
Glucagon	P (Hep or EDTA)		*pg/mL*		*ng/L*
			30–210	× 1	30–210
		Average:	75 ± 4 (SEM)		75 ± 4 (SEM)
		Big glucagon:	113 ± 79		113 ± 79
		Proglucagon:	11 ± 16		11 ± 16
		Glucagon:	31 ± 29		31 ± 29
		Small glucagon:	26 ± 18		26 ± 18

	Amf	(Mostly big glucagon)			
		Midgestation:	43 ± 10 (SE)		43 ± 10 (SE)
		Term:	117 ± 38		117 ± 38
Glucose	S, fasting		*mg/dL*		*mmol/L*
		Cord:	45–96	× 0.0555	2.50–5.33
		Premature:	20–60		1.11–3.33
		Neonate:	30–60		1.67–3.33
		Newborn,			
		1 d:	40–60		2.22–3.33
		>1 d:	50–80		2.78–4.44
		Child:	60–100		3.33–5.55
		Adult:	70–105		3.89–5.83
		>60 y:	80–115		4.44–6.38
		>70 y:	83–110		4.61–6.10
	WB (Hep)	Adult:	65–95		3.61–5.27
	CSF	Infant, child:	60–80		3.33–4.44
	U	Adult:	40–70		2.22–3.89
Quan., enzymatic	U	<0.5 g/d		× 5.55	<2.8 mmol/d
Qual.		Negative			Negative
Glucose-6-Phosphate Dehydrogenase (G-6-PD) in Erythrocytes *WHO and ICSH*	WB (ACD, EDTA, or Hep)	12.1 ± 2.09 U/g Hb (SD)		× 0.0645	0.78 ± 0.13 MU/mol Hb
		351 ± 60.6 U/10^{12} RBC		× 10^{-3}	0.35 ± 0.06 nU/RBC
		4.11 ± 0.71 U/mL RBC		× 1	4.11 ± 0.71 kU/L RBC
Glucose, 2 h Postprandial	S	<120 mg/dL		× 0.0555	<6.7 mmol/L
		Diabetes: *see Glucose Tolerance Test, Oral*			

			mg/dL Normal	*mg/dL* Diabetic		*mmol/L* Normal	*mmol/L* Diabetic
Glucose Tolerance Test (GTT)		Adults,					
		Fasting:	70–105	>140	× 0.0555	3.9–5.8	>7.8
Oral	S	60 min:	120–170	⩾200		6.7–9.4	⩾11.1
		90 min:	100–140	⩾200		5.6–7.8	⩾11.1
		120 min:	70–120	⩾140		3.9–6.7	⩾7.8
IV	S	5 min:	<250			<13.88	
		90 min: at or below fasting concentration					
		or K = >1.5%					

Clinical Chemistry and Toxicology (*Continued*).

Test	Specimen	Reference Range		Conversion Factor	Reference Range (International Units)
Glucose Tolerance Test (GTT) with Cortisone *Dose: 50 mg, 85 and 2 h before test*	P (F^-/Ox): baseline, 1, 1½, 2 h after glucose	Glucose,	*mg/dL*		*mmol/L*
		Fasting:	70–105	× 0.0555	3.89–5.83
		1 h:	<200		<11.10
		1½ h:	<200		<11.10
		2 h:	<140		<7.77
Glutamine	CSF		*mg/dL ± SD*		*mmol/L ± SD*
		Newborn–15 d:	9.7 ± 2.9	× 0.06842	0.66 ± 0.20
		15 d–6 mo:	8.6 ± 2.7		0.59 ± 0.18
		6–12 mo:	7.1 ± 2.1		0.49 ± 0.14
		12–30 mo:	5.4 ± 1.8		0.37 ± 0.12
		Adult:	6–16		0.41–1.10
γ-Glutamyltransferase (GGT) *37°C, aca*	S	M:	9–50 U/L		Same
		F:	8–40 U/L		
Glutathione, Reduced (GSH)	WB (ACD, EDTA, or Hep)	6.57 ± 1.04 μmol/g Hb (SD)		× 0.0645	0.42 ± 0.07 mol/mol Hb
		190 ± 30.16 μmol/10^{12} RBC		× 1	190 ± 30 amol/RBC
		2.23 ± 0.35 μmol/mL RBC		× 1	2.23 ± 0.35 mmol/L RBC (Conv. factor based on hemoglobin, M.W. 64,500)
Glutathione Reductase in Erythrocytes *ICSH, 37°C*	WB (ACD, EDTA, or Hep)	Adult (reaction without added flavin adenine dinucleotide, FAD):			
		7.18 ± 1.09 U/g Hb (SD)		× 0.0645	0.46 ± 0.07 MU/mol Hb
		208 ± 31.6 U/10^{12} RBC		× 10^{-3}	0.21 ± 0.03 nU/RBC
		2.44 ± 0.37 U/mL RBC		× 1	2.44 ± 0.37 kU/L RBC
		Adult (reaction using FAD):			
		10.4 ± 1.5 U/g Hb (SD)		× 0.0645	0.67 ± 0.10 MU/mol Hb
		302 ± 43.5 U/10^{12} RBC		× 10^{-3}	0.30 ± 0.04 nU/RBC
		3.54 ± 0.51 U/mL RBC		× 1	3.54 ± 0.51 kU/L RBC

Glycerol, Free	P (EDTA)	3–10 y:	0.56–2.14 mg/dL	× 0.1086	0.061–0.232 mmol/L
		11–80 y:	0.29–1.72 mg/dL		0.032–0.187 mmol/L
Glycine	U, 24 h		*mg/d*		*mmol/d*
		10 d–7 wk:	15–59	× 0.01332	0.20–0.79
		3–12 y:	12–107		0.16–1.43
		Adult:	59–294		0.79–3.92
		or 60 ± 24 mg/g creatinine (SD)		× 1.51	or 90.6 ± 36.2 mmol/mol creatinine (SD)
Glycolic Acid	U, 24 h	Adult:	15–60 mg/d	× 0.0131	0.20–0.79 mmol/d
Gold	S	<10 µg/dL		× 0.0508	<0.51 µmol/L
		Therap.:	38–500 µg/dL		1.93–25.4 µmol/L
	U, 24 h	<1 µg/d		× 5.08	<5.08 nmol/d
Gonadotropins, *see Pregnancy Tests and Chorionic Gonadotropin. β-Subunit*					
Growth Hormone (hGH, Somatotropin)	S or P (EDTA or Hep)		*ng/mL*	× 1	*µg/L*
		Cord:	10–50		10–50
		Newborn:	10–40		10–40
		Child:	<1–10		<1–10
		(occasional values up to 20)			
		Adult, M:	<2		<2
		F:	<10		<10
		>60 y, M:	0.4–10		0.4–10
		F:	1–14		1–14
	Amf	20 wk:	10		10
		Term:	30		30
Growth Hormone–Arginine Stimulation Test *Dose, adult: 30 g arginine HCl, IV, within 30 min; child: 0.5 g/kg*	S: baseline, 30-min intervals for 2 h	Fasting: <5 ng/mL; rise to >7 ng/mL during test (peak range 8–35 ng/mL) at 30–60 min		× 1	Fasting: <5 µg/L; rise to >7 µg/L during test (peak range 8–35 µg/L) at 30–60 min

Clinical chemistry and toxicology (*Continued*).

Test	Specimen	Reference Range	Conversion Factor	Reference Range (International Units)
Growth Hormone–Glucagon Stimulation Test *Dose: 1 mg glucagon, IM or SC*	S: baseline then hourly for 3–4 h	>7 ng/mL after stimulation or >5 ng/mL rise above baseline	× 1	>7 μg/L after stimulation or >5 μg/L rise above baseline
Growth Hormone–L-Dopa Stimulation Test *Dose, adult: 500 mg L-dopa, orally: child: 10 mg/kg*	S: baseline, 30, 60, 90, 120, and 180 min after L-dopa	Peak: >7 ng/mL or >5 ng/mL rise above baseline	× 1	>7 μg/L or >5 μg/L above baseline
Haptoglobin	S			
RID		83–267 mg/dL	× 10	830–2670 mg/L
Hemoglobin binding capacity		40–180 mg Hb/dL	× 0.155	6.20–27.9 μmol Hb/L
Nephelometry		26–185 mg/dL	× 10	260–1850 mg/L
HDL/Cholesterol (HDL-C)	S or P (EDTA)	*mg/dL* *M* *F*		*mmol/L* *M* *F*
		Mean: 45 55		1.17 1.42
		Range,	× 0.0259	
		Cord blood: 5–50 5–50		0.13–1.30 0.13–1.30
		0–14 y: 30–65 30–65		0.78–1.68 0.78–1.68
		15–19 y: 30–65 30–70		0.78–1.68 0.78–1.81
		20–29 y: 30–70 30–75		0.78–1.81 0.78–1.94
		30–39 y: 30–70 30–80		0.78–1.81 0.78–2.07
		>40 y: 30–70 30–85		0.78–1.81 0.78–2.20
		Values for Blacks ~10 mg/dL higher		

Test	Specimen		Conventional		Factor	SI	
			HDL-C, % of Total Chol			*Fraction HDL-C of Chol*	
		CHD Risk	M	F		M	F
		Dangerous:	<7	<12	× 0.01	<0.07	<0.12
		High:	7–15	12–18		0.07–0.15	0.12–0.18
		Average:	15–25	18–27		0.15–0.25	0.18–0.27
		Below average:	25–37	27–40		0.25–0.37	0.27–0.40
		Protection probable:	>37	>40		>0.37	>0.40
Hematocrit	WB (EDTA)		*% Packed Red Cell Volume (V Red Cells/V Whole Blood × 100)*			*Volume Fraction (V Red Cells/V Whole Blood)*	
		Cord blood:	42–60		× 0.01	0.42–0.60	
		1–3 d (cap):	45–67			0.45–0.67	
		1 wk:	42–66			0.42–0.66	
		2 wk:	39–63			0.39–0.63	
		1 mo:	31–55			0.31–0.55	
		2 mo:	28–42			0.28–0.42	
		3–6 mo:	29–41			0.29–0.41	
		0.5–2 y:	33–39			0.33–0.39	
		2–6 y:	34–40			0.34–0.40	
		6–12 y:	35–45			0.35–0.45	
		12–18 y, M:	37–49			0.37–0.49	
		F:	36–46			0.36–0.46	
		18–49 y, M:	41–53			0.41–0.53	
		F:	36–46			0.36–0.46	
Hemoglobin	WB (EDTA)		*g/dL*			*mmol/L*	
		Cord:	13.5–20.0		× 0.155	2.09–3.10	
		1–3 d (cap):	14.5–22.5			2.25–3.49	
		1 wk:	13.5–21.5			2.09–3.33	
		2 wk:	12.5–20.5			1.94–3.18	
		1 mo:	10.0–18.0			1.55–2.79	
		2 mo:	9.0–14.0			1.40–2.17	
		3–6 mo:	9.5–13.5			1.47–2.09	
		0.5–2 y:	10.5–13.5			1.63–2.09	
		2–6 y:	11.5–13.5			1.78–2.09	
		6–12 y:	11.5–15.5			1.78–2.40	
		12–18 y, M:	13.0–16.0			2.02–2.48	
		F:	12.0–16.0			1.86–2.48	
		18–49 y, M:	13.5–17.5			2.09–2.71	
		F:	12.0–16.0			1.86–2.48	

Clinical chemistry and toxicology (*Continued*).

Test	Specimen	Reference Range		Conversion Factor	Reference Range (International Units)
	P (EDTA, ACD, or Hep)	1–4 mg/dL		× 0.155	0.16–0.62 μmol/L
	S	<3 mg/dL with butterfly setup and 18-g needle			<0.47 μmol/L with butterfly setup and 18-g needle
	U, fresh, random	Negative			Negative
Hemoglobin A_{Ic}	WB (Hep, EDTA, or Ox)				
Electrophoresis		5.6–7.5% of total Hb		× 0.01	Fraction of Hb:
Column		6–9% of total Hb			0.056– 0.075
					0.06–0.09
Hemoglobin A_2 (HbA_2)	WB (EDTA or Ox)	Adult:	1.5–3.5% (2 SD)	× 0.01	0.015–0.035 (2 SD)
		Lower in infants <1 y			
		β-Thalassemia trait:	3.75–6.5% (2 SD)		0.038–0.065 (2 SD)
					Hb Fraction
Hemoglobin (Hb) Electrophoresis	WB (EDTA, Cit, or Hep)	HbA:	>95%	× 0.01	>0.95
		HbA_2:	1.5–3.5%		0.015–0.035
		HbF:	<2%		<0.02
Hemoglobin F	WB (EDTA)		*% HbF*		*Mass Fraction HbF*
Alkali denaturation (White)		1 d:	77.0 ± 7.3	× 0.01	0.77 ± 0.073
		5 d:	76.8 ± 5.8		0.768 ± 0.058
		3 wk:	70.0 ± 7.3		0.70 ± 0.073
		6–9 wk:	52.9 ± 11.0		0.529 ± 0.11
		3–4 mo:	23.2 ± 16.0		0.232 ± 0.16
		6 mo:	4.7 ± 2.2		0.047 ± 0.022
		8–11 mo:	1.6 ± 1.0		0.016 ± 0.010
		Adult:	<2.0		<0.020

Hemoglobin H (HbH) *Isopropanol precipitation*	WB (ACD, EDTA, or Hep)	No precipitation at 40 min			No precipitation at 40 min
Hemopexin	S	Fetus, term:	>30% of mean adult conc. or 18% of maternal conc.	× 0.01	Fraction of adult conc: >0.30 Fraction of maternal conc.: 0.18
		Maternal:	>1.5 times that of non-pregnant adults		Same
		Adult:	50–115 mg/dL	× 0.01	0.50–1.15 g/L
	U	Mean:	0.2 mg/d		0.2 mg/d
Hexachlorophene	WB		*mg/L*		*μmol/L*
		Infant:	<0.182	× 2.46	<0.448
		Adult:	<0.089		<0.219
		After use:	0.1–0.655		0.246–1.611
	Milk	<0.009 mg/L			<0.022
	Fat	<0.05 mg/kg		× 2.46	<0.123 μmol/kg
Homocystine	U, random	Negative			Negative
Homogentisic Acid	U, random	Negative			Negative
Homovanillic Acid (HVA)	U, 24 h	Child:	3–16 μg/mg creatinine	× 0.621	1.86–9.94 mmol/mol creatinine
		Adult:	<15 mg/d	× 5.49	<82 μgmol/d
Hydrogen Sulfide	WB (F^-/Ox)	<0.05 mg/L		× 29.3	<1.5 μmol/L
		Toxic:	>0.90 mg/L		>26.4 μmol/L
β-Hydroxybutyric Acid	S or P	Undetectable			Undetectable

Clinical chemistry and toxicology (*Continued*).

Test	Specimen	Reference Range		Conversion Factor	Reference Range (International Units)
17-Hydroxycorticosteroids (17-OHCS)	U, 24 h		*mg/d*		*μmol/d*
		0–1 y:	0.5–1.0	× 2.76	1.4–2.8
		Child:	1.0–5.6		2.8–15.5
		Adult, M:	3.0–10.0		8.2–27.6
		F:	2.0–8.0		5.5–22
					(Conversion based on hydrocortisone, M.W. 362)
		or 3–7 mg/g creatinine		× 0.312	or 0.9–2.5 mmol/mol creatinine
	Amf	Increases 4–6-fold throughout pregnancy			Same
5-Hydroxyindoleacetic Acid (5-HIAA)					
Qual.	U, random	Negative (<25 mg/d)		× 5.2	Negative (<130 μmol/d)
Quant.	U, 24 h	2–8 mg/d		× 5.2	10.4–41.6 μmol/d
17-Hydroxyprogesterone (17-OHP)	S		*ng/mL*		*nmol/L*
		M, Pub, stage I:	0.1–0.3	× 3.03	0.30–0.91
		Adult:	0.2–1.8		0.61–5.45
		F, Pub, stage I:	0.2–0.5		0.61–1.52
		Follicular:	0.2–0.8		0.61–2.42
		Luteal:	0.8–3.0		2.42–9.10
		Postmenopausal:	0.04–0.5		0.12–1.52
		Values are highest at birth but decrease rapidly during 1st week of life			
Hydroxyproline	S		*mg/dL*		*μmol/L*
		Premature, 1 d:	0.52 ± 0.52	× 76.3	40 ± 40
		6–18 y, M:	0–0.66		0–50
		F:	0–0.58		0–44
		Adult, M:	0–0.55		0–42
		F:	0–0.46		0–34

	U, 24 h		*mg/d*		*μmol/d*
		1–5 y:	20–65	× 0.0076	0.15–0.49
		6–10 y:	35–99		0.27–0.75
		11–14 y:	63–180		0.48–1.37
		18–21 y:	20–55		0.15–0.42
		>21 y:	15–43		0.11–0.33
		Free hydroxyproline: 2–5% of total		× 0.01	Free hydroxyproline fraction of total: 0.02–0.05
Immunglobulin A (IgA)					
Nephelometric	S		*mg/dL*		*g/L*
		Cord:	0–5	× 0.01	0–0.05
		Newborn:	0–2.2		0–0.02
		4–6 mo:	3–82		0.03–0.82
		6 mo-2 y:	14–108		0.14–1.08
		2–6 y:	23–190		0.23–1.90
		6–12 y:	29–270		0.29–2.70
		12–16 y:	81–232		0.81–2.32
		Adult:	76–390		0.76–3.90
		>60 y, M:	90–410		0.90–4.10
		F:	50–373		0.50–3.73
RIA	CSF		*mg/dL*	× 10	*mg/L*
		15–20 y:	0.07 ± 0.04 (SD)		0.7 ± 0.4 (SD)
		21–40 y:	0.07 ± 0.03		0.7 ± 0.3
		41–60 y:	0.01 ± 0.03		1.0 ± 0.3
		61–87 y:	0.11 ± 0.06		1.1 ± 0.6
Immunoglobulin D (IgD)	S	Newborn:	<1.0 mg/dL	× 10	<10 mg/L
		Adult:	0–8 mg/dL		0–80 mg/L
Immunoglobulin E (IgE)	S		*IU/mL*	× 1	*kIU/L*
		Adult:	0–380		0–380
		>60 y, M:	0–250		0–250
		F:	0–175		0–175

Clinical chemistry and toxicology (*Continued*).

Test	Specimen	Reference Range		Conversion Factor	Reference Range (International Units)
Immunoglobulin G					
(IgG)			*mg/dL*	× 0.01	*g/L*
Nephelometric	S	Cord:	760–1700		7.6–17.0
		Newborn:	700–1480		7.0–14.8
		½–6 mo:	300–1000		3.0–10.0
		6 mo-2 y:	500–1200		5.0–12.0
		2–6 y:	500–1300		5.0–13.0
		6–12 y:	700–1650		7.0–16.5
		12–16 y:	700–1550		7.0–15.5
		Adult:	650–1500		6.5–15.0
		(higher in Blacks)			
			mg/dL		*mg/L*
RIA	CSF	15–20 y:	3.5 ± 2.0 (SD)	× 10	35 ± 20 (SD)
		21–40 y:	4.2 ± 1.4		42 ± 14
		41–60 y:	4.7 ± 1.0		47 ± 10
		61–87 y:	5.8 ± 1.6		58 ± 16
Immunoglobulin G/ Albumin Ratio	CSF and S	0.3–0.6			0.3–0.6
Immunoglobulin G Synthesis Rate	CSF and S	−9.9 to + 3.3 mg/d			− 9.9 to + 3.3 mg/d
Immunoglobulin M					
(IgM)	S		*mg/dL*		*mg/L*
Nephelometric: Std: Beckman; Atlantic Antibodies; WHO		Cord:	4–24	× 10	40–240
		Newborn:	5–30		50–300
		½–6 mo:	15–109		150–1090
		6 mo-2 y:	43–239		430–2390
		2–6 y:	50–199		500–1990
		6–12 y:	50–260		500–2600

		12–16 y:	45–240		450–2400
		Adult:	40–345		400–3450
		Results vary with std. preparation			
			mg/dL		*mg/L*
	CSF	15–20 y:	0.02 ± 0.009 (SD)	× 10	0.2 ± 0.09 (SD)
		21–40 y:	0.016 ± 0.003		0.16 ± 0.03
		41–60 y:	0.017 ± 0.004		0.17 ± 0.04
		61–87 y:	0.017 ± 0.005		0.17 ± 0.05
Insulin (12 h Fasting)	S		*μIU/mL*		*mIU/L*
		Newborn:	3–20	× 1.0	3–20
		Adult:	6–24		6–24
		>60 y:	6–35		6–35
	Amf	<16 wk:	Undetectable		Undetectable
		Term:	11.3 (mean)	× 1	11.3 (mean)
Insulin Antibodies	S	Undetectable			Undetectable
Insulin and Glucose Suppression Test	S, every 6–12 h	>50 mg glucose/dL during a 72-h period of fasting, with values slightly lower in females		× 0.0555	>2.8 mmol glucose/L during a 72 h period of fasting, with values slightly lower in females
		Insulin: <4 μIU/mL or undetectable		× 1	Insulin: <4 mU/L or undetectable
		Normal fasting insulin-glucose ratio: <0.3			Normal fasting insulin-glucose ratio: <5.4
Insulin with Oral Glucose Tolerance Test	S	*Min*	*Insulin, μIU/mL*		*mIU/L*
		0:	6–24	× 1	6–24
		30:	25–231		25–231
		60:	18–276		18–276
		120:	16–166		16–166
		180:	4–38		4–38

Clinical chemistry and toxicology (*Continued*).

Test	Specimen	Reference Range	Conversion Factor	Reference Range (International Units)
Insulin Tolerance Test *Dose: 0.1–0.15 U/kg, IV*	S	*Glucose*: Decrease ~50% of the fasting level by 30 min and return to normal fasting limits by 90–120 min	× 0.01	Fractional decrease in glucose ~ 0.50 of the fasting level by 30 min and return to normal fasting limits by 90–120 min
		hGH: Increase of >5 ng/mL within 60 min of hypoglycemia	× 1	*hGH*: Increase of >5 μg/L within 60 min of hypoglycemia
		Cortisol: Increase of >6 μg/dL with peak of >20 μg/dL	× 27.59	*Cortisol*: Increase of >165 nmol/L with peak of >552 nmol/L
Intrinsic Factor, *see Vitamin B_{12} Intrinsic Factor*				
Insulin Clearance Test	S and U	*(mL/min)/1.73 m²* M F		*(mL/s)/m²* M F
		20–29 y: 90–174 84–156	× 0.00963	0.87–1.68 0.81–1.50
		30–39 y: 88–168 82–150		0.85–1.62 0.79–1.44
		40–49 y: 78–162 82–146		0.75–1.56 0.79–1.41
		50–59 y: 68–152 66–142		0.65–1.46 0.63–1.37
		60–69 y: 57–137 58–130		0.55–1.32 0.56–1.25
		70–79 y: 42–122 45–121		0.40–1.17 0.43–1.17
		80–89 y: 39–105 39–105		0.38–1.01 0.38–1.01
Iron *ICSH*	S	*μg/dL*		*μmol/L*
		Newborn: 100–250	× 0.179	17.90–44.75
		Infant: 40–100		7.16–17.90
		Child: 50–120		8.95–21.48
		Adult, M: 65–170		11.64–30.43
		F: 50–170		8.95–30.43
		Strongly method dependent		

Iron-Binding Capacity, Total (TIBC)	S	Infant:	100–400 µg/dL	× 0.179	17.90–71.60 µmol/L
		Thereafter:	250–450 µg/dL		44.75–80.55 µmol/L
Iron Saturation	S	20–55%		× 0.01	Fraction saturation 0.20–0.55
Isocitrate Dehydrogenase (ICD) 30°C	S	1.2–7.0 U/L			1.2–7.0 U/L
Isoleucine	S		*mg/dL*	× 76.3	*µmol/L*
		Premature, 1 d:	0.52 ± 0.26 (SD)		40 ± 20 (SD)
		Newborn, 1 d:	0.35–0.69		27–53
		1–3 mo:	0.77 ± 0.18 (SD)		59 ± 14 (SD)
		2–6 mo:	0.50–1.61		38–123
		9 mo–2 y:	0.34–1.23		26–94
		3–10 y:	0.37–1.10		28–84
		6–18 y:	0.50–1.24		38–95
		Adult:	0.48–1.28		37–98
	U, 24 h		*mg/d*		µmol/d
		10 d–7 wk:	trace–0.4	× 7.62	trace–3
		3–12 y:	2–7		15–53
		Adult:	2–24		15–183
		or 3 ± 1 mg/g creatinine		× 0.86	or 2.6 ± 0.9 mmol/mol creatinine
17-Ketogenic Steroids (17-KGS)	U, 24 h		*mg/d*		µmol/d
		0–1 y:	<1.0	× 3.467	<3.5
		1–10 y:	<5		<17
		11–14 y:	<12		<42
		Adult, M:	5–23		17–80
		F:	3–15		10–52
		>70 y, M:	3–15		10–52
		F:	3–13		10–45
					(Conversion based on dehydroepiandrosterone, M.W. 288)

Clinical chemistry and toxicology (*Continued*).

Test	Specimen	Reference Range		Conversion Factor	Reference Range (International Units)
Ketose Bodies					
Qual.	S	Negative			Negative
	U, random	Negative			Negative
Quant.	S	0.5–3.0/mg/dL		× 10	5–30 mg/L
17-Ketosteroids	U, 24 h		*mg/d*		*μmol/d*
(17 KS), Total		14 d–2 y:	⩽1	× 3.467	⩽3.5
Zimmerman reaction		2–6 y:	⩽2		⩽7
		6–10 y:	1–4		3.5–14
		10–12 y:	1–6		3.5–21
		12–14 y:	3–10		10–35
		14–16 y:	5–12		17–42
		Adult,			
		M, 18–30 y:	9–22		31–76
		M, >3 y:	8–20		28–70
		F:	6–15		21–52
		Decreases with age			Decreases with age
GLC		Adult, M:	5.0–12.0		17–42
		F:	3.0–10.0		10–35
					(Conversion based on dehydroepiandrosterone, M.W. 288)
17-Ketosteroids (17 KS)					
Fractions	U, 24 h		*mg/d*		*μmol/d*
Androsterone		0–1 y:	<0.1	× 3.44	<0.34
		1–5 y:	<0.3		<1.03
		6–9 y:	0.1–1.0		0.34–3.44
		10–15 y, M:	0.2–2.0		0.69–6.88
		F:	0.5–3.0		1.72–10.32
		Adult, M:	2.2–5.0		7.57–17.20
		F:	0.5–2.4		1.72–8.26

Dehydroepiandro-sterone	0–5 y:	<0.1	× 3.47	<0.35
	6–9 y:	<0.2		<0.69
	10–15 y:	<0.4		<1.39
	Adult, M:	<2.3		<7.98
	F:	<1.5		<5.21
Etiocholanolone	0–1 y:	<0.1	× 3.44	<0.34
	1–2 y:	<0.4		<1.38
	3–5 y:	<0.7		<2.41
	6–9 y:	0.3–1.0		1.03–3.44
	10–15 y, M:	0.1–1.6		0.34–5.50
	F:	0.7–3.1		2.41–10.66
	Adult, M:	1.9–4.7		6.54–16.17
	F:	1.1–3.5		3.78–12.04
11-β-Hydroxyandro-sterone	0–2 y:	<0.3	× 3.26	<0.98
	3–5 y:	<0.4		<1.30
	6–9 y:	0.4–1.0		1.30–3.26
	10–15 y, M:	0.1–1.1		0.33–3.59
	F:	0.2–1.0		0.65–3.26
	Adult, M:	0.5–1.3		1.63–4.24
	F:	0.2–0.6		0.65–1.96
11-β-Hydroxyetiocho-lanolone	0–2 y:	<0.1	× 3.26	<0.33
	3–5 y:	<0.4		<1.30
	6–9 y:	0.1–0.5		0.33–1.63
	10–15 y, M:	<0.3		<0.98
	F:	0.1–0.5		0.33–1.63
	Adult, M:	0.3–0.7		0.98–2.28
	F:	0.2–0.6		0.65–1.96
11-Ketoandrosterone	≤15 y:	<0.1	× 3.27	<0.33
	Adult, M:	0.2–1.0		0.65–3.27
	F:	0.2–0.8		0.65–2.62
11-Ketoetiocho-lanolone	0–2 y:	<0.1	× 3.27	<0.33
	3–5 y:	<0.4		<1.30
	6–9 y:	0.1–0.7		0.33–2.29
	10–15 y, M:	0.2–0.6		0.65–1.96
	F:	0.1–0.6		0.33–1.96
	Adult, M:	0.2–1.0		0.65–3.27
	F:	0.2–0.8		0.65–2.62

Clinical chemistry and toxicology (*Continued*).

Test	Specimen	Reference Range		Conversion Factor	Reference Range (International Units)
17-Ketosteroids (17 KS) Fractions	U, 24 h				
Beta-Alpha ratio		<0.2			<0.2
Alpha-Beta ratio		>5			>5
L-Lactate			*mg/dL*		*mmol/L*
	P (NaF)	Venous:	4.5–19.8	× 0.111	0.5–2.2
		Arterial:	4.5–14.4		0.5–1.6
	WB (Hep)	At bed rest,			
		Venous:	8.1–15.3		0.9–1.7
		Arterial:	<11.3		<1.25
	U, 24 h	496–1982 mg/d		× 0.0111	5.5–22 mmol/d
	CSF	<25.2 mg/dL		× 0.111	<2.8 mmol/L
Qual.	Gastf	Negative			Negative
Lactate Dehydrogenase (LDH)					
Total (L → P), 30°C	S		*U/L*		Same
		Newborn:	160–450		
		Neonate:	300–1500		
		Infant:	100–250		
		Child:	60–170		
		Adult:	45–90		
		>60 y:	55–100		
Total (P → L), 30°C	CSF	~10% of serum value	150–320	× 0.01	~0.10 fraction of serum value
			% of Total		*Fraction of Total*
Isoenzymes, Agarose	S	Fraction 1:	14–26	× 0.01	0.14–0.26
		Fraction 2:	29–39		0.29–0.39
		Fraction 3:	20–26		0.20–0.26
		Fraction 4:	8–16		0.08–0.16
		Fraction 5:	6–16		0.06–0.16

Test	Specimen	Reference Range (Conventional)			Factor	Reference Range (SI)	
Lactate Dehydrogenase (LDH) in Erythrocytes	WB (ACD, EDTA, or Hep)	Adult:					
		200 ± 26.5 U/g Hb (SD)			× 0.0645	12.9 ± 1.7 MU/mol Hb	
		5800 ± 768 U/10^{12} RBC			× 10^{-3}	5.80 ± 0.77 nU/RBC	
		68.0 ± 9.01 U/mL RBC			× 1	68.0 ± 9.01 kU/L RBC	
						(Conv. factor based on hemoglobin, M.W. 64,500)	
Lactate/Pyruvate Ratio	WB (Hep)	10/1				10/1	
Lactose	S	<0.5 mg/dL			× 29.21	<14.6 µmol/L	
	U	12–40 mg/dL			× 29.21	350–1168 µmol/L	
LDL-Cholesterol (LDL-C) *Calculated*	S or P (EDTA)		*mg/dL*			*mmol/L*	
			M	*F*		*M*	*F*
		Cord blood:	10–50	10–50	× 0.0259	0.26–1.30	0.26–1.30
		0–19 y:	60–140	60–150		1.55–3.63	1.55–3.89
		20–29 y:	60–175	60–160		1.55–4.53	1.55–4.14
		30–39 y:	80–190	70–170		2.07–4.92	1.81–4.40
		40–49 y:	90–205	80–190		2.33–5.31	2.07–4.92
		50–59 y:	90–205	90–220		2.33–5.31	2.33–5.70
		60–69 y:	90–215	100–235		2.33–5.57	2.59–6.09
		>70 y:	90–190	95–215		2.33–4.92	2.46–5.57
		Recommended (desirable) range for adults: 65–175 mg/dL				1.68–4.53	
Lead	WB (Hep)		µg/dL			µmol/L	
		Child:	<30		× 0.0483	<1.45	
		Adult:	<40			<1.93	
		Toxic:	≥100			≥4.83	
	U, 24 h	<80 µg/L			× 0.00483	<0.39 µmol/L	
Lecithin-Cholesterol Acyltransferase *37°C*	P (Hep, EDTA, or Cit) or S	(92 ± 14.2 µmol/h)/L (SD)			× 0.0167	153 ± 0.24 U/L plasma (SD)	
Lecithin/Sphingomyelin (L/S) Ratio	Amf	2.0–5.0 indicates probable fetal lung maturity; >3.0 in diabetics				Same	
Lecithin Phosphorus	Amf	>0.10 mg/dL indicates probable adequate fetal lung maturity			× 0.3229	>0.33 mmol/L indicates probable adequate fetal lung maturity	

Clinical chemistry and toxicology (*Continued*).

Test	Specimen	Reference Range		Conversion Factor	Reference Range (International Units)
Leucine			*mg/dL*		*μmol/L*
		Premature, 1 d:	0.92 ± 0.33 (SD)	× 76.3	70 ± 25 (SD)
		Newborn, 1 d:	0.62 ± 1.43		47 ± 109
		1–3 mo:	1.36 ± 0.39		104 ± 30
		9 mo–2 y:	0.59–2.03		45–155
		3–10 y:	0.73–2.33		56–178
		6–18 y:	1.03–2.28		79–174
		Adult:	0.98–2.29		75–175
	U, 24 h		*mg/d*		*μmol/d*
		10 d–7 wk:	0.9–2.0	× 7.624	7–15
		3–12 y:	3–11		23–84
		Adult:	3–70		23–533
		or 4 ± 2 mg/g creatinine		× 0.86	or 3.4 ± 1.7 mmol/mol creatinine
Leukocyte Count (WBC Count)	WB (EDTA)		*Cells × 10^3/μL*		*Cells × 10^9/L*
		Birth:	9.0–30.0	× 10^6	9.0–30.0
		24 h:	9.4–34.0		9.4–34.0
		1 mo:	5.0–19.5		5.0–19.5
		1–3 y:	6.0–17.5		6.0–17.5
		4–7 y:	5.5–15.5		5.5–15.5
		8–13 y:	4.5–13.5		4.5–13.5
		Adult:	4.5–11.0		4.5–11.0
	CSF	0–5 mononuclear cells/μL			0–5 × 10^6 cells/L
Lipase	S				
Tietz method		<1.0 unit/mL		× 278	<278 U/L
BMD turbidimetric		Adult:	10–150 U/L		Same
		>60 y:	18–180 U/L		
β-Lipoprotein (LDL, Low-Density Lipoprotein)	S, 12–14 h fasting	28–53% of total lipoproteins		× 0.01	Mass fraction of total: 0.28–0.53

Test	Specimen	Conventional units		Factor	SI units
Lipoprotein Electrophoresis	S	Distinct β-band: negligible chylomicron and pre-β bands			
Long-Acting Thyroid Stimulating Hormone (LATS)	S	Undetectable			Undetectable
Luteinizing Hormone (hLH)	S or P (Hep); avoid EDTA		*mIU/mL*		*IU/L*
		1–3 mo, M:	22.3 ± 13.4 (SD)	× 1	22.3 ± 13.4 (SD)
		F:	17.4 ± 9.6		17.4 ± 9.6
		3–5 mo, M:	15.5 ± 11.8		15.5 ± 11.8
		F:	13.2 ± 7.6		13.2 ± 7.6
		5–7 mo, M:	17.1 ± 8.0		17.1 ± 8.0
		F:	13.4 ± 8.0		13.4 ± 8.0
		7–12 mo, M:	24.0 ± 18.3		24.0 ± 18.3
		Prepuberty, phase I, M:	3.9 ± 2.1		3.9 ± 2.1
		M, 10–13 y:	4–12		4–12
		12–14 y:	6–12		6–12
		12–17 y:	6–16		6–16
		15–18 y:	7–19		7–19
		Adult:	6–23		6–23
		F, 8–12 y:	2.0–11.5		2.0–11.5
		9–14 y:	2.0–14.0		2.0–14.0
		12–18 y:	3.0–29.0		3.0–29.0
		Follicular:	5–30		5–30
		Midcycle:	75–150		75–150
		Luteal:	3–40		3–40
		Postmenopausal:	30–200		30–200
	U		*IU/d*		
		1 wk–2 y:	0.05–3.3		Same
		2–5 y:	0.07–1.2		
		5–8 y:	0.25–2.2		
		8–11 y:	0.19–2.2		
		11–13 y:	0.48–11.28		
		13–15 y:	2.6–27.6		
		15–17 y:	4.6–24.0		
		Adult, M:	13–60		
		F:			
		Follicular:	7.2–23.5		

Clinical chemistry and toxicology (*Continued*).

Test	Specimen	Reference Range		Conversion Factor	Reference Range (International Units)
Lysozyme (Muramidase)	S or P (EDTA)	5–15 μg/mL		× 1	5–15 mg/L
Macroamylase	S	Present in ~1% of healthy subjects with normal serum amylase activity and in 2.5% of patients with abnormal activity			Same
Magnesium	S		*mEq/L*		*mmol/L*
		Newborn, 2–4 d:	1.0–1.8	× 0.5	0.5–0.9
		5 mo–6 y:	1.65±0.23(2 SD)		0.83 ± 0.12 (2 SD)
		6–12 y:	1.56 ± 0.18		0.78 ± 0.09
		12–20 y:	1.56 ± 0.21		0.78 ± 0.11
		Adult:	1.3–2.1		0.65–1.05
		(Higher in females during menses)			
	U, 24 h	6.0–10.0 mEq/d			3.00–5.00 mmol/d
Melanin	U, random	Negative			Negative
Mercury	WB (EDTA)	<5.0 μg/dL		× 0.0499	<0.25 μmol/L
	U, 24 h	<20 μg/L		× 0.00499	<0.1 μmol/L
		Toxic: >150 μg/L			>0.75 μmol/L
Metanephrine, Total	U, 24 h		*μg/mg creatinine*		*mmol/mol creatinine*
		<1 y:	0.001–4.60	× 0.547	0.0006–2.64
		1–2 y:	0.27–5.38		0.15–3.09
		2–5 y:	0.35–2.99		0.20–1.72
		5–10 y:	0.43–2.70		0.25–1.55
		10–15 y:	0.001–1.87		0.0006–1.07
		15–18 y:	0.001–0.67		0.0006–0.38
		Adult:	0.05–1.20		0.03–0.69
Methanol	WB (F^-/Ox)		*mg/L*		*mmol/L*
			<1.5	× 0.0312	<0.05

Test	Specimen		Conventional	Factor	SI
		Toxic:	>200		>6.24
	U	Occup. exp.:	<50		<1.56
	Br	<0.8 ppm		× 0.0312	<0.02
		Occup. exp.:	<2.5 ppm		<0.08
Methemoglobin (MetHb, Hemiglobin)	WB (EDTA, Hep, or ACD)	0.06–0.24 g/dL or		× 155	9.3–37.2 µmol/L*
		0.78 ± 0.37% of total Hb (SD)		× 0.01	Mass fraction of total Hb: 0.0078 ± 0.0037 (SD) (*Conv. factor based on hemoglobin, M.W. 64,500)
Methionine	S		*mg/dL*		*µmol/L*
		Premature, 1 d:	0.52 ± 0.07 (SD)	× 67.1	35 ± 5 (SD)
		Newborn, 1 d:	0.13–0.61		9–41
		1–3 mo:	0.31 ± 0.13 (SD)		21 ± 9 (SD)
		2–6 mo:	0.24–0.73		16–49
		9 mo–2 y:	0.04–0.43		3–29
		3–10 y:	0.16–0.24		11–16
		6–18 y:	0.24–0.55		16–37
		Adult:	0.09–0.60		6–40
	U, 24 h		*mg/d*		*µmol/d*
		10 d–7 wk:	0.8–2.0	× 6.70	5–13
		3–12y:	3–14		20–94
		Adult:	trace-9.0		trace-60
		or 4.5 ± 2.5 mg/g creatinine (SD)		× 0.76	or 3.4 ± 1.9 mmol/mol creatinine (SD)
Metyrapone (Metopyrone) Stimulation Test	S	11-Deoxycortisol:	>7.0 µg/dL	× 28.86	11-Deoxycortisol: >200 nmol/L
		Cortisol:	<8 µg/dL	× 27.59	Cortisol: <220 nmol/L
Dose, adult: 750 mg q 4 h × 6: child: 300 mg/m^3	U, 24 h	17-KGS:	2.5–3-fold rise, but at least 10 mg/d	× 3.467	17-KGS: 2.5–3-fold rise but at least 35 µmol/d*
		17-KS:	>2× base level		Same
		17-OHCS:	3–5× base level		Same (* Conv. factor based on DHEA, M.W. 288)

Chemistry and toxicology (*Continued*).

Test	Specimen	Reference Range	Conversion Factor	Reference Range (International Units)
Metyrapone (Metopyrone) Stimulation Test (*continued*)				
Single Dose Metyrapone Test Dose: 30 mg/kg orally with milk or snack at midnight	S, 0800 h	11-Deoxycortisol: >7 μg/dL	× 28.86	>200 nmol/L
Microsomal Antibodies, Thyroid, *see Thyroid Microsomal Antibodies*				
Molybdenum	S	0.58 ± 0.21 ng/mL (SD)	× 10.42	6.04 ± 2.19 nmol/L (SD)
Mucopolysaccharide Screen (MPS)	U, random	Negative		Negative
Myelin Basic Protein	CSF	<4 ng/mL	× 1	<4 μg/L
Myoglobin	S	M: 49 ± 17 μg/L (SD) F: 35 ± 14 μg/L Increases slightly with age		Same
	U, random	Negative		Negative
Niacin	U, 24 h	0.3–1.5 mg/d (mean: 0.6)	× 8.113	2.43–12.17 μmol/d (mean: 4.87)
Nickel	S or P (Hep)	*μg/dL* 0.11–0.46	× 170	*nmol/L* 18.7–78.2
	WB (Hep)	M: 0.45 ± 0.14 (SD) F: 0.53 ± 0.11		76.5 ± 23.8 (SD) 90.1 ± 18.7
	U, 24 h	M: 2.6±1.3 μg/d(SD) F: 2.2 ± 0.8 μg/d	× 17	44.2 ± 22.1 nmol/d (SD) 37.4 ± 13.6 nmol/d
	F	260±120 μg/d(SD)	× 0.017	4.4 ± 2.1 μmol/d (SD)

Test	Specimen	Reference range		Factor	SI reference range
	H	M: F:	0.24±0.09 μg/kg 0.19±0.04 μg/kg	× 17	4.1 ± 1.5 nmol/kg 3.2 ± 0.7 nmol/kg
Nitrites	U	Negative Toxic:	 Nitrites detected		Same
Nitrogen, Total	F	Infants: Adults:	0.11–0.52 g N/d <2 g N/d	× 71.4	7.9–37 mmol N/d <143 mmol N/d
Nonprotein Nitrogen (NPN)	WB (Ox) S	<50 mg/dL <35 mg/dL		× 0.714	<35.7 mmol/L <25.0 mmol/L
Normetanephrine, Total	P (EDTA and Na metabisulfite)	Normotensive: 1.2 ± 0.1 ng/mL (SEM) Primary hypertensive: 2.5 ± 0.2 ng/mL (SEM)		× 5.46	6.55 ± 0.55 nmol/L 13.65 ± 1.09 nmol/L
Occult Blood	F, random	Negative (<2 mL blood/150 g stool per d)		× 6.67	Negative (<13.3 mL blood/kg stool per d)
Qual.	U, random	Negative			Negative
Oleic Acid-^{125}I Absorption Test *Dose: 50 μCi in milk*	P F, 72 h	>1.7% of administered dose/L after 4–6 h Less than 5% of administered dose in 72 h specimen		× 0.01 × 0.01	Fraction of administered dose: >0.017 Fraction of administered dose: <0.05
Orosomucoid, *see* a_i*-acid Glycoprotein*					
Osmolality	S	Neonate: Child, adult: >60 y:	May be as low as 266 mOsmol/kg 275–295 mOsmol/kg 280–301 mOsmol/kg		Same
	U, random	50–1400 mOsmol/kg, depending on fluid intake			

Clinical chemistry and toxicology (*Continued*).

Test	Specimen	Reference Range		Conversion Factor	Reference Range (International Units)
Osmolality (*continued*)	U, random	After 12 h fluid restriction: >850 mOsmol/kg			Same
	U, 24 h	~300–900 mOsmol/kg			
Osmolality Ratio, Urine/Serum	U and S	1.0–3.0 >3.0 after 12 h fluid restriction			Same
Oxalate	S	1.0–2.4 μg/mL		× 11.4	11–27 μmol/L
		Ethylene glycol poisoning:	>20 μg/mL		>228 μmol/L
	U, 24 h	8–40 mg/d		× 11.4	91–456 μmol/d
		Ethylene glycol poisoning:	>150 mg/d		>1710 μmol/d
Oxygen, P_{50}	WB (Hep)	Newborn:	18–24 mm Hg	× 0.133	2.39–3.19 kPa
		Adult, adjusted to pH (P) 7.4:	25–29 mm Hg		3.33–3.86 kPa
Oxygen, Partial Pressure (pO_2)	WB, arterial (Hep)		*mm Hg*		*kPa*
		Birth:	8–24	× 0.133	1.1–3.2
		5–10 min:	33–75		4.4–10.0
		30 min:	31–85		4.1–11.3
		>1 h:	55–80		7.3–10.6
		1 d:	54–95		7.2–12.6
		Thereafter:	83–108		11.04–14.36
		(Decreases with age and high altitude)			
Oxygen Saturation	WB, arterial (Hep)				Fraction saturated:
		Newborn:	40–90%	× 0.01	0.40–0.90
		Thereafter:	95–98%		0.95–0.98
Oxytocin	P (EDTA)	<3.2 μIU/mL		× 1	<3.2 mIU/L
pO_2, see Oxygen, Partial Pressure					

Palmitic Acid, Total	Amf	Fetal maturity:	>11.5 mg/L	× 3.90	>44.9 µmol/L
		Fetal maturity:	>8.0 mg/L		>31.2 µmol/L
Pancreatic Polypeptide	S		*hPP pmol/L*		Same
		Age	*mean ± SE*		
		20–29	*12.9 ± 1.0*		
		30–39	*27.4 ± 2.9*		
		40–49	*39.3 ± 3.1*		
		50–59	*43.1 ± 6.7*		
		60–69	*49.3 ± 6.7*		
Pantothenic Acid	WB (NaCit) or S	Total:	1.03–1.83 µg/mL	× 4.56	4.70–8.34 µmol/L
Parathyroid Hormone (hPTH)	S	Varies with laboratory,			
		Mayo Clinic. Bioscience:			
		N-terminal	230–630 pg/mL	× 1	230–630 ng/L
		C-terminal	430–1860 pg/mL		430–1860 ng/L
		Nichols Institute:			
		C-terminal	40–100 µLEq/mL		40–100 mLEq/L
		Immuno Nuclear:		× 100	
		Midmolecule	0.29–0.85 ng/mL		29–85 pmol/L
		Higher in pregnancy			
Pentachlorophenol (PCP)	P (EDTA)		*mg/L*		*µmol/L*
			<1	× 3.75	<3.8
		Occup. exp.:	<20		<75.0
		Toxic:	>30		>112
	U		<0.6		<2.3
		Occup. exp.:	<39		<146
		Toxic:	>60		>225
Pentoses	U, 24 h	*Total Pentoses*			
		Fruit-free diet:	(2–5 mg/kg)/d	× 6.66	(13.3–33.3 µmol/kg)/d
			or 225 mg/d	× 0.00666	1.50 mmol/d
		Slightly higher in children			

Clinical chemistry and toxicology (*Continued*).

Test	Specimen	Reference Range		Conversion Factor	Reference Range (International Units)
Pentoses (*continued*)	U, 24 h				
		L-Xylulose:	<60 mg/d	× 6.66	<400 μmol/d
		D-Ribose:	<15 mg/d	×6.66	<100 μmol/d
		D-Ribulose:	traces		
	S	L-Xylulose:	<2 mg/dL	× 66.6	<133.2 μmol/L
Pepsinogen (PG I)	S		*ng/mL ± SEM*		*μg/L ± SEM*
		Premature:	22 ± 2	× 1	22 ± 2
		Cord:	26 ± 2		26 ± 2
		<1 y:	77 ± 5		77 ± 5
		1–2 y:	98 ± 8		98 ± 8
		3–6 y:	92 ± 12		92 ± 12
		7–10 y:	95 ± 8		95 ± 8
		11–14 y:	107 ± 11		107 ± 11
		19–38 y:	133 ± 9		133 ± 9
		Women at delivery:	127 ± 11		127 ± 11
pH (37°C)	WB, arterial (Hep)				
		Premature, 48 h:	7.35–7.50		Same
		Birth, full term:	7.11–7.36		
		5–10 min:	7.09–7.30		
		30 min:	7.21–7.38		
		>1 h:	7.26–7.49		
		1 d:	7.29–7.45		
		Therafter:	7.35–7.45		
		or H^+ conc.:	36–44 nEq/L	× 1	36–44 nmol/L
	U, random	Newborn/neonate:	5–7		Same
		Thereafter:	4.5–8		
		Average	~6		
	Serf (Plf, Pericf, Ascf)	6.8–7.6			
	Synf	Parallels serum			
	CSF	7.35–7.40			

Test	Specimen		Conventional	Factor	SI
	Semf	7.2–8.0 (average: 7.8)			
	F	7.0–7.5			
		(May be acid with high lactose intake)			
Phenols	U		*mg/L*		*μmol/L*
		Phenol:	5–8	× 10.6	53–85
		p-Cresol:	20–200	× 9.25	185–1850
		Toxic,			
		Phenol:	>10	× 10.6	>106
		o-Cresol:	>2	× 9.25	>19
		m-Cresol:	>2	× 9.25	>19
		p-Cresol:	>200	× 9.25	>1850
Phenolsulfonphthalein	U, timed		*% Dose Excreted*		*Fraction of Dose Excreted*:
Test (PSP Test) *Dose: 1 mL (6 mg). IV, 30 min after patient has voided and drunk 600 mL water*		15 min:	28–51	× 0.01	0.28–0.51
		30 min:	13–24		0.13–0.24
		60 min:	9–17		0.09–0.17
		120 min:	3–10		0.03–0.10
		Total 2 h:	63–84		0.63–0.84
Phenylalanine	S		*mg/dL*		*mmol/L*
		Premature:	2.0–7.5	× 0.06054	0.12–0.45
		Newborn:	1.2–3.4		0.07–0.21
		Adult:	0.8–1.8		0.05–0.11
	U, 24 h		*mg/d*		*μmol/d*
		10 d–7 wk:	1–2	× 6.05	6–12
		3–12 y:	4–18		24–109
		Adult:	trace-17		trace-103
		or 6 ± 2 mg/g creatinine (SD)		× 0.68	or 4.1 ± 1.4 mmol/mol creatinine (SD)
Phenylpyruvic Acid *Qual.*	U, random	Negative $FeCl_3$ test			Negative by $FeCl_3$ test
Phosphatase, Acid					
Prostatic (RIA)	S	<3.0 ng/mL		× 1	<3.0 μg/L
Roy, Brower, and Hayden, 37°C		0.11–0.60 U/L			0.11–0.60 U/L

Clinical chemistry and toxicology (*Continued*).

Test	Specimen	Reference Range		Conversion Factor	Reference Range (International Units)
Phosphatase, Alkaline	S		*U/L*		Same
p-Nitrophenyl phosphate, carbonate buffer, 30°C		Infant:	50–165		
		Child:	20–150		
		Adult:	20–70		
		>60 y:	30–75		
Bowers and McComb, 30°C					
IFCC, 30°C		Adult:	25–90		
		M:	30–90		
		F:	20–80		
Phosphatidylglycerol (PG)	Amf	Absent:	Fetal immaturity		Same
		Present:	Fetal maturity		
Phosphofructokinase (PFK) in Erythrocytes *IFCC, 30°C*	WB (ACD, EDTA, or Hep)	9.05 ± 1.89 U/g Hb (SD)		× 0.0645	0.58 ± 0.12 MU/mol Hb
		262 ± 55 U/10^{12} RBC		× 10^{-3}	0.26 ± 0.05 nU/RBC
		3.08 ± 0.64 U/mL RBC		× 1	3.08 ± 0.64 kU/L RBC
		Lower in newborns			
Phospholipids, Total	S or P (EDTA)		*mg/dL*		*g/L*
		Newborn:	75–170	× 0.01	0.75–1.70
		Infant:	100–275		1.00–2.75
		Child:	180–295		1.80–2.95
		Adult:	125–275		1.25–2.75
		>65 y:	196–366		1.96–3.66
Phosphorus, Inorganic	S		*mg/dL*		*mmol/L*
		Cord:	3.7–8.1	× 0.323	1.20–2.62
		24 h:	3.5–8.6		1.13–2.78
		24–48 h:	5.5–9.5		1.78–3.07
		Infant:	4.5–6.5		1.45–2.10
		Child:	4.5–5.5		1.45–1.78
		Thereafter:	2.7–4.5		0.87–1.45
		>60 y, M:	2.3–3.7		0.74–1.20
		F:	2.8–4.1		0.90–1.32

Test	Specimen	Reference Range (Conventional)		Factor	Reference Range (SI)
	U, 24 h	Adults on diet containing 0.9–1.5 g P and 10 mg Ca/kg: <1.0 g/d		× 32.3	Adults on diet containing 29–48 mmol P and 0.25 mmol Ca/kg: <32.3 mmol/d
		On nonrestricted diet:	0.4–1.3 g/d		On nonrestricted diet: 12.9–42.0 mmol/d
Placental Lactogen (hPL)	S		*μg/mL*		*mg/L*
		Nonpregnant F:	<0.5	× 1	<0.5
		Pregnancy (wk),			
		22:	1.0–3.8		1.0–3.8
		26:	1.5–4.5		1.5–4.5
		30:	2.8–5.8		2.8–5.8
		34:	3.4–6.9		3.4–6.9
		38:	3.6–8.2		3.6–8.2
		42:	3.0–8.0		3.0–8.0
		In diabetic patients, mean values at term: 11.0 ± 1.0			11.0 ± 1.0
	Amf	Rises slowly during pregnancy			
		<20 wk:	0.3–0.4 μg/mL(mean)	× 1	0.3–0.4 mg/L (mean)
		36–40 wk:	0.4–0.6 μg/mL(mean)	× 1	0.4–0.6 mg/L (mean)
	T, Placent.	300 μg/g		× 1	300 mg/kg
Plasma Volume	P (Hep)	M:	25–43 mL/kg	× 0.001	0.025–0.043 L/kg
		F:	28–45 mL/kg		0.028–0.045 L/kg
Porphobilinogen (PBG)					
Quant.	U, 24 h	0–2.0 mg/d		× 4.42	0–8.8 μmol/d
Qual.	U, random	Negative			Negative
Postheparin Lipolytic	P (Hep)		*(μmol FFA/min)/mL*		*U/L*
Activity		TG < 200 mg/dL:	0.24–0.57	× 1000	240–570
		TG > 200 mg/dL:	0.06–0.71		60–710
Potassium	S		*mEq/L*		*mmol/L*
		Premature,			
		Cord:	5.0–10.2	× 1	5.0–10.2
		48 h:	3.0–6.0		3.0–6.0

Clinical chemistry and toxicology (*Continued*).

Test	Specimen	Reference Range		Conversion Factor	Reference Range (International Units)
Potassium (*continued*)					
		Newborn,	*mEq/L*		*mmol/L*
		Cord:	5.6–12.0	× 1	5.6–12.0
		Newborn:	3.7–5.9		3.7–5.9
		Infant:	4.1–5.3		4.1–5.3
		Child:	3.4–4.7		3.4–4.7
		Thereafter:	3.5–5.1		3.5–5.1
	P (Hep)	M:	3.5–4.5		3.5–4.5
		F:	3.4–4.4		3.4–4.4
	U, 24 h	25–125 mEq/d; varies with diet			25–125 mmol/d; varies with diet
	CSF	70% of plasma level; 2.5–3.2 mEq/L, rise with plasma hyperosmolality		× 0.01 × 1	0.70 plasma level fraction; 2.5–3.2 mmol/L, rises with plasma hyperosmolality
	F, 24 h	~5 mEq/d		× 1	~5 mmol/d
	Gastf	~ 10 mmol/L; parietal and nonparietal juice have the same conc.		× 1	~ mmol/L; parietal and nonparietal juice have the same conc.
	RBC	~105 mEq/L		× 1	~105 mmol/L
	Sal	Without stimulation:	19–23 mEq/L	× 1	19–23 mmol/L
		With stimulation:	18–19 mEq/L		18–19 mmol/L
	Swt	5–17 mEq/L		× 1	5–17 mmol/L
Pregnancy Tests					
Chorionic Gonadotropin (hCG)					
Tube Test					
Qual.	S or U	Negative Positive by 4th–8th d after expected menstrual period			Same
Semiquant.	S or U, 24 h	Peak values up to 120,000 mIU/mL		× 1	Peak values up to 120,000 IU/L

Test	Specimen	Reference range (conventional)		Factor	Reference range (SI)
Chorionic Gonadotropin (β-hCG), see Chorionic Gonadotropin, β-Subunit					
Radio Receptor Assay *(RRA)* *Qual.*	S	Negative; pregnancy can be detected <10 d after conception			Same
Pregnanediol	U, 24 h		*mg/d*		*μmol/d*
		<2 y:	<0.1	× 3.12	<0.3
		3–5 y:	<0.3		<0.9
		6–9 y:	<0.5		<1.6
		M, Adult:	0.1–0.7		0.3–2.2
		F, 10–15 y:	0.1–1.2		0.3–3.7
		Adult,			
		Follicular:	<1.0		<3.1
		Luteal:	2–7		6.2–21.8
		Postmenopausal:	0.2–1.0		6.2–3.1
		Pregnancy (wk),			
		16:	5–21		16–65
		20:	6–26		19–81
		24:	12–32		37–100
		28:	19–51		59–160
		32:	22–66		69–206
		36:	13–77		41–240
		40:	23–63		72–197
Pregnanetriol	U, 24 h		*mg/d*		*μmol/d*
		2 wk–2 y:	0.02–0.2	× 2.97	0.06–0.59
		2–5 y:	<0.5		<1.49
		5–15 y:	<1.5		<4.46
		>15 y:	<2.0		<5.94
Pregnenolone	S	Adult:	0.3–2.0 ng/mL	× 3.16	0.95–6.32 nmol/L
Progesterone	S		*ng/mL*		*nmol/L*
		M, Pub. stage I:	0.11–0.26	× 3.18	0.35–0.83
		Adult:	0.12–0.3		0.38–0.95

Clinical chemistry and toxicology (*Continued*).

Test	Specimen	Reference Range		Conversion Factor	Reference Range (International Units)
Progesterone (*continued*)			*ng/mL*		*nmol/L*
		F, Pub. stage I:	0–0.3	× 3.18	0–0.95
		II:	0–0.46		0–1.46
		III:	0–0.6		0–1.91
		IV:	0.05–13.0		0.16–41.3
		Follicular:	0.02–0.9		0.06–2.86
		Luteal:	6.0–30.0		19.1–95.4
Progesterone Receptor Assay (PRA)	T, tumor		*fmol/mg protein*		*nmol/kg protein*
		Normal, or benign and nonresponsive tumor:	≤5	× 1	≤5
		Positive:	>10		>10
Proinsulin	S	<30% of total immunoreactive insulin-like material, or <0.2 ng/mL		× 0.01	Fraction of immunoreactive insulin-like material: 0.30, or <0.2 μg/L
Prolactin (hPRL)	S		*ng/mL*		*μg/L*
		Adults, M:	<20	× 1	<20
		F, Folicular:	<23		<23
		Luteal:	5–40		5–40
		Pregnancy,			
		1st trimester:	<80		<80
		2nd trimester:	<160		<160
		3rd trimester:	<400		<400
		Newborn:	>10-fold adult levels		
Prolactin-Insulin Stimulation Test *Dose, adult: 0.5 g arginine HCl/kg, IV, over 30 min*	S	Peak values:	1.4–19.0×baseline within 35–75 min after stimulation		Same

Test	Specimen		Conventional	Factor	SI
Properdin	S		*mg/dL ± SD*		*mg/L ± SD*
		Cord:	1.5 ± 0.1	× 10	15 ± 1
		1 mo:	1.4 ± 0.4		14 ± 4
		6 mo:	1.9 ± 0.3		19 ± 3
		Adult:	2.8 ± 0.4		28 ± 4
Prostaglandins, E	P (Hep)	25–200 pg/mL		× 2.82	71–564 pmol/L
F		25–150 pg/mL			71–423 pmol/L
Protein					
Total	S		*g/dL*		*g/L*
		Premature:	3.6–6.0	× 10	36–60
		Newborn:	4.6–7.0		46–70
		Cord:	4.8–8.0		48–80
		1 wk:	4.4–7.6		44–76
		7 mo–1 y:	5.1–7.3		51–73
		1–2 y:	5.6–7.5		56–75
		⩾3 y:	6.0–8.0		60–80
		Adult,			
		Ambulatory:	6.4–8.3		64–83
		Recumbent:	6.0–7.8		60–78
		>60 y:	lower by ~0.2		~2
Electrophoresis		Albumin,	*g/dL*		*g/L*
		Adult:	3.5–5.0		35–50
		>60 y:	3.7–4.7		37–47
		α_1-Globulin,			
		Adult:	0.1–0.3		1–3
		>60 y:	0.2–0.5		2–5
		α_2-Globulin,			
		Adult:	0.6–1.0		6–10
		>60 y:	0.5–1.1		5–11
		β-Globulin,			
		Adult:	0.7–1.1		7–11
		>60 y:	0.5–1.2		5–12
		γ-Globulin,			
		Adult:	0.8–1.6		8–16
		>60 y:	0.6–1.6		6–16

Clinical chemistry and toxicology (*Continued*).

Test	Specimen	Reference Range		Conversion Factor	Reference Range (International Units)
Protein (*continued*)					
Total	U, 24 h	1–14 mg/dL		× 10	10–140 mg/L
		50–80 mg/d (at rest)			Same
		<250 mg/d after intense exercise			
Electrophoresis			*Average % of Total Protein*		*Fraction of Total*
		Albumin	37.9	× 0.01	0.379
		α_1-Globulin	27.3		0.273
		α_2-Globulin	19.5		0.195
		β-Globulin	8.8		0.088
		γ-Globulin	3.3		0.033
Total	CSF, lumbar				*mg/L*
Column		8–32 mg/dL		× 10	80–320
Turbidimetry			*>mg/dL*		
		Premature:	15–130		150–1300
		Full-term newborn:	40–120		400–1200
		<1 mo:	20–80		200–800
		Thereafter:	15–40		150–400
Electrophoresis			*% of Total*		*Fraction of Total*
		Prealbumin:	2–7	× 0.01	0.02–0.07
		Albumin:	56–76		0.56–0.76
		α_1-Globulin:	2–7		0.02–0.07
		α_2-Globulin:	4–12		0.04–0.12
		β-Globulin:	8–18		0.08–0.18
		γ-Globulin:	3–12		0.03–0.12
Electrophoresis	Synf	Albumin:	63		0.63
		α_1-Globulin:	7		0.07
		α_2-Globulin:	7		0.07
		β-Globulin:	9		0.09
		γ-Globulin:	14		0.14
		Fibrinogen:	0		0

Prothrombin Time	WB (NaCit)				
One-stage (Quick)		In general:	11–15 s (varies with type of thromboplastin)		Same
		Newborn:	Prolonged by 2–3 s		
Two-stage modified (Ware and Seegers)		18–22 s			
Protoporphyrin	WB (Hep or EDTA)	<50 μg/dL RBC		× 0.0178	<0.89 μmol/L RBC
	F, 24 h	≤60 μg/g dry wt or <1500 μg/d		× 0.00178	≤0.11 mmol/kg dry wt or <2.67 μmol/d
Pseudocholinesterase (PChE), *see Cholinesterase II*					
Pyruvic Acid	WB (Hep)	0.3–0.9 mg/dL		× 0.114	0.03–0.10 mmol/L
	U	88.1 mg/d		× 0.0114	1 mmol/d
	CSF	0.5–1.7 mg/dL		× 0.114	0.06–0.19 mmol/L
Renal Plasma Flow (RPF)	P and U	M:	560–830 mL/min	× 0.01667	9.34–13.84 mL/s
		F:	490–700 mL/min		8.17–11.67 mL/s
		or (390 mL/min)m^2 body surface			or (6.50 mL/s)m^2 body surface
		>40 y:	decreases~75 mL/decade		
Renin	P (EDTA)	*Normal sodium diet:*			
			(ng/h)/mL ± SE		μg·h^{-1}·L^{-1} ± *SE*
		Supine:	1.6 ± 1.5	× 1	1.6 ± 1.5
		Standing (4 h):	4.5 ± 2.9		4.5 ± 2.9
		Low sodium:			
		Supine:	3.2 ± 1.1		3.2 ± 1.1
		Standing (4 h):	9.9 ± 4.3		9.9 ± 4.3
Reverse Triiodothyronine (rT_3)	S		*ng/dL*		*nmol/L*
		1–5 y:	15–71	× 0.0154	0.23–1.09
		5–10 y:	17–79		0.26–1.22
		10–15 y:	19–88		0.29–1.36
		Adults:	30–80		0.46–1.23

Clinical chemistry and toxicology (*Continued*).

Test	Specimen	Reference Range		Conversion Factor	Reference Range (International Units)
Riboflavin (Vitamin B_2)	U, random		*μg/g creatinine*		*μmol/mol creatinine*
		1–3 y:	500–900	× 0.3	150–270
		4–6 y:	300–600		90–180
		7–9 y:	270–500		81–150
		10–15 y:	200–400		60–120
		Adult:	80–269		24–81
		Pregnancy:	90–120		27–36
Schilling Test (Intrinsic Factor Test) *Dose: 0.5–1.0* μCi ^{58}*Co-Vitamin* B_{12}	U, 24 h	>7.5% of dose		× 0.01	Fraction of dose: 0.075
Secretin	S or P (Hep or EDTA)	37 ± 8 pg/mL (SD)		× 1	37 ± 8 ng/L (SD)
Selenium	WB (Hep)	10–34 μg/dL Serum approx. 20% lower		× 0.127	1.27–4.32 μmol/L
	U, 24 h	10–100 μg/L		× 0.0127	0.13–1.27 μmol/L
Serotonin	WB (EDTA)	39–361 mg/mL		× 0.00568	0.22–2.05 μmol/L
	Pit	~314 ng/10^9 platelets		× 0.00568	~1.78 amol/platelet
Sodium	S or P (Hep)		*mEq/L*		*mmol/L*
		Premature, Cord:	116–140	× 1	116–140
		48 h:	128–148		128–148
		Newborn, Cord:	126–166		126–166
		Newborn:	134–144		134–144
		Infant:	139–146		139–146
		Child:	138–145		138–145
		Thereafter:	136–146		136–146
	U, 24 h	40–220 mEq/d (diet dependent)		× 1	40–220 mmol/d
	Swt	10–40 mEq/L		× 1	10–40 mmol/L

Test	Specimen	Conventional			Factor	SI	
		Cystic fibrosis:		>70 mEq/L		>70 mmol/L	
Somatomedin C	P (EDTA)	0.4–2.0 IU/mL			× 1000	400–2000 IU/L	
Specific Gravity	U, random	Newborn:		1.012		Same	
		Infant:		1.002–1.006			
		Adult:		1.002–1.030			
		After 12 h fluid restriction:		>1.025			
	U, 24 h	1.015–1.025					
Sucrose	S or P	Mean:	0.06 mg/dL		× 29.21	1.75 µmol/L	
	U	Mean:	2.2 mg/dL			64.26 µmol/L	
Sulfhemoglobin	WB (EDTA, Hep or ACD)	≤1.0% of total Hb			× 0.01	≤0.010 of total Hb (mass fraction)	
Testosterone, Free	S		*ng/dL* (mean ± *SE)*	*% of Total*		*pmol/L (mean ± SE)*	*Fraction of Total*
		Cord,					
		M:	1.0 ± 0.4	2.9 ± 0.6	× 34.7	34.7 ± 13.9	0.029 ± 0.006
		F:	0.89 ± 0.29	3.0 ± 0.5	and	30.9 ± 10.1	0.03 ± 0.005
		1–15 d,			× 0.01		
		M:	0.8 ± 0.8	1.3 ± 0.2		27.8 ± 27.8	0.013 ± 0.002
		F:	0.14 ± 0.06	1.2 ± 0.2		4.9 ± 2.1	0.012 ± 0.002
		Prepubertal,					
		M:	0.04 ± 0.01	0.7 ± 0.2		1.4 ± 0.35	0.007 ± 0.002
		F:	0.04 ± 0.01	0.7 ± 0.1		1.4 ± 0.35	0.007 ± 0.001
		Adult,					
		M:	7.9 ± 2.3	1.4 ± 0.3		274 ± 80	0.014 ± 0.003
		F:	0.31 ± 0.07	0.9 ± 0.2		10.8 ± 2.4	0.009 ± 0.002
Testosterone, Total	S			*ng/dL ± SD*		*nmol/L ± SD*	
		Cord, M:		39 ± 11	× 0.0347	1.35 ± 0.38	
		F:		30 ± 7		1.04 ± 0.24	
		1–15 d, M:		68 ± 60		2.36 ± 2.08	
		F:		12 ± 6		0.42 ± 0.21	
		1–3 mo, M:		208 ± 68		7.22 ± 2.36	
		F:		9 ± 4		0.31 ± 0.14	

Clinical chemistry and toxicology (*Continued*).

Test	Specimen	Reference Range		Conversion Factor	Reference Range (International Units)
Testosterone, Total					
(*continued*)			*ng/dL ± SD*		*nmol/L ± SD*
	S	3–5 mo, M:	95 ± 53		0.30 ± 1.84
		F:	6.7 ± 2.7		0.23 ± 0.09
		5–7 mo, M:	23 ± 18		0.80 ± 0.62
		F:	6.8 ± 3.1		0.24 ± 0.11
		7–12 mo, M:	6.6 ± 4.6		0.23 ± 0.16
		F:	5.5 ± 2.8		0.19 ± 0.10
		Prepubertal, M:	6.6 ± 2.5		0.23 ± 0.09
		F:	6.6 ± 2.5		0.23 ± 0.09
		Adult, M:	572 ± 135		19.85 ± 4.68
		F:	37 ± 10		1.28 ± 0.35
		Pregnancy: (Level unrelated to sex of fetus)	114 ± 38		3.96 ± 1.32
	U, 24 h		*μg/kg Body Weight*		*nmol/kg Body Weight*
		Pubertal stage I, M:	0.25	× 3.47	0.87
		F:	0.16		0.56
		II, M:	0.34		1.18
		F:	0.16		0.56
		III, M:	0.37		1.28
		F:	0.16		0.56
			μg/d		*nmol/d*
		20–50 y, M:	50–135	× 3.47	173–470
		F:	2–12		7–42
		>50 y, M:	40–60		139–210
		F:	2–8		7–28

Test	Specimen	Reference range	ng/dL Median	ng/dL Range	Factor	nmol/L Median	nmol/L Range
	Amf	Fetal age (wk)					
		9–12, M:	5.0	2.0–72.6	× 0.0347	0.17	0.07–2.52
		F:	2.7	1.3–4.0		0.09	0.05–0.14
		12–16, M:	25.0	7.0–72.4		0.87	0.24–2.51
		F:	2.6	1.3–10.0		0.09	0.05–0.35
		16–19, M:	19.3	8.4–23.0		0.67	0.29–0.80
		F:	2.9	1.0–9.0		0.10	0.03–0.31
		28–34, M:	12.3	84.0–26.4		0.43	0.92–2.91
		34–40, M:	18.0	2.0–16.0		0.62	0.07–0.56
		F:	3.4	2.2–10.2		0.12	0.08–0.35
Tetrahydrocortisol (THF)	U, 24 h	Adult:	0.5–1.5 mg/d		× 2.72	Adult: 1.4–4.1 µmol/d	
Tetrahydrodeoxy-cortisol	U, 24 h	<1000 µg/d			× 0.0029	<2.9 µmol/d	
		10-fold increase over baseline after metyrapone				Same	
Thallium	WB (NaHep)	0.5 µg/dL			× 48.9	24.5 nmol/L	
		Toxic:	10–800 µg/dL		× 0.0489	0.5–39.1 µmol/L	
	U, 24 h	<2.0 µg/L			× 4.89	<9.78 nmol/L	
		Toxic:	1.0–20.0 mg/L			4.9–97.8 µmol/L	
Thyroglobulin (Tg)	S	<50 ng/mL			× 1	<50 µg/L	
Thyroid Antibodies	S	Adult:	≤1:10 dilution			Same	
		Child:	≤1:4				
Thyroid Microsomal Antibodies	S	Nondetectable (hemagglutination) or <1:10 (IFA)				Same	

Clinical chemistry and toxicology (*Continued*).

Test	Specimen	Reference Range		Conversion Factor	Reference Range (International Units)
Thyroid Stimulating	S or P		*μIU/mL*		*mIU/L*
Hormone (hTSH)		Cord:	3–12	× 1	3–12
		Newborn:	3–20		3–20
		Child:	4.5 ± 3.6 (SD)		4.5 ± 3.6 (SD)
		Adult:	<10		<10
		>60 y, M:	2–7.3		2–7.3
		F:	2–16.8		2–16.8
Thyroid Stimulating Hormone–Response to TRH *Dose, adult: 400–500 μg TRH (Thypinone). IV, rapid; child: 7 μg/kg*	S	30 min after stimulation:	*μIU/mL*		*mIU/L*
		Child:	11–35	× 1	11–35
		Adult, M:	15–30		15–30
		F:	20–40		20–40
Thyroid Uptake of Radioactive Iodine, ^{131}I, ^{125}I, or ^{123}I					*Activity Fraction*
		2 h:	<6%	× 0.01	<0.06
		6 h:	3–20%		0.03–0.20
		24 h:	8–30%		0.08–0.30
Thyroid Uptake of $^{99m}TcO_4^-$		Uptake ratio:	<1.15 in euthyroid		<1.15
Thyrotropin Releasing Hormone (hTRH)	P	Newborn, 30 min after delivery:	78 pg/mL (mean), falling to normal at 24 h	× 1	78 ng/L (mean)
		Adult:	5–60 pg/mL		5–60 ng/L

	U, 24 h	Adult, M:	195 ng/d (mean)		Same
		F:	119 ng/d (mean)		
Thyrotropin Releasing Hormone Stimulation Test *Dose, adult: 500 µg TRH, IV*	S	TSH within 30 min,			TSH within 30 min,
		<40 y:	>6 µIU/mL rise		<40 y: >6 mIU/L rise
		>40 y, M:	>2 µIU/mL rise		>40 y, M: >2 mIU/L rise
		hPRL:	3–5-fold rise above baseline (diminishes with age)		hPRL: 3–5-fold rise above baseline (diminishes with age)
Thyroxine Binding Globulin (TBG)	S		*mg/dL*		*mg/L*
		Cord:	1.4–9.4	× 10	14–94
		1–4 wk:	1.0–9.0		10–90
		1–12 mo:	2.0–7.6		20–76
		1–5 y:	2.9–5.4		29–54
		5–10 y:	2.5–5.0		25–50
		10–15 y:	2.1–4.6		21–46
		Adult:	1.5–3.4		15–34
		Pregnancy, last 5 mo:	5.6–10.2		56–102
		As T_4 binding capacity, Adult:	10–25 µg/dL		As T_4 binding capacity, Adult: 100–250 µg/L
Thyroxine, Free (FT_4)	S	0.8–2.4 ng/dL		× 12.9	10.3–31.0 pmol/L
Thyroxine Index, Free, *See Free Thyroxine Index*					
Thyroxine Ratio, Effective (ETR)		0.86–1.13		× 1	0.86–1.13
Thyroxine/TBG Ratio	S	0.2–0.5 T_4 (µg/dL)/TBG (µg/mL)		× 12.9	2.6–6.4 T_4 (nmol/L)/TBG (mg/L)

Clinical chemistry and toxicology (*Continued*).

Test	Specimen	Reference Range		Conversion Factor	Reference Range (International Units)
Thyroxine (T_4), Total	S		*μg/dL*		*nmol*L
		Cord:	8–13	12.9	103–168
		Newborn:	11.5–24		148–310
		Neonate:	9–18		116–232
		Infant:	7–15		90–194
		1–5 y:	7.3–15		94–194
		5–10 y:	6.4–13.3		83–172
		Adult:	5–12		65–155
		>60 y, M:	5–10		65–129
		F:	5.5–10.5		71–135
		Pregnancy, last 5 mo:	6.1–17.6		79–227
Transcortin	S		*mg/dL*		*mg/L*
		M:	1.5–2.0	× 10	15–20
		F, Follicular:	1.7–2.0		17–20
		Luteal:	1.6–2.1		16–21
		Postmenopausal:	1.7–2.5		17–25
		Pregnancy, 21–28 wk:	4.7–5.4		47–54
		33–40 wk:	5.5–7.0		55–70
Transferrin	S		*mg/dL*		*g/L*
Nephelometric		Newborn:	130–275	× 0.01	1.30–2.75
		Adult:	220–400		2.20–4.00
		>60 y:	180–380		1.80–3.80
Transketolase					
Ribose/sedoheptulose, 37°C	WB (Hep)	(9–12 μmol/h)/mL whole blood		× 16.67	150–200 U/L whole blood
		If Hct is abnormal: (2.1–2.4 μmol/h)/10^9 red cells		× 0.0167	0.035–0.040 nU/red cell

Test	Specimen		mg/dL M	mg/dL F	Factor	mmol/L M	mmol/L F
Triglycerides (TG) *Fluorometric; colorimetric*	S, ≥12-h fast		*M*	*F*		*M*	*F*
		Cord blood:	10–98	10–98	× 0.0113	0.11–1.11	0.11–1.11
		0–5 y:	30–86	32–99		0.34–0.97	0.36–1.12
		6–11 y:	31–108	35–114		0.35–1.22	0.40–1.29
		12–15 y:	36–138	41–138		0.41–1.56	0.46–1.56
		16–19 y:	40–163	40–128		0.45–1.84	0.45–1.45
		20–29 y:	44–185	40–128		0.50–2.09	0.45–1.45
		30–39 y:	49–284	38–160		0.55–3.21	0.43–1.81
		40–49 y:	56–298	44–186		0.63–3.37	0.50–2.10
		50–59 y:	62–288	55–247		0.70–3.25	0.62–2.79
		Values decrease slightly after age 60 Levels for Blacks: 10–20 mg/dL lower				Levels for Blacks: 0.11–0.23 mmol/L lower	
		Recommended (desirable) levels for adults:					
		Male:	40–160 mg/dL			0.45–1.81 mmol/L	
		Female:	35–135 mg/dL			0.40–1.53 mmol/L (Conv. factor based on triolein, M.W. 885)	
Triiodothyronine, Free	S		*mean pg/dL*			*mean pmol/L*	
		Cord:	130 ± 10 (SE)		× 0.0154	2.0 ± 0.15 (SE)	
		1–3 d:	410 ± 20			6.31 ± 0.31	
		6 wk:	400 ± 20			6.16 ± 0.31	
		Adult (20–50 y):	230–660 pg/dL			3.54–10.16 pmol/L	
			% of Total			*Fraction of Total*	
Triiodothyronine Resin Uptake Test (T_3RU)	S	Newborn:	25–37		× 0.01	0.25–0.37	
		Adult:	24–34			0.24–0.34	
		>60 y, M:	24–32			0.24–0.32	
		F:	22–32			0.22–0.32	

Clinical chemistry and toxicology (*Continued*).

Test	Specimen	Reference Range		Conversion Factor	Reference Range (International Units)
Triiodothyronine, Total	S		*ng/dL*		*nmol/L*
T_3 (RIA)		Cord:	30–70	× 0.0154	0.46–1.08
		Newborn:	65–275		0.98–4.26
		1–5 y:	100–260		1.54–4.00
		5–10 y:	90–240		1.39–3.70
		10–15 y:	80–210		1.23–3.23
		Adult:	120–195		1.85–3.00
		>60 y, M:	105–175		1.62–2.69
		F:	108–205		1.66–3.16
Triolein-^{131}I Absorption Test	P	>1.7% of administered dose/L after 4–6 h		× 0.01	Fraction of administered dose: 0.017/L
Dose: 50 μCi in milk	F, 72 h	<5% of administered dose in 72 h specimen			Fraction of administered dose: <0.50/72 h
Tubular Reabsorption of Phosphate (TRP)	U, 4 h (0800–1200 h) and S	82–95%		× 0.01	Fraction: 0.82–0.95
Tyrosine	S		*mg/dL*		*mmol/L*
Fluorometric		Premature:	7.0–24.0	× 55.2	386–1325
		Newborn:	1.6–3.7		88–204
		Adult:	0.8–1.3		44–72
Urea, *see Urea Nitrogen*					
Urea Nitrogen	S		*mg/dL*		*mmol urea/L*
		Cord:	21–40	× 0.357	7.5–14.3
		Premature (1 wk):	3–25		1.1–8.9
		Newborn:	4–12		1.4–4.3
		Infant/child:	5–18		1.8–6.4
		Adult:	7–18		2.5–6.4
		>60 y:	8–21		2.9–7.5
		Higher after protein intake			

Test	Specimen	Group	Conventional units	Factor	SI units
Urea Nitrogen/Creatinine Ratio	S	12/1 to 20/1			12/1 to 20/1
Uric Acid					
Phosphotungstate	S		*mg/dL*		*mmol/L*
		Adult, M:	4.5–8.2	× 0.059	0.27–0.48
		F:	3.0–6.5		0.18–0.38
		>60 y, M:	4.2–8.0		0.25–0.47
		F:	3.2–7.3		0.19–0.43
Uricase		Child:	2.0–5.5		0.12–0.32
		Adult, M:	3.5–7.2		0.21–0.42
		F:	2.6–6.0		0.15–0.35
	U, 24 h		*mg/d*		*mmol/d*
		Free purine diet, M:	<420	× 0.0059	<2.48
		F:	slightly lower		slightly lower
		Low purine diet, M:	<480		<2.83
		F:	<400		<2.36
		High purine diet:	<1000		<5.90
		Average diet:	250–750		1.48–4.43
Urine Volume	U, 24 h		*mL/d*		Same
		Newborn (1–2 d):	30–60		
		Infant, 3–10 d:	100–300		
		10–60 d:	250–450		
		60–365 d:	400–500		
		Child, 1–3 y:	500–600		
		3–5 y:	600–700		
		5–8 y:	650–1000		
		8–14 y:	800–1400		
		Adult, M:	800–1800		
		F:	600–1600		
		Older adult:	250–2400		
		(varies with water intake and other factors)			

Clinical chemistry and toxicology (*Continued*).

Test	Specimen	Reference Range		Conversion Factor	Reference Range (International Units)
Urobilinogen	U, 2 h	0.1–0.8 EU*/2 h			Same
	U, 24 h	0.5–4.0 EU/d			
	F	75–275 EU/100 g		× 10	750–2750 EU*/kg
		75–400 EU/d			75–400 EU/d
		40–280 mg/d		× 1.69	67–473 μmol/d
		*Ehrlich Unit			
Uroporphyrin	U, 24 h	<50 μg/d		× 1.2	<60 nmol/d
	F, 24 h	10–40 μg/d			12–48 nmol/d
	RBC (Hep or EDTA)	Negative			Negative
Valine	S		*mg/dL*		*μmol/L*
		Premature, 1 d:	1.52 ± 0.59 (SD)	× 1	130 ± 50 (SD)
		Newborn, 1 d:	0.94–2.88		80–246
		1–3 mo:	2.27 ± 0.57 (SD)		194 ± 49 (SD)
		9 mo–2 y:	0.67–3.07		57–262
		3–10 y:	1.50–3.31		128–283
		6–18 y:	1.83–3.37		156–288
		Adult:	1.65–3.71		141–317
	U, 24 h		*mg/d*		*μmol/d*
		10 d–7 wk:	1–3	× 8.53	9–26
		3–12 y:	2–6		17–51
		Adult:	2–12		17–102
		or 4 ± 1 mg/g creatinine (SD)		× 0.97	or 3.9 ± 1.0 mmol/mol creatinine (SD)

Test	Specimen		Conventional Units	Factor	SI Units
Vanillylmandelic Acid (Vanillmandelic Acid)	U, 24 h		*mg/d*		*μmol/d*
		Newborn:	<1.0	× 5.05	<5.1
		Neonate:	<1.0		<5.1
		Infant:	<2.0		<10.1
		Child:	1–5		5.1–25.3
		Adolescent:	1–5		5.1–25.3
		Thereafter:	2–7		10.1–35.4
		or 1.5–7 μg/mg creatinine		× 0.571	or 0.86–4.00 mmol/mol creatinine
Vasoactive Intestinal Polypeptide (VIP)	P (Hep)	20–53 pg/mL		× 1	20–53 ng/L
Viscosity	S	1.10–1.22 Centipoise		× 1	1.10–1.22 Centipoise
Vitamin A	S		*μg/dL*		*μmol/L*
		Newborn:	35–75	× 0.0349	1.22–2.62
		Child:	30–80		1.05–2.79
		Adult:	30–65		1.05–2.27
Vitamin A Tolerance Test *Dose: 5000 U vit. A in oil/kg orally*	S	3 and/or 6 h: 200–600 μg vit. A/dL		× 0.0349	7–21 μmol/L
Vitamin B_2, *see Riboflavin*					
Vitamin B_6	P (EDTA)	3.6–18 ng/mL		× 4.046	14.6–72.8 nmol/L
Vitamin B_{12}, True	S	100–700 pg/mL		× 0.738	74–516 pmol/L
		>60 y:	110–800 pg/mL		81–590 pmol/L
Vitamin B_{12}, Intrinsic Factor	Gastf	50–400% enhancement of $^{57}Co\text{-}B_{12}$ uptake by GPIMH* *Guinea pig intestinal mucosal homogenate		× 0.01	Fractional increase in $^{57}Co\text{-}B_{12}$ uptake by GPIMH*: 0.50–4.00

Clinical chemistry and toxicology (*Continued*).

Test	Specimen	Reference Range		Conversion Factor	Reference Range (International Units)
Vitamin C *Dinitrophenylhydrazine, colorimetric*	P (Ox, Hep, or EDTA)	0.6–2.0 mg/dL		× 56.78	34–114 μmol/L
	Buffy coat (Hep)	20–53 μg/10^8 WBC		× 0.568	11.4–30.1 amol/cell
Vitamin C Saturation Test *Dose: 0.5–2.0 g ascorbate orally over a period of 4 d*	U, 24 h	60–80% of test dose excreted		× 0.01	Fraction test dose excreted: 0.60–0.80
Vitamin D_3, 1,25-dihydroxy	S	25–45 pg/mL		× 2.4	60–108 pmol/L
Vitamin D_3, 25-hydroxy	P (Hep)	Summer: Winter:	15–80 ng/mL 14–42 ng/mL	× 2.496	37.4–200 nmol/L 34.9–105 nmol/L
Vitamin E	S	5.0–20 μg/mL		× 2.32	11.6–46.4 μmol/L
Xylene	WB (F/Ox)	Negative			Negative
		Occup. exp.: Toxic:	<1 mg/L >3 mg/L	× 9.42	<9.4 *μmol/L* >28.3 *μmol/L*
Xylose Absorption	WB (NaF)		*mg/dL*		*mmol/L*
Test		Child, 1 h (5 g dose): Adult, 2 h (25 g dose):	>20 >25	× 0.0666	>1.33 >1.67
	U, 5 h	Child: 16–33% of ingested dose		× 0.01	Fraction ingested dose: 0.16–0.33
		Adult,	*g/5 h*		*mmol/5 h*
		5 g dose: 25 g dose: >65 y:	>1.2 >4.0 >3.5	× 6.66	>8.00 >26.64 >23.31
Zinc	S	70–150 μg/dL		× 0.153	10.7–22.9 μmol/L

Reprinted with permission from *Textbook of Clinical Chemistry*, N. W. Tietz (Ed.), WB Saunders Co., Philadelphia, PA.

APPENDIX B

Drugs–Therapeutic and Toxic Ranges

Doses for drugs listed as part of the protocol for laboratory tests, as well as their therapeutic and toxic ranges, are those commonly accepted on the basis of present knowledge. The constant acquisition of new knowledge makes it necessary to confirm and compare information supplied in this appendix with data furnished by manufacturers; additional experience with these drugs may lead to revised values. It should also be considered that there are significant differences in drug response among individuals. Where no therapeutic or toxic level is given, it was felt by the authors that there are presently no reliable data available.

Data collected for therapeutic monitoring requires careful coordination between the time of sampling and drug administration. Therefore, recommendations have been made regarding the optimal time for sampling of many drugs. Hours in parenthesis indicate the minimum sampling times. The interested reader can read about the identity, toxicology and side effects of each drug in the current edition of the *Physicians Desk Reference*.

For convenience and to preserve space, we have used standard abbreviations commonly used in laboratory medicine. Less common abbreviations and some non-standard abbreviations are given below.

Abbreviations

EDTA	ethylenediaminetetraacetate, acetic acid	prem.	premature
		S	serum
Hep	heparin	Therap.	therapeutic
Occup. exp.	occupational exposure	U	urine
P	plasma	WB	whole blood

Drug	Specimen	Reference Range		Conversion Factor	Reference Range (International Units)
Acetaminophen	S or P (Hep or EDTA)	Therap.:	10–30 μg/mL	× 6.62	66–199 μmol/L
		Toxic:	>200 μg/mL		>1324 μmol/L
Amikacin	S or P (EDTA)	Therap.,	*μg/mL*		*μmol/L*
		Peak:	25–35	× 1.71	43–60
		Trough (less severe infection):	1–4		1.7–6.8
		(life-threatening infection):	4–8		6.8–13.7
		Toxic,			
		Peak:	>35–40		>60–68
		Trough:	>10–15		>17–26
ε-Aminocaproic Acid	S or P (Hep or EDTA); trough	Therap.:	>130 μg/mL	× 7.62	>991 μmol/L
Amitriptyline	S or P (Hep or EDTA); trough (>12 h after dose)	Therap.:	120–250 ng/mL	× 3.61	433–903 nmol/L
		Toxic:	>500 ng/mL		>1805 nmol/L

Amobarbital, quant.	S	Therap.:	1–5 μg/mL	× 4.42	4–22 μmol/L
		Toxic:	>10 μg/mL		>44 μmol/L
Amphetamine	S or P (Hep or EDTA)	Therap.:	20–30 ng/mL	× 7.40	148–222 nmol/L
		Toxic:	>200 ng/mL		>1480 nmol/L
Bromide	S	Therap.:	750–1500 μg/mL	× 0.0125	9.4–18.7 mmol/L
		Toxic:	>1250 μg/mL		>15.6 mmol/L
Caffeine	S or P (Hep or EDTA)	Therap.:	3–15 μg/mL	× 5.15	15–77 μmol/L
		Toxic:	>50 μg/mL		>258 μmol/L
Carbamazepine	S or P (Hep or EDTA); trough	Therap.:	8–12 μg/mL	× 4.23	34–51 μmol/L
		Toxic:	>15 μg/mL		>63 μmol/L
Carbenicillin	S or P (Hep or EDTA)	Therap.:	Dependent on minimum inhibition conc. of specific organism		Same
		Toxic:	>250 μg/mL (neurotoxicity)	× 2.64	>660 μmol/L

Drugs — therapeutic and toxic (*Continued*).

Drug	Specimen	Reference Range		Conversion Factor	Reference Range (International Units)
Chloral Hydrate	S	As trichloroethanol: Therap.: Toxic:	 2–12 μg/mL >20 μg/mL	× 6.69	13–80 μmol/L >134 μmol/L
Chloramphenicol	S or P (Hep or EDTA); trough	Therap.: Toxic:	10–25 μg/mL >25 μg/mL	× 3.09	31–77 μmol/L >77 μmol/L
Chlordiazepoxide	S or P (Hep or EDTA); trough	Therap.: Toxic:	700–1000 ng/mL >5000 ng/mL	× 0.0033	2.34–3.34 μmol/L >16.7 μmol/L
Chlorpromazine	S or P (Hep or EDTA); trough	Therap.: Toxic:	50–300 ng/mL >750 ng/mL	× 3.14	157–942 nmol/L >2355 nmol/L
Cimetidine	S or P (Hep or EDTA); trough	Therap.:	>1.0 μg/mL	× 3.96	>4.0 μmol/L
Clonazepam	S or P (Hep or EDTA); trough	Therap.: Toxic:	15–60 ng/mL >80 ng/mL	× 3.17	48–190 nmol/L >254 nmol/L
Clonidine	S or P (Hep or EDTA)	Therap.:	1.0–2.0 ng/mL	× 4.35	4.4–8.7 nmol/L

Clorazepate	S or P (Hep or EDTA)	As desmethyldiazepam: Therap.:	0.12–1.0 μg/mL	× 3.01	0.36–3.01 μmol/L
Cocaine	S or P (Hep or EDTA); on ice	Therap.: Toxic:	100–500 ng/mL >1000 ng/mL	× 3.3	330–1650 nmol/L >3300 nmol/L
Desipramine	S or P (Hep or EDTA); trough (≥12 h after dose)	Therap.: Toxic:	75–160 ng/mL >1000 ng/mL	× 3.75	281–600 nmol/L >3750 nmol/L
Desmethylmethsuximide	S	Therap.: Toxic:	10–40 μg/mL >40 μg/mL	× 5.29	53–212 μmol/L >212 μmol/L
Diazepam	S or P (Hep or EDTA); trough	Therap.: Toxic:	100–1000 ng/mL >5000 ng/mL	× 0.0035	0.35–3.51 μmol/L >17.55 μmol/L
Digitoxin	S or P (Hep or EDTA); ≥6 h after dose	Therap.: Toxic:	20–35 ng/mL >45 ng/mL	× 1.31	26–46 nmol/L >59 nmol/L
Digoxin	S or P (Hep or EDTA); ≥12 h after dose		*ng/mL*		*nmol/L*
		Therap., CHF: Arrhythmias:	 0.8–1.5 1.5–2.0	 × 1.28	 1.0–1.9 1.9–2.6
		Toxic, Adult: Child:	 >2.5 >3.0		 >3.2 >3.8
Diphenylhydantoin, *see Phenytoin*					

Drugs — therapeutic and toxic (*Continued*).

Drug	Specimen	Reference Range		Conversion Factor	Reference Range (International Units)
Disopyramide	S or P (Hep or EDTA); trough	Therap.,	*μg/mL*		*μmol/L*
		Arrhythmias,			
		Atrial:	2.8–3.2	× 2.95	8.3–9.4
		Ventricular:	3.3–7.5		9.7–22
		Toxic:	>7		>20.7
Doxepin	S or P (Hep or EDTA); trough (≥12 h after dose)	Therap.:	30–150 ng/mL	× 3.58	107–537 nmol/L
		Toxic:	>500 ng/mL		>1790 nmol/L
Ethchlorvynol	S or P (Hep or EDTA)	Therap.:	2–8 μg/mL	× 6.92	14–55 μmol/L
		Toxic:	>20 μg/mL		>138 μmol/L
Ethosuximide	S or P (Hep or EDTA); trough	Therap.:	40–100 μg/mL	× 7.08	283–708 μmol/L
		Toxic:	>150 μg/mL		>1062 μmol/L
Fenoprofen	P (EDTA)	Therap.:	20–65 μg/mL	× 4.12	82–268 μmol/L
Furosemide	S	Therap.: 30 min after last dose	1–2 μg/mL	× 3.023	3–6 μmol/L
Gentamicin	S or P (EDTA)	Therap.,	μg/mL		*μmol/L*
		Peak (less		× 2.09	
		severe infection):	5–8		10.4–16.7
		(severe infection):	8–10		16.7–20.9
		Trough (less			
		severe infection):	<1		<2.1
		(moderate infection):	<2		<4.2
		(severe infection):	<2–4		<4.2–8.4

		Toxic,			
		Peak:	>10–12		>21–25
		Trough:	>2–4		>4.2–8.4
Glutethimide	S	Therap.:	2–6 μg/mL	× 4.60	9–28 μmol/L
		Toxic:	>5 μg/mL		>23 μmol/L
Imipramine	S or P (Hep or EDTA); trough (⩾12 h after dose)	Therap.:	125–250 ng/mL	× 3.57	446–893 nmol/L
		Toxic:	>500 ng/mL		>1785 nmol/L
Isoniazid	S or P (Hep or EDTA)	Therap.:	1–7 μg/mL	× 7.29	7–51 μmol/L
		Toxic:	20–710 μg/mL		146–5176 μmol/L
Kanamycin	S or P (EDTA)	Therap.,	*μg/mL*		μmol/L
		Peak:	25–35	× 2.06	52–72
		Trough (less severe infection):	1–4		2–8
		(life threatening infection):	4–8		8–16
		Toxic,			
		Peak:	>35–40		>72–82
		Trough:	>10–15		>21–31
Lidocaine	S or P (Hep or EDTA); ⩾45 min following bolus dose		μg/mL		*μmol/L*
		Therap.:	1.5–6.0	× 4.27	6.4–26
		Toxic,			
		CNS, cardiovascular depression:	6–8		26–34.2
		Seizures, obtundation, decreased cardiac output:	>8		>34.2

Drugs – therapeutic and toxic (*Continued*).

Drug	Specimen	Reference Range		Conversion Factor	Reference Range (International Units)
Lithium	S or P (Hep or EDTA); ⩾12 h after last dose	Therap.: Toxic:	0.6–1.2 mEq/L >2 mEq/L	× 1	0.6–1.2 mmol/L >2 mmol/L
Lorazepam	S or P (Hep or EDTA)	Therap.:	50–240 ng/mL	× 3.11	156–746 nmol/L
Lysergic Acid Diethylamide	P (EDTA) U	After hallucinogenic dose: 0.005–0.009 μg/mL 0.001–0.050 μg/mL		× 3090	15.5–27.8 nmol/L 3.1–154 nmol/L
Meperidine	S or P (Hep or EDTA)	Therap.: Toxic:	70–500 ng/mL >1 μg/mL	× 4.04 × 4043	283–2020 nmol/L >4043 nmol/L
Meprobamate	S	Therap.: Toxic:	6–12 μg/mL >60 μg/mL	× 4.58	28–55 μmol/L >275 μmol/L
Methadone	S or P (Hep or EDTA)	Therap.: Toxic:	100–400 ng/mL >2000 ng/mL	× 0.00323	0.32–1.29 μmol/L >6.46 μmol/L
Methaqualone	S or P (Hep or EDTA)	Therap.: Toxic:	2–3 μg/mL >10 μg/mL	× 4.00	8–12 μmol/L >40 μmol/L
Methotrexate	S or P (Hep or EDTA)	Therap.: Toxic, 1–2 wk after low-dose therapy: >9.1 ng/mL; 48 h after high-dose therapy: 454 ng/mL	variable	× 2.20	variable >20 nmol/L >1000 nmol/L

Methsuximide (N-desmethyl methsuximide)	S	Therap.: Toxic:	10–40 µg/mL >40 µg/mL	× 5.29	53–212 µmol/L >212 µmol/L
Methyldopa	P (EDTA)	Therap.: Toxic: (not well defined)	1–5 µg/mL >7 µg/mL	× 4.73	4.7–23.7 µmol/L >33 µmol/L
Methyprylon	S	Therap.: Toxic:	8–10 µg/mL >50 µg/mL	× 5.46	43–55 µmol/L >273 µmol/L
Morphine	S or P (Hep or EDTA)	Surgical anesthesia: Toxic:	65–80 ng/mL 200–5000 ng/mL	× 3.50	227–280 nmol/L 700–17,500 nmol/L
N-Acetylprocainamide	S or P (Hep or EDTA); trough	Therap.: Toxic:	5–30 µg/mL >40 µg/mL	× 3.61	18–108 µmol/L >144 µmol/L
Nitroprusside	S or P (EDTA)	As thiocyanate: Therap.:	6–29 µg/mL	× 17.2	103–499 µmol/L
Normethsuximide	S	Therap.: Toxic:	10–40 µg/mL >40 µg/mL	× 5.29	53–212 µmol/L >212 µmol/L
Nortriptyline	S or P (Hep or EDTA); trough (≥12 h after dose)	Therap.: Toxic:	50–150 ng/mL >500 ng/mL	× 3.80	190–570 nmol/L >1900 nmol/L
Oxazepam	S or P (Hep or EDTA)	Therap.:	0.2–1.4 µg/mL	× 3.49	0.70–4.9 µmol/L

Drugs — therapeutic and toxic (*Continued*).

Drug	Specimen	Reference Range		Conversion Factor	Reference Range (International Units)
Paraldehyde	S or P (Hep or EDTA)	Therap.,	*μg/mL*		*μmol/L*
		Sedation:	10–100	× 7.57	76–757
		Anesthesia:	>200		>1514
		Toxic:	200–400		1514–3028
		Lethal:	>500		>3785
			μg/mL		*μmol/L*
Paraquat	WB (EDTA)	Toxic:	0.1–1.6	× 3.89	0.39–6.2
	U	Occup. exp.:	0.3		1.17
		Toxic:	0.9–64		3.50–249
Pentobarbital	S or P (Hep or EDTA); trough	Therap.,	*μg/mL*		*μmol/L*
		Hypnotic:	1–5	× 4.42	4–22
		Therap. coma:	20–50		88–221
		Toxic:	>10		>44
Phenacetin	P (EDTA)	Therap.:	1–20 μg/mL	× 5.58	6–112 *μmol*/mL
		Toxic:	50–250 μg/mL		279–1395 μmol/mL
Phencyclidine	S or P (Hep or EDTA)	Toxic:	90–800 ng/mL	× 4.11	370–3288 nmol/L
Phenobarbital	S or P (Hep or EDTA); trough		*μg/mL*		*μmol/L*
		Therap.:	15–40	× 4.31	65–170
		Toxic,			
		Slowness, ataxia, nystagmus:	35–80		151–345
		Coma with reflexes:	65–117		280–504
		Coma without reflexes:	>100		>430

Phensuximide (both parent and N-desmethyl metabolites)	S or P (Hep or EDTA)	Therap.:	40–60 µg/mL	× 5.71	228–324 µmol/L
Phenylbutazone	P (EDTA)	Therap.: (not well defined)	50–100 µg/mL	× 3.08	162–324 µmol/L
		Toxic:	>100 µg/mL		>324 µmol/L
Phenytoin	S or P (Hep or EDTA); trough	Therap.:	10–20 µg/mL	× 3.96	40–79 µmol/L
		Toxic:	>20 µg/mL		>79 µmol/L
Primidone	S or P (Hep or EDTA); trough	Therap.:	5–12 µg/mL	× 4.58	23–55 µmol/L
		Toxic:	>15 µg/mL		>69 µmol/L
Procainamide	S or P (Hep or EDTA); trough	Therap.:	4–10 µg/mL	× 4.23	17–42 µmol/L
		Toxic:	>10–12 µg/mL		>42–51 µmol/L
		Also consider effect of metabolite (NAPA)			
Propoxyphene	P (EDTA)	Therap.:	0.1–0.4 µg/mL	× 2.95	0.3–1.2 µmol/L
		Toxic:	>0.5 µg/mL		>1.5 µmol/L
Propranolol	S or P (Hep or EDTA); trough	Therap.:	59–100 ng/mL	× 3.86	193–386 nmol/L
Protriptyline	S or P (Hep or EDTA); trough (⩾12 h after dose)	Therap.:	70–250 ng/mL	× 3.80	266–950 nmol/L
		Toxic:	>500 ng/mL		>1900 nmol/L

Drugs — therapeutic and toxic (*Continued*).

Drug	Specimen	Reference Range		Conversion Factor	Reference Range (International Units)
Quinidine	S or P (Hep or EDTA); trough	Therap.:	2–5 μg/mL	× 3.08	6–15 μmol/L
		Toxic:	>6 μg/mL		>18 μmol/L
Salicylates	S or P (Hep or EDTA); trough	Therap.:	150–300 μg/mL	× 7.24	1086–2172 μmol/L
		Toxic:	>300 μg/mL		>2172 μmol/L
Secobarbital	S	Therap.:	1–2 μg/mL	× 4.20	4.2–8.4 μmol/L
		Toxic:	>5 μg/mL		>21.0 μmol/L
Theophylline	S or P (Hep or EDTA)	Therap.,	*μg/mL*		*μmol/L*
		Bronchodilator:	8–20	× 5.55	44–111
		Prem. apnea:	6–13		33–72
		Toxic:	>20		>110
Thiocyanate	S or P (EDTA)		*μg/mL*		*μmol/L*
		Nonsmoker:	1–4	× 17.2	17–69
		Smoker:	3–12		52–206
		Therap. after nitroprusside infusion:	6–29		103–499
	U	Nonsmoker:	1–4 mg/d	× 17.2	17–69 μmol/d
		Smoker:	7–17 mg/d		120–292 μmol/d

Thiopental	S or P (Hep or EDTA); trough		*μg/mL*		*μmol/L*
		Hypnotic:	1.0–5.0	× 4.13	4.1–20.7
		Coma:	30–100		124–413
		Anesthesia:	7–130		29–536
		Toxic conc.:	>10		>41
Thioridazine	S or P (Hep or EDTA)	Therap.:	1.0–1.5 μg/mL	× 2.70	2.7–4.1 μmol/L
		Toxic:	>10 μg/mL		>27 μmol/L
Tobramycin	S or P (Hep or EDTA)	Therap.,	*μg/mL*		μmol/L
		Peak (less severe infection):	5–8	× 2.14	11–17
		(severe infection):	8–10		17–21
		Trough (less severe infection):	<1		<2
		(moderate infection):	<2		<4
		(severe infection):	<2–4		<4–9
		Toxic,			
		Peak:	>10–12		>21–26
		Trough:	>2–4		>4–9
Valproic Acid	S or P (Hep or EDTA); trough	Therap.:	50–100 μg/mL	× 6.93	347–693 μmol/L
		Toxic:	>100 μg/mL		>693 μmol/L
Vancomycin	S or P (Hep or EDTA); trough	Therap.: Not well established			
		Toxic:	>80–100 μg/mL	× 1	>18–100 mg/L
Warfarin	S or P (Hep or EDTA)	Therap.:	1–10 μg/mL	× 3.24	3–32 μmol/L

References

Beutler, E.: Hemolytic Anemia in Disorders of Red Cell Metabolism. New York. Plenum Publishing Company, 1978.

Brown, S. S., Mitchell, F. L., and Young, D.S., Eds.: Chemical Diagnosis of Disease. Amsterdam, Elsevier/North-Holland Biomedical Press, 1979.

Gilman, A. G., Goodman, L., and Gilman, A., Eds.: The Pharmacological Basis of Therapeutics. 6th ed. New York. Macmillan, 1980.

Mabry, C., and Tietz, N. W.: Tables of normal laboratory values. In Nelson Textbook of Pediatrics. 12th ed. R. E. Behrman, and V. C. Vaughan, III, Eds. Philadelphia, W. B. Saunders Company, 1983.

Tietz, N. W., Ed.: Clinical Guide to Laboratory Tests. Philadelphia, W. B. Saunders Company, 1983.

Tietz, N. W.: Reference ranges and laboratory values of clinical importance. In Cecil Textbook of Medicine. 17th ed. J. B. Wyngaarden and L. H. Smith, Jr., Eds. Philadelphia, W. B. Saunders Company, 1985.

Tietz, N. W., and Blackburn, R. H., Eds.: Reference Ranges and General Information Clinical Laboratories, A. B. Chandler Medical Center, University of Kentucky, Lexington, Kentucky, 1984.

APPENDIX C

Select Bibliography

Source Books on Biological Monitoring

This chronological list of books gives a good indication of the historical development of the field of biological monitoring in addition to providing the major source materials. Foreign publications are also cited.

1. Elkins, H. B. 1950. *The Chemistry of Industrial Toxicology*, John Wiley and Sons, New York, pp. 1–406.
2. Teisinger, J.; Skramovsky, S.; and Srbova, J. 1956. *Chemical Methods for the Investigation of Biological Material in Industrial Toxicology*, Praha Statni zdravotnicke nakladatelstvi, Prague, Czechoslovakia, pp. 1–128 (in Czech).
3. Dutkiewicz, T.; Piotrowski, J.; and Kesy-Dobrowska, I. 1964. *Chemical Investigation of Biological Material in Industrial Toxicology*, Warszawa Panstw. zaklad wydawnictw lekarskich, Warsaw, Poland, pp. 1–248 (in Polish).
4. Parke, D. V. 1968. *The Biochemistry of Foreign Compounds*, 1st ed., Pergamon Press, New York.
5. Gadaskina, I. D., and Filov, V. A. 1971. *Biotransformation and Determination of Industrial Organic Poisons*, Medicina, Leningrad, pp. 1–221 (in Russian).
6. Linch, A. L. 1974. *Biological Monitoring for Industrial Chemical Exposure Control*, CRC Press, Cleveland, OH.
7. Doss, M. 1976. *Porphyrins in Human Diseases*, Karger, Basel, Switzerland.
8. Henschler, D. 1976. *Analyses of Biological Material*, Vol. 2, *Analytical Methods for Examination of Substances Harmful to the Health of Workers*, Verlag Chemie, Weinheim, Germany (in German).
9. Waritz, R. S. 1979. Biological indicators of chemical dosage and burden. In *Patty's Industrial Hygiene and Toxicology*, Vol. 3, L. J. Cralley, and L. V. Cralley (eds.), John Wiley and Sons, New York, pp. 257–318.
10. Strik, J. J. T. W. A., and Koeman, J. H., (eds.). 1979. *Chemical Porphyria in Man*, Elsevier/North-Holland Biomedical Press, New York.
11. Berlin, A.; Wolff, A. H.; and Hasegawa, Y. (eds.). 1979. *The Use of Biological Specimens for the Assessment of Human Exposure to Environmental Pollutants*, Martinus Nijhoff Publishers, The Hague, The Netherlands.

12. Dubach, U. C., and Schmidt, V. (eds.). 1979. *Diagnostic Significance of Enzymes and Proteins in Urine*, H. Huber Publishers, Bern, Switzerland.
13. Holmstedt, B.; Lauwerys, R.; Mercier, M.; and Roberfroid, M. (eds.). 1980. *Mechanisms of Toxicity and Hazard Evaluation*, Elsevier/North-Holland Biomedical Press, New York.
14. Bardodej, Z.; David, A.; Sedivec, V.; Skramovsky, S.; and Teisinger, J. 1980. *Exposure Tests in Industrial Toxicology*, Avicenum, Prague, Czechoslovakia (in Czech).
15. Hodgson, E., and Guthrie F. E. (eds.). 1980. *Introduction to Biochemical Toxicology*, Elsevier, New York.
16. Sugimura, T.; Kondo, S.; and Takebe, H. (eds.). 1982. *Environmental Mutagens and Carcinogens*, Alan R. Liss, New York.
17. Hayes, W. 1982. *Pesticides Studied in Man*, Williams and Wilkins, Baltimore, MD.
18. Lauwerys, R. R. 1983. *Industrial Chemical Exposure: Guidelines for Biological Monitoring*, Biomedical Publications, Davis, CA.
19. Fiserova-Bergerova, V. (ed.). 1983. *Modeling of Inhalation Exposure to Vapors: Uptake, Distribution, and Elimination*, Vol. 1, CRC Press, Boca Raton, FL.
20. Berlin, A., and Yodaiken, R. E. 1983. *Assessment of Toxic Substances at the Workplace*, Martinus Nijhoff Publishers, The Hague, The Netherlands.
21. Berlin, A.; Draper, M.; Hemminki, K.; and Vainio, H. 1984. *Monitoring Human Exposure to Carcinogenic and Mutagenic Agents*, IARC Publication 59, Lyon, France.
22. Aitio, A.; Riihimaki, V.; and Vainio, H. 1984. *Biological Monitoring and Surveillance of Workers Exposed to Chemicals*, Hemisphere Publishing, Washington, DC.
23. Teisinger, J. (ed.). 1984. *Exposure Tests in Industrial Toxicology*, Verlag Volk und Gesundheit, Berlin, Germany (in German).
24. Eastham, R. D. 1985. *Biochemical Values in Clinical Medicine*, 7th Ed., John Wright and Sons, Bristol, United Kingdom.
25. Wilson, A. F. (ed.). 1985. *Pulmonary Function Testing Indications and Interpretations*, Grune and Stratton, Orlando, FL.
26. van Heemstra-Lequin, E. A. H., and van Sittert, N. J. 1986. Biological Monitoring of Workers Manufacturing, Formulating and Applying Pesticides. *Toxicology Letters*, Vol. 33, Elsevier, Amsterdam, The Netherlands.
27. Sheldon, L.; Umana, M.; Bursey, J.; Gutknecht, W.; Handy, R.; Hyldburg, P.; Michael, L.; Moseley, A.; Raymer, J.; Smith, D.; Sparacino, C.; and Warner, M. 1986. *Biological Monitoring Techniques for Human Exposure to Industrial Chemicals: Analysis of Human Fat, Skin, Nails, Blood, Urine, and Breath*, Noyes Publications, Park Ridge, NJ.
28. Carson, B. L.; Ellis H. V., III; and McCann, J. L. 1986. *Toxicology and Biological Monitoring of Metals in Humans: Including Feasibility and Need*, Lewis Publishers, Chelsea, MI.
29. Liu, P. I. 1986. *Blue Book of Diagnostic Tests*, W. B. Saunders, Philadelphia, PA.
30. Wallach, J. 1986. *Interpretation of Diagnostic Tests*, 4th ed., Little, Brown, Boston, MA.
31. Sorsa, M., and Norppa, H. (eds.). 1986. *Monitoring of Occupational Genotoxicants*, Alan R. Liss, New York.
32. Tietz, N. W. (ed.). 1986. *Textbook of Clinical Chemistry*, W. B. Saunders, Philadelphia, PA.
32. Silbergeld, E. K., and Fowler, B. A. 1987. Mechanisms of Chemical-Induced Porphyrinopathies, *Annals of the New York Academy of Sciences, Vol. 514.*
33. Ho, M. H., and Dillon, H. K. 1987. *Biological Monitoring of Exposure to Chemicals: Organic Compounds*, John Wiley and Sons, New York.

34. Foa, V.; Emmett, E. A.; Maroni, M.; and Colombi, A. (eds.). 1987. *Occupational and Environmental Chemical Hazards: Cellular and Biochemical Indices for Monitoring*, John Wiley and Sons, New York.
35. Notten, W. R. F.; Herber, R. F. M.; Hunter, W. J.; Monster, A. C.; and Zielhuis, R. L. (eds.). 1988. *Health Surveillance of Individual Workers Exposed to Chemical Agents*, Spinger-Verlag, Berlin, Germany.
36. Fischbach, F. T. 1988. *A Manual of Laboratory Diagnostic Tests*, 3rd ed., J. B. Lippincott, Philadelphia, PA.
37. Kneip, T. J., and Crable, J. V. (eds.). 1988. *Methods for Biological Monitoring: A Manual for Assessing Human Exposure to Hazardous Substances*, American Public Health Association, Washington, DC.
38. Baselt, R. C. 1988. *Biological Monitoring Methods for Industrial Chemicals*, 2nd ed., PSG Publishing, Littleton, MA.
39. Clarkson, T. W. (eds.). 1988. *Biological Monitoring of Toxic Metals*, Plenum Press, New York.
40. Prasad, A. S. (ed.). 1988. *Essential and Toxic Trace Elements in Human Health and Disease*, Alan R. Liss, New York.
41. Wang, R. G. M.; Franklin, C. A.; Honeycutt, R. C.; and Reinert, J. C. 1989. *Biological Monitoring for Pesticide Exposure: Measurement, Estimation and Risk Reduction*, American Chemical Society Symposium Series, Vol. 382, American Chemical Society, Washington, DC.
42. National Research Council. 1989. *Biologic Markers in Reproductive Toxicology*, National Academy Press, Washington, DC.
43. National Research Council. 1989. *Biologic Markers in Pulmonary Toxicology*, National Academy Press, Washington, DC.
44. Cella, J. H., and Watson, J. 1989. *Nurse's Manual of Laboratory Tests*, F. A. Davis Co., Philadelphia, PA.
45. Fiserova-Bergerova, V., and Ogata, M. (eds.). 1990. *Biological Monitoring of Exposure to Industrial Chemicals*, American Conference of Governmental Industrial Hygienists, Cincinnati, OH.

Continuing Series of Publications on Biological Monitoring

46. Biological Exposure Indices Committee of the American Conference of Governmental Industrial Hygienists. *Documentation of the Biological Exposure Indices*, American Conference of Governmental Industrial Hygienists, Cincinnati, OH. Expanded and revised yearly.
47. Alessio, L.; Berlin, A.; Roi, R.; and Boni, M. (eds.). *Biological Indicators for the Assessment of Human Exposure to Industrial Chemicals*, Commission of the European Communities, Luxembourg, Luxembourg. Published yearly since 1983 in the form of monographs.
48. Henschler, D., and Lehnert, G. (eds.). *Arbeitsmedizinisch-Toxikologische Begrundung von BAT-Werten*, VCH-Verlag, Weinheim, Germany. Published yearly since 1984.

APPENDIX D

Contributors

SHANE QUE HEE

Shane Que Hee has been Associate Professor of Environmental Health Sciences at the UCLA School of Public Health since 1989, and Vice Chair there since 1991. Before then he was Associate Professor of Environmental Health at the University of Cincinnati Medical Center from 1984 to 1989, and was Assistant Professor there from 1978 to 1984. He obtained a Ph.D. in Chemistry and Chemical Engineering from the University of Saskatchewan in Canada in 1976, a Master of Science degree in Physical Chemistry from the University of Queensland, Australia in 1971, and an Honors Bachelor of Science degree in Chemistry from the latter university in 1968.

Dr. Que Hee has had over 80 publications in such diverse areas as environmental analytical chemistry, environmental hygiene sampling and analytical chemistry, biological monitoring, microanalytical methods, direct-reading devices, toxic interactions between chemicals, organic and inorganic analytical methods development, and screening bioassays. He has had published a book on the phenoxy herbicides, and has consulted with many agencies on the environmental and toxic effects of chemicals. He served on the peer review panel of the Hazardous Substances Data Base of the National Library of Medicine between 1985 and 1989, has written reviews for many journals, and is a member of several editorial boards.

STANLEY BAUER

Dr. Bauer is Associate Director for Clinical Pathology at the Beth Israel Medical Center, New York, NY and Associate Professor of Pathology at the Mount Sinai School of Medicine. Dr. Bauer was previously Director of Pathology at the Bronx-Lebanon Hospital, Bronx, New York and Professor of Pathology and Laboratory Medicine at the Albert Einstein College of Medicine. He received his M.D. from the Chicago Medical School in 1954 and his B.S. in Pharmacy from Rutgers University, New Brunswick, NJ.

Dr. Bauer has been active in many areas of clinical pathology and is a member of the Board of Directors of the National Committee for Clinical Laboratory Standards. He was chairman of the Taskforce on the Protection of Laboratory Workers of the NCCLS, which published a guideline on the protection of laboratory workers from infectious disease transmitted by blood, body fluids, and tissues. Dr. Bauer has been a pioneer in the use of Zidovudine in the chemoprophylaxis of laboratory acquired HIV infection due to accidental exposure.

AMIT BHATTACHARYA

Dr. Amit Bhattacharya holds a Ph.D. degree in biomedical engineering and an M.S. in fluid mechanics/heat transfer, both from the University of Kentucky in Lexington, KY. He holds the rank of Associate Professor of Environmental Health and Industrial Engineering at the University of Cincinnati in Cincinnati, OH.

Dr. Bhattacharya has made contributions in the areas of heat stress, occupational biomechanics/ergonomics, physiological/biomechanical effects of external vibration, development of countermeasures for cardiovascular deconditioning resulting from weightlessness, and development of noninvasive, sensitive techniques for the quantification of postural imbalance. His research in the area of noninvasive quantification of postural balance for use in detecting chemical toxicity recently received national recognition when he was invited by the National Institute of Environmental Health Sciences (NIEHS) to present a hands-on demonstration of this technique during National Medical Research Day at the U.S. House of Representatives and at the Earth-Tech '90 Show (both in Washington, DC). Dr. Bhattacharya serves on the editorial board of the *Journal of Orthopaedic and Sports Physical Therapy* and is a current member of the Safety and Occupational Health Study Section for the National Institute for Occupational Safety and Health (NIOSH).

ATTAR S. CHAWLA

Attar S. Chawla is a Research Scientist with the Bureau of Radiation and Medical Devices, Health and Welfare Canada in Ottawa. At the Bureau he is responsible for biomaterials, explanted medical devices, and evaluation of failed medical devices.

Dr. Chawla obtained a Ph.D. degree in polymer science from McGill University, Montreal in 1970. After graduation he spent a year at the University of Waterloo as a postdoctoral fellow. He returned to McGill University as a research associate and moved on to become Assistant Professor of Physiology. In addition to his teaching duties he headed the Biomaterials Section of the Artificial Cells and Organs Research Center. He left McGill University in 1982 to join the Bureau of Radiation and Medical Devices.

His research interests are in the area of biomaterials, medical devices, and artificial internal organs. He has published over 30 scientific papers and is on the editorial boards of two scientific journals. He is a member of various national and international standards committees.

I. HINBERG

Dr. Hinberg received a B.Sc. in Chemistry from McGill University and a Ph.D. in Biophysical Chemistry from the University of Ottawa. After completing a postdoctoral fellowship in Biochemical Engineering at the University of Waterloo, he joined Polymeric Enzymes, Inc., where, as Director of Research, he designed a variety of new *in vitro* diagnostic devices.

Dr. Hinberg joined the Bureau of Radiation and Medical Devices in February 1975 as a Research Scientist. He planned, organized, and coordinated the Bureau's *in vitro* diagnostics program. He is now Head of the Research and Development Section, where he manages a multidisciplinary team of ten scientists. He has provided scientific leadership for the Bureau's research in Clinical Chemistry, Biophysics, Ergonomics, Electrophysiology, and Materials Science.

Dr. Hinberg represents the Bureau on a variety of national and international organizations. He is Chairman of the Department's Task Force on Sale of Devices to the Public. He is also Chairman of the Canadian Standards Association's Biomedical Laboratory Technology Committee. He is the Canadian representative on the International Working Group on Medical Device Testing.

Dr. Hinberg is actively involved in research on home-use and doctor's-office devices. He has developed guidelines for several classes of these devices and techniques for testing their clinical reliability in the hands of the intended user. He has published many articles on this topic.

JOHN McCUE

John McCue has been the editor for science and medicine with the New England Book Co. since leaving his post as Assistant Professor of Chemistry and Public Health at Salem State College in 1989. Before this, he served as Research Director at the Gibson Institute for Medical Research (1978–80) and as Senior Scientist for the development of therapeutics with the Cutter Group of Bayer, AG (1981–86).

Dr. McCue received his Ph.D. in chemistry from the University of California at Santa Barbara in 1976, was a postdoctorial fellow in hematology and biochemistry at the University of California Medical School in San Francisco (1976–77), and earned his M.P.H. degree from Harvard University in 1981. His work has appeared in various medical journals, and most recently in the monograph *Blood Separation and Plasma Fractionation*, published by Wiley-Liss, Inc. (1991). In addition, Dr. McCue was editor for the monograph *HIV*, published by the New England Book Co. (1991).

MICHAEL A. PEREIRA

Michael A. Pereira has been Vice-President of Toxicology for Environmental Health Research and Testing, Cincinnati, OH since 1986. Before then, he was Chief of the Bioassay Branch of the U.S. Environmental Protection Agency, Health Effects Research Laboratory. He obtained from the Ohio State University a B.S. in Microbiology in 1967 and a Ph.D. in Pharmacology in 1971.

He has published over 80 journal articles and 19 book chapters in areas of toxicology and chemical carcinogenesis that include: dosimetry, exposure assessment, and indicators of biological responses to chemical exposures in humans; mechanisms of carcinogens, mutagens, tumor initiators, and tumor promoters; determination of the human health hazard of toxic substances and complex mixtures of environmental samples such as drinking water, wastewater and reuse, and diesel exhaust; and biochemical and molecular pharmacology and toxicology. These studies have been performed in humans, in laboratory animals, and *in vitro* in prokaryotes and mammalian cells in culture. He has edited the publication of a workshop and of a symposium, and has reviewed publications for many toxicology and cancer research journals. He is a member of the AACR, AALAS, ACS, ACT, ASPET, EMS, and SOT and has held the position of Secretary-Treasurer (1988–90) and Councilor (1990–present) of the Carcinogenesis Specialty Section of SOT.

J. THOMAS PIERCE

J Thomas Pierce, Ph.D. 1978, is the staff industrial hygienist Center for Environmental and Occupational Health, University of Kansas Medical Center. He was formerly Chairman and Professor, Department of Safety Science and Technology, Central Missouri State University, and Director and Associate Professor, Industrial Hygiene Curriculum, Medical College of Virginia, Virginia Commonwealth University (1988–90). Dr. Pierce previously served as Associate Professor of Industrial Hygiene, and created the Occupational and Environmental Health Laboratory at the University of North Alabama.

In 1983, Dr. Pierce was named an Environmental Science and Engineering Fellow of the American Association for the Advancement of Science and the U.S. Environmental Protection Agency. He is board-certified in chemical aspects and comprehensive practice in industrial hygiene, and general toxicology (American Board of Toxicology).

EVELYN R. WARING

Evelyn Waring, RN, BSN, CSPI, has been the Director of the Virginia Poison Center at Virginia Commonwealth University since 1986. Prior to that time, she held a clinical teaching position in pediatric nursing services at the Children's Medical Center in that University (1984–86). After she received a Bachelor of Science with Distinction in Nursing from the University of Virginia in 1979, she practiced nursing in adult critical care.

She has published an article on injury epidemiology, and maintains membership in the American Association of Poison Control Centers. She lectures extensively in undergraduate health sciences programs and to health-care professionals on topics of acute human toxicology.

Index